# Stewart's Clinical Removable Partial Prosthodontics
## Third Edition

# Stewart's
# Clinical Removable
# Partial Prosthodontics

*Third Edition*

**Rodney D. Phoenix,** DDS, MS, FACP
Associate Professor
University of Texas Health Science Center
San Antonio, Texas

**David R. Cagna,** DMD, MS, FACP
Associate Professor
University of Texas Health Science Center
San Antonio, Texas

**Charles F. DeFreest,** DDS, FACP
Colonel
United States Air Force Dental Corps

Quintessence Publishing Co, Inc

Chicago, Berlin, Tokyo, Copenhagen, London, Paris, Milan, Barcelona, Istanbul, São Paulo, New Delhi, Moscow, Prague, and Warsaw

**Library of Congress Cataloging-in-Publication Data**

Phoenix, Rodney D.
  Stewart's clinical removable partial prosthodontics.— 3rd ed. /
Rodney D. Phoenix, David R. Cagna, Charles F. DeFreest.
     p. ; cm.
Rev. ed. of: Clinical removable partial prosthodontics / Kenneth L.
Stewart, Kenneth D. Rudd, William A. Kuebker. 2nd ed. c1992.
Includes bibliographical references and index.
  ISBN 0-86715-417-9 (hardcover)
1. Partial dentures, Removable.
  [DNLM: 1. Denture, Partial, Removable.  WU 515 P574s 2002] I. Title:
Clinical removable partial prosthodontics. II. Cagna, David R. III.
DeFreest, Charles F. IV. Stewart, Kenneth L. Clinical removable partial
prosthodontics. V. Title.
  RK665 .S73 2002
  617.6'92—dc21

                                    2002013928

©2003 Quintessence Publishing Co, Inc

Quintessence Publishing Co, Inc
4350 Chandler Drive
Hanover Park, IL 60133
www.quintpub.com

Editor: Kathryn O'Malley
Cover and Internal Design: Dawn Hartman
Production: Dawn Hartman and Patrick Penney

Printed in China

# In Memoriam

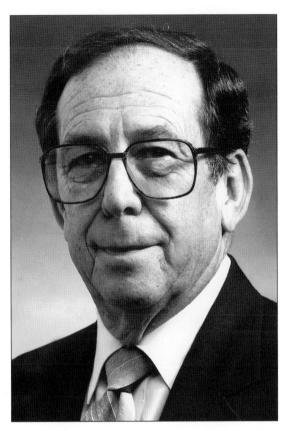

**Kenneth Lowe Stewart**
**1925–1996**

A talented clinician, inspirational teacher, and trusted
colleague, his memory and beliefs will live forever through
his students and the many lives he touched.

# Table of Contents

# Preface

On August 1, 1996, dentistry lost one of its giants. Dr Kenneth Stewart died following an extended battle with cancer. Although saddened by this loss, we are extremely grateful for the opportunity to have known and worked with Dr Stewart, an extremely bright and talented practitioner and a gentleman in every sense of the word. He was exceptionally generous with his time and his knowledge, and he wanted only the best for his students, friends, and family.

In 1983, Dr Stewart collaborated with Drs William Kuebker and Kenneth Rudd to publish *Clinical Removable Partial Prosthodontics*, a textbook that took a new, more practical approach to presenting removable partial denture treatment. Unlike previous texts in the field, the book was arranged in the sequence of patient treatment, allowing students and practitioners to achieve a basic understanding of all aspects of removable partial denture therapy and then apply these concepts in a clinical situation. When Drs Kuebker and Rudd approached us with the opportunity to author a new edition of this text, we gratefully accepted. This text, *Stewart's Clinical Removable Partial Prosthodontics*, is the culmination of our efforts.

Like the preceding editions, this book is intended for dental students, residents, and practitioners. It is presented in chronological sequence—procedure by procedure. Each chapter is intended to build upon the information presented in previous chapters, thereby providing a firm foundation in removable partial denture design, construction, and placement. The text is supported by numerous photographs and diagrams designed to facilitate understanding.

This text is intended to provide readers with a clear understanding of removable partial denture concepts and procedures. It is also our hope that it will lead to improved patient treatment and years of enjoyable dental practice.

We would like to thank the family of Dr Kenneth Stewart. They have been extremely supportive of our efforts, and for this we are grateful. We also would like to thank Dr William Kuebker and Dr Kenneth Rudd for their contributions to dentistry, for their mentorship, and for the opportunity to author this textbook.

We would like to acknowledge the practitioners who have contributed to previous editions of this book: Drs James Brudvik, John Jones, Madeline Kurrasch, Merrill Mensor, Steven Parel, and Richard Seals. Their efforts have been instrumental in the continued success of this textbook. We also would like to thank Drs James Brudvik, Raymond Koeppen, Michael Mansueto, and Ronald Verrett for their contributions to the current edition of this textbook. They are among the most talented practitioners in contemporary dentistry, and their support and friendship are very much appreciated.

We also would like to recognize the efforts of Christina Elliott. She has served in numerous capacities, from proofreader to cheerleader. Her input was invaluable, and her support was directly responsible for the timely completion of this text.

We would be remiss if we did not thank our instructors and mentors through the years. The countless hours they spent with us are very much appreciated.

Finally, our heartfelt thanks go to our families and friends, particularly our wives and children. Without their support, none of this would have been possible.

# Contributors

**James S. Brudvik,** DDS, FACP
Professor Emeritus of Prosthodontics
University of Washington School of Dentistry
Seattle, Washington

**Raymond G. Koeppen,** DDS, MS, FACP
Colonel
United States Air Force Dental Corps

**Michael A. Mansueto,** DDS, MS, FACP
Assistant Professor
University of Texas Health Science Center
San Antonio, Texas

**Ronald G. Verrett,** DDS, MS, FACP
Assistant Professor
University of Texas Health Science Center
San Antonio, Texas

# Introduction and Classification

## ⌑ Terminology

Several efforts have been made to standardize dental terminology, beginning with Dr Louis Ottofy's compilation of accepted dental terms in 1923.[1] This document greatly improved communication within the dental profession. As the dental profession matured, new materials and techniques were introduced. Increasing dental knowledge gave rise to recognized dental specialties, and dental terminology continued to evolve. The greatest advance in prosthodontic terminology was made in 1956 when the Academy of Denture Prosthetics published the *Glossary of Prosthodontic Terms*. Since that time, the publication has been updated on a regular basis. Currently, the Glossary is published in the *Journal of Prosthetic Dentistry* every 2 years.

To ensure that the terminology used throughout this book will be understood by all readers, definitions of some of the most frequently encountered words are provided in this section. In addition, the terms used in this book are limited to those that are recognized as acceptable.

## *Branches of prosthodontics*

The art or science of replacing absent body parts is termed *prosthetics*, and any artificial part is called a *prosthesis*. As applied to dentistry, the terms *prosthodontics* and *dental prosthesis* are used. Prosthodontics is the branch of dental art and science that deals with the replacement of missing teeth and oral tissues to restore and maintain oral form, function, appearance, and health. There are three major divisions of prosthodontics: fixed prosthodontics, removable prosthodontics, and maxillofacial prosthodontics (Fig 1-1). Despite the importance of dental implants, the authors of this text do not consider implantology a major division of prosthodontics. Instead, implants are considered adjuncts in fixed, removable, and maxillofacial therapy.

According to the *Glossary of Prosthodontic Terms*, fixed prosthodontics is the branch that deals with the replacement and/or restoration of teeth by artificial substitutes that are not readily removed from the mouth.[2] This book discusses fixed prosthodontics only as it relates to removable partial dentures. The glossary defines maxillofacial prosthodontics as the

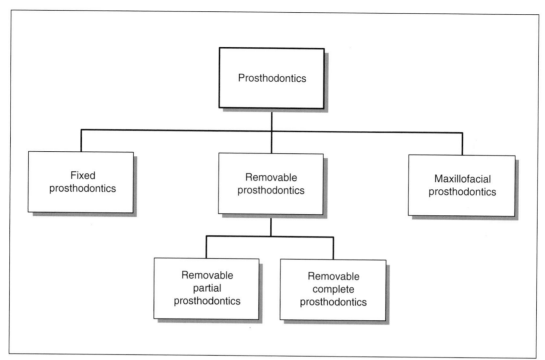

**Fig 1-1** Branches of prosthodontics.

branch of prosthodontics concerned with the restoration and/or replacement of stomatognathic and associated facial structures that have been affected by disease, injury, surgery, or congenital defect.[2] Removable prosthodontics is devoted to replacement of missing teeth and contiguous tissues with prostheses designed to be removed by the wearer. It includes two disciplines: removable complete and removable partial prosthodontics. This book deals with the latter.

## Terms related to dental prostheses

As previously noted, a prosthesis is an artificial replacement for a missing body part. A dental prosthesis is an artificial replacement of one or more teeth and/or associated structures. In clinical applications, dental prostheses may be supported by teeth, residual ridges, dental implants, or a combination thereof. Consequently, practitioners must be familiar with the associated terminology.

The terms *abutment* and *retainer* are central to a discussion of dental prostheses. An abutment is any tooth or dental implant that supports a dental prosthesis. In contrast, a retainer is the portion of a fixed or removable partial denture that attaches the prosthesis to an abutment (Fig 1-2). Hence, an abutment

is part of the patient's oral cavity (eg, a tooth or implant), while a retainer is part of the prosthesis.

Traditionally, fixed partial dentures have been attached to abutments using dental cements, while removable partial dentures have been attached to abutments by other means. In removable partial denture prosthodontics, there are two principle types of retainers. They are termed *extracoronal retainers* and *intracoronal retainers*. Extracoronal retainers consist of two fingers of metal (ie, clasps) that lie on the surface of a clinical crown (Fig 1-3). One finger of metal is termed a *retentive clasp*, while the other is termed a *reciprocal clasp*. The retentive clasp is located in an undercut area of the clinical crown and resists displacement of the prosthesis away from the underlying hard and soft tissues. The reciprocal clasp is located in a non-undercut area and serves as a bracing or stabilizing element for the prosthesis. The resultant assembly is termed an *extracoronal retainer* because the retentive and reciprocal components lie on the external surfaces of an abutment.

Unlike extracoronal retainers, intracoronal retainers are contained entirely within the contours of a clinical crown (Fig 1-4). Consequently, the use of intracoronal retainers generally requires the fabrication of two or more specially designed, complete-coverage crowns. In most instances, retention of intracoronal removable

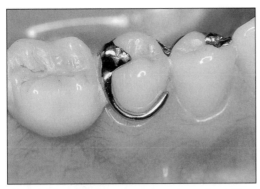

**Fig 1-2** The abutment is any tooth or dental implant that supports a prosthesis. The retainer is the portion of the prothesis that attaches the prosthesis to an abutment.

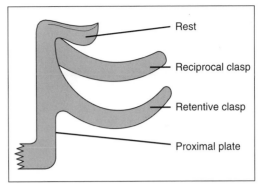

**Fig 1-3** Components of an extracoronal retainer usually include a rest, retentive and reciprocal clasps, and a proximal plate.

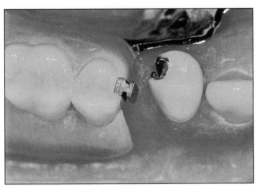

**Fig 1-4** An intracoronal retainer lies within the contours of the clinical crown. An intracoronal retainer consists of a matrix or "female" component *(right)* and a patrix or "male" component *(left).*

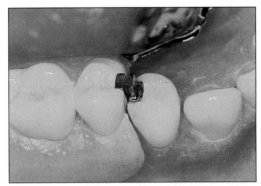

**Fig 1-5** When joined, matrix and patrix components form a closely fitting retentive assembly.

partial dentures is dependent upon exact parallelism of the retentive assemblies. Each assembly consists of two parts, commonly termed *matrix* ("female"), and *patrix* ("male"). Figure 1-5 illustrates the joining of a patrix and matrix to form a functional retentive unit. When a dislodging force is applied to the removable partial denture, binding occurs between the external walls of the patrix and the internal walls of the matrix. This binding results in retention of the prosthesis.

Another method for categorizing removable partial dentures relates to the manner of their support. A partial denture that receives support from natural teeth at each end of the edentulous space or spaces is a *tooth-supported removable partial denture* (Fig 1-6). Although the denture base contacts the adjacent soft tissues, the prosthesis does not receive significant vertical support from the residual ridge.

A second category of removable partial dentures includes those that extend anteriorly or posteriorly and are supported by teeth at only one end (Fig 1-7). These are called *extension base removable partial dentures* or *tooth-tissue–supported removable partial dentures*. The majority of these are *distal extension removable partial dentures*. Distal extension removable partial dentures are supported by teeth at the anterior aspect of the edentulous space and by tissues of the edentulous ridge posteriorly.

In certain instances, the terms *interim*, *transitional*, and *treatment* are applied to specific types of removable partial dentures. An interim removable partial denture is a provisional prosthesis intended to improve esthetics and function until a more definitive form of treatment can be rendered. A transitional removable partial denture may be used when loss of additional teeth is inevitable, but immediate extraction is not advisable or desirable. Artificial teeth may be added to a transitional removable partial denture as natural teeth are extracted. A transitional removable partial denture may be worn during the healing process and replaced

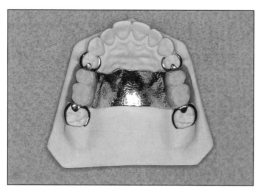

**Fig 1-6** A tooth-supported removable partial denture.

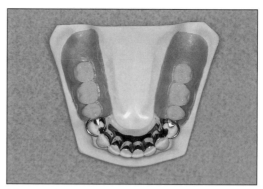

**Fig 1-7** A tooth-tissue–supported (extension base) removable partial denture.

with a definitive prosthesis when extraction sites have stabilized. A treatment denture may be used as a carrier for treatment material, as a protective covering for a surgical site, or as a matrix for soft tissue healing. In most instances, treatment dentures are used in conjunction with resilient tissue conditioners. The resultant prostheses provide cushioning effects for the underlying soft tissues and promote improved tissue health. Interim, transitional, and treatment prostheses are intended for short-term applications and should never be used for prolonged treatment. The use of such prostheses over extended periods may cause irreparable damage to a patient's remaining teeth, soft tissues, and bone.

Other terms of interest include *model* and *cast*. While *cast* may be used as a verb (to cast an inlay) or as an adjective (a cast framework), it is most often used as a noun to describe an accurate, positive reproduction of a maxillary or mandibular dental arch. Certain adjectives are commonly used to provide a more specific meaning for the term (eg, diagnostic cast, master cast, refractory cast). The term *model* is used to describe a reproduction for demonstration or display purposes. The term *model* does not imply dimensional or spatial accuracy. Hence, a model should be a reasonable facsimile of an object, but need not be an accurate reproduction such as that required for construction of a successful prosthesis.

Terms related to clinical applications also must be considered. Undoubtedly the most defined term in prosthodontics is *centric relation*, closely followed by *maximal intercuspal position* and *centric occlusion position*. The basic definition of centric relation is the physio-

logic relationship of the mandible to the maxilla when both condyles are properly related to their articular discs and the condyle-disc assemblies are stabilized against the posterior slopes of the articular eminences. This relationship may occur at varying degrees of mandibular opening, but must precede the downward and forward movement (ie, translation) of the condyles. This definition may be embellished in many ways, but if the basic premise of a bone-to-bone relationship is maintained, acceptance of this simple concept can avoid confusion. Maximal intercuspal position may be defined as the most complete interdigitation of the teeth independent of condylar position. Hence, maximum intercuspation is a maxillomandibular relationship determined by tooth-to-tooth relationships. Centric occlusion position represents the first contact of the teeth that occurs when the mandibular condyles are in centric relation. Therefore, centric occlusion position is a maxillomandibular relationship dictated by bone-to-bone relationships (Fig 1-8).

Other key terms relate to the displacement resistance exhibited by a prosthesis. The most important of these are *retention*, *support*, and *stability*. For purposes of this discussion, retention may be defined as resistance to displacement away from the teeth and soft tissues of the dental arch; support may be defined as resistance to displacement toward the teeth and soft tissues of the dental arch; and stability may be defined as resistance to displacement in a mediolateral or anteroposterior direction (Fig 1-9).

Those terms that deal directly with the components of a removable partial denture will not be presented here, but will be covered in subsequent chapters.

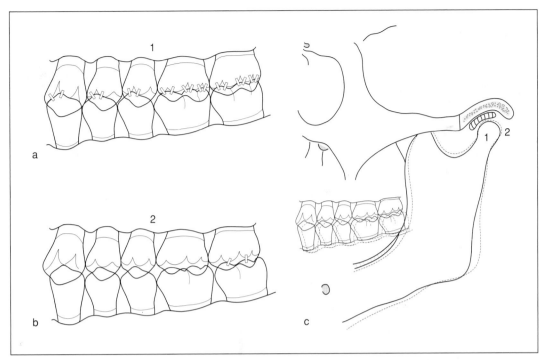

**Fig 1-8** *(a)* Maximal intercuspal position is the most complete interdigitation of the teeth and is independent of condylar position. *(b)* Centric occlusion position is the first contact of the teeth that occurs when the mandibular condyles are in their centric relation positions. *(c)* Maximum intercuspation and centric relation can be coincident if the occlusion is appropriately developed or properly adjusted. This would occur with the teeth in position 1 and the temporomandibular joints in position 2.

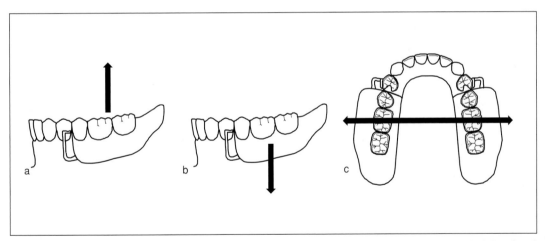

**Fig 1-9** *(a)* Retention may be defined as resistance to displacement away from the underlying hard and soft tissues. *(b)* Support may be defined as resistance to displacement toward the associated tissues. *(c)* Stability may be defined as resistance to displacement in a mediolateral or anteroposterior direction.

## ❑ Treatment of Partially Edentulous Patients

When all factors are favorable, the treatment of choice for a partially edentulous patient is placement of a fixed partial denture, and the advent of dental implants has provided a number of new options for carrying out this treatment modality. However, not all patients are candidates for dental implant therapy. Contraindications for dental implant therapy include unfavorable regional anatomy, uncontrolled systemic disease, high-dose head and neck radiation, and extreme surgical risk. Moreover, there are contraindications associated with any type of fixed partial denture therapy, as outlined in the following section.

## Contraindications for fixed partial denture therapy

### Age of patient

Most patients younger than 18 years are poor candidates for fixed partial dentures because of large dental pulps and lack of clinical crown height. Tooth reduction sufficient to reestablish normal coronal anatomy in the cast restoration often compromises the health of the pulpal tissues. Consequently, an interim partial denture should be considered for patients younger than 18 years.

### Length of edentulous span

One of the rules of dentistry that has most successfully passed the test of time is that of Dr Irvin Ante. Ante's Law states that the periodontal membrane area of the abutment teeth for a fixed partial denture must be equal to or greater than the periodontal membrane area of the teeth being replaced.[3] Although other conditions may modify this rule to some degree, exceeding the rule by a margin of any significance is almost certain to create problems.

### Loss of supporting tissues

When a large amount of the edentulous ridge has been lost, the practitioner must fabricate a prosthesis that restores function and provides support for the lips and cheeks. In addition, the prosthesis must allow access for oral hygiene. Replacement of missing tissues with a fixed partial denture generally makes it difficult for the patient to maintain a healthy oral environment. In contrast, restoration with a removable partial denture allows the patient to remove the prosthesis from the mouth. This facilitates cleaning of the prosthesis and permits increased access to the remaining teeth and soft tissues.

## Rationale for removable partial denture therapy

As stated by Dr M. M. DeVan, the primary purpose of removable partial denture therapy must always be "the preservation of that which remains, and not the meticulous replacement of that which has been lost."[4] After it has been determined that this purpose can be satisfied, one should consider the additional purposes of removable partial denture therapy: maintaining or improving phonetics, establishing or increasing masticatory efficiency, stabilizing dental relationships, and developing the required esthetics.

If, on the other hand, it is indicated that the health of all or part of the remaining oral structures will be compromised, alternative forms of treatment must be considered. For too many years, removable partial dentures were considered stepping stones on the road to complete dentures. With the materials, equipment, and techniques currently available, this type of thinking must be relegated to the past. Removable partial denture therapy is an acceptable form of treatment that provides an increased spectrum of restorative options.

## Indications for removable partial denture therapy

### Long-span edentulous area

The teeth adjacent to a long-span edentulous area support a removable partial denture in much the same manner that they would support a fixed partial denture. However, a removable denture receives additional support and stabilization from the tissues of the residual ridge and from the abutment teeth on the opposite side of the arch. Without this distribution of forces, the leverage and torque on the abutment teeth would be excessive.

### No abutment tooth posterior to the edentulous space

Where there is no tooth posterior to the edentulous space to act as an abutment, the choice of replacements is limited. Fixed partial dentures that are supported at only one end (ie, cantilevered fixed partial dentures) produce harmful torquing forces (Fig 1-10). These forces often produce bone resorption, tooth mobility, and restoration failure.

In some instances, one or more dental implants may be placed in the edentulous area, and the arch may be restored with a fixed partial denture. When placement of implants is not possible, the only practical treatment involves placement of a removable partial denture.

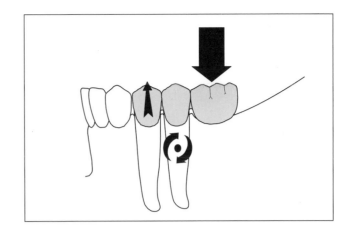

**Fig 1-10** When a load *(large arrow)* is applied to a fixed partial denture that is supported only at one end, harmful torquing forces *(small arrows)* can result.

### Reduced periodontal support for remaining teeth

In mouths where bony support for the remaining teeth has been severely compromised, prospective abutments may be unable to support fixed prostheses. In these situations, removable partial dentures can derive appreciable support from the remaining teeth and residual ridges. Hence, the total support that must be provided by the abutment teeth is diminished.

### Need for cross-arch stabilization

When stabilization of the remaining teeth is needed to offset mediolateral and anteroposterior forces (eg, after treatment of advanced periodontal disease), cross-arch stabilization frequently is required. A fixed partial denture can provide excellent anteroposterior stabilization, but limited mediolateral stabilization. Because removable partial dentures are bilateral prostheses, cross-arch stabilization is enhanced.

### Excessive bone loss within the residual ridge

When a missing tooth is replaced by a fixed partial denture, the artificial tooth (pontic) is positioned so its neck lightly contacts the mucosa over the edentulous ridge. When trauma, surgery, or abnormal resorptive patterns have caused excessive bone loss, a clinician also must deal with replacement of ridge contours. With the advent of successful regenerative therapies (eg, bone grafting, guided tissue regeneration), it may be possible to restore optimum dimensions to severely resorbed residual ridges. But for patients in whom regenerative therapy is not a viable option, denture bases can be used to restore missing portions of the dental arches. Therefore, properly contoured denture bases may be used to support the lips and cheeks, and to reestablish desirable facial contours.

### Physical or emotional problems exhibited by patients

The lengthy preparation and construction procedures for fixed partial dentures can be trying, especially for patients with physical or emotional problems. In many instances, removable partial denture therapy is indicated to minimize patient-dentist contact time. Treatment should be designed to prevent further oral deterioration and continued until the underlying physical or emotional problems are resolved or appropriately managed. Treatment selection should not compromise the fit and function of the completed reconstruction.

### Esthetics of primary concern

In some instances, a practitioner is faced with the option of fixed versus removable partial denture therapy. It is often possible to attain a more pleasing appearance by using one or more denture teeth on a denture base. This is particularly true when the practitioner must simulate the appearance of diastemata, dental crowding, dental rotation, or extreme changes in the soft tissue architecture (eg, recreation of papillae to avoid the appearance of dark interdental spaces). Denture teeth on a denture base also may permit the practitioner to more effectively satisfy a patient's phonetic and functional requirements.

## Immediate need to replace extracted teeth

The replacement of teeth immediately following extraction is most readily accomplished using a removable prosthesis. Unlike fixed restorations, properly designed removable partial dentures may be altered rather easily. Acrylic resin denture bases may be relined as ridge resorption occurs. When the edentulous area has stabilized, definitive treatment can be undertaken with fixed or removable partial dentures.

## Patient desires

Patients sometimes insist on removable prostheses in place of fixed prostheses *(1)* to avoid operative procedures on sound, healthy teeth; *(2)* to avoid the placement of one or more implants; and *(3)* for economic reasons. Patients who have had unpleasant experiences with previous dental procedures often object strenuously to the tooth reduction required for fixed prosthesis fabrication. Other patients are hesitant to undergo surgical procedures associated with implant placement. A third category of patients needs and desires replacement, but cannot afford fixed or implant-borne prostheses. Differences in these forms of treatment should be explained to patients. It should never be implied that patients opting for removable partial denture therapy will receive inadequate treatment. Successful removable partial denture therapy should be expected if fundamental principles are observed.

## Unfavorable maxillomandibular relationships

Difficulties are often encountered in patients with unfavorable maxillomandibular relationships. These unfavorable relationships include disharmonies in arch size, shape, and position. A common scenario involves a patient with few serviceable teeth and a moderate-to-severe Class 2 skeletal relationship. Because of the difficulties associated with complete denture therapy in such a patient, every attempt should be made to retain the teeth that may support removable partial dentures. Failure to retain such teeth may result in extremely difficult restorative situations.

# Classification of Partially Edentulous Arches

During the early 1900s, dental practitioners began devising methods for the classification of partially edentulous arches. While numerous classification systems were proposed, few met the needs of the profession. Some classification systems were overly simplified, while others were immensely complex. It was decided that for a classification system to be acceptable, it should

1. Allow visualization of the type of partially edentulous arch being considered
2. Permit differentiation between tooth-supported and tooth-tissue–supported partial dentures
3. Serve as a guide to the type of design to be used
4. Be universally accepted

## *Kennedy Classification System*

The most widely used method for classification of partially edentulous dental arches was proposed by Dr Edward Kennedy of New York in 1925.[5] Although relatively simple, the system can easily be applied to nearly all semi-edentulous conditions.

The Kennedy Classification System is composed of four major categories, denoted Class I through Class IV. The numeric sequence of the classification system was based partly on the frequency of occurrence, with Class I arches being most common and Class IV arches least common.

- Kennedy Class I arch: Characterized by bilateral edentulous areas located posterior to the remaining natural teeth (Figs 1-11 and 1-12).
- Kennedy Class II arch: Displays a unilateral edentulous area located posterior to the remaining natural teeth (Figs 1-13 and 1-14).
- Kennedy Class III arch: Presents a unilateral edentulous area with natural teeth both anterior and posterior to it (Figs 1-15 and 1-16).
- Kennedy Class IV arch: Displays a single, bilateral edentulous area located anterior to the remaining natural teeth. It is important to note that the edentulous space must cross the dental midline (Figs 1-17 and 1-18).

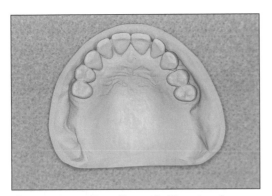

**Fig 1-11** A maxillary Kennedy Class I arch.

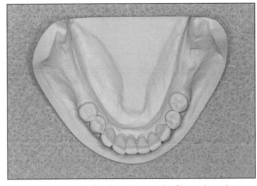

**Fig 1-12** A mandibular Kennedy Class I arch.

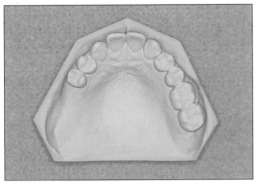

**Fig 1-13** A maxillary Kennedy Class II arch.

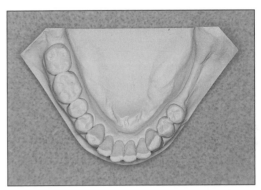

**Fig 1-14** A mandibular Kennedy Class II arch.

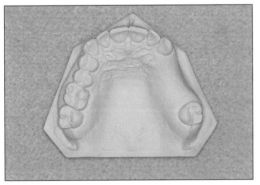

**Fig 1-15** A maxillary Kennedy Class III arch.

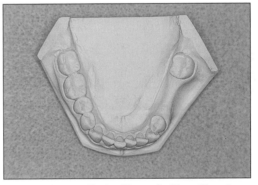

**Fig 1-16** A mandibular Kennedy Class III arch.

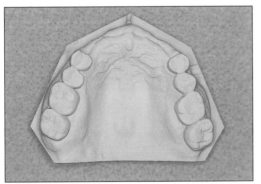

**Fig 1-17** A maxillary Kennedy Class IV arch.

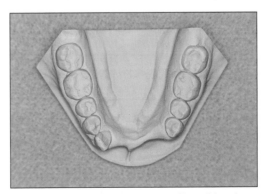

**Fig 1-18** A mandibular Kennedy Class IV arch.

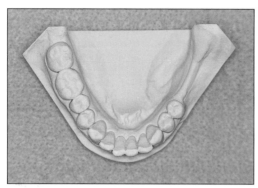

**Fig 1-19** A representative mandibular Kennedy Class II arch with no modification spaces.

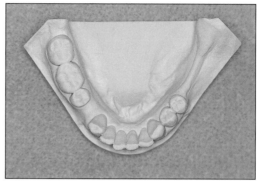

**Fig 1-20** A mandibular Kennedy Class II arch with a one-tooth modification space (Kennedy Class II, Modification 1).

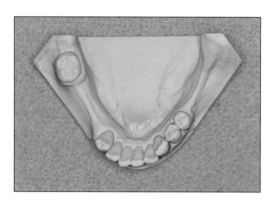

**Fig 1-21** A mandibular Kennedy Class II arch with a three-tooth modification space (Kennedy Class II, Modification 1).

## Modification spaces

Each Kennedy classification, except Class I, refers to a single edentulous area. In reality, additional areas of edentulism may occur within a dental arch (Figs 1-19 to 1-21). Kennedy referred to each additional edentulous area—not each additional missing tooth—as a modification space (see Figs 1-20 and 1-21). Dr Kennedy included the number of modification areas in the classification (eg, Class I, Modification 1; Class II, Modification 3).

## Applegate's rules for classification

While the Kennedy system provided a method for classification of partially edentulous arches, there was some uncertainty regarding its application. In 1954, Dr O. C. Applegate provided the following rules to govern application of the Kennedy system[6]:

1. Classification should follow rather than precede extractions that might alter the original classification (Fig 1-22).
2. If the third molar is missing and not to be replaced, it is not considered in the classification (Fig 1-23).
3. If a third molar is present and is to be used as an abutment, it is considered in the classification (Fig 1-24).
4. If a second molar is missing and is not to be replaced (that is, the opposing second molar is also missing and is not to be replaced), it is not considered in the classification (Fig 1-25).
5. The most posterior edentulous area(s) always determines the classification (Fig 1-26).
6. Edentulous areas other than those determining the classification are referred to as modification spaces and are designated by their number (Fig 1-27).

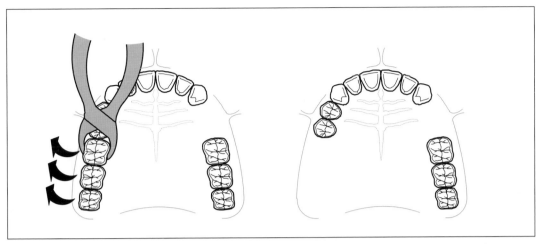

**Fig 1-22** If extractions are to be performed, classification should follow rather than precede the extractions. In this instance, the indicated extractions yield a Kennedy Class II, Modification 1 arch.

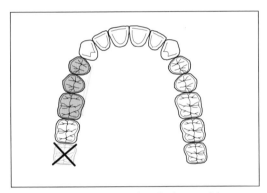

**Fig 1-23** If a third molar is missing and is not to be replaced, it is not considered in the classification. For purposes of this discussion, each tooth that is missing and to be replaced is shaded. Each tooth that is missing and not to be replaced is identified with an *X*. Hence, the illustration represents a Kennedy Class III arch.

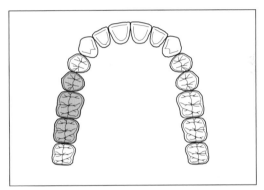

**Fig 1-24** If a third molar is present and is to be used as an abutment, it is considered in the classification. Consequently, this illustration represents a Kennedy Class III arch.

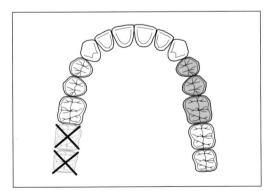

**Fig 1-25** If a second molar is missing and is not to be replaced, it is not considered in the classification. This illustration represents a Kennedy Class III arch.

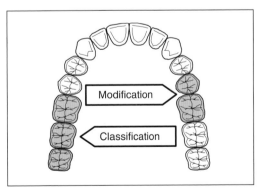

**Fig 1-26** The most posterior edentulous area(s) always determines the classification. As a result, this pattern of edentulism represents a Kennedy Class II, Modification 1 arch.

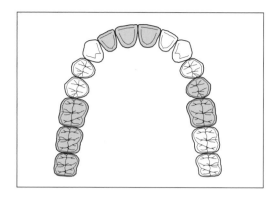

**Fig 1-27** Edentulous areas other than those determining the classification are referred to as modification spaces and are designated by their number. This illustration represents a Kennedy Class II, Modification 2 arch.

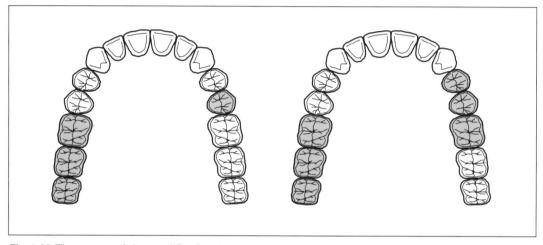

**Fig 1-28** The extent of the modification is not considered; only the number of additional edentulous areas is important. Consequently, both illustrations represent Kennedy Class II, Modification 1 arches.

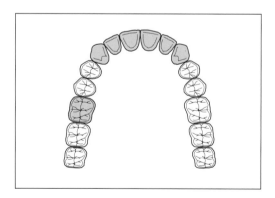

**Fig 1-29** There can be no modification areas in Class IV arches. Any edentulous area lying posterior to the single bilateral area determines the classification. This illustration depicts a Kennedy Class III, Modification 1 arch.

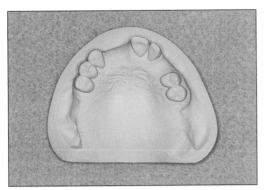

**Fig 1-30** A maxillary Kennedy Class I, Modification 2 arch.

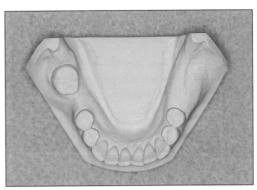

**Fig 1-31** A mandibular Kennedy Class II, Modification 1 arch.

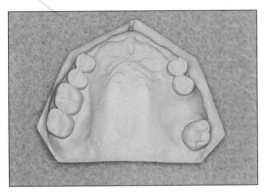

**Fig 1-32** A maxillary Kennedy Class III, Modification 1 arch.

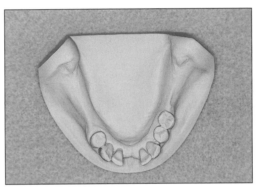

**Fig 1-33** A mandibular Kennedy Class I, Modification 1 arch.

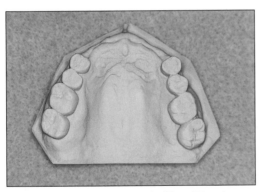

**Fig 1-34** A maxillary Kennedy Class IV arch.

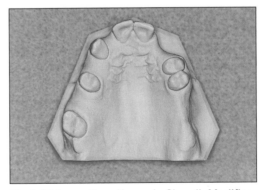

**Fig 1-35** A maxillary Kennedy Class II, Modification 4 arch.

7. The extent of the modification is not considered, only the number of additional edentulous areas (Fig 1-28).

8. There can be no modification areas in Class IV arches. Any edentulous area lying posterior to the single bilateral area determines the classification (Fig 1-29).

Properly classified maxillary and mandibular arches are presented in Figs 1-30 to 1-35.

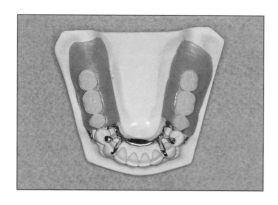

**Fig 1-36** A Kennedy Class I removable partial denture must derive support from the teeth and soft tissues.

## ☐ Fundamental Design Considerations

Any discussion of removable partial denture design should be preceded by a basic understanding of oral biomechanics. Support for removable partial dentures may be derived from the remaining teeth, the hard and soft tissues of the residual ridge, or both. As might be expected, there is a significant difference in the support that can be derived from these structures.

Teeth are connected to the surrounding bone via thin periodontal ligaments. Under function, healthy teeth may be displaced as much as 0.2 mm. In contrast, soft tissues overlying residual bone generally may be displaced 1.0 mm or more. As a result, there may be a significant difference in the support provided by the teeth and the tissues of the residual ridge. It is important to understand this difference when designing removable partial prostheses.

A practitioner also must consider the components that prevent displacement of removable partial dentures away from the underlying oral tissues. In removable partial denture design, the components responsible for retention of the prosthesis are termed *direct retainers* and *indirect retainers*. These components will be discussed more fully in subsequent chapters.

### Class I removable partial dentures

Kennedy Class I removable partial dentures present significant challenges for patients and dentists alike. Because Class I removable partial dentures exhibit bilateral extension bases, they must derive support from the remaining teeth and residual ridges (Fig 1-36). To

preserve the remaining teeth and residual ridges, removable partial dentures must provide an equitable distribution of forces. Concentration of forces upon the remaining teeth may produce rapid destruction of the periodontal tissues and potential abutment loss. Concentration of forces upon the residual ridges may produce rapid destruction of the associated tissues and an accompanying decrease in ridge height. Consequently, practitioners must carefully consider the effects of removable partial denture design upon the remaining oral structures. The following features must be included in the design of Class I removable partial dentures: provision of optimum support for the distal extension denture bases, incorporation of flexible direct retention, and provision of indirect retention.

### Optimum support for distal extension denture bases

All portions of a residual ridge that are capable of providing support should be covered by an accurately fitting denture base. Broad coverage permits a favorable distribution of stresses, often described as a *snowshoe effect* (Fig 1-37). Inadequate soft tissue coverage can lead to stress concentration, breakdown of underlying bone, and a decrease in ridge volume. Adequate support of a distal extension base is often so critical that a second impression of the residual ridge is required. The technique and rationale for this procedure are covered in chapter 12.

### Flexible direct retention

The soft tissues are displaceable and allow vertical movement of the denture bases upon loading (Fig 1-38). Ver-

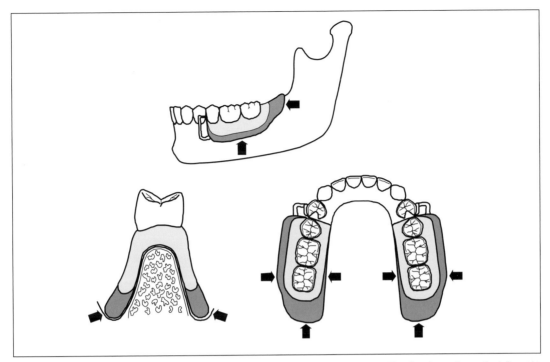

**Fig 1-37** Full extension of the denture base permits a more favorable distribution of applied forces. The lightly shaded area depicts an underextended denture base. The darker shading depicts a denture base that has been fully extended.

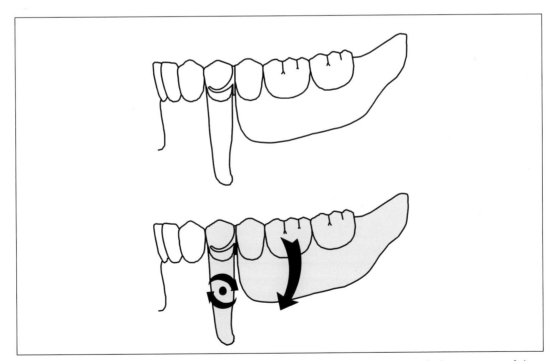

**Fig 1-38** Because the soft tissues are displaceable, loading often produces vertical movement of denture bases. Flexible direct retention must be utilized to prevent the application of harmful torquing forces to the abutments.

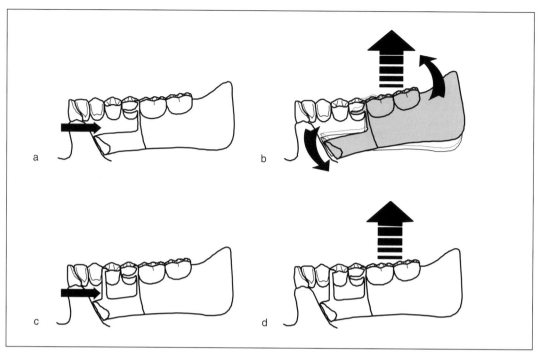

**Fig 1-39** Indirect retention must be provided in Class I applications. *(a)* An extension base removable partial denture that lacks appropriate indirect retention *(arrow)*. *(b)* When the denture base moves away from the underlying soft tissues *(large arrow)*, uncontrolled rotation of the removable partial denture occurs *(small arrows)*. *(c)* Indirect retention has been provided *(arrow)*. *(d)* When an unseating force is applied to the denture base *(arrow)*, the indirect retainer resists rotation.

tical displacement of the denture bases may result in the application of stresses to the most posterior abutments. Improperly designed direct retainers may magnify these stresses. The resultant "rocking" forces may damage the associated periodontal tissues and produce mobility of the abutment teeth. Therefore, direct retainers must permit dissipation of forces resulting from denture base movement. Each direct retainer should be designed to flex or move into an area of greater undercut as forces are applied to the removable partial denture. Clasp design is a key factor in successful removable partial denture service.

## Indirect retention

In some instances, sticky foods may lift denture bases away from the supporting tissues. This displacement produces rotation of the removable partial denture around the most posterior abutment (Fig 1-39). Rotation must be controlled to prevent damage to the remaining teeth and oral tissues. To accomplish this objective, auxiliary rests should be placed as far as is

practical from the fulcrum line. Because the auxiliary rests minimize rotation and aid in retention of the associated prosthesis, they are termed *indirect retainers*. The concept of indirect retention is discussed in detail in chapter 3.

## *Class III removable partial dentures*

Class III removable partial dentures (Fig 1-40) do not have the same design requirements as Class I removable partial dentures. Because Class III removable partial dentures are supported by teeth or dental implants at both ends of an edentulous space, denture bases generally do not rotate or lift away from the underlying tissues. Therefore, compensation for rotational forces is not needed.

There a few things that should be kept in mind when designing a Class III removable partial denture. First, support should be provided entirely by the abutment teeth. Due to the favorable distribution of abutments, Class III removable partial dentures often

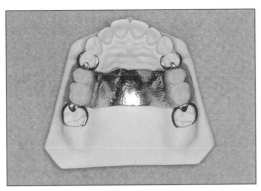

**Fig 1-40** Representative Class III removable partial denture (Kennedy Class III, Modification 1).

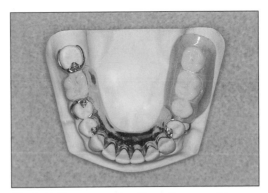

**Fig 1-41** Representative Class II removable partial denture (Kennedy Class II, Modification 1).

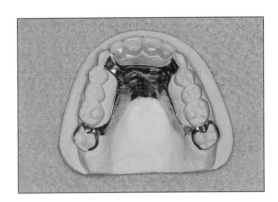

**Fig 1-42** Representative Class IV removable partial denture.

function like fixed prostheses. Residual ridges should be used for support only when edentulous spans are long or abutments display decreased periodontal support.

It is also important to remember that appropriate direct retention must be incorporated into the design. Class III removable partial dentures do not tend to move in function. Consequently, a wide variety of retentive elements may be used in Class III applications. Direct retention is needed only to prevent dislodgement of the prosthesis. The characteristics of commonly used clasping assemblies will be discussed in chapter 3.

Finally, one must keep in mind that indirect retention generally is not necessary. Since Class III removable partial dentures do not tend to move or rotate in function, there is no need for indirect retention. However, if direct retention cannot be obtained on one or more abutment teeth, indirect retention may be required.

## Class II removable partial dentures

A Class II removable partial denture must embody features of both Class I and Class III designs (Fig 1-41). The unilateral distal extension side must be designed as a Class I removable partial denture, whereas the tooth-supported side must be designed as a Class III removable partial denture. The prosthesis must include a well-adapted denture base, properly designed direct retention, and appropriately positioned indirect retention.

## Class IV removable partial dentures

A Class IV design should be regarded as a Class I removable partial denture in reverse, particularly if the edentulous span is lengthy (Fig 1-42). As previously noted, the prosthesis must include a well-adapted denture base, properly designed direct retention, and appropriately positioned indirect retention.

## ☐ References

1. Ottofy, L. Standard Dental Dictionary. Chicago: Laird and Lee, 1923: IX.

2. Glossary of Prosthodontic Terms, ed 4. St. Louis: Mosby, 1977.

3. Ante IH. The fundamental principles, design and construction of crown and bridge prosthesis. Dent Items Interest 1928;1:215–232.

4. DeVan MM. The nature of the partial denture foundation: Suggestions for its preservation. J Prosthet Dent 1952;2:210–218.

5. Kennedy E. Partial denture construction. Dent Items Interest 1928;1:3–8.

6. Applegate OC. Essentials of Removable Partial Prosthesis, ed 1. Philadelphia: Saunders, 1954.

## ☐ Bibliography

Akers PE. A new and simplified method of partial denture prosthesis. J Am Dent Assoc 1925;12:711–715.

Applegate OC. The rationale of partial denture choice. J Prosthet Dent 1960;10:891–907.

Avant WE. A universal classification for removable partial denture situations. J Prosthet Dent 1966;16:533–539.

Boucher CO (ed). Current Clinical Dental Terminology: A Glossary of Accepted Terms in All Disciplines of Dentistry, ed 2. St. Louis: Mosby, 1974.

Cummer WE. Partial denture service. In: Textbook of Prosthetic Dentistry. Philadelphia: Lea & Febiger, 1942.

Friedman J. The ABC classification of partial denture segments. J Prosthet Dent 1953;3:517–524.

Godfrey RJ. A classification of removable partial dentures. J Am Coll Dent 1951;18:5–13.

Heartwell CM Jr. Syllabus of Complete Dentures, ed 3. Philadelphia: Lea & Febiger, 1980.

Mauk EH. Classifications of mutilated dental arches requiring treatment by removable partial dentures. J Am Dent Assoc 1942;29:2121–2131.

Miller EL. Systems for classifying partially dentulous arches. J Prosthet Dent 1970;24:25–40.

Öwall BE, Taylor RL. A survey of dentition and removable partial dentures constructed for patients in North America. J Prosthet Dent 1989;61:465–470.

Skinner CN. A classification of removable partial dentures based upon the principles of anatomy and physiology. J Prosthet Dent 1959;9:240–246.

Terkla L, Lacy W. Partial Dentures, ed 3. St. Louis: Mosby, 1963.

# Major Connectors, Minor Connectors, Rests, and Rest Seats

Each component of a removable partial denture has a name that is descriptive of its function. For example, a major connector serves as the principal method for connecting the opposing sides of a removable partial denture. A minor connector joins smaller components to the major connector. A rest contacts the surface of the abutment tooth to prevent movement of the removable partial denture toward the underlying tissues. A clasp assembly grasps an abutment tooth and resists removal of the prosthesis. Components of a clasp assembly are further classified as retentive and reciprocal elements based upon their primary functions. Retentive clasps are designed to keep a removable partial denture in position, while reciprocal clasps are intended to brace abutment teeth upon insertion and removal of the prosthesis. Representative components are displayed in Figs 2-1 to 2-13.

Every removable partial denture will have some or all of the following components:

- Major connector
- Minor connectors
- Rests
- Direct retainers/clasps

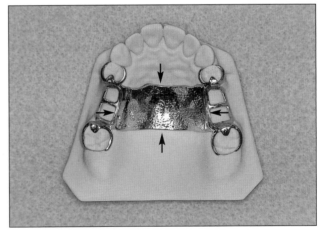

**Fig 2-1** A major connector *(arrows)* is a relatively large, rigid band of metal that joins components on the right and left sides of a removable partial denture.

- Indirect retainers
- One or more denture bases in conjunction with prosthetic teeth

The first three components are considered in this chapter, while the remaining components are presented in chapter 3.

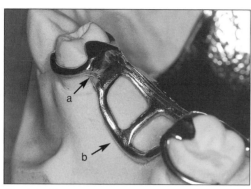

**Fig 2-2** Minor connectors join smaller components to the major connector. Minor connectors include proximal plates (a) and resin-retaining elements (b).

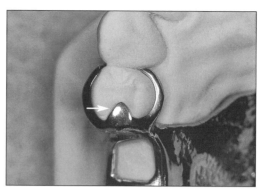

**Fig 2-3** A rest *(arrow)* contacts the surface of an abutment tooth to prevent movement of the prosthesis toward the underlying oral tissues. Properly positioned rests maintain the correct placement of the removable partial denture and prevent damage to the hard and soft tissues.

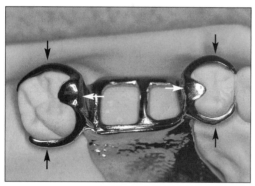

**Fig 2-4** Clasp assemblies *(arrows)* grasp the associated abutments and resist removal of the prosthesis.

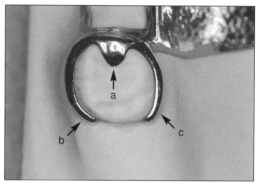

**Fig 2-5** A circumferential clasp assembly includes a rest (a), a retentive arm (b), and a reciprocal arm (c).

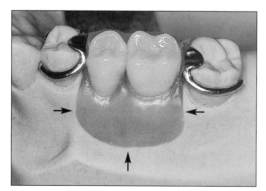

**Fig 2-6** A denture base *(arrows)* spans an edentulous area and provides a platform for prosthetic teeth.

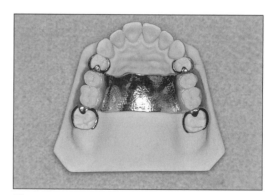

**Fig 2-7** A representative maxillary removable partial denture.

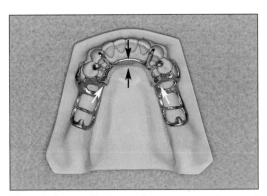

Fig 2-8 A mandibular major connector *(arrows)* must not interfere with function of the tongue or the associated soft tissues. Consequently, the major connector must follow a curved path in crossing the anterior mandible.

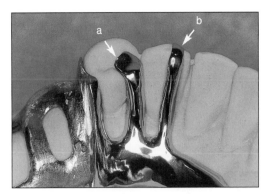

Fig 2-9 An occlusal rest (a) occupies a position on the occlusal surface of a posterior tooth, while an incisal rest (b) traverses the incisal edge of an anterior tooth.

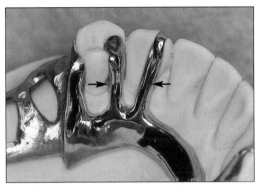

Fig 2-10 Struts *(arrows)* that connect occlusal and incisal rests to the remainder of the prosthesis are classified as minor connectors.

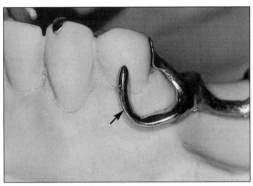

Fig 2-11 Infrabulge clasps *(arrow)* are frequently used to provide retention. Such clasps approach the undercut from an apical direction.

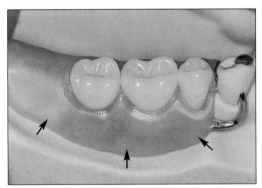

Fig 2-12 In some instances, a denture base *(arrows)* must derive at least part of its support from the tissues of the underlying ridge. These denture bases are commonly referred to as extension bases.

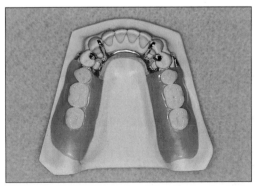

Fig 2-13 A representative mandibular removable partial denture.

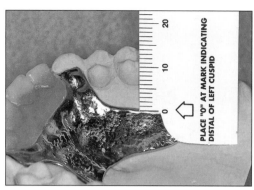

**Fig 2-14** In the maxillary arch, borders of a major connector should be positioned at least 6 mm from the free gingival margins. Otherwise the major connector should be carried onto the lingual surfaces of the teeth in the form of plating.

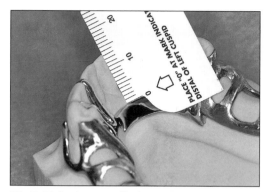

**Fig 2-15** In the mandibular arch, borders of the major connector should be positioned at least 3 mm from the free gingival margins. Otherwise the major connector should be carried onto the lingual surfaces of the teeth in the form of plating.

## ⌑ Major Connectors

A major connector joins the components on one side of the arch with those on the opposite side. Therefore, all components are attached to the associated major connector either directly or indirectly.

To function effectively and minimize potentially damaging effects, all major connectors must

1. Be rigid
2. Provide vertical support and protect the soft tissues
3. Provide a means for obtaining indirect retention where indicated
4. Provide a means for placement of one or more denture bases
5. Promote patient comfort

The first requirement for all major connectors is *rigidity*. Structural rigidity permits broad distribution of applied forces. Hence, occlusal loads may be transmitted to abutment teeth, other teeth included in the partial denture design, the associated soft tissues, and underlying bone. Other components of a removable partial denture such as retentive clasps, occlusal rests, and indirect retainers can be effective only if the major connector is rigid.

A flexible major connector may cause severe damage to the hard and soft tissues of the oral cavity. Flexibility allows forces to be concentrated on individual

teeth and segments of the residual ridges. This may lead to tooth mobility or tooth loss. The concentration of forces upon small segments of the residual ridges may cause resorption of the hard and soft tissues. This may result in decreased ridge height and decreased support for the associated denture bases.

The second fundamental requirement of a major connector is that it must not permit impingement upon the free gingival margins of the remaining teeth. The marginal gingivae are highly vascular and susceptible to injury from sustained pressure. For this reason, care should be exercised during the design and fabrication of removable partial dentures.

In the maxillary arch, the borders of a major connector should be located at least 6 mm from the free gingival margins (Fig 2-14). In the mandibular arch, the borders of a major connector should be positioned at least 3 mm from the free gingival margins (Fig 2-15). The borders should run parallel to the gingival margins of the remaining teeth (Fig 2-16). If the gingival margins must be crossed, they should be crossed at right angles to minimize coverage of the delicate marginal tissues (Fig 2-17).

Where the major connector crosses a gingival margin, relief (ie, space) must be provided between the metal and soft tissues. If relief is not provided, inflammation of the soft tissues will result.

In addition to the aforementioned requirements, a major connector also must provide a means for obtaining indirect retention where indicated. A remov-

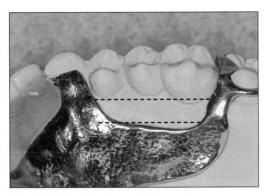

**Fig 2-16** The borders of the major connector should run parallel to the gingival margins of the remaining teeth.

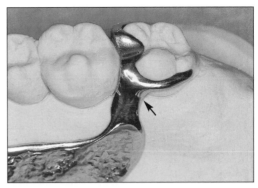

**Fig 2-17** Gingival margins should be crossed at right angles *(arrow)* to minimize coverage of the delicate marginal tissues.

able partial denture that is not supported at each end of an edentulous space tends to rotate about a fulcrum line. The most common method for controlling this movement is through the use of one or more indirect retainers. For practical purposes, indirect retainers will always take the form of rests. When properly positioned, these rests can minimize the rotational movements of a prosthesis.

It is important to note that a major connector should never be considered an indirect retainer. Although a major connector may play an auxiliary role in resisting rotation of the prosthesis, it is the action of the rests and rest seats that is responsible for indirect retention. A major connector that is not properly rested will undergo rotation and may cause orthodontic movement of the associated teeth.

A fourth requirement for major connectors involves the proper placement of denture bases. Generally, the type of major connector will be dictated by the number and location of edentulous areas. Certain major connectors are indicated for anterior tooth replacement, while others are not. Some major connectors may be selected for tooth-supported removable partial dentures, but not for tooth-tissue–supported applications. In each instance, a major connector must allow appropriate placement of the associated denture base(s).

Finally, a major connector must promote patient comfort. Consequently, the edges of a major connector should be contoured to blend with the oral tissues.

This is particularly true for major connectors that cross the anterior palate. The anterior border of a maxillary major connector should not end on the anterior slope of a prominent ruga (Fig 2-18a). The additional thickness produced by metal coverage will create a noticeable prominence on this section of the palate, and may interfere with the patient's comfort and speech. Instead, the anterior border of the major connector should be terminated on the posterior slope of a prominent ruga (Fig 2-18b). In this manner, the edge of the prosthesis may be blended with the existing soft tissue contours. Posterior borders must also be placed with regard for patient comfort and function.

It is good design policy to make the major connector as symmetrical as possible. In addition, the borders of a maxillary major connector should cross the palatal midline at right angles (Fig 2-19). Tissues covering the maxillary midline are often thin and susceptible to irritation. By crossing the maxillary midline at right angles, the length of the crossing may be minimized and the potential for irritation reduced.

Tori also should be avoided if possible (Fig 2-20). In the maxillary arch, a major connector may cover a small torus if its surgical removal is impossible and if it cannot be avoided by altering the design of the major connector. If a maxillary torus must be covered, relief should be provided. Avoiding a mandibular torus is much more complicated. Therefore, as a rule, mandibular tori should be surgically removed.

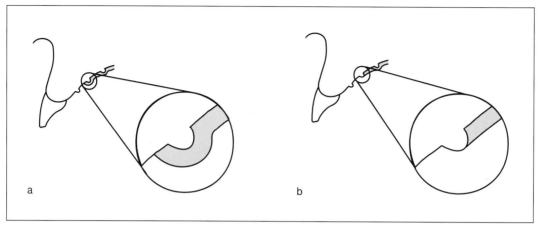

**Fig 2-18** *(a)* The anterior border of a maxillary major connector should not end on the anterior slope of a prominent ruga. This produces a noticeable prominence that may interfere with the patient's comfort and speech. *(b)* The anterior border of the major connector should be terminated on the posterior slope of a prominent ruga. In this manner, the edge of the prosthesis may be blended with the existing soft tissue contours.

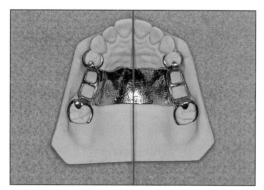

**Fig 2-19** The borders of a maxillary major connector should always cross the palatal midline at 90 degrees.

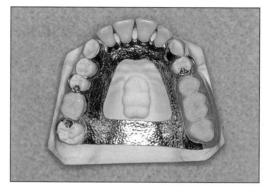

**Fig 2-20** Coverage of tori should be avoided if possible. The tissues covering tori are extremely thin and susceptible to irritation.

In addition to the previous considerations, a major connector should exhibit smooth, rounded contours (Fig 2-21). Sharp angles and corners may cause patient discomfort and produce areas of stress concentration within a removable partial denture framework. Areas of stress concentration may lead to structural fatigue and prosthesis fracture.

A removable partial denture also must be designed to be as self-cleansing as possible. Therefore, a major connector must not create food entrapment areas. In most instances, it is best to avoid covering the lingual surfaces of teeth with the metal of the major connector. However, when freeing the gingival margin will result in a design that may cause the entrapment of food or other debris, the area may be covered with a thin

layer of metal. It is important to note that food entrapment is most frequently encountered when an attempt is made to free the gingival margin around a single tooth. Care should be taken to avoid such contours.

When it is necessary to extend components of a removable partial denture framework onto the teeth, embrasures should be used to disguise the thickness of the metal (Fig 2-22).

These design considerations are fundamental to all major connectors. The importance of each requirement depends on the type of partially edentulous arch that is being treated. Hence, the type of major connector should be selected on the basis of an individual patient's needs. Specific design concerns and

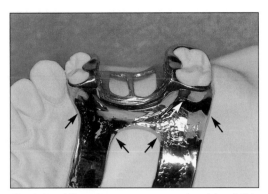

**Fig 2-21** All major connectors should exhibit smooth, rounded contours *(arrows)*. Sharp angles may produce patient discomfort and also concentrate stress.

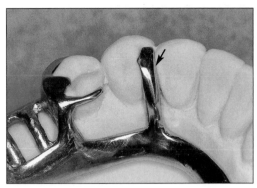

**Fig 2-22** When partial denture components must be extended onto the teeth, embrasures *(arrow)* may be used to disguise the thickness of the metal framework.

types of major connectors are presented in the following sections.

## Maxillary major connectors

### Special structural requirements

All maxillary major connectors should display minor elevations at those borders that contact the palatal soft tissues (Fig 2-23). The elevations are termed *bead lines* and are intended to slightly displace the adjacent soft tissues. This displacement produces a mechanical seal and prevents food particles from collecting under the major connector. In addition, these elevations provide excellent visual finish lines for technicians who finish and polish removable partial denture frameworks.

Bead lines must be scribed on the surface of the master cast before duplication in investment material. These lines are best prepared with a small spoon excavator or round bur rotating at slow speed. Each bead line should have a width and depth of 0.5 to 1.0 mm. The bead line should fade out approximately 6 mm from the gingival margins of the remaining teeth. The depth of the beading also should be reduced in areas of thin tissue coverage such as the midpalatine raphe or a palatal torus. When the partial denture is not in the mouth, the outline of the beading should be evident in the palatal soft tissues, but there should be no evidence of irritation or inflammation.

Except in the presence of a palatal torus or a prominent median suture line, relief should not be used under a maxillary major connector. The intimate contact between the palatal soft tissues and the metal connector enhances the retention and stability of the denture. To maintain this intimate metal–soft tissue contact, the tissue side of the major connector is not brought to a high finish during polishing procedures. Electrolytic polishing is sufficient to produce a smooth, well-finished surface without disturbing the accuracy of the casting.

### Types of maxillary major connectors

The following six types of maxillary major connectors are used in removable partial denture therapy:

1. Palatal bar
2. Palatal strap
3. Anteroposterior palatal bar
4. Horseshoe
5. Anteroposterior palatal strap
6. Complete palate

**Palatal bar** The palatal bar is a narrow half oval with its thickest point at the center. The bar is gently curved and should not form a sharp angle at its junction with the denture base (Fig 2-24).

*Advantages of the palatal bar.* For many years, the palatal bar was one of the most widely used maxillary major connectors. Today, palatal bar major connectors are used primarily in interim applications. The palatal bar has few advantages and should be avoided.

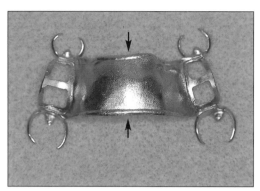

**Fig 2-23** Maxillary major connectors should display minor elevations *(arrows)* at those borders that contact the palatal tissues. These elevations are termed *bead lines* and are intended to prevent the collection of food particles under the prosthesis.

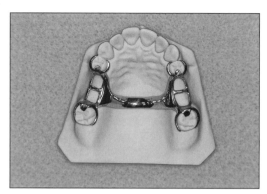

**Fig 2-24** Palatal bar major connector.

*Disadvantages of the palatal bar.* To provide the necessary rigidity, a palatal bar major connector must be bulky. Consequently, patients find the palatal bar uncomfortable. Moreover, because of its narrow anteroposterior width, a palatal bar derives little vertical support from the bony palate. As a result, a palatal bar major connector must derive nearly all of its support from rests on the remaining teeth.

If used, the palatal bar should be limited to short-span Class III applications (eg, replacing one or two teeth on each side of the arch). In addition, the palatal bar should not be placed anterior to the second premolar position, otherwise its bulk may produce noticeable discomfort and alteration of speech.

**Palatal strap** The palatal strap is the most versatile maxillary major connector. The palatal strap consists of a wide band of metal with a thin cross-sectional dimension (Fig 2-25). Because of its minimal depth, this major connector may be used to cross the palate in an unobtrusive manner. Nevertheless, the anteroposterior dimension of a palatal strap major connector should not be less than 8 mm to avoid compromise of its rigidity (Fig 2-26).

The width of a palatal strap major connector should be increased as the edentulous space increases in length. This increase in width not only ensures rigidity, but also permits greater support from the hard palate. The wider the palatal strap becomes, the more

it resembles a complete palate major connector. While a wide palatal strap may be used for unilateral distal extension partial dentures (ie, Kennedy Class II), it should not be used for bilateral distal extension applications (ie, Kennedy Class I).

*Advantages of the palatal strap.* Because the palatal strap is located in two or more planes, it offers great resistance to bending and twisting forces. This theory is similar to the "L-beam" principle used in building construction. Simply stated, forces transmitted on different planes are counteracted more easily.

Because the palatal strap is inherently strong, it can be kept relatively thin. Since this configuration offers little interference with normal tongue action, palatal strap major connectors are well accepted by patients. In addition, the increased tissue coverage helps distribute applied stresses over a larger area.

*Disadvantages of the palatal strap.* In some instances, a patient may complain of excessive palatal coverage. Frequently, this complaint can be traced to improper positioning of the strap borders. Therefore, the anterior border of the major connector should be positioned posterior to the palatal rugae if possible. If this is not possible, the anterior border should be terminated on the posterior slopes of prominent rugae (see Fig 2-18). The posterior border of the major connector should be positioned anterior to the junction of the hard and soft palates.

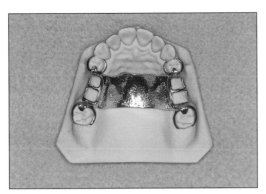

Fig 2-25 Palatal strap major connector.

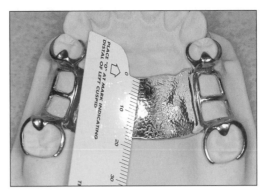

Fig 2-26 The anteroposterior dimension of a palatal strap major connector should never be less than 8 mm.

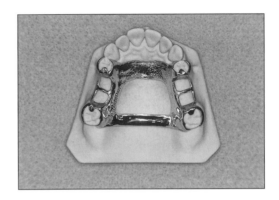

Fig 2-27 Anteroposterior palatal bar major connector.

The increased soft tissue coverage associated with a wide palatal strap also may predispose the patient to papillary hyperplasia. This condition is seen when the partial denture is worn 24 hours a day and normally is accompanied by poor oral hygiene. In many cases, the occurrence of papillary hyperplasia may be traced to inadequate patient instruction. Therefore, it is essential that each removable partial denture patient be provided with thorough oral and written instructions regarding the wear, care, and cleaning of oral prostheses.

**Anteroposterior palatal bar** The anteroposterior palatal bar displays characteristics of palatal bar and palatal strap major connectors (Fig 2-27). The anterior bar is relatively flat. Its cross-sectional shape is similar to that of a palatal strap. Borders of the anterior bar are positioned on the appropriate slopes of prominent rugae, thereby allowing it to blend with the contours of the anterior palate. The posterior bar

is a half oval, similar to the palatal bar major connector. The two bars are joined by flat longitudinal elements on each side of the palate. This configuration gives the effect of a circle and is considerably more rigid than any of the individual elements. The two bars, lying in different planes, produce a structurally strong L-beam effect.

*Advantages of the anteroposterior palatal bar.* As previously noted, the main advantage of an anteroposterior palatal bar is its rigidity. The anteroposterior palatal bar minimizes soft tissue coverage, yet provides exceptional resistance to deformation.

The anteroposterior palatal bar may be used when support is not a major consideration and when the anterior and posterior abutments are widely separated. Anteroposterior palatal bar major connectors also may be chosen for patients with large palatal tori that cannot be removed for health reasons.

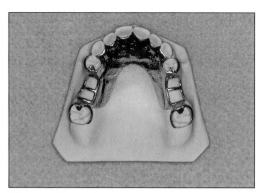

**Fig 2-28** Horseshoe major connector.

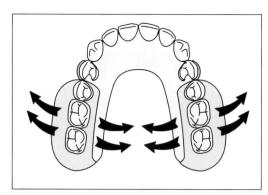

**Fig 2-29** A horseshoe major connector has a tendency to flex or deform when a load is placed. Therefore, it is a poor choice for most maxillary applications.

*Disadvantages of the anteroposterior palatal bar.* The anteroposterior palatal bar is frequently uncomfortable. The bulk and contour of the connector may be bothersome to the tongue and may interfere with phonetics. Moreover, because of its limited contact with the palatal tissues, the anteroposterior palatal bar derives little support from the bony palate. Consequently, its use may be contraindicated in patients with reduced periodontal support.

As a general rule, the anteroposterior palatal bar should not be considered the first choice for a maxillary major connector. It should be selected only after other choices have been considered and eliminated.

**Horseshoe connector** The horseshoe connector consists of a thin band of metal running along the lingual surfaces of the remaining teeth and extending onto the palatal tissues for 6 to 8 mm (Fig 2-28).

The medial borders of this connector should be placed at the junction of the horizontal and vertical slopes of the palate. Rigidity can be increased by extending the borders slightly onto the horizontal surfaces of the hard palate.

The connector should display symmetry and should extend to the same height on both sides. All borders of the connector should be gently curved and smooth.

*Advantages of the horseshoe connector.* This major connector is used primarily when several anterior teeth

are being replaced. It is a reasonably strong connector that can derive some vertical support from tissues of the hard palate.

In the presence of a prominent median suture line or an inoperable torus, this major connector may offer distinct advantages. The horseshoe connector may be designed to avoid bony prominences without sacrificing vertical support.

*Disadvantages of the horseshoe connector.* When vertical force is applied to one or both ends of a horseshoe major connector, there is a tendency for the connector to flex or deform (Fig 2-29). Therefore, it is a poor choice for distal extension partial dentures. For the same reason, this is not a good connector when cross-arch stabilization is required. The horseshoe connector displays limited resistance to flexing, and noticeable movement can occur at the open end. This may result in the concentration of forces and damage to the associated abutments.

To avoid the tendency to flex, the metal crossing the anterior palate must be thicker than that used in most other major connectors. This places the greatest bulk of metal in an area that is critical to patient comfort and phonetics. As a result, the horseshoe connector should be considered only if more rigid connectors cannot be used.

**Anteroposterior palatal strap** The anteroposterior palatal strap is a structurally rigid major connector

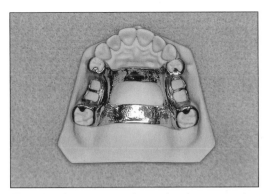

**Fig 2-30** Anteroposterior palatal strap major connector.

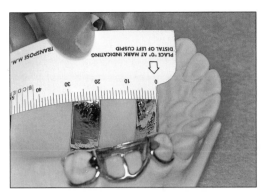

**Fig 2-31** Both the anterior and posterior straps of an anteroposterior palatal strap major connector should be at least 8 mm in width.

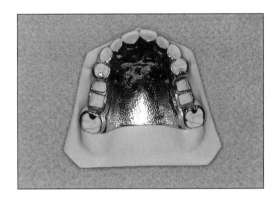

**Fig 2-32** Complete palate major connector.

that may be used in most maxillary partial denture applications (Fig 2-30). This major connector is particularly indicated when numerous teeth are to be replaced, or when a palatine torus is present.

Each strap should be at least 8 mm in width and relatively thin in cross section (Fig 2-31). Borders of the major connector should be kept 6 mm from the free gingival margins or should extend onto the lingual surfaces of the remaining teeth. Palatal borders should exhibit smooth, gentle curves.

When anterior teeth are not being replaced, the anterior strap should be in the farthest posterior position possible. Appropriate placement promotes patient comfort and minimizes interference with speech. The posterior strap also should be in a posterior position, but should not contact the tissues of the movable soft palate. The open area in the palatal region should be at least 20 × 15 mm. Otherwise, another type of major connector should be chosen (eg, wide palatal strap, complete palate, modified complete palate).

*Advantages of the anteroposterior palatal strap.* The anteroposterior palatal strap is a rigid connector that derives good support from the tissues of the hard palate despite its open design. The corrugated contour of the metal over the rugae adds strength to the connector and allows the metal to be made relatively thin (< 1 mm). The structural encirclement produced by the anterior and posterior straps contributes to the rigidity of the connector. The shape of this connector also provides a definite L-beam effect, thereby increasing the resistance to flexure.

*Disadvantages of the anteroposterior palatal strap.* Even though the metal over the rugae area may be thinner than in some other major connectors, interference with phonetics may occur in some patients. In addition, the extensive length of borders may cause irritation to the tongue.

**Complete palate** The complete palate provides the ultimate rigidity and support (Fig 2-32). It also provides the greatest amount of tissue coverage. Hence, the need for maximum support and rigidity should be determined before this connector is selected.

As noted for other types of major connectors, the anterior border of a complete palate must be kept 6 mm from the marginal gingivae, or it must cover the cingula of the anterior teeth. The posterior border should extend to the junction of the hard and soft palates.

The posterior palatal seal that is employed with complete dentures should not be used with a removable partial denture framework. In a removable partial denture, it is not possible to produce a peripheral seal similar to that produced by border molding a complete denture. Attempts to use a posterior palatal seal not only fail to accomplish the desired purpose, but also place unnecessary forces on the abutments due to rebound of the underlying soft tissues.

A slight mechanical seal may be formed by ensuring the presence of a bead line along the posterior border of the major connector. This gently rounded elevation prevents debris from collecting beneath the major connector. Intimate contact of the cast metal palate with the underlying soft tissues aids retention through the action of adhesive and cohesive forces.

*Advantages of the complete palate.* Complete palatal coverage is advantageous when all posterior teeth are to be replaced. Complete palatal coverage also may be indicated when the remaining teeth are periodontally compromised. In such applications, the vertical support provided by a complete palate can be extremely beneficial. Complete palatal coverage permits distribution of applied forces to the remaining teeth, as well as to the palatal tissues.

When minimal ridge height is available, a complete palate can provide additional stabilization for the prosthesis. Undesirable lateral or horizontal forces may be dissipated by intimate contact between the major connector and the underlying soft tissues.

A cast metal palate can be produced as a uniformly thin plate that reproduces the anatomic contours of the palate. As a result, the complete palate generally is comfortable and exerts little or no effect upon phonetics. In addition, the coverage of multiple palatal planes provides an L-beam effect and makes the complete palate an extremely rigid major connector.

An all-metal connector also enhances thermal conductivity. This characteristic permits stimulation of the underlying soft tissues and may contribute to long-term tissue health. This advantage is lost when acrylic resin is used.

Metal also exhibits a less porous surface than that of commonly used acrylic resins. Consequently, the surface of a metal framework is more resistant to colonization by potentially harmful microorganisms such as *Candida albicans.*

*Disadvantages of the complete palate.* Because of the extensive tissue coverage, adverse soft tissue reactions may occur in conjunction with complete palate major connectors. These reactions generally are characterized by soft tissue hyperplasia and accompanied by poor oral hygiene and prolonged periods of denture wear.

Occasionally, problems with phonetics may be encountered. This may be related to the extensive soft tissue coverage exhibited by complete palate major connectors.

### Review of structural requirements for maxillary major connectors

1. The borders must be placed a minimum of 6 mm from gingival margins or extended onto the lingual surfaces of the teeth (see Fig 2-14). The location is determined by the need for support, stabilization, and/or oral hygiene.
2. Relief is normally not required under maxillary major connectors.
3. Borders that extend onto the anterior palate should blend with the palatal anatomy. This may be accomplished by positioning borders on the appropriate slopes of the rugae (see Fig 2-18).
4. The anterior and posterior elements of an anteroposterior palatal strap should be at least 8 mm wide (see Fig 2-31). The posterior strap should be located in the farthest posterior position possible without contacting the movable soft palate.
5. All borders should taper slightly toward the underlying soft tissues.
6. Both anterior and posterior borders should cross the maxillary midline at right angles, never diagonally (see Fig 2-19).

7. For those major connectors that present open central areas, the medial borders should be positioned at the junction of the horizontal and vertical surfaces of the palate. For gently curved palates, the proper locations must be approximated. Appropriate placement is necessary to minimize patient awareness and potential discomfort.

8. Thickness of the metal should be uniform throughout the palate.

9. Borders of the metal framework should be gently curved, never angular (see Fig 2-21).

10. The metal should be smooth but not highly polished on the tissue side (ie, intaglio).

11. All borders that contact soft tissues should display bead lines (see Fig 2-23). The bead lines should become less distinct as they approach the gingival margins of the teeth.

### Review of indications for maxillary major connectors

1. If the periodontal support of the remaining teeth is weak, more of the palate should be covered. A wide palatal strap or a complete palate is indicated.

2. If the remaining teeth have adequate periodontal support and little additional support is needed, a palatal strap or anteroposterior palatal bar may be used.

3. For long-span distal extension bases where rigidity is critical, an anteroposterior palatal strap or complete palate is indicated.

4. When anterior teeth must be replaced, an anteroposterior palatal strap, complete palate, or horseshoe major connector may be used. The final selection must be based on modifying factors such as number and location of missing posterior teeth, periodontal support of remaining teeth, and type of opposing occlusion.

5. If a torus is present and is not to be removed, an anteroposterior palatal strap, anteroposterior palatal bar, or horseshoe major connector may be used. Final selection must be based on modifying factors.

6. A horseshoe connector should be used very sparingly. Flexure of this major connector may permit the concentration of forces upon individual teeth or localized segments of the maxillary arch.

7. A palatal bar is rarely indicated.

## Mandibular major connectors

### Special structural requirements

In general, mandibular major connectors are long and relatively narrow. Therefore, special consideration must be given to the design of such connectors. Mandibular connectors must be rigid without being so bulky that they compromise patient comfort. Furthermore, mandibular major connectors must not impinge upon the movable floor of the mouth, the associated frena, or mandibular tori.

Unlike maxillary major connectors, for which relief is infrequently required, mandibular major connectors may require relief between a mandibular removable partial denture and the underlying soft tissues. The amount of relief is dependent upon several factors. For an entirely tooth-supported prosthesis, little or no relief is needed because the denture does not tend to move in function. For a distal extension removable partial denture, however, a moderate amount of relief my be indicated because this type of prosthesis tends to rotate during function. Relief prevents the margins of the major connector from lacerating the sensitive lingual mucosa as a result of this movement.

The slope of the anterior ridge also influences the amount of relief needed (Fig 2-33). If the soft tissues are vertical, or nearly so, only minimal relief is required. Tissues that slope toward the tongue require the greatest amount of relief because any movement of the connector will bring it into contact with the adjacent soft tissues. If the anterior ridge is undercut, sufficient space may be created when the technician blocks out the undercut area. Specific recommendations for the placement of relief are presented in chapter 10.

It is important to note that bead lines are not used in conjunction with mandibular major connectors. Contact with the friable mucosa of the mandibular arch may cause irritation, ulceration, and patient discomfort.

### Types of mandibular major connectors

The following four types of mandibular major connectors are used in removable partial denture therapy:

1. Lingual bar
2. Lingual plate

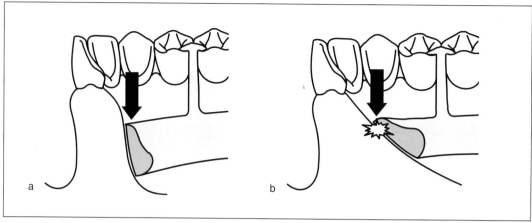

**Fig 2-33** *(a)* If the lingual soft tissues are vertical, or nearly vertical, minimal relief may be used. *(b)* Tissues that slope toward the tongue require the greatest amount of relief because any movement of the major connector will bring it into contact with the adjacent soft tissues.

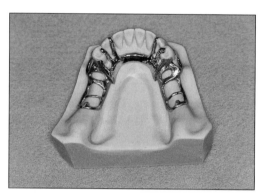

**Fig 2-34** Lingual bar major connector.

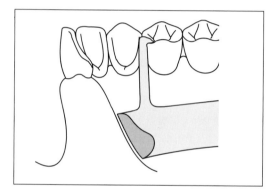

**Fig 2-35** A lingual bar major connector is half-pear shaped when viewed in cross section. The broadest portion of the bar is located nearest the floor of the mouth.

3. Double lingual bar (Kennedy bar)
4. Labial bar

Lingual bar and lingual plate major connectors are used in the overwhelming majority of removable partial denture applications. Double lingual bar and labial bar major connectors are used for special applications in which lingual bars and lingual plates are contraindicated. Although additional configurations may be employed, these major connectors are relatively rare and are not included in this discussion.

**Lingual bar** The lingual bar is perhaps the most frequently used mandibular major connector (Fig 2-34).

Because of its simplicity in design and construction, a lingual bar should be used unless one of the other connectors offers a definite advantage. A lingual bar is indicated for all tooth-supported removable partial dentures unless there is insufficient space between the marginal gingivae and the floor of the mouth.

When viewed in cross section, a lingual bar is half-pear shaped. The broadest portion of the bar is located at its inferior border, nearest the floor of the mouth (Fig 2-35). If additional rigidity is desired, the thickness of the bar may be increased during the waxing process. However, care must be taken to avoid making the bar so bulky that it interferes with patient comfort and function.

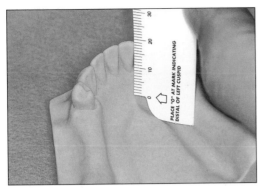

**Fig 2-36** Placement of a lingual bar requires at least 8 mm of space between the gingival margins and the floor of the mouth. This permits the major connector to have a minimum height of 5 mm and allows 3 mm of space between the gingival margins and the superior border of the bar.

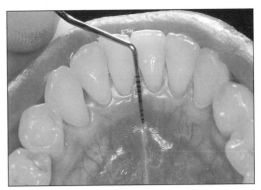

**Fig 2-37** A periodontal probe may be used to measure from the gingival margins to the floor of the mouth.

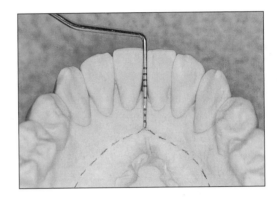

**Fig 2-38** Intraoral measurements (see Fig 2-37) may be transferred to the corresponding dental cast.

The normal thickness of a lingual bar is that of a 6-gauge half-pear-shaped wax or plastic pattern. The resultant casting will be relatively rigid unless the span is extremely long. If there is concern that the bar will not be rigid, wax may be added to the half-pear shape to increase its thickness. If space is available, the height of the bar also may be increased.

Availability of space is a key factor in determining whether a lingual bar can be used. To accommodate a lingual bar, at least 8 mm of vertical space must be present between the gingival margins of the teeth and the floor of the mouth (Fig 2-36). This permits the major connector to have a minimum height of 5 mm and allows 3 mm of space between the gingival margins and the superior border of the bar. Failure to provide 3 mm of space may lead to irritation of the adjacent soft tissues.

In a clinical setting, the available space may be determined using a periodontal probe. The patient should be instructed to elevate and protrude the tongue so that its tip touches the vermilion border of the upper lip. This activates the floor of the mouth and raises the tissues to the height that occurs during function. While the patient maintains this position, a periodontal probe can be positioned gently in the oral cavity (Fig 2-37). The tip of the probe should rest on the floor of the mouth, and readings should be taken at the most apical portion of each gingival margin. Subsequently, these readings should be transferred to the diagnostic cast or master cast (Fig 2-38). The lingual bar should be located in the most apical position the movable soft tissues will allow.

The presence of mandibular tori complicates the design, fabrication, and placement of lingual bar

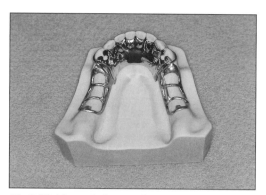

**Fig 2-39** Lingual plate major connector.

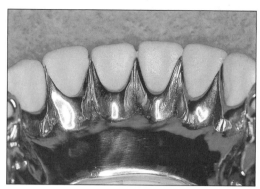

**Fig 2-40** The superior border of a lingual plate major connector should display a scalloped appearance.

major connectors. Surgical removal of mandibular tori usually is required for successful removable partial denture therapy. If mandibular tori cannot be surgically removed, another type of mandibular major connector should be considered. In most instances, the soft tissues over lingual tori are thin and respond to minimal pressure with ulceration and pain. Attempting to construct a lingual bar by avoiding the tori or by trying to gain adequate relief for the tori usually makes the prosthesis bulky and uncomfortable. In addition, it may jeopardize the rigidity of the major connector.

*Advantages of the lingual bar.* In addition to its simplicity, a lingual bar has minimal contact with the remaining teeth and soft tissues. As a result, there is decreased plaque accumulation and increased soft tissue stimulation. These factors may be critical in the long-term maintenance of teeth and soft tissues and should not be overlooked by the practitioner.

*Disadvantages of the lingual bar.* The greatest disadvantage is that if extreme care is not taken in the design and construction of a lingual bar, the resultant framework may not be rigid. This may result from improper waxing procedures or aggressive finishing of the cast framework. In either instance, the major connector can become too thin and too flexible. This permits the concentration of potentially destructive forces upon individual teeth and segments of the mandibular arch.

**Lingual plate** The structure of a lingual plate is basically that of a half-pear-shaped lingual bar with a thin, solid piece of metal extending from its superior border (Fig 2-39). This thin projection of metal is carried onto the lingual surfaces of the teeth and presents a scalloped appearance.

The inferior border of a lingual plate should be positioned as low in the floor of the mouth as possible, but should not interfere with the functional movements of the tongue and soft tissues. The inferior portion of the lingual plate may be slightly less bulky than the corresponding portion of a lingual bar, but no compromise in rigidity should be made.

The superior border of a lingual plate must be contoured to intimately contact the lingual surfaces of the teeth above the cingula. In addition, the lingual plate must completely close the interproximal spaces to the level of the contact points. Sealing these spaces from the lingual aspect prevents food from being packed into these areas. As a result of this contouring, the lingual plate should display a scalloped appearance (Fig 2-40). The superior margins of the scalloped metal should be knife edged to avoid a "ledging" effect on the lingual surfaces of the teeth. Ledging occurs when metal margins are thick or linear and produces unnatural contours, which are annoying to the tongue.

When a patient exhibits open embrasures or the anterior teeth are widely spaced, modifications to the lingual plate may be indicated. "Step backs" can be designed to avoid an unwanted display of metal (Fig

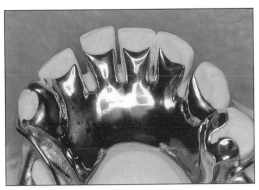

**Fig 2-41** A lingual plate may include "step backs" to minimize or eliminate the appearance of metal.

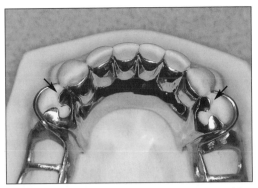

**Fig 2-42** A lingual plate must be supported by rests *(arrows)* located no farther posterior than the mesial surfaces of the first premolars.

2-41). To accomplish this, the superior border of a lingual plate should cover the cingulum of the individual tooth. The border should extend toward the contact area of the tooth and then turn apically, following the line angle to the level of the gingiva. The metal should cross the free gingival margin at a right angle, assume a gently curved path to the line angle of the adjacent tooth, and follow the line angle toward the contact area. The potential danger in using this approach is making the step back so severe that the connector may not be rigid. To ensure rigidity of the major connector, the inferior border of the lingual plate should be made thicker.

It is important to note that an anterior lingual plate must always be supported by rests located no farther posterior than the mesial fossae of the first premolars (Fig 2-42). Failure to provide these rests may result in pronounced rotation of the framework and labial displacement of the remaining anterior teeth.

*Advantages of the lingual plate.* There are a number of indications for using a lingual plate major connector. In many instances, a lingual plate must be used because there is insufficient vertical space for a lingual bar. This lack of space may be related to gingival recession, high muscle attachments, or high frenum attachments on the lingual aspect of the mandibular arch. When properly contoured, a lingual plate provides exceptional rigidity yet does not interfere with the functional movements of the tongue and the floor of the mouth.

A lingual plate also may be indicated when the remaining teeth have lost much of their periodontal support and require splinting. In this application, a lingual plate may be used to stabilize the remaining teeth and to distribute applied forces over the remaining teeth and soft tissues.

When one or more anterior teeth are periodontally compromised but may provide service for a time, these teeth may be supported by a lingual plate until extraction is necessary. As teeth are lost, retentive loops may be soldered to the lingual plate and prosthetic teeth may be added to the removable partial denture. This permits placement of prosthetic teeth without the expense of remaking the prosthesis.

When posterior teeth have been lost and there is a need for additional indirect retention, the use of a lingual plate may be advantageous. While a lingual plate does not serve as an indirect retainer, it may contribute to indirect retention if it is properly rested at each end.

Lingual plate major connectors also may be indicated for patients with conditions that prevent the removal of existing mandibular tori. Moderate relief must be provided during framework fabrication to prevent irritation of the fragile soft tissues that cover such tori.

One of the greatest advantages of the lingual plate major connector is its exceptional rigidity. In addition, patients often consider a well-fitting lingual plate more comfortable than a lingual bar.

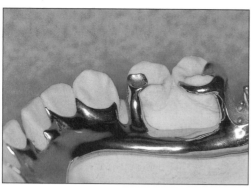

**Fig 2-43** In certain applications, the lingual surfaces of the anterior teeth may be covered, while the lingual surfaces of one or more posterior teeth may be left uncovered.

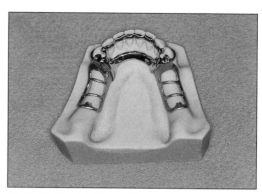

**Fig 2-44** Double lingual bar major connector.

*Disadvantages of the lingual plate.* The lingual plate's extensive coverage may contribute to decalcification of enamel surfaces and irritation of the soft tissues in patients with poor oral hygiene. Consequently, a thorough examination is essential to recognize those patients for whom a lingual plate is contraindicated.

A lingual plate generally contacts the anterior teeth, but also may extend posteriorly. In such applications, the lingual surfaces of the anterior teeth usually are covered, while the lingual surfaces of one or more posterior teeth may be left uncovered (Fig 2-43). This is an acceptable approach as long as the resultant contours are self-cleansing. If spaces are too small, they may act as food traps. Extreme care must be taken to ensure that a lingual plate major connector does not create additional oral hygiene challenges for a patient.

### Double lingual bar (Kennedy bar)

A double lingual bar displays characteristics of both lingual bar and lingual plate major connectors (Fig 2-44). The position and contour of the upper and lower borders of a double lingual bar are similar to those of a lingual plate. Unlike those of a lingual plate, however, the upper and lower components of a double lingual bar are not joined by a continuous sheet of metal. As a result, the lingual surfaces of the teeth and the interproximal soft tissues are largely exposed.

The lower component of this major connector should display the same structural characteristics as does a lingual bar. It should be half-pear shaped in cross section, with its greatest diameter at the inferior

margin. The upper bar should be half oval in cross section. This bar should be 2 to 3 mm in height and 1 mm thick. The upper bar should not run straight across the lingual surfaces of the teeth but should present a scalloped appearance.

The two bars should be joined by rigid minor connectors at each end. The minor connectors should be located in the interproximal spaces to disguise the thickness of the metal and to be less noticeable to the tongue.

Rests should be placed at each end of the upper bar and should be located no farther posterior than the mesial fossae of the first premolars. Placement of these rests is intended to prevent the bar from moving inferiorly and causing orthodontic movement of the remaining anterior teeth.

A double lingual bar is indicated primarily when contact with the remaining mandibular anterior teeth is indicated, but open embrasures exist. The upper bar should exhibit a scalloped contour that extends from the contact points to the cingula. The major connector should not be evident when the patient is viewed in a frontal plane.

*Advantages of the double lingual bar.* When properly supported by rests at each end, a double lingual bar effectively extends indirect retention in an anterior direction. It also contributes to horizontal stabilization of the prosthesis, since stress is transferred to those teeth contacted by the removable partial denture.

Because the gingival tissues and the interproximal embrasures are not covered, a free flow of saliva is per-

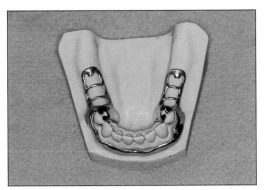

**Fig 2-45** Labial bar major connector.

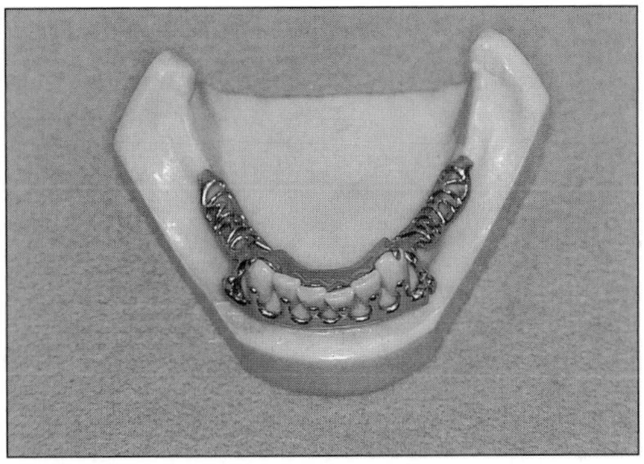

**Fig 2-46** The Swing-Lock removable partial denture represents a useful modification of the labial bar concept. The labial component functions as a gate that may be closed and locked to provide retention.

mitted and the marginal gingiva receives natural stimulation. These factors may be critical in the long-term health of the remaining teeth and oral tissues.

*Disadvantages of the double lingual bar.* The principal disadvantage of a double lingual bar is its tendency to trap debris. This arises from the marked crowding often exhibited by mandibular anterior teeth. Crowding produces undercuts and makes accurate adaptation of the upper bar extremely difficult. If the bar does not maintain intimate contact with tooth surfaces, food entrapment and patient discomfort will generally occur. Hence, the selection of a double lingual bar in preference to a lingual plate is questionable.

Patients also may find a double lingual bar irritating to the tongue. The presence of multiple borders and the thickness of the upper bar are often annoying. As a result, a modified lingual plate major connector may be preferred.

**Labial bar** As its name suggests, a labial bar runs across the mucosa on the facial surface of the mandibular arch (Fig 2-45). Like other mandibular major connectors, a labial bar displays a half-pear shape when viewed in cross section. But, because of its placement on the external curvature of the mandible, a labial bar is longer than a corresponding lingual bar, double lingual bar, or lingual plate. To ensure rigidity, the height and thickness of a labial bar must be greater than those described for a lingual bar.

The only justification for using a labial bar is the presence of a gross uncorrectable interference that makes the placement of a lingual major connector impossible. Interferences that commonly lead to the selection of a labial bar are *(1)* malpositioned or lingually inclined teeth and *(2)* large mandibular tori that preclude the use of a lingual bar or lingual plate. Every attempt should be made to correct the condition by extraction of severely malpositioned teeth, orthodontic correction of lingually inclined teeth, placement of crowns, or surgical intervention to remove tori. Because of the position and bulk of a labial bar, the probability of successful treatment with this type of major connector is extremely limited.

The Swing-Lock removable partial denture represents a useful modification of the labial bar (Fig 2-46). In this application, the labial component does not serve as a major connector. Instead, the modified labial bar has a hinge at one end and a locking device at the opposite end. This permits an opening and closing action similar to a gate. The framework may be positioned in the mouth with the gate in the open position. Upon complete seating of the prosthesis, the gate may be closed. This permits the removable partial denture to reach otherwise inaccessible undercuts on the labial surfaces of the teeth. Use of the Swing-Lock removable partial denture is discussed at length in chapter 19.

*Advantages of the labial bar.* When the remaining mandibular teeth are tipped so far lingually that a more conventional major connector cannot be used, a labial bar may be considered. Nevertheless, every possible means of avoiding the use of a labial bar should be entertained before it is incorporated into the design of a partial denture.

*Disadvantages of the labial bar.* Patient acceptance of labial bar major connectors generally is poor. The bulk of the major connector distorts the lower lip unless the lip is relatively immobile, and the mere presence of metal between the gingival tissues and the lip causes significant discomfort. In addition, the labial vestibule usually is not deep enough to permit a sufficiently rigid connector without encroaching on the free gingival margins.

### Review of indications for mandibular major connectors

1. For a tooth-supported removable partial denture, the lingual bar normally is the mandibular major connector of choice.
2. When there is insufficient room between the floor of the mouth and the gingival margins (< 8 mm), a lingual plate should be used. This major connector also is indicated for patients with large inoperable tori and patients with high lingual frenum attachments.
3. When the anterior teeth have reduced periodontal support and require stabilization, a lingual plate is recommended.
4. When the anterior teeth exhibit reduced periodontal support and large interproximal spaces, a modified lingual plate (ie, step-back design) or double lingual bar should be used.
5. When a removable partial denture will replace all mandibular posterior teeth, a lingual plate should be used.
6. A labial bar is rarely indicated.

## ⌑ Minor Connectors

The primary function of a minor connector is to join the remaining components of a removable partial denture to the major connector. Minor connectors also are responsible for distribution of applied forces to the supporting teeth and oral tissues. Therefore, rigidity is an essential characteristic of all minor connectors. The broad distribution of forces prevents any one tooth or any one portion of an edentulous ridge from bearing a destructive amount of stress. In contrast, bending or deformation of a minor connector may result in stress concentration and damage to the supporting teeth and soft tissues.

### Types of minor connectors

There are four categories of minor connectors. They may be described as follows:

1. Minor connectors that join clasp assemblies to major connectors (Fig 2-47)
2. Minor connectors that join indirect retainers or auxiliary rests to major connectors (Fig 2-48)
3. Minor connectors that join denture bases to major connectors (Fig 2-49)
4. Minor connectors that serve as approach arms for vertical projection or bar-type clasps (Fig 2-50)

### Minor connectors that join clasp assemblies to major connectors

Minor connectors that join clasp assemblies to major connectors must be rigid, because they support the active components of the removable partial denture, the retentive clasps. They also support the rests, which prevent vertical movement of a prosthesis toward the underlying tissues. As a result, minor connectors must have sufficient bulk to ensure rigidity, but they must be positioned so they do not irritate the oral tissues.

Most minor connectors that support clasp assemblies are located on proximal surfaces of teeth adjacent to edentulous areas. These minor connectors should be broad buccolingually, but thin mesiodistally (Fig 2-51). This shape makes it easier to place a prosthetic tooth in a natural position.

In many instances, a clasp assembly must be positioned on a tooth that is not adjacent to an edentulous space. When this occurs, a minor connector should be positioned in the associated lingual embrasure (Fig 2-52). This results in a sufficient bulk of metal without encroaching on the tongue space. Hence, the minor connector may be rigid yet unobtrusive. A minor connector should never be positioned on the convex lingual surface of a tooth where its bulk will be evident.

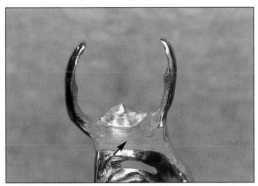

**Fig 2-47** A minor connector *(arrow)* that joins a clasp assembly to the associated major connector.

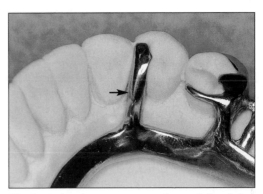

**Fig 2-48** A minor connector *(arrow)* that joins an indirect retainer to the major connector.

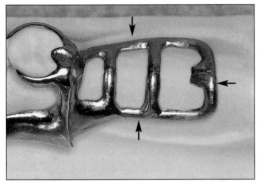

**Fig 2-49** A minor connector *(arrows)* that joins a resin denture base to the major connector.

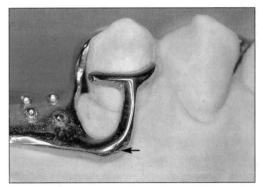

**Fig 2-50** A minor connector *(arrow)* that serves as the approach arm for a bar-type clasp.

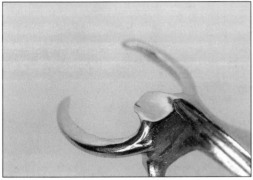

**Fig 2-51** A minor connector that joins a clasp assembly to the major connector must be broad buccolingually, but thin mesiodistally. This allows the minor connector to be strong, yet does not interfere with prosthetic tooth placement.

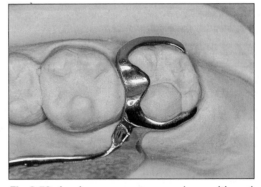

**Fig 2-52** A minor connector may be positioned in a lingual embrasure to disguise its thickness.

### Minor connectors that join indirect retainers or auxiliary rests to major connectors

Minor connectors that support indirect retainers or auxiliary rests are often used in removable partial denture therapy. These minor connectors should form right angles with the corresponding major connectors, but junctions should be gently curved to prevent stress concentration (Fig 2-53). As previously noted, minor connectors should be positioned in lingual embrasures to disguise their bulk and promote patient comfort.

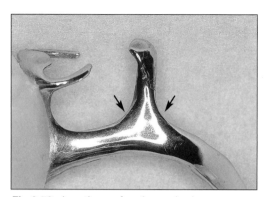

**Fig 2-53** Junctions of major and minor connectors should be gently curved *(arrows)* to prevent stress concentration and promote patient comfort.

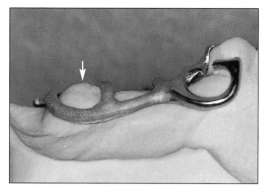

**Fig 2-54** In the maxillary arch, a distal extension base must extend into the pterygomaxillary notch. To provide appropriate mechanical support for the denture base, the minor connector should extend beyond the most prominent portion of the tuberosity *(arrow)*.

### Minor connectors that join denture bases to major connectors

Minor connectors that join the denture base to the major connector may be described as follows:

1. Open construction
2. Mesh construction
3. Bead, wire, or nailhead components on a metal base

These minor connectors must be strong enough to anchor a denture base to the removable partial denture framework. They must be rigid enough to resist fracture and displacement. In addition, these components must provide minimal interference with the arrangement of artificial teeth.

In the maxillary arch, a distal extension base must extend the entire length of the ridge and should cover the tuberosity. Consequently, the minor connector should be extended as far posteriorly as is practical. In many instances, the minor connector may extend beyond the most prominent portion of the tuberosity (Fig 2-54). In other cases, the minor connector must be terminated anterior to this area.

In the mandibular arch, a distal extension base must cover the retromolar pad. Therefore, the minor connector should extend two thirds the length of the edentulous ridge (Fig 2-55). This provides adequate support and retention for the associated resin base.

**Open construction** Open construction consists of longitudinal and transverse struts that form a ladder-like network (Fig 2-56).

Placement of the longitudinal and transverse struts is a critical factor in prosthetic tooth arrangement. In the mandibular arch, one longitudinal strut should be positioned buccal to the crest of the ridge and the other lingual to the ridge crest. In the maxillary arch, one longitudinal strut should be positioned buccal to the ridge crest. The border of the major connector generally will act as the second longitudinal strut.

Positioning of a longitudinal strut along the crest of the ridge must be avoided. This not only interferes with the placement of artificial teeth, but also predisposes the denture base to fracture.

Transverse struts also must be positioned to facilitate the placement of artificial teeth. When there is adequate room for the placement of teeth, the number of cross struts is not critical. When vertical space is minimal, improperly placed struts may create difficulties in tooth placement. Ideally, transverse struts should be designed to pass between the necks of the artificial teeth. This aids in tooth arrangement and often results in improved esthetics.

During the framework fabrication process, those areas of a master cast that are to feature open retention must be relieved with an appropriate thickness of wax. Relief provides space between the completed minor connector and the tissues of the residual ridge.

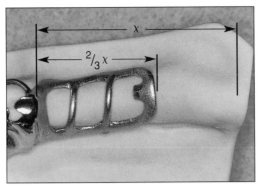

Fig 2-55 In the mandibular arch, a distal extension base must cover the retromolar pad. To provide appropriate mechanical support, the associated minor connector should be two thirds the length of the edentulous ridge.

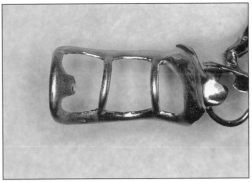

Fig 2-56 Open retention consists of longitudinal and transverse struts that form a ladderlike network.

Fig 2-57 Mesh construction may be compared to a rigid metallic screen.

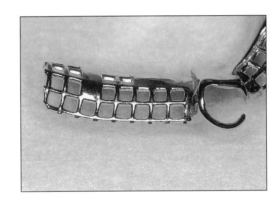

The space permits an acrylic resin to encircle the longitudinal and transverse struts, thereby providing retention for the denture base.

Open construction can be used whenever multiple teeth are to be replaced. Studies have shown that this form of minor connector provides the strongest attachment of acrylic resin to the removable partial denture framework. It also facilitates relining and rebasing of removable partial dentures.

**Mesh construction** A mesh minor connector may be compared to a rigid metallic screen (Fig 2-57). Channels that pass through the connector are intended to permit acrylic resin penetration. This allows resin encirclement of the minor connector and mechanical retention of the denture base.

Relief and border extension for a mesh minor connector should be identical to those described for open construction.

The main drawback of a mesh minor connector is the difficulty it presents during the packing of acrylic resin. Increased pressure is needed to force resin through the small holes in the minor connector. Insufficient packing pressure may result in inadequate resin penetration and a weak attachment to the framework. Studies have shown that the smaller the openings in this minor connector, the weaker the attachment.

Mesh construction also may interfere with the arrangement of prosthetic teeth. Mesh must cover the entire ridge crest and cannot be limited to those areas between the necks of artificial teeth. As a result, the ridge lap areas of artificial teeth may require significant reduction to facilitate proper arrangement. When restorative space is minimal, this reduction may be significant and may result in compromised esthetics.

Mesh construction may be used whenever multiple teeth are to be replaced. Nevertheless, open construction is preferred.

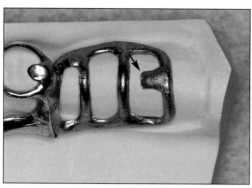

**Fig 2-58** A cast stop *(arrow)* is essential to prevent displacement or deformation of the metal framework during resin-packing procedures.

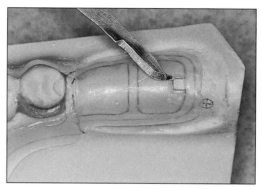

**Fig 2-59** A cast stop is created by removing a small square of relief wax at the appropriate position on the cast.

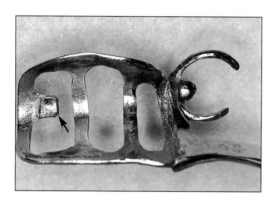

**Fig 2-60** The cast stop *(arrow)* projects from the tissue surface of the minor connector to contact the dental cast.

**The importance of cast stops** As previously noted, relief is provided beneath minor connectors of open construction and mesh construction. This relief provides space between the minor connector and the underlying master cast (or residual ridge). This space permits resin to encircle the minor connector and provides a mechanism for attachment of the denture base to the framework. While this method works quite well for tooth-supported removable partial dentures, it must be modified for distal extension applications.

In a distal extension prosthesis, the use of relief produces a minor connector that is supported at only one end. As a result, the minor connector may bend when a load is applied. Since considerable force is applied during the packing and processing of acrylic resin, the probability of bending is increased during these procedures. To prevent bending, a small area at the free end of the minor connector should contact the master cast (Fig 2-58). This portion of the minor connector is termed a *cast stop*.

A cast stop is created by removing a small square of relief wax (2 × 2 mm) where the posterior strut of

the minor connector crosses the center of the ridge (Fig 2-59). This depression is incorporated into the refractory cast. During the waxing process, this depression is filled with wax. Upon casting the framework and returning it to the master cast, the cast stop should contact the surface of the master cast (Fig 2-60). Because the minor connector is supported at both ends, bending of the framework can be minimized or eliminated.

As might be expected, the role of cast stops is quite important in removable partial denture construction.

**Bead, nailhead, or wire construction** Bead, nailhead, or wire components are often used in conjunction with metal denture bases. The metal bases are cast to fit directly against the underlying soft tissues. Hence, no relief is provided beneath these minor connectors. Resin is attached to the free surface of such bases, and retention is gained by encompassment of surface projections.

Projections may be created by placing resin beads on the appropriate segments of the wax pattern, in-

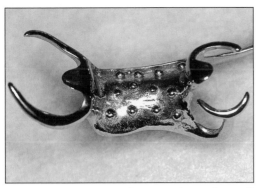

**Fig 2-61** Bead retention consists of small spheres on a cast metal base.

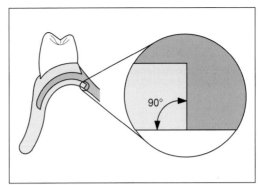

**Fig 2-62** A butt joint should be used to join acrylic resin and metal components at the internal surface of a removable partial denture. Each internal finish line should display an angle of 90 degrees.

vesting the completed pattern, eliminating the pattern materials via heat application, and casting the framework (Fig 2-61). Nailheads may be produced in a similar manner. Projections also may be added by casting or soldering irregular wire forms to a metal base.

The primary advantage of a metal base is related to improved hygiene and thermal stimulation. Disadvantages include difficulty in adjusting and relining cast metal bases. Furthermore, the attachment of resin is relatively weak.

Bead, nailhead, and wire construction should be limited to short-span, tooth-supported applications in patients with well-healed ridges.

**Attachment of minor connectors to major connectors** A minor connector that supports an acrylic resin denture base must be joined to the major connector with sufficient bulk to avoid fracture. In addition, each acrylic resin denture base must join the major connector in a smooth, even fashion. Any irregularity or "step" between the two surfaces will irritate the tongue or the soft tissues of the ridge. Consequently, the interfacial geometry and material properties must be considered.

Currently, acrylic resin is used to construct the overwhelming majority of denture bases. Because acrylic resin gains its strength with increasing bulk, it should not be finished to a thin edge. If this is attempted, the material may chip or fracture. This can create unhygienic and potentially irritating conditions.

To prevent the acrylic resin from becoming too thin, the design of the resin-metal interface must be

considered. Ideally, a butt joint should be provided so the acrylic resin can blend evenly with the major connector (Fig 2-62).

Because acrylic resin is processed completely around open minor connectors and mesh minor connectors, resin-metal interfaces must be created on both the internal and external surfaces of the associated major connectors. For metal base minor connectors, acrylic resin is processed only on the external surface. Therefore, resin-metal joints should be created only at the external surfaces. These interfaces are referred to as *finish lines*. If they are located on the outer surfaces of major connectors, they are called *external finish lines*. If they are positioned on the inner or tissue surfaces, they are termed *internal finish lines*.

*Internal finish lines.* Internal finish lines are formed as a result of relief wax placed on the edentulous ridges of a master cast prior to duplication (Fig 2-63). The relief wax (24 to 26 gauge) creates an elevated area on the resultant refractory cast. As previously noted, this elevation is necessary to create space for acrylic resin beneath open and mesh connectors.

The margins of the relief wax establish internal finish lines in the completed metal framework (Fig 2-64). The margins of the relief wax should be sharp and well defined.

*External finish lines.* External finish lines also must be sharp and should be slightly undercut to help lock the acrylic resin to the major connector. The internal angle

43

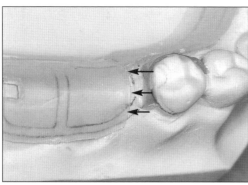

**Fig 2-63** Internal finish lines result from relief wax placed on the master cast prior to duplication. *Arrows* indicate the presence of a well-defined vertical wall, which will produce an internal finish line.

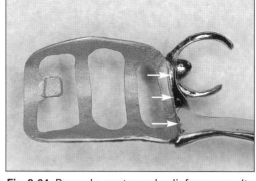

**Fig 2-64** Properly contoured relief wax results in a sharply defined internal finish line.

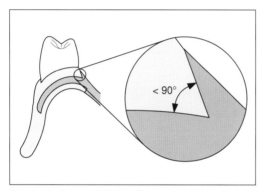

**Fig 2-65** External finish lines should be slightly less than 90 degrees. This results in improved mechanical retention for acrylic resin components.

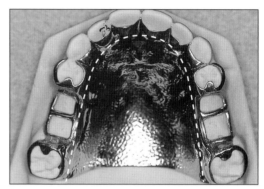

**Fig 2-66** When possible, an external finish line should follow an arc established by the lingual surfaces of the remaining teeth *(broken line)*. This disguises the position of the external finish line and results in improved patient comfort.

formed at the junction of the major and minor connectors should be less than 90 degrees (Fig 2-65).

An external finish line is formed by the placement and carving of wax during framework fabrication. It should originate at the lingual extent of the rest seat and continue down the lingual aspect of the minor connector. The external finish line should be well defined along its entire length. The contour of the external finish line should be consistent with the contours of the major connector. Transition from the external finish line to a denture base should be smooth and flowing.

When viewed from an occlusal perspective, the external finish line should follow an arc established by the lingual surfaces of the remaining teeth (Fig 2-66). This permits the development of contours that are not irritating to the patient.

### Minor connectors that serve as approach arms for vertical projection or bar-type clasps

Approach arms for vertical projection or bar-type clasps are the only minor connectors that are not required to be rigid (Fig 2-67). These components support direct retainers (clasps) and therefore must exhibit some degree of flexibility.

A minor connector of this type approaches the tooth from an apical direction rather than from an occlusal direction. The approach arm should display a smooth, even taper from its origin to its terminus. It must not cross a soft tissue undercut, and for this reason its use is contraindicated in some instances. This minor connector is considered in greater depth in chapter 3.

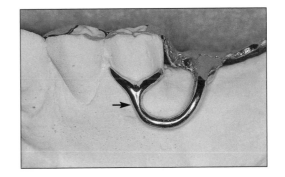

**Fig 2-67** Approach arms *(arrow)* for bar-type clasps are the only minor connectors that are not required to be rigid.

## ▣ Rests and Rest Seats

Forces that are applied to a removable partial denture must be transferred to the supporting teeth and tissues in an atraumatic fashion. The components of a removable partial denture that transfer forces down the long axes of the abutment teeth are called *rests*. The prepared surfaces of the teeth into which rests fit are called *rest seats*.

The relationship between a rest and a rest seat must be such that forces transmitted from the prosthesis to an abutment are directed apically down the long axis of the tooth (Fig 2-68). In this manner, stress can be absorbed by the fibers of the periodontal ligament without damaging the ligament or the supporting bone.

In the case of a tooth-supported removable partial denture, all the stresses are transferred to the abutment teeth. In a tooth-tissue–supported removable partial denture, only a portion of the stresses are transferred to the teeth, while the edentulous ridge must absorb the remainder of the load.

In addition to transferring forces, each rest should serve as a vertical stop for the prosthesis (Fig 2-69). Firm, positive contact between a rest and rest seat minimizes vertical displacement of the prosthesis and prevents injury to the soft tissues.

A rest also must maintain the retentive clasp in its proper position. If the clasp is not supported, it will lose its ability to retain the prosthesis in its intended position (Fig 2-70).

A rest that is part of a retentive clasp assembly is referred to as a *primary rest*. A rest that is responsible for additional support or indirect retention is called an *auxiliary rest* or *secondary rest*.

Primary rests prevent vertical movement of a prosthesis toward the tissues and also help transmit applied forces to the supporting teeth. The transmission of lateral forces may be increased by deepening the accompanying rest seats, but this should be done only for entirely tooth-supported prostheses. In all other applications, rest seats should be shallow and saucer shaped, and should function as ball-and-socket joints (Fig 2-71). This geometry permits dissipation of potentially harmful lateral forces.

Auxiliary or secondary rests are used as indirect retainers in extension base removable partial dentures (Class I, Class II, and long-span Class IV applications). These rests are placed anterior or posterior to the axis of rotation to prevent the extension bases from lifting away from the underlying ridges (Fig 2-72). A more complete discussion of indirect retention and its importance is presented in chapter 3.

While there are a variety of rests that may be used in removable partial denture therapy, this text focuses on three major forms. These are

1. Occlusal rests—so named because they are seated on the occlusal surfaces of posterior teeth
2. Lingual or cingulum rests—those seated on the lingual surfaces of anterior teeth, usually maxillary canines
3. Incisal rests—those seated on the incisal edges of anterior teeth

Characteristics of each of the rests and their respective rest seats are covered in the following paragraphs. Techniques for the preparation of rest seats are presented in chapter 9.

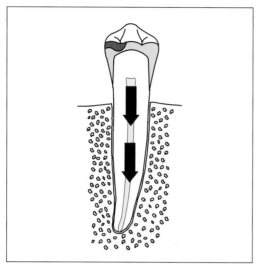

**Fig 2-68** A rest and rest seat should direct forces along the long axis of the associated abutment *(arrows)*.

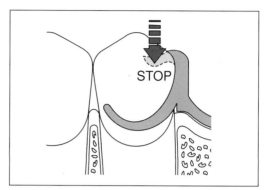

**Fig 2-69** A rest must prevent apical displacement of the prosthesis. If this is not accomplished, the underlying hard and soft tissues may be damaged.

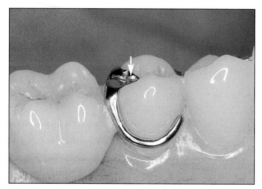

**Fig 2-70** Each clasp assembly must include a rest *(arrow)*. The rest is responsible for maintaining the retentive clasp in its proper position. If this is not accomplished, the clasp assembly will not function as intended.

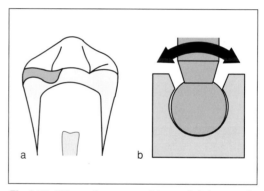

**Fig 2-71** When the removable partial denture is in position, the rest seat and rest *(a)* should function as a ball-and-socket joint *(b)*.

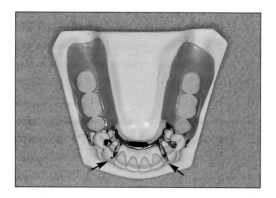

**Fig 2-72** Auxiliary or secondary rests *(arrows)* are used as indirect retainers in extension base removable partial dentures. Because of their positions, these rests resist displacement of extension bases away from the underlying soft tissues.

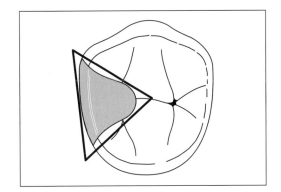

**Fig 2-73** The outline form of an occlusal rest seat should be roughly triangular, with the base of the triangle located at the marginal ridge and the rounded apex directed toward the center of the occlusal surface.

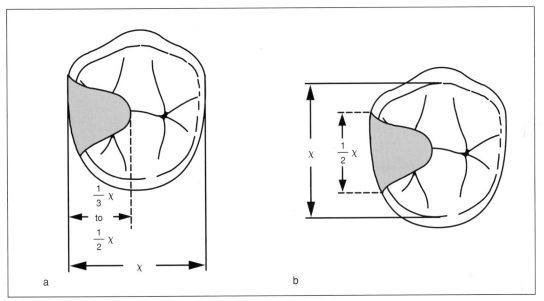

**Fig 2-74** An occlusal rest seat should occupy one third to one half the mesiodistal diameter of the abutment (a) and approximately one half the buccolingual width of the tooth measured from cusp tip to cusp tip (b).

## Occlusal rests and rest seats

It is essential that a rest seat be prepared in the occlusal surface of each tooth that is to receive an occlusal rest. A rest should never be placed on a tooth that has not been adequately prepared.

The outline form of an occlusal rest seat should be triangular, with the base of the triangle located at the marginal ridge and the rounded apex directed toward the center of the tooth (Fig 2-73).

If there is one descriptive phrase that can be applied to occlusal rest seats, it is "smooth gentle curves." Sharp angles, walls, and ledges must be avoided. Any portion of the rest seat that restricts movement of the rest may transmit undesirable horizontal forces to the tooth.

The shape of the rest seat should follow the outline of the mesial or distal fossa for the chosen abutment. The rest seat should occupy one third to one half the mesiodistal diameter of the tooth and approximately one half the buccolingual width of the tooth measured from cusp tip to cusp tip (Fig 2-74).

The floor of the occlusal rest seat must be inclined slightly toward the center of the tooth. The enclosed angle formed by a line dropped down the proximal surface of the tooth parallel to the long axis of the tooth and the floor of the rest seat must be less than 90 degrees so that the transmitted occlusal forces can

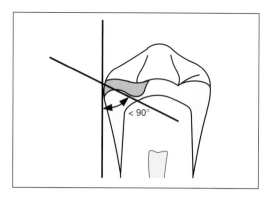

**Fig 2-75** The enclosed angle formed by a line dropped down the proximal surface of the tooth and the floor of the rest seat must be less than 90 degrees. This permits forces to be transmitted along the long axis of the abutment.

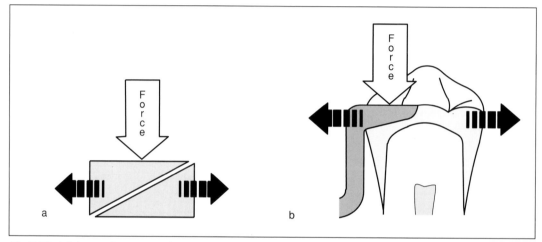

**Fig 2-76** (a) An angle greater than 90 degrees transmits destructive horizontal forces and creates an inclined plane effect. (b) The latter phenomenon may result in migration of the affected abutment.

be directed along the vertical axis of the tooth (Fig 2-75). An angle greater than 90 degrees not only will not transmit the forces vertically, but will create an inclined plane effect (Fig 2-76). This inclined plane effect can produce slippage of the prosthesis away from the abutment teeth. In addition, it can cause orthodontic movement of abutment teeth, with concurrent pain and bone loss.

When viewed in cross section, the deepest part of an occlusal rest seat should be located near the center of the mesial or distal fossa. From its depth, the floor of the rest seat should rise gently toward the marginal ridge (Fig 2-77).

The most common mistake in occlusal rest seat preparation is insufficient reduction of the marginal ridge. This leads to construction of a rest that is extremely thin and subject to fracture. An occlusal rest must be at least 0.5 mm thick at its thinnest point and should be between 1.0 and 1.5 mm thick where it crosses the marginal ridge (Fig 2-78). Techniques for the preparation and assessment of rest seats are presented in chapter 9.

## Occlusal rests on amalgam restorations

Placing occlusal rests on large amalgam restorations is hazardous at best. The primary reason for attempting

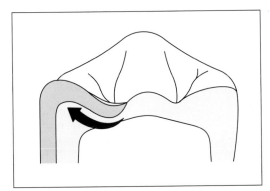

**Fig 2-77** The deepest portion of an occlusal rest should be located near the center of the mesial or distal fossa. From this point, the rest seat should rise gently toward the marginal ridge.

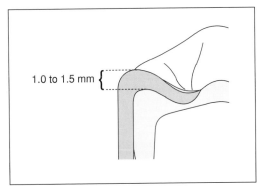

**Fig 2-78** An occlusal rest should be at least 0.5 mm thick at its thinnest point and 1.0 to 1.5 mm thick where it crosses the marginal ridge.

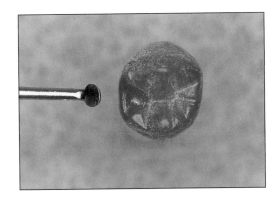

**Fig 2-79** When a cast restoration is planned for an abutment, an appropriate rest seat should be carved into the wax pattern.

this is economics, since an amalgam restoration costs less than a comparable cast gold restoration. However, when one considers the potential disadvantages of the procedure, this justification is hardly logical.

The unfavorable flow characteristics and poor tensile characteristics of amalgam increase the probability of restoration failure. In addition, replacement of a defective restoration under an existing removable partial denture is difficult and the result is usually less than optimal. Retreatment may require restoration of the abutment as well as fabrication of a new removable partial denture. This is both costly and inefficient, and should be avoided.

While conservative amalgam restorations may be used to support removable partial dentures, the treat-

ing practitioner must carefully consider the potential advantages and disadvantages of such treatment. The patient also should be informed of treatment options and their implications. The practitioner and patient should then agree on an acceptable treatment plan.

### Occlusal rests on gold restorations

When a cast gold restoration is planned for an abutment tooth, the wax pattern should display ideal contours. An appropriate rest seat should be carved into the wax pattern (Fig 2-79). Upon completion of the casting process, restoration contours should be refined in preparation for delivery. The technique for this procedure is discussed in chapter 7.

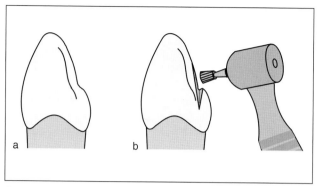

**Fig 2-80** The normal morphology of a maxillary canine *(a)* facilitates preparation of a lingual or cingulum rest seat *(b)*.

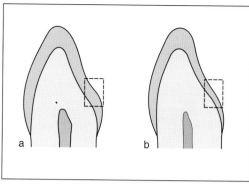

**Fig 2-81** Unlike a maxillary canine *(a)*, a mandibular canine *(b)* does not exhibit a sufficient thickness of lingual enamel to allow preparation of a lingual or cingulum rest seat. (*Boxes* denote areas of proposed tooth preparation.)

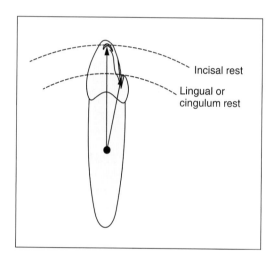

**Fig 2-82** Because it is located closer to the rotational center of an abutment, a lingual or cingulum rest is preferred to an incisal rest.

## Lingual or cingulum rests and rest seats

Lingual or cingulum rests are used primarily on maxillary canines. The normal morphology of a maxillary canine permits preparation of a satisfactory rest seat with minimal tooth reduction (Fig 2-80).

The thickness of enamel on the lingual surface of a mandibular canine rarely allows a lingual rest to be used (Fig 2-81). Lingual rests on incisors are also rare. The main indication for their use is missing canines. In this instance, multiple incisors should receive lingual rests to distribute the stresses over a number of teeth because a single incisor seldom offers adequate support.

Although a lingual rest may be used successfully, an occlusal rest in the mesial fossa of the first premolar is preferred if the occlusion permits. An occlusal rest is located in a more favorable orientation (nearly horizontal), and the accompanying rest seat is easier to prepare.

However, a lingual rest is preferred to an incisal rest. A lingual rest is located closer to the rotational center of the supporting tooth and does not tend to tip the tooth (Fig 2-82). The longer lever arm associated with an incisal rest magnifies the rotational movement of the prosthesis and may result in significant tooth movement. Since a lingual rest is confined to the lingual surface of an anterior tooth, it permits improved esthetics. Because of the configuration of the lingual rest, it is also less subject to breakage and distortion.

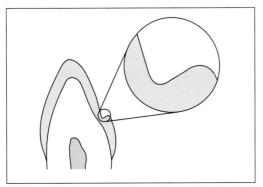

Fig 2-83 A lingual or cingulum rest seat should be V shaped when viewed in cross section. This geometry prevents migration of the abutment away from the removable partial denture framework.

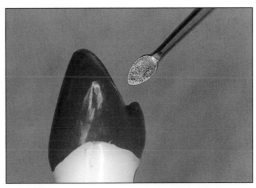

Fig 2-84 When a rest seat is to be placed on an anterior tooth requiring a cast restoration, a lingual or cingulum rest should be used. Hence, a properly contoured rest seat should be placed into the wax pattern.

The form of a lingual rest seat should be V shaped when viewed in cross section (Fig 2-83). The preparation should display a relatively upright lingual wall that originates at the level of the cingulum and extends incisally. The remaining wall should originate at the crest of the cingulum and incline labiogingivally toward the center of the tooth. This wall must provide a definite seat for the rest and must prevent the migration of the abutment away from the framework.

When viewed from the lingual aspect, the outline form of a lingual rest seat should be crescent shaped. This geometry provides some freedom of movement in a mesiodistal direction. Hence, the rest and rest seat may function as a ball-and-socket assembly.

Sharp line angles and corners must be avoided because they complicate the fit of the cast framework and may serve as stress concentrators.

Placement of lingual rest seats in enamel surfaces is a sound practice provided the following circumstances exist:

1. The cingulum is prominent enough to permit appropriate tooth recontouring.
2. The patient practices good oral hygiene.
3. The caries index is low.

### Lingual rest seats on cast restorations

When a crown is to be placed on an anterior tooth and a rest seat is required, the rest seat should be placed in the wax pattern (Fig 2-84). The cingulum of the restoration should be accentuated to allow development of a rest seat that will direct occlusal forces along the long axis of the tooth.

### *Incisal rests and rest seats*

Incisal rests and rest seats are less desirable than lingual rests and rest seats for anterior teeth. Nevertheless, they may be used successfully if abutments are sound and cast restorations are not indicated (Fig 2-85). If a cast restoration is planned for an anterior abutment, an incisal rest is never indicated. A lingual rest should be incorporated into the restoration instead.

Incisal rests are most frequently used on mandibular canines, but may be used on maxillary canines. They are not indicated on incisors except under unusual circumstances. If stabilization of incisors is indicated and placement of a fixed restoration is not warranted, incisal rests may be incorporated into a lingual plate to support these teeth.

Incisal rests should be positioned near the incisal angles of abutment teeth. Whether they are designed for mesioincisal or distoincisal angles depends on the prescribed clasping system. If an individual tooth is not to be clasped, yet requires an incisal rest, the rest should be placed where it will exert the least impact upon esthetics. In most instances, this requires that

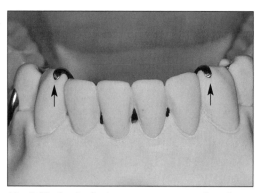

**Fig 2-85** An incisal rest seat approaches from the lingual surface, crosses the incisal edge, and extends onto the facial surface of an abutment *(arrows)*.

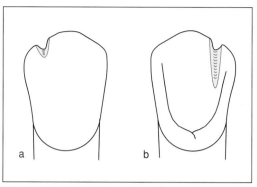

**Fig 2-86** An incisal rest seat should appear as a small, V-shaped notch located 1.5 to 2.0 mm from the proximal-incisal angle of the tooth. Facial *(a)* and lingual *(b)* views are provided.

the rest be placed at the distoincisal surface of the abutment.

An incisal rest seat should appear as a small, V-shaped notch located approximately 1.5 to 2.0 mm from the proximal-incisal angle of the tooth (Fig 2-86). The deepest part of the preparation should be toward the center of the tooth mesiodistally. The notch should be rounded and should extend slightly onto the facial surface to provide a positive seat for the rest.

The enamel on the lingual surface should be prepared as a shallow depression to accommodate the minor connector and avoid annoying the tongue. Because of the greater length of this minor connector, care must be taken to ensure its rigidity.

## ▣ Bibliography

Anderson JN. Dimensions of cast palatal and lingual bars. Dent Pract Dent Rec 1958;8:270–274.

Applegate OC. The partial denture base. J Prosthet Dent 1955;5:636–648.

Askinas SW. Facings in removable partial dentures. J Prosthet Dent 1975;33:633–636.

Beck HO. Alloys for removable partial dentures. Dent Clin North Am 1960;4:591–596.

Ben-Ur Z, Matalan S, Aviv I, Cardash HS. Rigidity of major connectors when subjected to bending and torsion forces. J Prosthet Dent 1989;62:557–562.

Berg T, Caputo AA. Anterior rests for maxillary removable partial dentures. J Prosthet Dent 1978;39:139–146.

Buckner H, LaVelle WE. Metal backings for denture teeth. J Prosthet Dent 1974;32:579–581.

Campbell LD. Subjective reactions to major connector designs for removable partial dentures. J Prosthet Dent 1977;37:506–517.

Cecconi BT. Effect of rest design on transmission of forces to abutment teeth. J Prosthet Dent 1974;32:141–151.

Cecconi BT. Lingual bar design. J Prosthet Dent 1973;29:635–639.

Dirksen LC, Compagna SJ. Mat surface and rugae reproduction for upper partial denture casting. J Prosthet Dent 1954;4:67–72.

Dunny JA, King GE. Minor connector design for anterior acrylic resin bases: A preliminary study. J Prosthet Dent 1975;34:496–502.

Fisher RL, Jaslow C. The efficiency of an indirect retainer. J Prosthet Dent 1975;33:24–30.

Henderson D. Major connectors for mandibular removable partial dentures. J Prosthet Dent 1973;30:532–548.

Henderson D. Major connectors—United it stands. Dent Clin North Am 1973;17:661–668.

Laney WR, Desjardins RP. Comparison of base metal alloys and Type IV gold alloys for removable partial denture framework. Dent Clin North Am 1973;17:611–630.

LaVere AM, Krol AJ. Selection of a major connector for the extension base removable partial denture. J Prosthet Dent 1973;30:102–105.

MacKinnon KP. Indirect retention in partial denture construction. Dent J Aust 1955;27:221–225.

Seidin A. Occlusal rests and rest seats. J Prosthet Dent 1958;8:431–440.

Skinner FW, Chung P. The effect of surface contact in the retention of a denture. J Prosthet Dent 1951;1:229–235.

Wallace DH. The use of gold occlusal surfaces in complete and partial dentures. J Prosthet Dent 1964;14:326–333.

# Direct Retainers, Indirect Retainers, and Tooth Replacements

## ⊔ Direct Retainers

A removable partial denture must include components that prevent displacement of the prosthesis from the patient's mouth during function. The components of a removable partial denture that engage abutments and resist dislodging forces are called *direct retainers*. Strict criteria guiding the design and fabrication of direct retainers must be observed. This ensures effective prosthesis retention and minimizes the transmission of detrimental forces to the associated abutments and supporting tissues. In general, there are two types of direct retainers: intracoronal direct retainers and extracoronal direct retainers (Fig 3-1).

### Intracoronal direct retainers

The first intracoronal direct retainer was introduced by Herman E. S. Chayes in 1906.[1] As its name implies, an intracoronal direct retainer resides within the normal contours of an abutment and functions to retain and stabilize a removable partial denture. The retainer consists of two distinct components (Figs 3-2 to 3-4). The first component, or *matrix*, is a metal receptacle con-

tained within the normal clinical contours of a fixed restoration. The second component, or *patrix*, is attached to the associated removable partial denture.

When two or more intracoronal attachments are used in a single removable partial denture, the precise parallelism of all matrix and patrix components is essential. Parallelism results in a well-defined path of insertion and removal and in mechanical binding when off-axis forces are applied to the prosthesis. This binding phenomenon is considered the major factor contributing to retention. Nevertheless, friction between the matrix and patrix components also may provide measurable resistance to displacement.

Intracoronal direct retainers may be subdivided into two categories based on their method of fabrication and the tolerance of fit between components. If components are fabricated in metal using high-precision manufacturing techniques, the intracoronal retainers are considered *precision attachments* (see Figs 3-2 to 3-4). These attachments usually exhibit long, parallel walls and exceptional surface adaptation.

A second category of intracoronal attachments displays a less intimate fit between matrix and patrix components. These are termed *semiprecision attach-*

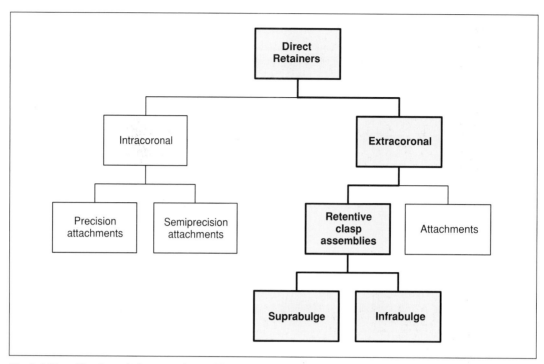

**Fig 3-1** Classification of direct retainers. The shaded boxes indicate areas that will be covered in depth in this chapter.

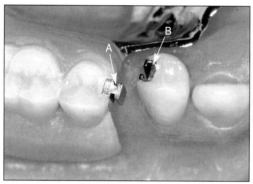

**Fig 3-2** Clinical example of a precision attachment, intracoronal, direct retainer demonstrating the patrix (A) extending from the removable partial denture and the matrix (B) housed within the normal clinical contours of the abutment crown.

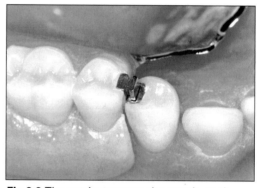

**Fig 3-3** The patrix engages the matrix as the removable partial denture is initially seated.

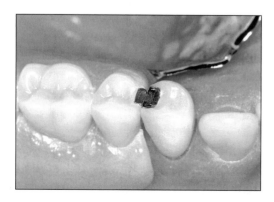

**Fig 3-4** The interlocking relationship of the precision attachment, intracoronal, direct retainer is clearly illustrated with the removable partial denture completely seated in the patient's mouth.

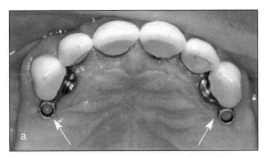 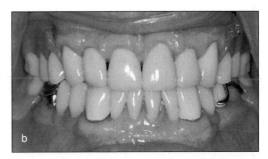

**Fig 3-5** The extracoronal attachment system *(arrows)* used in this maxillary removable partial denture *(a)* provided adequate retention of the prosthesis while eliminating the display of objectionable metallic components *(b)*.

*ments.* Components usually originate as wax or plastic patterns, which are subsequently cast in metal. Unlike precision attachments, semiprecision attachments often display gently tapering walls.

## Extracoronal direct retainers

Extracoronal direct retainers consist of components that reside entirely outside the normal clinical contours of abutment teeth. They serve to retain and stabilize removable partial dentures when dislodging forces are encountered. Extracoronal direct retainers may be divided into two distinct subcategories: *extracoronal attachments* and *retentive clasp assemblies.*

### Extracoronal attachments
Extracoronal attachments were first introduced by Henry R. Boos in the early 1900s and were later modified by F. Ewing Roach (1908).[2] As previously noted, extracoronal attachments are located outside the normal clinical contours of abutment crowns (Fig 3-5).

Like their intracoronal counterparts, extracoronal attachments derive their retention from closely fitting components termed *matrices* and *patrices.* Many of these attachments permit vertical movement of prostheses during occlusal loading. This mechanical accommodation is intended to minimize the transfer of potentially damaging forces to the abutments. This concept has led to "stress breaking" or "stress directing" theories of removable partial denture design. A more extensive description of these theories is presented in chapter 20.

### Retentive clasp assemblies
Retentive clasp assemblies represent the most common method for extracoronal direct retention. These assemblies probably date to the mid-1700s or early 1800s, but first appeared in the dental literature with Dr W. G. A. Bonwill's description in 1899.[3]

The retentive element of an individual clasp assembly is a metal clasp arm that displays a limited amount of flexibility. This flexibility allows the tip of the retentive clasp to pass over the greatest diameter of an abutment and contact the surface of the tooth as it converges apically (Fig 3-6). To understand the mechanics of such a retainer, the practitioner must understand two important concepts—the path of insertion and removal for the prosthesis, and the height of contour for each abutment.

To properly design a removable partial denture, the practitioner must consider the path along which the prosthesis will be inserted and removed from its fully seated position. Upon insertion, the clasp arms will contact the axial surfaces of the abutments. With continued seating, the retentive clasp arms will flex as they pass over the greatest convexities of the abutments. Once the point of greatest tooth convexity is reached, further placement of the prosthesis allows each retentive clasp arm to return to its "unstrained" or "passive" state. This places the retentive terminus in an undercut relative to the path of insertion and removal (Fig 3-7). If this is not the case, the clasp assembly will not contribute to optimal retention of the prosthesis.

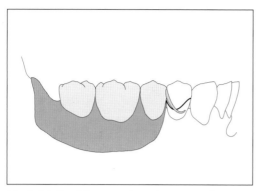

**Fig 3-6** A flexible, retentive clasp arm, direct retainer is engaging the first premolar. A retentive clasp arm is designed so that its terminus contacts the abutment apical to the height of contour (designated by the black survey line on the abutment). This design prevents displacement of the removable partial denture during function.

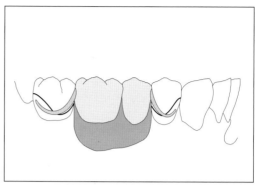

**Fig 3-7** Flexible, retentive clasp arm, direct retainers engage the first premolar and second molar. With the prosthesis fully seated, the clasp arm termini rest passively against the abutments apical to the heights of contour (designated by the black survey lines on the abutments).

Forces such as gravity or the pull of sticky foods acting to dislodge a removable partial denture typically occur perpendicular to the occlusal plane. To most effectively resist dislodging forces, abutments must provide undercut axial surfaces when the dental arch is oriented with the occlusal plane parallel to the horizon (Fig 3-8).

Proper use of a dental surveyor is the only reliable method of effectively analyzing teeth for their potential contributions to retention of a removable partial denture. This indispensable tool was first introduced in 1918 by A. J. Fortunati and was made commercially available when the Ney Company produced Weinstein and Roth's surveyor in 1923. A practitioner must understand the use of a dental surveyor and its role in identifying tooth contours that are favorable for removable partial denture retention. The dental literature contains numerous reports addressing optimal relationships between tooth contours and prosthesis retention. One of the earliest discussions was provided by J. H. Prothero.[4] In 1916, Prothero introduced the "cone theory" of clinical crown anatomy and provided a conceptual basis for mechanical retention. According to Prothero's explanation, the contours of a clinical crown resemble two cones sharing a common base (Fig 3-9). The line formed at the junction of these cones represents the greatest diameter of the tooth. This diameter is commonly referred to as the *height of contour*, a term first used by Dr Edward Kennedy in 1928.[5]

Practically speaking, the height of contour resides at the junction of the occlusal and cervical convergence. It represents the greatest axial diameter of the clinical crown when viewed along the proposed path of insertion. Any alteration in the proposed path of insertion, as represented by tilting the dental cast on the surveying table, will alter the perceived height of contour (Figs 3-10 and 3-11). Therefore, the chosen path of insertion and removal will always define the height of contour and the associated areas of undercut.

A clasp terminus designed to contact the abutment surface apical to the height of contour will resist displacement in an occlusal direction. Resistance to displacement is encountered because the clasp arm must undergo "deflection" or "bending" to pass over the height of contour. Therefore, retention of the removable partial denture is determined, in part, by the location of the clasp terminus relative to the height of contour.

To facilitate discussion and application of Prothero's cone theory, M. M. DeVan introduced the terms *suprabulge* and *infrabulge*.[6] These terms are extremely useful in discussions of coronal form, clasp form, and clasp placement. Hence, their im-

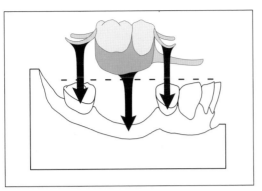

**Fig 3-8** Forces acting to dislodge a removable partial denture typically occur perpendicular to the occlusal plane *(broken line)*. To effectively resist dislodgement, the path of prosthesis insertion and removal *(arrows)* should also be perpendicular to the occlusal plane.

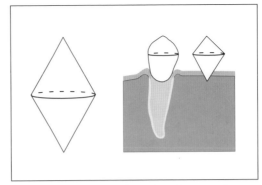

**Fig 3-9** Illustration of Prothero's cone theory. Conceptually, the axial contour of an abutment resembles two cones sharing a common base. The top cone represents the occlusal convergence contour while the bottom cone represents the apical convergence contour. The line formed at the junction of the two cones represents the height of contour.

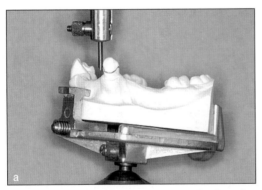

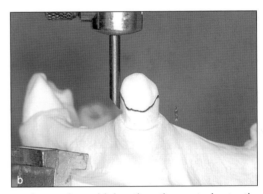

**Fig 3-10** *(a)* This mandibular cast is tilted so that the anterior teeth are higher than the posterior teeth. *(b)* A carbon marker placed in the vertical arm of a dental surveyor represents the path of insertion and removal of the prosthesis. The carbon marker is used to trace a line that represents the abutment's height of contour.

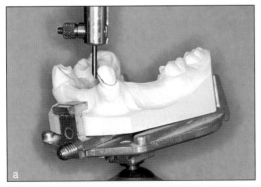

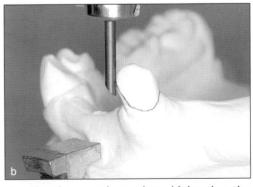

**Fig 3-11** *(a)* The same cast used in Fig 3-10 is now tilted so that the posterior teeth are higher than the anterior teeth. *(b)* The carbon marker now traces a distinctly different line on the abutment. The line (height of contour) is dependent on the orientation of the occlusal plane (the tilt of the cast) relative to the vertical arm of the dental surveyor. Therefore, the path of insertion and removal, represented by the vertical arm of the surveyor, will always define the height of contour.

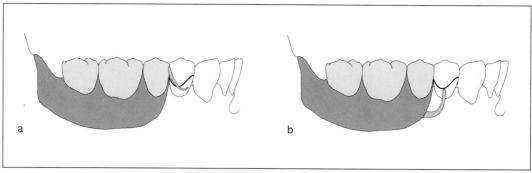

**Fig 3-12** The terms *suprabulge* and *infrabulge* are useful when considering clasp design. *(a)* A suprabulge retentive clasp arm originates from the removable partial denture occlusal to the height of contour. *(b)* In contrast, an infrabulge retentive clasp arm originates from a position apical to the height of contour.

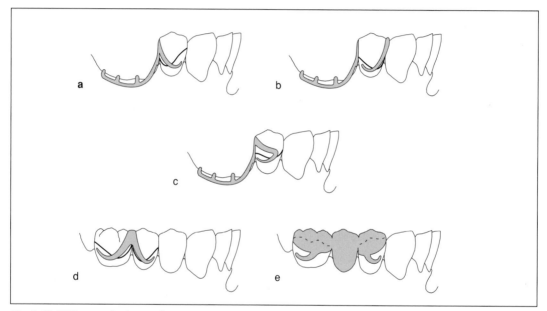

**Fig 3-13** Different designs of suprabulge direct retainers include the *(a)* simple circlet clasp, *(b)* reverse circlet clasp, *(c)* C-clasp, *(d)* embrasure clasp, and *(e)* onlay clasp. All of these designs involve retentive clasp arms that originate occlusal to the height of contour.

portance should not be overlooked (Fig 3-12). According to DeVan's descriptions, the portion of an abutment that converges toward the occlusal or incisal surface is considered the suprabulge aspect of the abutment. The portion of the clinical crown that converges apically from the height of contour is considered the infrabulge aspect of the abutment. A tooth surface or region is considered retentive if it resides apical to the height of contour or in an infrabulge location. As a result, infrabulge locations are designated as *undercut* relative to the height of contour.

As an extension of DeVan's concepts, professionals have defined two basic categories of retentive clasp assemblies: circumferential or suprabulge direct retainers (Figs 3-13 and 3-14) and vertical projection, bar-type, or infrabulge direct retainers (Fig 3-15). A suprabulge direct retainer is frequently referred to as an *Akers clasp* after Dr Polk E. Akers, who improved and standardized its construction.[7]

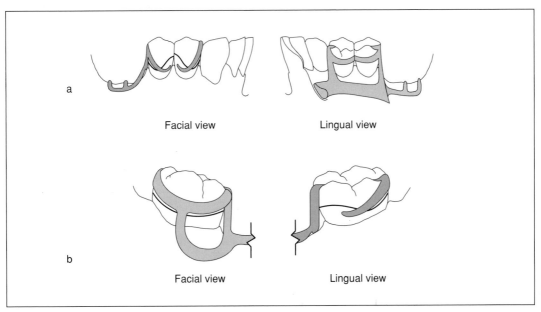

**Fig 3-14** Additional designs of suprabulge direct retainers include the *(a)* multiple circlet clasp and *(b)* ring clasp.

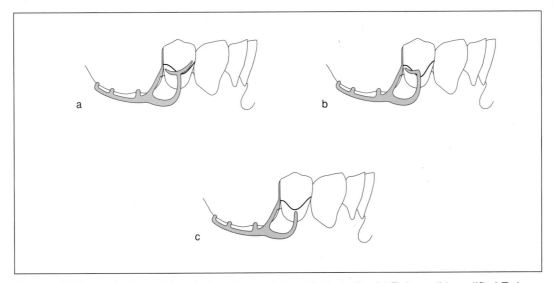

**Fig 3-15** Different designs of infrabulge direct retainers include the *(a)* T-clasp, *(b)* modified T-clasp, and *(c)* I-clasp. All of these designs involve clasp arms that originate apical to the height of contour.

*Roach clasp*

An infrabulge or bar-type direct retainer is often called a *Roach clasp* after Dr F. Ewing Roach, an early proponent of this design element.[8] However, the authors prefer the use of descriptive terms rather than eponyms. Therefore, the two basic categories of direct retainers will be designated *suprabulge direct retainers* and *infrabulge direct retainers*.

**Structure of a clasp assembly** To function effectively, a retentive arm must be accompanied by other structural elements. When combined, these structural elements form a clasp assembly. A properly designed clasp assembly has the following parts: *(1)* a rest, *(2)* a retentive arm, *(3)* a reciprocal element, and *(4)* one or more minor connectors (Fig 3-16).

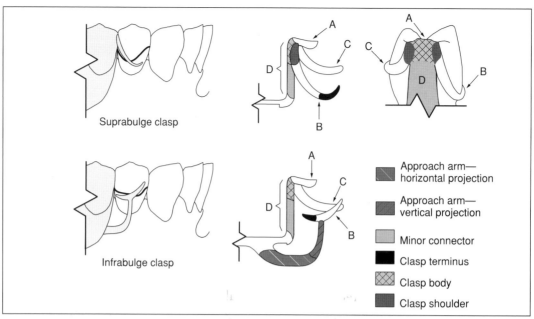

**Fig 3-16** A properly constructed suprabulge or infrabulge clasp assembly must incorporate the following components: a rest (A), a retentive clasp (B), a reciprocal element (C), and one or more minor connectors (D). Specific design features of the various components include vertical and horizontal approach arms, clasp termini, clasp bodies, and clasp shoulders.

The component of a clasp that provides vertical support for the prosthesis is called a *rest* (see Fig 3-16). The portion of the abutment tooth prepared to receive the rest is a *rest seat*. In most instances, rest seats are located on the occlusal surfaces of premolars and molars, the cingula of maxillary canines, or the incisal edges of mandibular incisors. Properly prepared rest seats and the corresponding rests serve to: *(1)* resist displacement of the prosthesis toward the supporting tissues and *(2)* transmit functional forces parallel to the long axes of the abutments. Since forces acting on a removable partial denture may be substantial, the structural integrity of each rest is critical. Therefore, each rest must be rigidly joined to the remainder of the framework in order to resist fracture. It is interesting to note that a clear description of the occlusal rest appeared as early as 1817, but it was not until Dr W. G. A. Bonwill (1899) and Dr James H. Prothero (1916) emphasized the significance of the rest that it received due recognition.[3,4]

A retentive arm is the only portion of a removable partial denture that contacts the surface of an abutment apical to the height of contour (see Fig 3-16). There are two basic forms of retentive arms.

They are termed *suprabulge clasp arms* and *infrabulge clasp arms* (see Fig 3-12). These arms differ primarily in their approach to the undercut region of an abutment. Simply stated, a suprabulge clasp arm approaches the undercut region of an abutment from an occlusal or incisal direction, while an infrabulge clasp arm approaches the undercut region from an apical direction.

A suprabulge clasp arm (see Fig 3-16) originates from a minor connector occlusal or incisal to the height of contour. The portion of the clasp arm that arises from the minor connector is known as the *shoulder*. From the shoulder, the clasp arm follows a gently curving pathway on the surface of the abutment (Fig 3-17). The clasp arm passes over the height of contour, and its tip contacts a precisely measured undercut. This portion of the clasp is known as the *terminus*.

The shoulder comprises the proximal third of the clasp arm. For cast clasps, the shoulder segment is rigid because of its cross-sectional form, dimensions, and metallurgical properties. This rigidity requires that the shoulder be positioned at or occlusal to the height of contour. The midsection of the clasp arm extends from the shoulder.

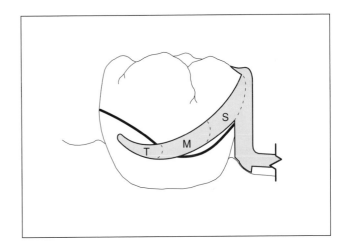

**Fig 3-17** Three distinct segments make up the suprabulge retentive clasp arm. The rigid clasp shoulder (S) originates from the minor connector and projects across the axial surface of the abutment. The relatively flexible midsection of the clasp arm (M) continues along the abutment surface and approaches the height of contour. The flexible clasp terminus (T) crosses apical to the height of contour, contacting the abutment on a surface undercut relative to the path of prosthesis insertion and removal.

Because of the gently tapering character of a retentive arm, the cross-sectional area of the midsection is slightly smaller than that of the shoulder. Consequently, the midsection is somewhat flexible. The clasp terminus displays a smaller cross-sectional area than the midsection, and therefore permits the greatest amount of flexure. The clasp terminus is the only part of a removable partial denture to contact the abutment tooth apical to the height of contour when the prosthesis is fully seated.

An infrabulge clasp arm consists of two distinct segments: the approach arm and the terminus (see Fig 3-16). The approach arm is a minor connector that originates from the framework, travels horizontally along the surface of the mucosa, and then turns vertically to cross the free gingival margin at 90 degrees. The terminus arises from the vertical portion of the approach arm and engages a measured undercut on the surface of the abutment. As for a suprabulge clasp, the terminus of an infrabulge clasp is the only component of a removable partial denture to contact the abutment apical to the height of contour. Flexibility of an infrabulge clasp is primarily related to its length, but the cross-sectional form, taper, and metallurgical properties also impact clasp flexibility.

The component of a clasp assembly that braces an abutment during prosthesis insertion and removal is called a *reciprocal element* (see Fig 3-16). The reciprocal element may be a cast clasp, a lingual plate, or a combination of mesial and distal minor connectors. Regardless of form, the recipro-

cal element must contact the abutment tooth at or occlusal to the height of contour.

The mechanism of action for a reciprocal element is relatively uncomplicated. As the retentive arm passes over the height of contour, the arm displays a slight amount of flexure. This flexure places lateral stress on the abutment. If this stress is not counteracted, it may cause lateral displacement of the abutment and significant damage to the supporting periodontium. To prevent these effects, a rigid reciprocal element must be used. The reciprocal element should be placed on the tooth surface opposite the retentive arm (eg, if the retentive arm is positioned on the facial surface of the abutment, the reciprocal element should be placed on the lingual surface, and vice versa).

During insertion of the prosthesis, the reciprocal element should contact the abutment slightly before the retentive arm contacts the abutment. Contact of the reciprocal element should be maintained while the retentive terminus passes over the height of contour and into the prescribed undercut (Fig 3-18).

If the retentive terminus contacts the abutment before the reciprocal element contacts the abutment, damaging non-axial forces may be applied to the abutment (Fig 3-19). For this reason, the abutment surface that will be contacted by the reciprocal element should be parallel to the removable partial denture's path of insertion and removal. The surface of the abutment can be prepared to produce the desired result (Fig 3-20).

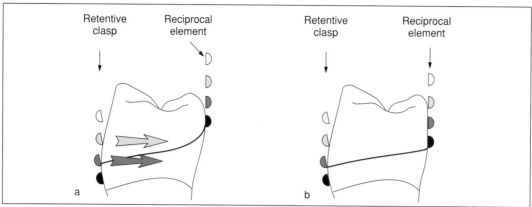

**Fig 3-18** Illustration of the relationship between the retentive clasp arm and the reciprocal element while the clasp assembly is inserted. In each diagram, a retentive clasp and reciprocal element pair move apically from the starting position *(white)*, to first tooth contact *(light gray)*, to deformation of the retentive clasp *(dark gray)*, and finally to complete seating *(black)*. *(a)* When incorrectly related, the retentive clasp contacts the abutment and begins to deform before the reciprocal element contact can resist lingual displacement of the tooth. In this situation, the abutment will incur lingually directed stress *(light and dark gray arrows)* until the reciprocal element contacts the tooth *(black)* to resist displacement. *(b)* When correctly related, the retentive clasp and reciprocal element contact the tooth simultaneously. The reciprocal element maintains contact with the abutment until the removable partial denture is completely seated. When this relationship exists, ideal design positions the retentive clasp terminus in the gingival third of the abutment and the reciprocal element at the junction of the middle and apical thirds of the tooth.

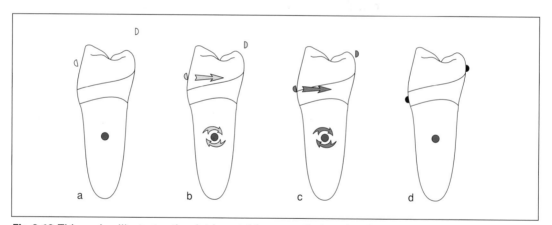

**Fig 3-19** This series illustrates the detrimental force applied to the abutment when the vertical position of the retentive clasp is incorrectly related to the reciprocal element. *(a)* The removable partial denture is in position prior to seating. *(b)* As the prosthesis is seated, the retentive clasp contacts the abutment first, causing the tooth to be lingually displaced *(light gray arrows)*. *(c)* With additional prosthesis seating, the retentive clasp deforms as it passes over the height of contour, causing further lingual displacement of the abutment *(dark gray arrows)*. *(d)* It is only when the removable partial denture is nearly seated that the reciprocal element finally engages the abutment, counteracting the displacing stress on the tooth.

When considering clasp assemblies, one must not overlook the importance of minor connectors. As might be expected, minor connectors often join elements of a clasp assembly to other components of a removable partial denture (see Fig 3-16). Hence, minor connectors must be rigid. Depending on the philosophy of design, a minor connector may serve as: *(1)* a guiding plate to direct insertion and removal of the removable partial denture, *(2)* a reciprocal element to counteract non-axial forces produced by a retentive clasp, or *(3)* an approach arm for an infrabulge clasp.

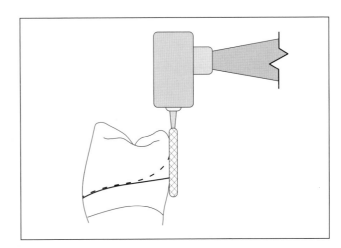

**Fig 3-20** The abutment surface to be contacted by the reciprocal element can be made parallel to the path of insertion and removal by subtle, but precise, tooth preparation. This will move the height of contour to a more apical location *(solid line)*, permitting the appropriate vertical relationship between the retentive clasp and reciprocal element.

**Requirements of a clasp assembly** All clasp assemblies must be designed so that they satisfy the following six requirements: *(1)* retention, *(2)* support, *(3)* stability, *(4)* reciprocation, *(5)* encirclement, and *(6)* passivity.

*Retention.* Retention is the quality of the clasp assembly that resists forces acting to dislodge components away from the supporting tissues. No single component of a clasp assembly is solely responsible for prosthesis retention. Rather, it is effective design and accurate construction that make the removable partial denture retentive. Each part contributes some critical feature. For example:

1. The retentive arm must be designed so that only the clasp terminus engages the prescribed undercut.
2. The accompanying rest must provide support so the clasp terminus is maintained in an optimal location.
3. The minor connector must be sufficiently rigid to ensure proper stability and function of parts of the clasp assembly.
4. The reciprocal element must contact the abutment slightly before the retentive element contacts the tooth, and it must maintain contact until the prosthesis is fully seated to protect the abutment from potentially destructive lateral forces.
5. Components must provide sufficient encirclement to prevent movement of the abutment away from

the associated clasp assembly, otherwise retention will be lost.
6. Indirect retainers must resist forces acting to dislodge the prosthesis from its fully seated position (these forces may result from the actions of sticky foods, gravity, etc).

To assume that retention is provided solely by the retentive arm or any other single element of the clasp assembly is to misunderstand the coordinated function of a well-designed removable partial denture.

The amount of retention provided by a clasp assembly is dependent upon many factors. These include the type of clasp used, flexibility of the retentive arm, and the axial convergence of tooth surfaces apical to the height of contour. As a general rule, the amount of retention designed into a removable partial denture should always be the minimum necessary to resist reasonable dislodging forces. A rigid clasp flexing over the height of contour may transfer harmful stresses to an abutment during insertion, removal, and functional movement of the prosthesis. Consequently, the characteristics of each clasp assembly should be carefully considered during the design process.

Dr K. J. Anusavice defines maximum flexibility as the strain occurring when a material is stressed to its proportional limit.[9] Maximum flexibility of a retentive clasp arm may be defined as the greatest

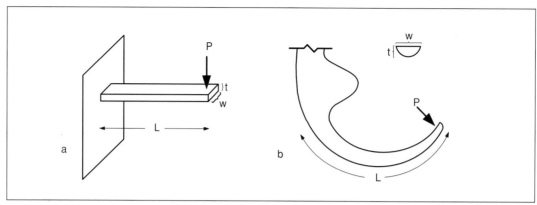

**Fig 3-21** (a) A theoretically ideal, uniform cantilever beam. Here, L is the beam length, w is the beam width, t is the beam thickness, and P is a load applied to the beam. (b) When beam principles are applied to a removable partial denture clasp, the clasp's length (L), thickness (t), and width (w) are measured as illustrated. The applied load (P) corresponds to the force causing deflection of the clasp as it passes over the height of abutment contour as the prosthesis is seated.

amount of displacement that can occur without causing permanent deformation of the clasp arm. The flexibility of the retentive clasp arm may be influenced by length, cross-sectional form, cross-sectional diameter, longitudinal taper, clasp curvature, and metallurgical characteristics of the alloy. These factors are summarized in the following paragraphs.

*Clasp flexibility increases as clasp length increases.* When assessing the impact of clasp length on flexibility, the practitioner should consider the mathematical formula for deflection of a uniform cantilever beam. This formula may be expressed as:

$$D = \frac{4PL^3}{Ewt^3}$$

where D = deflection, P = applied force, L = length, E = modulus of elasticity, w = beam width, and t = beam thickness (Fig 3-21).

Although direct application of this theory does not fully explain the clinical behavior of a clasp arm, its consideration may permit better understanding of clasp performance. From a theoretical perspective, flexibility or deflection of the clasp is directly proportional to the cube of its length. Scientific investigation supports the concept that increasing the length of a clasp arm produces a significant increase in flexibility. By increasing the

flexibility of the clasp, the horizontal stresses imparted to an abutment during placement, withdrawal, and movement of the prosthesis may be reduced. Nevertheless, the flexibility should not be so great that the retentive characteristics of the clasp are lost.

*Clasp flexibility increases as cross-sectional dimensions decrease* (Fig 3-22). Review of the cantilever beam equation reveals that deflection is inversely proportional to the cube of the beam's thickness. Therefore, as the thickness of a beam is increased, deflection upon loading is significantly decreased. The cantilever beam equation also reveals an inverse relationship between beam width and deflection. Hence, an increase in beam width yields a moderate decrease in deflection. From these observations, it should be evident that beam thickness has a much greater effect upon deflection than does beam width. Studies evaluating the flexibility of half-round cast clasps have shown a width-to-thickness ratio of 2:1 to be optimal. It is important, however, to realize that altering the clasp length is a more efficient method of increasing clasp flexibility than is altering clasp diameter.

*A uniformly tapered clasp is more flexible than a nontapered clasp of the same proximal dimensions.* Uniform longitudinal taper is an essential feature of retentive clasps. The taper should be consistent for both width and thickness. The cross-sectional dimen-

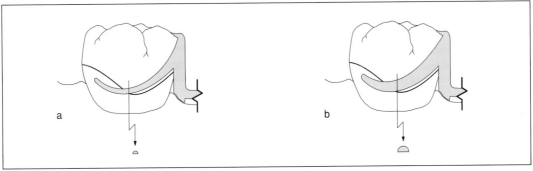

**Fig 3-22** As the cross-sectional dimensions of the retentive clasp arm decrease, the flexibility of the clasp increases. Therefore, a smaller-diameter clasp *(a)* will be more flexible than a larger-diameter clasp *(b)*.

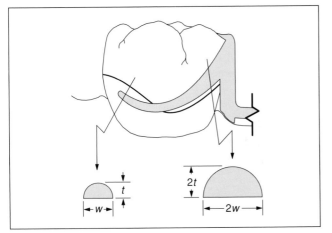

**Fig 3-23** To achieve the ideal uniform taper for optimal retentive clasp arm flexibility, the cross-sectional dimension of the clasp shoulder should be twice that of the clasp terminus.

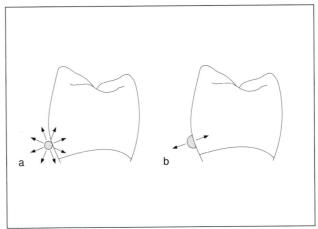

**Fig 3-24** When viewed in cross-section, a round clasp *(a)* is able to flex in all directions, while a half-round clasp *(b)* is restricted to bidirectional flexure.

sions at the shoulder of the clasp should be twice the cross-sectional dimensions at the clasp terminus (Fig 3-23). Evidence indicates that a tapered clasp arm is approximately twice as flexible as a clasp arm that does not exhibit a tapered design.

*A circular cross-sectional clasp form imparts omnidirectional flexure, while a half-round form allows only bidirectional flexure* (Fig 3-24). Because of its cross-sectional form, a round clasp may flex in all spatial planes. Consequently, a clasp exhibiting a circular cross-sectional form may permit dissipation of detrimental forces during functional movement of the prosthesis. A half-round clasp typically flexes in a plane that is perpendicular to the flat surface of the clasp. Therefore, stress dissipation is somewhat limited. As a re-

sult, a retentive clasp with a circular cross-sectional form provides some advantages.

*Curvature of a clasp in more than one spatial plane reduces the clasp's flexibility.* Deflection of a curved beam is less than that of a straight beam of similar length and material because curvature makes the beam more rigid. When contouring a wrought-wire clasp arm, the operator should ensure that the clasp arm remains in a single plane of space. Multiple bends, especially those placing the clasp arm in multiple planes of space, may produce permanent deformation of the microstructure and lead to increased rigidity.

*The metallurgical properties of an alloy influence clasp flexibility.* Alloys exhibiting higher elastic moduli ex-

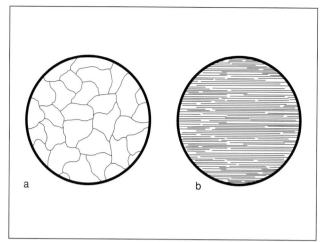

**Fig 3-25** Metallographic comparison of the microstructure of cast metal *(a)* and wrought metal *(b)* alloys. Most cast metals display distinct polycrystalline microscopic configurations. Distinct crystals, or grains, are evident in a photomicrograph and meet at identifiable grain boundaries. The photomicrograph of a wrought metal reveals a significantly different grain structure. When cast metal is cold worked and drawn through dies to form wire, the grain structure elongates and is oriented in the direction of the cold-working process. This very distinct microstructure contributes to the clinically identifiable physical and performance characteristics of wrought-wire clasps.

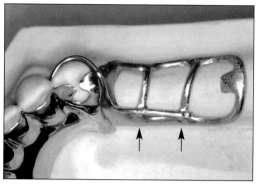

**Fig 3-26** To avoid the detrimental effects of high temperatures, wrought-wire clasps should be soldered *(arrows)* to the framework following casting. Care should be taken to place the solder joint as far from the retentive clasp arm as possible. This minimizes the adverse effects of crystallization and prolongs clasp life.

hibit greater stiffness, while alloys displaying lower elastic moduli exhibit greater flexibility. This is particularly important in removable partial denture construction. Because cobalt-chromium and nickel-chromium alloys have higher elastic moduli than do gold alloys, clasps made from chromium-containing alloys are more rigid. While this rigidity may be helpful in some instances, it is undesirable in other applications. In many instances, a practitioner may desire clasping materials with greater flexibility. Gold alloys provide such flexibility, but are quite expensive. As a result, the practitioner may choose a wrought-wire alloy when increased flexibility is required.

Wrought wire is produced by drawing a cast metal through a die. This process produces elongation of the alloy's crystalline microstructure (Fig 3-25), and alters the physical properties of the original alloy. The elongated crystalline structure of wrought wire imparts greater flexibility than a conventional crystalline structure.

Unfortunately, the flexibility of wrought wire may be diminished if the material is allowed to recrystallize. This may occur as a result of (1) cold working or (2) heating a wrought structure. Cold working is produced by the repeated bending of a wrought wire. This process leads to localized crystallization of the wire and predisposes the wire to fracture. It is similar to the failure that occurs when a wire clothes hanger is repeatedly bent and straightened.

Heating may occur when a molten alloy is cast directly to a wrought wire during framework construction. High temperatures produce crystallization of the wire and result in a noticeable decrease in flexibility. To avoid clinical difficulties, wrought-wire clasps should be attached to metal frameworks using common soldering procedures. Solder joints should be located as far from proximal plates as possible (Fig 3-26). If this is not done, crystallization may occur at areas of pronounced displacement and may result in accelerated clasp failure.

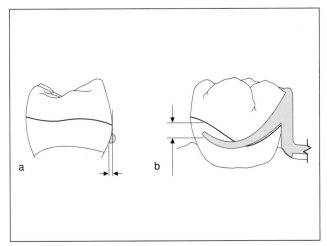

**Fig 3-27** The position of the retentive clasp terminus against the axial surface of an abutment influences the retentive force imparted by the clasp. This position is designated by both a horizontal *(a)* and a vertical *(b)* dimension. A dental surveyor must be used to identify the appropriate horizontal and vertical locations.

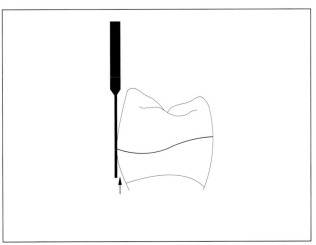

**Fig 3-28** The angular space *(arrow)* that results when the analyzing rod is positioned in a dental surveyor and placed against the abutment surface.

Location of each retentive clasp terminus relative to the height of contour may be described in two distinct dimensions: *(1)* a mediolateral or horizontal dimension and *(2)* an occluso-apical or vertical dimension (Fig 3-27). The position of a clasp terminus with regard to these dimensions will influence the retentive forces exerted by a clasp. Therefore, the position of each clasp terminus must be considered carefully during the design process. This process is accomplished using a dental surveyor.

With the cast properly oriented on the surveying table, the point of contact between the analyzing rod and the axial surface of the abutment defines the height of contour for that tooth. When the analyzing rod is replaced with a carbon marker, a line designating the height of contour can be traced onto the surface of the dental cast. This line is commonly called a *survey line* and separates the infrabulge and suprabulge portions of the abutment.

From a practical standpoint, the infrabulge or undercut portion of the abutment lies apical to the height of contour. When the analyzing rod is positioned in the surveyor and placed against the tooth surface, an angular space is formed apical to the height of contour (Fig 3-28). This angular space represents a mechanical undercut. Placement of a clasp terminus into a mechanical undercut forms the basis for removable partial denture design, construction, and service. The tool used to identify the proper position for each clasp terminus is called an undercut gauge (Fig 3-29). Undercut gauges are available in 0.010-, 0.020-, and 0.030-inch configurations.

The amount of undercut used in a given situation depends on a variety of factors, not the least of which are prevailing clinical conditions and the practitioner's philosophy of removable partial denture design. As might be expected, the degree of undercut used in removable partial denture therapy dramatically affects the resultant retentive force. While keeping all other clasp-related factors constant, positioning the clasp terminus at a greater horizontal undercut will result in increased retentive force (Fig 3-30).

The angle formed between the analyzing rod and the tooth surface apical to the height of contour is called the *angle of gingival convergence* (Fig 3-31). As the angle of gingival convergence becomes greater, the force required to remove the retentive clasp from the abutment also becomes greater. This may provide distinct advantages or disadvantages depending upon the clinical situation. If the abutment

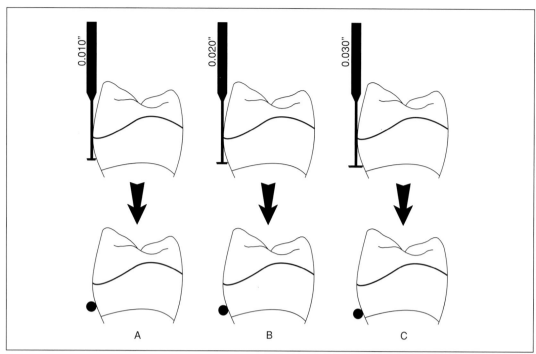

**Fig 3-29** The position of the terminus of a round retentive clasp arm is determined using undercut gauges in a dental surveyor. The undercut gauge used on abutment A positions the clasp in a 0.010-inch undercut. Abutment B has a clasp terminus located in a 0.020-inch undercut. Finally, the undercut gauge selected for abutment C locates the clasp terminus in a 0.030-inch undercut. Selection of an undercut gauge when designing a retentive clasp is based on both clinical and philosophic requirements of the case.

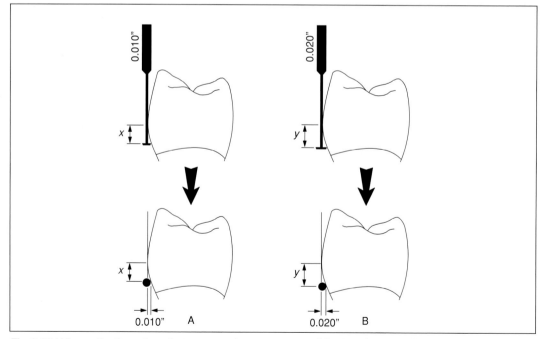

**Fig 3-30** When all other clasp factors remain constant, positioning the retentive clasp terminus at a greater horizontal undercut will result in increased retentive force. Therefore, a retentive clasp terminus positioned in a 0.020-inch horizontal undercut (B) will provide greater retentive force than will a clasp positioned in a 0.010-inch undercut (A).

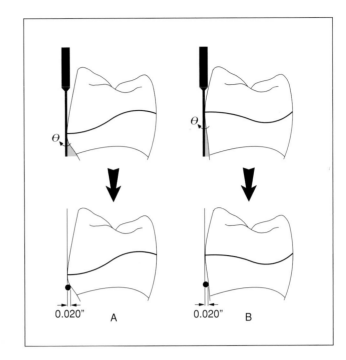

**Fig 3-31** When all other clasp factors remain constant, a retentive clasp engaging an abutment that possesses a greater angle of cervical convergence (θ) will possess increased retentive force. Therefore, the retentive clasp on abutment A provides greater retentive force than the retentive clasp on abutment B.

demonstrates a severe angle of gingival convergence, one of two treatment approaches should be considered. The first involves recontouring the tooth surface to reduce this angle. The second approach involves placing the associated clasp terminus into a smaller undercut (eg, engaging a 0.010-inch undercut rather than a 0.020-inch undercut). Both approaches are directed at maintaining an optimal retentive force for the chosen clasp assembly.

*Support.* Support is the quality of a clasp assembly that resists displacement of a prosthesis in an apical direction. The removable partial denture component that provides the greatest resistance to apical displacement is the rest. Other elements that contact the abutment occlusal to the height of contour (eg, a reciprocal element or shoulder of retentive clasp) also may contribute to the support function. However, in order to achieve effective support, a rest must contact the associated abutment at a properly prepared surface (ie, a rest seat).

Rest seats are primarily located on the occlusal surfaces of premolars and molars, the cingula of

maxillary canines, or the incisal edges of mandibular canines and incisors. Their importance with regard to the clinical success of removable partial dentures was emphasized by Dr W. G. A. Bonwill as early as 1899.[3]

A properly prepared rest seat and corresponding rest serve to *(1)* resist displacement of the prosthesis toward the supporting teeth and soft tissues, thereby ensuring that the clasp assembly maintains its intended relation to the abutment, and *(2)* transmit functional forces parallel to the long axes of the abutments. These factors are critical to the health and longevity of abutments.

*Stability.* Stability is the quality of a clasp assembly that resists displacement of a prosthesis in a horizontal direction. All framework components that are rigid and contact vertically oriented hard and soft tissues may contribute to the stability of a prosthesis. Within an individual clasp assembly, the greatest contributions to stability come from the reciprocal element, the shoulder(s) of a cast circumferential retentive clasp, and vertically oriented minor connectors. The

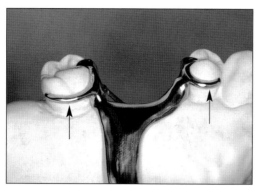

**Fig 3-32** Cast clasp arms *(arrows)* serve as the reciprocal elements for these first premolar and second molar clasp assemblies.

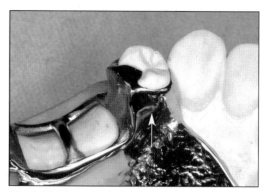

**Fig 3-33** Lingual plating *(arrow)* serves as the reciprocal element in this first premolar clasp assembly.

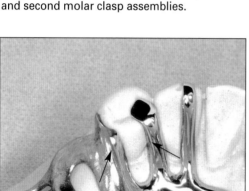

**Fig 3-34** The combination of mesial and distal minor connectors *(arrows)* serves as the reciprocal element for this first premolar clasp assembly.

retentive clasp terminus, which by definition must be flexible, does not effectively contribute to stability. In a similar fashion, a wrought-wire clasp with relative flexibility throughout its length, does not effectively augment stability.

*Reciprocation.* Reciprocation is the quality of a clasp assembly that counteracts lateral displacement of an abutment when the retentive clasp terminus passes over the height of contour. Lateral displacement of an abutment is potentially harmful to the supporting periodontal tissues. Therefore, lateral forces must be offset by components of the clasp assembly.

As previously noted, the retentive clasp must flex to pass over the height of contour. This results in the application of lateral forces to the abutment. To negate these forces, a clasp assembly must include a rigid component that resists lateral movement of the affected tooth. This component is known as a *reciprocal element* (see Fig 3-16). The

reciprocal element may be a cast clasp (Fig 3-32), lingual plating (Fig 3-33), or a combination of mesial and distal minor connectors (Fig 3-34). Regardless of form, the reciprocal element must be rigid and must contact the abutment tooth at or occlusal to the height of contour.

To optimize reciprocation, the axial surface of an abutment should be prepared parallel to the path of insertion and removal. Furthermore, the reciprocal element should contact the abutment at the junction of the gingival and middle thirds of the crown contours (Fig 3-35). This permits simultaneous contact of the retentive terminus and the reciprocal element during insertion and removal of the prosthesis (see Fig 3-18). If the retentive terminus contacts the abutment before the reciprocal element contacts the abutment, reciprocation will be ineffective. If the reciprocal element is positioned on a surface with a significant occlusal convergence, vertical movement of the prosthesis away from the supporting tissues will cause the recipro-

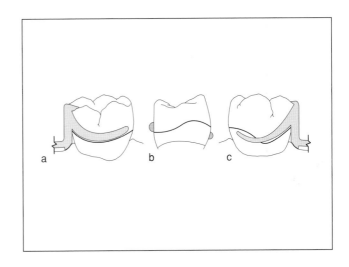

**Fig 3-35** The ideal location of the reciprocal clasp arm on the lingual surface of the abutment is illustrated. *(a)* The lingual view demonstrates the rigid reciprocal clasp arm contacting the abutment occlusal to the height of contour. *(b)* From a proximal view, it is apparent that the lingual surface of the abutment was prepared so that the reciprocal clasp could be located near the junction of the middle and gingival thirds of the tooth. *(c)* The facial view depicts optimal contour and position of the retentive clasp arm.

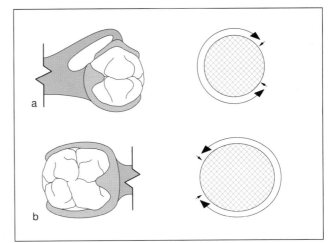

**Fig 3-36** Both the infrabulge *(a)* and suprabulge *(b)* clasp assemblies have been designed to provide encirclement. Direct contact over at least 180 degrees of the abutment's circumference prevents movement of the tooth away from the clasp assembly.

cal element to lose contact with the tooth. This will result in inadequate reciprocation and potential damage to the abutment. Consequently, the importance of reciprocation must not be overlooked.

*Encirclement.* Encirclement is the characteristic of a clasp assembly that prevents movement of an abutment away from the associated clasp assembly. Each clasp assembly must be designed to provide direct contact over at least 180 degrees of the tooth's circumference (Fig 3-36). This contact provides encirclement and prevents movement of the abutment away from the clasp assembly.

Encirclement may be provided in the form of continuous contact, as demonstrated by circumferential clasp assemblies. Encirclement also may be provided by discontinuous contact, as evidenced by infrabulge clasp assemblies (Fig 3-37). If discon-

tinuous encirclement is planned, the clasp assembly must contact the abutment tooth at three widely separated areas that encompass more than half the tooth's circumference. Inadequate encirclement may permit movement or "escape" of the abutment tooth from the confines of the clasp assembly during functional movement of the prosthesis (Fig 3-38).

*Passivity.* Passivity is the quality of a clasp assembly that prevents the transmission of adverse forces to the associated abutment when the prosthesis is completely seated. When fully seated, a clasp assembly should be passive. The retentive arm should be activated only when dislodging forces are applied to the removable partial denture. One of the major causes of discomfort in removable partial denture therapy is incomplete seating of a clasp as-

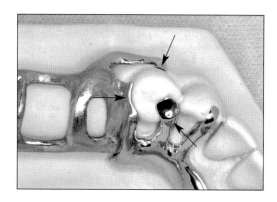

**Fig 3-37** Encirclement may be provided by discontinuous contact with the abutment surface. In order for discontinuous contact to be effective, it must occur at three widely separated areas *(arrows)* encompassing more than half the tooth's circumference.

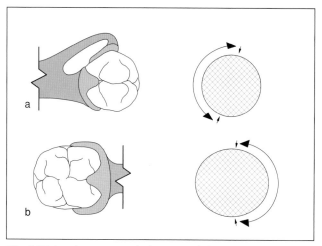

**Fig 3-38** Inadequate encirclement of the abutment by the infrabulge *(a)* or suprabulge *(b)* clasp assembly may result in the tooth moving away from the framework during displacement of the prosthesis.

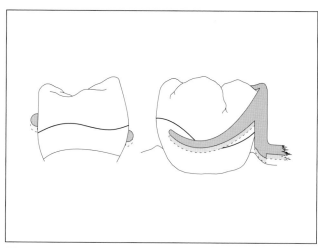

**Fig 3-39** The retentive clasp arm may remain active *(dark gray)* if the clasp assembly is not fully seated *(light gray)* on the abutment. Sustained, non-axial stress on the abutment may cause discomfort, damage to the abutment, or premature failure of the removable partial denture.

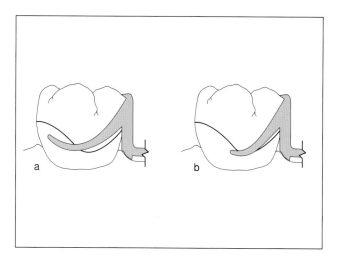

**Fig 3-40** The design of a retentive clasp arm should incorporate maximum clasp length for optimal flexibility. *(a)* Ideally, a suprabulge retentive clasp should originate from a proximal minor connector and extend across the abutment's facial surface, terminating at the opposite proximofacial line angle. *(b)* If the clasp is too short, it will lack the necessary flexibility.

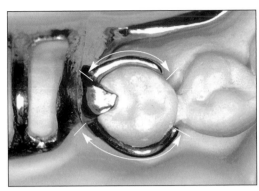

**Fig 3-41** Because of more favorable facial surface contours and the location of occlusal rest seats, clasp arms placed facially are typically longer than lingual clasp arms. The additional length resulting from facial clasp placement permits improved flexibility of the retentive clasp arm.

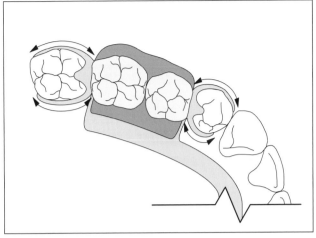

**Fig 3-42** The lingual surface of molar abutments permits relatively long clasp arms when compared with those of premolar abutments. Therefore, carefully designed and constructed lingual retentive clasps may be used on molar abutments.

sembly on the associated abutment. If the clasp assembly is not fully seated, the retentive terminus will not be positioned in its intended location. As a result, the clasp assembly will apply non-axial (ie, lateral) forces to the abutment. The sustained application of non-axial forces may result in significant dental discomfort, the potential for unintended tooth movement, or premature failure of the retentive arm due to metallurgical fatigue (Fig 3-39).

**Location of the retentive clasp terminus** In general, the retentive terminus for a suprabulge or infrabulge clasp arm should be located at the mesial or distal line angle of the corresponding abutment (Fig 3-40). The retentive clasp should be positioned on the facial surface of the abutment if appropriate contours are present. Facial placement permits increased length of the retentive arm and yields improved clasp flexibility. In contrast, lingual placement of the retentive arm results in decreased clasp length and an accompanying decrease in flexibility (Fig 3-41).

While facial placement of the retentive clasp arm is preferred, abutment contours sometimes favor lingual placement. Hence, the practitioner must consider additional factors. Placement of a retentive clasp on the lingual surface of a premolar

is contraindicated in most instances. Most premolars present limited mesiodistal dimensions. As a result, lingual retentive arms on premolars are relatively short and inflexible. This may result in ineffective clasping or the transfer of damaging horizontal forces to premolar abutments.

Unlike premolars, most molars provide significantly increased mesiodistal dimensions. As a result, lingual retentive elements can be used with molar abutments (Fig 3-42). This is particularly true of mandibular molar abutments. Mandibular molars have relatively large mesiodistal dimensions and commonly exhibit undercuts on their lingual surfaces. Therefore, mandibular molars may be clasped using facial or lingual retention, depending upon the locations of available undercuts.

When designing a removable partial denture, the practitioner also must consider the relationships of clasp assemblies to one another. If a retentive clasp on one side of the arch is positioned on the facial surface of an abutment, at least one retentive clasp on the contralateral side of the arch should be located on the facial surface of an abutment. In a similar manner, if lingual retention is used on one side of the arch, it should be opposed by lingual retention on the contralateral side of the arch. This geometry provides a more effective system of retention.

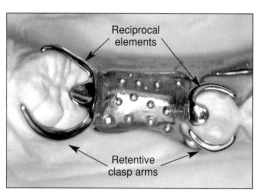

**Fig 3-43** When designing retentive clasp assemblies, it is important that each abutment receive one retentive clasp arm and one reciprocal element.

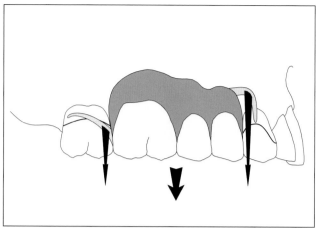

**Fig 3-44** A comparison of the retentive mechanics between the infrabulge I-bar clasp on the canine and the suprabulge circumferential clasp on the second molar reveals a striking difference. As the removable partial denture is displaced away from the supporting tissues *(arrows)*, the clasp termini move in an occlusal direction, flexing over the heights of contour of the abutments. Because it originates occlusal to the height of contour, the retentive terminus of the suprabulge clasp is "pulled" over the height of contour by the prosthesis. In contrast, origination of the infrabulge clasp apical to the height of contour requires it to be "pushed" over the abutment's height of contour.

It is important to remember that only one retentive clasp should be used on any abutment and that this retentive clasp must be opposed by a reciprocal element on the opposite side of the abutment (Fig 3-43). Therefore, if a retentive arm is placed on the facial surface of an abutment, a reciprocal element must be placed on the lingual surface of the abutment. Conversely, if a retentive arm is placed on the lingual surface of an abutment, a reciprocal element must be positioned on the facial surface of the abutment.

**Comparison of retention: Infrabulge vs suprabulge clasp assemblies** Practically speaking, a removable partial denture must provide sufficient retention to resist dislodging forces such as gravity or the pull of sticky foods. Retentive capacity beyond that required to resist normal dislodging forces may be detrimental to abutments and their supporting tissues. Therefore, a brief discussion of the retention provided by commonly used clasp assemblies is in order.

An infrabulge clasp approaches the associated undercut from an apical direction. Displacement of the clasp requires that the infrabulge retentive arm be "pushed" over the height of contour. In contrast, a suprabulge clasp approaches the associated undercut from an occlusal or incisal direction. Displacement occurs when the suprabulge clasp is "pulled" over the height of contour (Fig 3-44). As a result of these mechanical differences, there are accompanying differences in the retentive characteristics of infrabulge and suprabulge clasp assemblies.

An explanation of these differences was presented by Dr Eugene R. Stone in 1936.[10] Stone suggested that removal of an infrabulge clasp required significantly more force than did removal of a suprabulge clasp. This would be true if all factors were equal (ie, clasp length, flexibility, cross-sectional geometry, taper, material, depth of un-

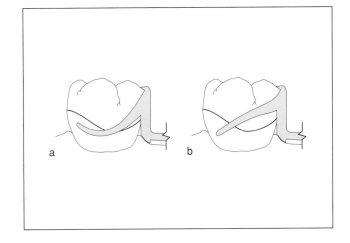

**Fig 3-45** *(a)* A properly designed suprabulge retentive arm should possess long, gently curving contours with the retentive terminus pointing toward the occlusal surface. *(b)* A short clasp that curves toward the gingiva is not acceptable.

dercut, and angle of gingival convergence). However, these factors are not equal in common clinical applications. In particular, the retentive arm of an infrabulge clasp is significantly longer than the retentive arm of a suprabulge clasp assembly. Consequently, the expected retentive force may be negated by the increased flexibility of the infrabulge arm. Therefore, achieving optimal retention when designing a removable partial denture is more dependent upon careful diagnosis and appropriate application of design principles than upon the specific clasp forms incorporated into the prosthesis.

**Cast circumferential clasp** The cast circumferential clasp design was introduced by Dr N. B. Nesbitt in 1916.[11] The clasp is remarkable for its simplicity and ease of construction. It is the design of choice for tooth-supported removable partial dentures because of its excellent support, bracing, and retentive properties.

A cast circumferential clasp displays close adaptation to the abutment and, therefore, minimizes the entrapment of food and debris. Nevertheless, the cast circumferential design has certain disadvantages that also must be considered. One of the primary disadvantages of the cast circumferential design is the large amount of tooth surface that is covered by the clasp assembly. If proper oral hygiene is not maintained, the underlying enamel is at increased risk for decalcification. When in place, the cast circumferential clasp also alters the gross morphology of the clinical crown. This may inter-

fere with food flow and bolus elimination during the masticatory process. As a result, the abutment and associated periodontium may be damaged.

*Design rules.* The following rules apply to cast circumferential clasp design:

1. A cast circumferential clasp should originate from a portion of the framework that lies above the height of contour. The retentive arm should extend cervically and circumferentially in a gently arcing manner. The terminal third of the retentive clasp should pass over the height of contour and enter the infrabulge portion of the abutment. It is important to note that only the apical border of the retentive clasp terminus should engage the desired undercut. The reciprocal element should be located at or slightly above the height of contour on the opposite surface of the tooth and should prevent lateral displacement of the abutment when the retentive clasp flexes over the height of contour.
2. The retentive terminus should be directed occlusally, never toward the gingiva. The long, curved clasp arm that results from this contour permits improved flexibility (Fig 3-45).
3. A cast circumferential clasp arm should terminate at the mesial line angle or distal line angle of the abutment, never at the midfacial or midlingual surfaces.
4. The retentive arm should be positioned as far apically on the abutment as is practical. The clasp arm should never violate the prescribed relationship to

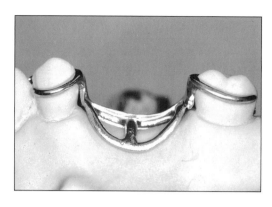

**Fig 3-46** Simple circlet, cast circumferential retentive clasps are present on facial surfaces of both the first premolar and second molar abutments.

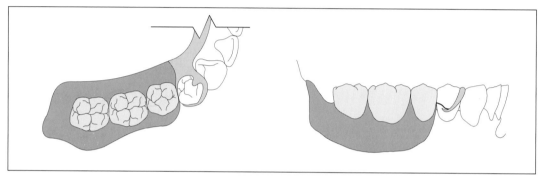

**Fig 3-47** Here, a reverse circlet, cast circumferential retentive clasp is used to engage a distofacial undercut. Frequently, this design is esthetically objectionable because the clasp traverses the abutment's mesial marginal ridge. It may be more appropriate to use an infrabulge clasp to engage the distofacial undercut in this situation.

the height of contour or impinge upon the free gingival margin. Proper placement of the retentive arm provides significant advantages with regard to mechanics and esthetics.

5. When designing the metal framework for an extension base removable partial denture, special consideration must be given to potentially detrimental forces associated with cast circumferential clasps. A cast circumferential clasp should not be used to engage *(a)* the mesiofacial surface of an abutment adjacent to a posterior edentulous space or *(b)* the distofacial surface of an abutment adjacent to an extensive anterior edentulous space. The biomechanical difficulties produced by such arrangements often lead to premature loss of abutments.

*Simple circlet design.* The simple circlet clasp design is versatile and widely used (Fig 3-46). It is generally considered the clasp of choice for tooth-supported removable partial dentures. A simple

circlet clasp usually originates on the proximal surface of an abutment adjacent to an edentulous area, with the clasp arms projecting away from the edentulous space. The terminus of the retentive arm engages an undercut that is remote from the edentulous space.

When a decision must be made between a simple circlet clasp and another design of apparently equal capabilities, the simple circlet clasp should be chosen. The simple circlet clasp fulfills the design requirements of support, stability, reciprocation, encirclement, and passivity. In addition, its uncomplicated design features make it easy to construct and relatively simple to repair.

As might be expected, the simple circlet design also displays limitations. Because of the half-round cross-sectional geometry of each clasp arm, adjustment is difficult. In most instances, a clasp can be adjusted only in a buccolingual direction (ie, perpendicular to the clasp's flat surface). Furthermore, the clasp assembly tends to increase the cir-

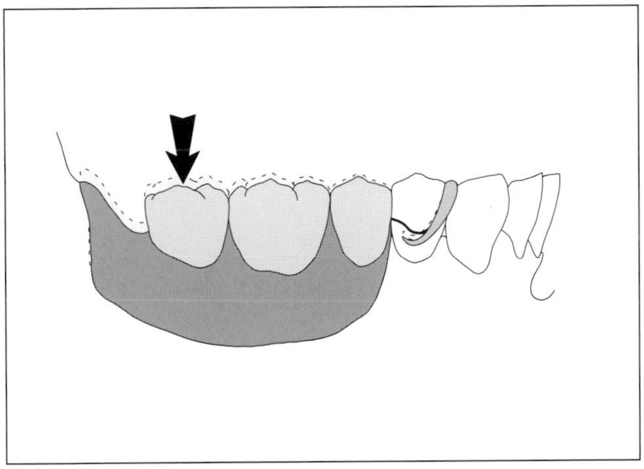

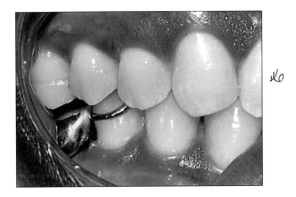

**Fig 3-48** The reverse circlet clasp may favorably control stresses delivered to the abutment upon loading of the removable partial denture *(arrow)*. As the extension base moves toward the underlying tissues, the clasp's retentive terminus moves into an area of greater undercut, minimizing torsional stress on the abutment.

**Fig 3-49** The reverse circlet clasp on the mandibular second premolar must cross the abutment's mesial marginal ridge and emerge onto the facial surface without interfering with normal occlusal contacts. Additionally, the clasp shoulder (not visible in the photograph) must possess adequate bulk for strength. In situations where inadequate occlusal clearance is available, use of the reverse circlet clasp may be contraindicated.

cumference of the clinical crown. This may interfere with the elimination of food from the occlusal table and may deprive the adjacent gingival tissues of essential physiologic stimulation. Increased tooth coverage may promote decalcification and compromise dental esthetics.

*Reverse circlet design.* A reverse circlet clasp is often used when the available undercut is located at the facial or lingual line angle adjacent to an edentulous space (Fig 3-47). The preferred method for engaging such an undercut involves the use of an infrabulge clasp that traverses the mucosa, turns vertically to cross the free gingival margin, and ultimately engages the undercut adjacent to the edentulous area. If, however, the anatomic contours of the hard and soft tissues apical to the abutment prohibit use of an infrabulge clasp, a reverse circlet clasp may be the retainer of choice.

In Kennedy Class I and Class II applications (ie, distal extension applications), the mesial-to-distal projection of a reverse circlet clasp may help control stresses transmitted to an abutment during functional movement of the prosthesis. As a distal extension base is loaded, the posterior aspect of the prosthesis moves toward the underlying tissues. At the same time, the tip of the retentive clasp moves into an area of greater undercut. Therefore, torsional stresses on the abutment are minimized (Fig 3-48). When a dislodging force is applied to the prosthesis, the retentive tip engages the undercut and the removable partial denture is retained.

The most significant problem associated with a reverse circlet design involves the strength of the resultant clasp assembly. The shoulder of a reverse circlet clasp originates from a minor connector that must traverse the marginal ridges of adjacent teeth (Fig 3-49). If these marginal ridges exhibit oc-

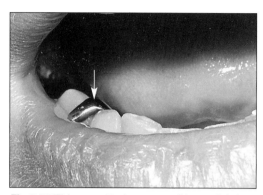

**Fig 3-50** This mandibular removable partial denture incorporates a reverse circlet clasp on the mandibular first premolar abutment *(arrow)*. The shoulder of the clasp extends over the abutment's mesial marginal ridge and the retentive terminus engages a distofacial undercut. Note the bulky, esthetically objectionable display of metal. Additionally, the clasp shoulder may interfere with normal occlusal contacts.

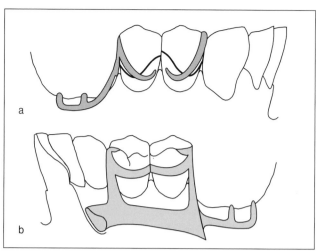

**Fig 3-51** A multiple circlet, cast circumferential retentive clasp assembly is present on the first and second premolar abutments. *(a)* The facial view demonstrates two simple circlet retentive arms. *(b)* The lingual view shows the joining of the terminal aspects of the reciprocal clasps. This clasp assembly design is typically considered when the primary abutment (first premolar) is periodontally compromised.

clusal contacts, it may be difficult to provide adequate room for clasp components without removing a significant amount of tooth structure from the abutments. Failure to remove adequate tooth structure often results in thin portions of the clasp assembly that are susceptible to fracture.

As might be expected, the lack of a rest adjacent to an edentulous space may allow the prosthesis to damage the associated soft tissues. The marginal gingiva also may be traumatized if food particles are forced between the proximal plate and the surface of the abutment. Food impaction may be eliminated by incorporating a disto-occlusal rest into the design. Unfortunately, addition of this rest will eliminate the releasing action of the retentive clasp terminus as the prosthesis moves during function.

Because a reverse circlet clasp is most commonly positioned at the mesio-occlusal surface of an abutment and crosses the facial surface from mesial to distal, it is a poor choice from an esthetic viewpoint. As a result, the reverse circlet clasp design is not the clasp of choice for canine and premolar abutments (Fig 3-50).

*Multiple circlet design.* A multiple circlet clasp design involves two simple circlet clasps joined at the terminal aspects of their reciprocal elements (Fig 3-51). This clasp design is primary indicated when the principal abutment tooth is periodontally compromised and stresses originating from prosthesis retention can be favorably distributed between multiple abutment teeth. The disadvantages of the multiple circlet clasp are the same as those discussed for simple circlet and reverse circlet clasps.

*Embrasure clasp design.* An embrasure clasp is essentially two simple circlets joined at their bodies (Figs 3-52 and 3-53). This design is most frequently used on the side of the arch where there is no edentulous space. Clasp arms originate from a minor connector that traverses the marginal ridges between teeth. Upon extension through the occlusal embrasure, retentive arms emerge to cross their respective facial surfaces and engage undercuts on the opposing line angles.

Occlusal rests must be used to support the embrasure portions of the clasp. Adequate preparation of the marginal ridges and adjacent facial in-

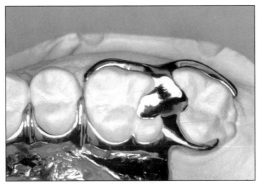

**Fig 3-52** This embrasure clasp assembly is designed for maxillary first and second molar abutments. On the first molar there is a simple circlet retentive clasp engaging a mesiofacial undercut, a distal rest, and a reciprocal plate. The second molar abutment exhibits a simple circlet retentive clasp engaging a distofacial undercut, a mesial rest, and a reciprocal clasp arm.

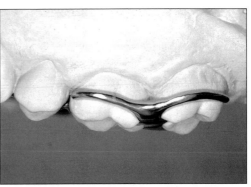

**Fig 3-53** Here, the same embrasure clasp assembly illustrated in Fig 3-52 is displayed from a facial view. Note that the simple circlet retentive clasps are joined at their bodies, forming a minor connector that traverses the occlusal embrasure between the first and second molars.

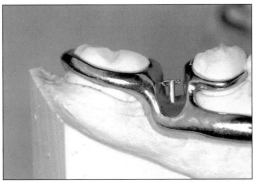

**Fig 3-54** A ring clasp assembly is used to engage a mesiolingual undercut on this mandibular second molar abutment that has tipped mesially and lingually following loss of the first molar. Viewed from the facial aspect, the clasp arm originates from a mesial minor connector and extends across the facial and distal surfaces of the tooth. Since no usable undercut exists on the facial tooth surface, the clasp arm is positioned occlusal to the height of contour.

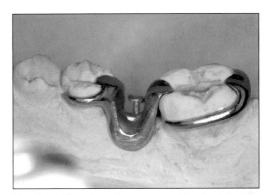

**Fig 3-55** The ring clasp assembly depicted in Fig 3-54 is viewed here from a lingual perspective. A distal rest on the second molar abutment is used to support the long clasp arm as it traverses the distal tooth surface. The retentive aspect of the clasp extends from the distal rest to engage a mesiolingual undercut.

clines must be accomplished to ensure a sufficient metal bulk for clasp strength. Fatigue failure of an embrasure clasp design is not uncommon, particularly when insufficient tooth preparation results in inadequate cross-sectional dimensions and compromised clasp strength. Therefore, the use of this clasp design should be avoided unless adequate tooth preparation can be achieved.

*Ring clasp design.* A ring clasp is most often indicated on a tipped mandibular molar (Figs 3-54 and 3-55). When the loss of mandibular posterior

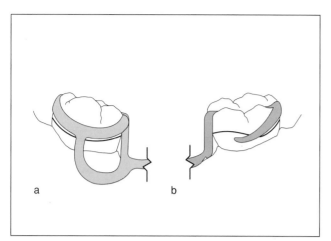

**Fig. 3-56** *(a)* To provide additional support for the long clasp arm of a ring clasp assembly, a facial bracing arm may be incorporated. The bracing arm originates from a mesial minor connector and joins the ring clasp as it crosses the facial surface. *(b)* This design helps to provide rigid and effective reciprocation for the lingually positioned retentive clasp.

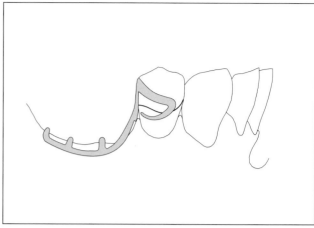

**Fig 3-57** The C-clasp design incorporates a retentive arm that originates from a proximal minor connector, extends across the abutment's facial surface, and curves back toward the clasp origin. The retentive clasp terminus is positioned in an appropriate undercut apical to the clasp's origin. This design must be accomplished carefully on mandibular posterior teeth to avoid interference with normal occlusal contacts.

teeth results in the absence of mesial proximal contact for a remaining molar, that molar tends to tip in a mesiolingual direction. At this inclination, the only available undercut is typically located at the mesiolingual line angle. The ring clasp permits engagement of this undercut through encirclement of the tooth. In most instances, the clasp originates from a mesial rest. The clasp arm then traverses the facial and distal surfaces of the tooth, remaining occlusal to the height of contour. At the middle of the lingual surface, the clasp arm passes apical to the height of contour and engages a measured undercut at the mesiolingual line angle.

Because of the length of the clasp arm, additional support must be available to ensure its rigidity. This support may be provided by an auxiliary bracing arm located at the facial aspect of the tooth (Fig 3-56). The bracing arm usually projects from the minor connector used to retain the acrylic resin denture base. The bracing arm runs horizontally across the mucosa apical to the abutment tooth and then turns occlusally to cross the free gingival margin and join the clasp arm at its midfacial aspect. Without this bracing element, the clasp assembly cannot provide effective reciprocation or cross-arch stability.

If desired, an additional rest may be placed on the disto-occlusal surface. This rest may provide additional support for the prosthesis and may improve the mechanical characteristics of the clasp assembly.

When using a ring clasp, the practitioner must cover an extensive amount of tooth structure. As a result, oral hygiene becomes more complicated and the likelihood of demineralization is increased. In addition, the ring clasp design significantly alters the functional contours of the abutment and may interfere with the elimination of food from the occlusal table. This alteration may result in insufficient stimulation of the associated soft tissues and adversely impact gingival health. From a structural standpoint, the ring clasp is susceptible to distortion and fracture. Correction of these problems is extremely difficult.

A ring clasp should not be considered when limited vestibular depth precludes placement of the auxiliary bracing arm. This clasp design is also contraindicated when the bracing arm must project across a soft tissue undercut area. As a general rule, the ring clasp should not be considered the clasp of choice when an alternative design is feasible.

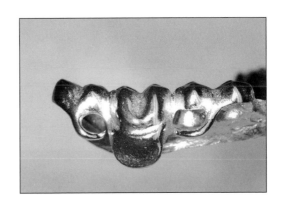

**Fig 3-58** Displayed here is a mandibular removable partial denture framework designed to incorporate an extensive onlay clasp assembly. The occlusal aspect of the onlay reestablishes a normal occlusal plane extending from the first premolar to the second molar. A missing first molar is restored with a full metal pontic. Retentive clasp arms engage a distofacial undercut on the second premolar and a mesiofacial undercut on the second molar. The onlay provides the necessary vertical support for the prosthesis by achieving intimate occlusal contact with the abutments.

*C-clasp design.* The C-clasp is also referred to as a "fishhook" or "hairpin" clasp. It is essentially a simple circlet clasp in which the retentive arm loops back to engage an undercut apical to the point of origin (Fig 3-57). As a result, the retentive arm has two horizontal components. The occlusal portion of the retentive arm should be considered a minor connector and must be rigid. The apical portion of the retentive arm must pass over the height of contour to engage the desired undercut. Hence, this portion of the clasp must be flexible. To achieve these objectives, the occlusal portion of the clasp arm should display consistent dimensions, while the apical portion of the clasp arm should be gently tapered.

To accommodate a C-clasp, the clinical crown must exhibit sufficient vertical height. There must be adequate space between the occlusal and apical aspects of the retentive arm to provide access for metal finishing procedures and to minimize the accumulation of food particles during mastication. The occlusal aspect of the retentive arm also should not interfere with the opposing teeth in maximum intercuspation.

Despite the best efforts of clinicians and laboratory personnel, a C-clasp design generally yields inadequate flexibility. As a result, the abutment may be subjected to harmful non-axial forces. The C-clasp also results in considerable coverage of the abutment surface. Hence, the accumulation of food and debris makes it inappropriate for patients who are particularly susceptible to caries de-velopment (eg, young patients and patients exhibiting poor oral hygiene). The excessive display of metal associated with this clasp often renders the C-clasp esthetically unacceptable. This is particularly true for canine and premolar teeth.

When the only available undercut is located at the line angle adjacent to the edentulous space, there are three clasp designs from which to choose: the infrabulge clasp, the reverse circlet clasp, and the C-clasp. The C-clasp is indicated when the soft tissue contour precludes use of a bar-type clasp and when the reverse circlet cannot be considered because of a lack of occlusal clearance.

*Onlay clasp design.* An onlay clasp consists of a rest that covers the entire occlusal surface and serves as the origin for buccal and lingual clasp arms (Fig 3-58). This clasp design is indicated when the occlusal surface of the abutment lies noticeably apical to the occlusal plane. The onlay rest serves as a vertical stop and also aids in the establishment of an acceptable occlusal plane (Figs 3-59 and 3-60).

Because of extensive tooth coverage, the onlay clasp should be prescribed only for caries-resistant patients. If the removable partial denture framework is to be constructed using a chrome alloy and is opposed by natural tooth structure, the occlusal surface of the onlay clasp should be veneered with acrylic resin or gold. Chrome alloys often induce rapid wear of enamel and dentin surfaces, while acrylic resin and gold display greater compatibility with natural tooth structure.

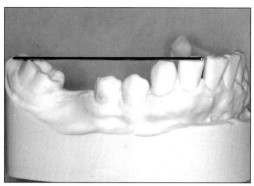

**Fig 3-59** The severe occlusal plane irregularity present on this mandibular cast is not typically amenable to conservative restorative therapy. The line extending from the canine to the second molar identifies a more desirable occlusal plane.

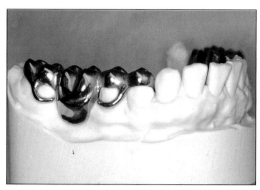

**Fig 3-60** This removable partial denture achieves both restoration of the missing first molar and establishment of a more desirable occlusal plane. Careful patient follow-up is indicated here to avoid wear of the opposing dentition and carious deterioration of the abutments.

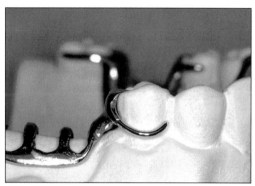

**Fig 3-61** A combination clasp assembly engages this mandibular second premolar abutment. A wrought-wire circumferential clasp originates from a distal guiding plate and extends across the facial tooth surface to engage a mesiofacial undercut.

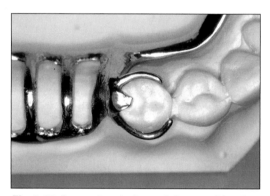

**Fig 3-62** An occlusal view of the combination clasp displayed in Fig 3-61 depicts a facial wrought-wire retentive clasp arm, a distal rest, and a lingual cast reciprocal clasp arm.

Although an onlay clasp may be used successfully, it is frequently more appropriate to restore the occlusal plane with one or more fixed restorations and consider a more conventional design for the removable prosthesis.

*Wrought-wire circumferential clasp.* Although used as early as 1847, the wrought-wire circumferential clasp did not gain wide acceptance until the "double-bow clasp" was introduced by Dr F. Ewing Roach in 1913.[12] In 1965, Dr O. C. Applegate introduced a modified wrought-wire clasp assembly known as the "combination clasp."[13]

The combination clasp consists of an occlusal rest, a cast metal reciprocal arm, and a wrought-wire retentive arm (Figs 3-61 and 3-62). The wrought-wire component is circular in cross section, thereby permitting flexure in all directions. This omnidirectional flexure allows the clasp to flex in all planes and can minimize the transfer of potentially harmful forces to the abutment (see Fig 3-24). The combination clasp is most frequently indicated on an abutment adjacent to a Kennedy Class I or Class II posterior edentulous area when the usable undercut is located at the mesiofacial line angle of the most posterior abutment. Masticatory

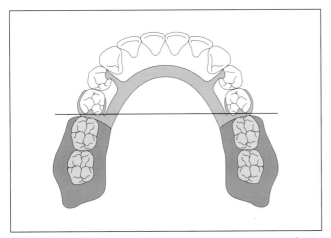

**Fig 3-63** Masticatory loading of the extension bases of this removable partial denture will result in prosthesis rotation around a fulcrum line that passes through the most posterior rests.

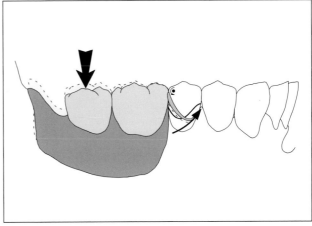

**Fig 3-64** As the distal extension base is loaded *(large arrow)*, the prosthesis rotates around a fulcrum that passes through the most posterior rests. This causes the wrought wire to move in an arcuate path that is directed mesially and occlusally *(small arrow)*.

loading causes the prosthesis to rotate around a fulcrum line that passes through the most posterior rests on either side of the arch. As the prosthesis rotates, the retentive clasp moves in an arcuate path that is directed occlusally (Figs 3-63 and 3-64). Omnidirectional flexure of the wrought-wire retentive arm permits partial dissipation of applied forces. Hence, the combination clasp is kinder to the associated abutment than a traditional half-round clasp arm would be (see Fig 3-24).

The improved flexibility of a wrought-wire retentive clasp also permits its placement into a slightly greater undercut. Consequently, a wrought-wire retentive arm can frequently be located in the apical third of the clinical crown, thereby producing a more esthetic result. As a result, a wrought-wire retentive clasp is often used on maxillary canine and premolar abutments.

Because of its cross-sectional geometry, wrought wire makes a very fine, linear contact with the surface of the abutment. Therefore, tooth coverage is markedly decreased. This minimal surface contact makes its use in caries-prone individuals somewhat more beneficial.

The main disadvantage of the combination clasp is that it involves additional steps during laboratory construction. It is also more prone to damage or breakage than is a cast clasp assembly. It is important to recognize that wrought wire is particularly susceptible to damage if the prosthesis is mishandled by the patient. Therefore, the patient should be instructed in proper care of the prosthesis. It is strongly recommended that the patient remove the partial denture by grasping the denture base and gently withdrawing the prosthesis from the mouth. The patient should avoid grasping the wrought-wire retentive arm, since this commonly results in distortion of the clasp and an accompanying loss of retention.

Because of the increased flexibility of the retentive clasp arm, the combination clasp assembly does not possess the bracing or stabilizing qualities of most circumferential clasps. Therefore, if stabilization is of primary importance, the combination clasp should not be the clasp assembly of choice.

**Infrabulge clasp** The infrabulge clasp design was introduced during the early 1900s, but did not receive widespread attention until 1930. At that time, Dr F. Ewing Roach presented his "bar-type" or "Roach" clasp and provided an appropriate rationale for its use.[8]

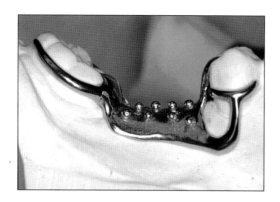

**Fig 3-65** This T-clasp originates from a minor connector and approaches the abutment from an apical direction. Therefore, upon removal of the prosthesis, the retentive terminus must be "pushed" over the abutment's height of contour.

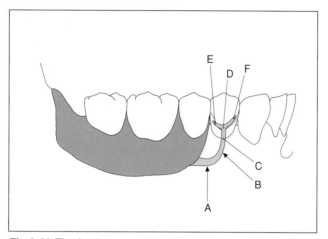

**Fig 3-66** The basic components and design features of a T-clasp include the horizontal projection portion of the approach arm (A), vertical projection aspect of the approach arm (B), location where the approach arm crosses perpendicular to the free gingival margin (C), point of first tooth contact at or occlusal to the height of abutment contour (D), terminus of the retentive clasp contacting the abutment apical to the height of contour (E), and encirclement portion of the clasp contacting the abutment occlusal to the height of contour (F). Note that the approach arm of the T-clasp is both long and gently tapering to maximize flexibility.

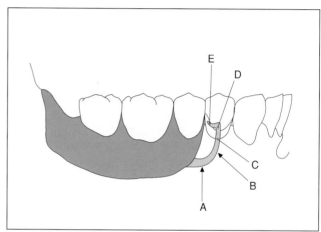

**Fig 3-67** The basic components and design features of a modified T-clasp include the horizontal projection portion of the approach arm (A), vertical projection aspect of the approach arm (B), location where the approach arm crosses perpendicular to the free gingival margin (C), point of first tooth contact at or occlusal to the height of abutment contour (D), and terminus of the retentive clasp contacting the abutment apical to the height of contour (E). Note that the approach arm of the modified T-clasp is both long and gently tapering to maximize flexibility.

An infrabulge clasp approaches the undercut region of an abutment from an apical direction (Fig 3-65). Therefore, an infrabulge clasp exhibits a "push" type of retention that is more effective than the "pull" retention associated with a suprabulge clasp.

Flexibility of the infrabulge clasp is controlled by the taper and length of the approach arm. The greater the length and the more marked the taper, the more flexible the clasp. Because an infrabulge clasp approaches the undercut from an apical direction, it is usually more esthetic than a supra-

bulge clasp. In addition, there are a variety of bar-type clasps that provide a wide range of adaptability. These clasps are described by their geometric shapes. Although a variety of clasps is included in this classification, this textbook deals primarily with four embodiments. These include: the T-clasp (Fig 3-66), the modified T-clasp (Fig 3-67), the Y-clasp (Fig 3-68), and the I-clasp or I-bar (Fig 3-69).

Among the disadvantages of infrabulge clasps is the tendency to accumulate food debris. In addition, the increased flexibility of the retentive arm does not contribute a great deal to the horizontal

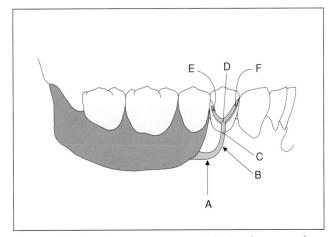

**Fig 3-68** The basic components and design features of an infrabulge Y-clasp include the horizontal projection portion of the approach arm (A), vertical projection aspect of the approach arm (B), location where the approach arm crosses perpendicular to the free gingival margin (C), point of first tooth contact at or occlusal to the height of abutment contour (D), terminus of the retentive clasp contacting the abutment apical to the height of contour (E), and encirclement portion of the clasp contacting the abutment occlusal to the height of contour (F). Note that the approach arm of the Y-clasp is both long and gently tapering to maximize flexibility.

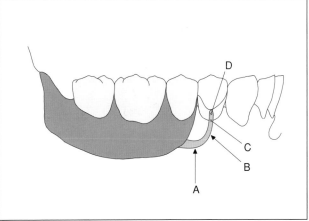

**Fig 3-69** The basic components and design features of an infrabulge I-clasp or I-bar include the horizontal projection portion of the approach arm (A), vertical projection aspect of the approach arm (B), location where the approach arm crosses perpendicular to the free gingival margin (C), and point of first tooth contact apical to the height of contour in the prescribed amount of undercut (D). Note that the approach arm of the I-clasp is both long and gently tapering to maximize flexibility.

stability of the prosthesis. Hence, additional bracing and stabilizing units may be required when an infrabulge clasp is used.

*Design rules.* The following design rules are applicable to infrabulge clasps:

1. The approach arm of an infrabulge clasp must not impinge on the soft tissues adjacent to the abutment. It is not desirable to provide relief under the approach arm, but the tissue surface of the approach arm should be smooth and well polished.
2. The approach arm should cross perpendicular to the free gingival margin. The sensitive periodontal tissues must be protected from irritation by inducing as little interference with normal function and contour as possible.
3. The approach arm should never be designed to "bridge" an area of soft tissue undercut since this will produce an increased risk of food entrapment and may result in irritation of the associated soft tissues (Fig 3-70).

4. To optimize flexibility, the approach arm should be uniformly tapered from its origin to the clasp terminus.
5. The clasp terminus should be positioned as far apically on the abutment as is practical. Proper placement of the clasp terminus yields a decrease in leverage-induced stresses resulting from movement of the prosthesis.
6. The minor connector that attaches the occlusal rest to the framework should be rigid and should contribute to the overall bracing and stabilization characteristics of the prosthesis.

*T-clasp design.* The T-clasp derives its name from the shape created where the retentive clasp arm joins the vertical aspect of the approach arm (see Fig 3-65). This clasp design is often used in Kennedy Class I or Class II partially edentulous situations when an undercut is located adjacent to the edentulous area. The approach arm typically originates from components located in the edentulous area and projects horizontally across the soft tissues. The approach

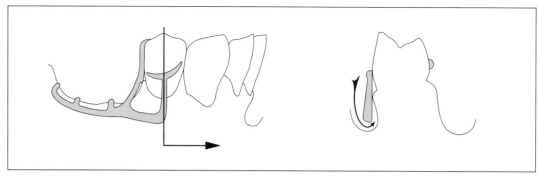

**Fig 3-70** An infrabulge clasp is not the design of choice when the approach arm must bridge an area of soft tissue undercut apical to the abutment *(a)* since there is an increased risk of food entrapment and soft tissue irritation *(b)*.

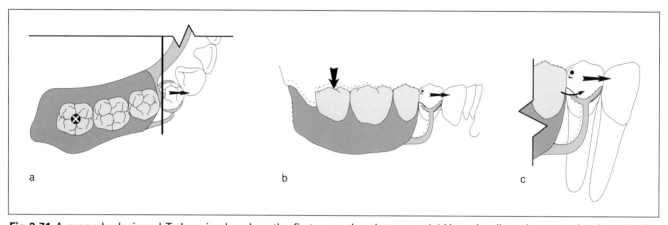

**Fig 3-71** A properly designed T-clasp is placed on the first premolar abutment. *(a)* Upon loading, the extension base is displaced toward the underlying tissues, causing the removable partial denture to rotate around a fulcrum line passing through the distal rest on the first premolar. *(b)* As prosthesis rotation occurs, the retentive terminus of the T-clasp moves mesially, engaging the abutment. Clasp engagement places mesially directed stress on the abutment. *(c)* The abutment tolerates this force, ie, is positionally stable, because of sound contact with the adjacent canine. Therefore, potentially harmful forces are minimized.

arm then turns vertically to cross the free gingival margin at 90 degrees and contact the abutment at the height of contour. From this point, two horizontal projections arise. One projection extends toward the edentulous area. This projection passes over the height of contour and enters a 0.010-inch undercut. The second projection extends in the opposite direction and remains occlusal/incisal to the height of contour. This projection improves bracing and stabilization provided by the clasp assembly. Both projections display a gentle curvature and point slightly toward the occlusal plane.

Upon loading of the extension base, the distal rest serves as a center of rotation. The tip of the retentive clasp moves apically and mesially. This minimizes potentially harmful torquing forces while transmitting a relatively small, mesially directed force to the abutment (Fig 3-71). The mesially directed force is well tolerated as a result of sound contact with the adjacent natural tooth.

It is important to realize that a T-clasp should never be used in a Kennedy Class I or Class II partially edentulous application if the only available undercut is located on the mesiofacial aspect of

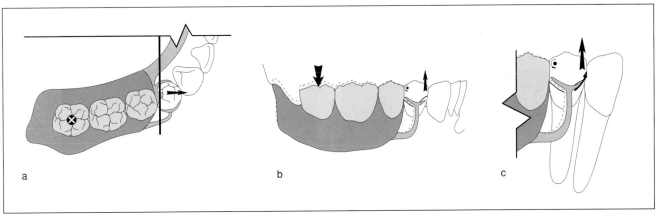

**Fig 3-72** An improperly designed T-clasp is placed on the first premolar abutment. Note that the clasp engages a mesiofacial undercut. *(a)* Upon loading, the extension base is displaced toward the underlying tissues, causing the removable partial denture to rotate around a fulcrum line passing through the distal rest on the first premolar. *(b)* As prosthesis rotation occurs, the retentive terminus of the T-clasp moves occlusally, engaging the abutment. Clasp engagement places occlusally directed stress on the abutment. *(c)* This stress is not counteracted, resulting in potentially harmful force being delivered to the abutment.

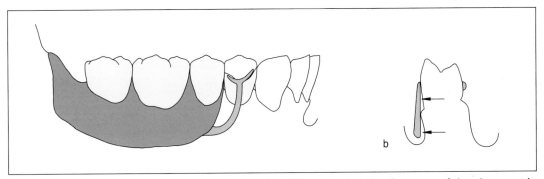

**Fig 3-73** *(a)* This T-clasp design is contraindicated. *(b)* When the height of contour of the abutment is located near the occlusal surface, space created between the vertical approach arm and the tooth surface *(top arrow)* may result in debris accumulation and patient discomfort.

the most posterior abutment. This configuration will prevent proper function of the clasp assembly and will result in the application of detrimental torquing forces to the abutment (Fig 3-72).

From a practical standpoint, a T-clasp should not be used if the approach arm must cross over an area of severe soft tissue undercut. The bridging effect produced by the clasp arm may result in noticeable food accumulation and irritation of the adjacent soft tissues.

A T-clasp is also contraindicated when the height of contour is located near the occlusal surface. Since the approach arm contacts the surface of the abutment only at the height of contour, the space created between the clasp arm and the tooth

surface may result in the accumulation of food particles and other debris (Fig 3-73).

A T-clasp may be esthetically superior to a suprabulge design because of the elimination of the clasp shoulder. However, the increased flexibility of an infrabulge clasp's approach arm detracts from the bracing qualities provided by the majority of cast suprabulge clasps.

*Modified T-clasp design.* The modified T-clasp is essentially a T-clasp that lacks the nonretentive, horizontal projection (Fig 3-74; see also Fig 3-67). As noted in the previous section, the approach arm originates from minor connector components located within the edentulous area. The approach

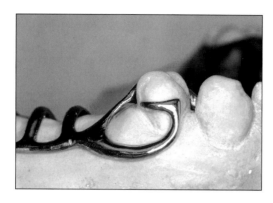

**Fig 3-74** The modified T-clasp placed on this second premolar abutment is similar to the T-clasp except that it lacks the mesial extension of the retentive clasp.

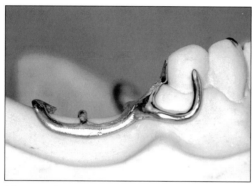

**Fig 3-75** The I-clasp, or I-bar, direct retainer derives its name from the linear configuration of the vertical approach arm.

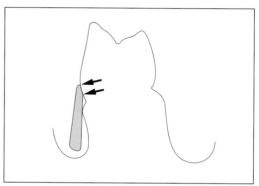

**Fig 3-76** As the I-clasp approaches the abutment from an apical direction, the clasp terminus makes first contact with the abutment surface at the measured undercut *(bottom arrow)*. Contact is then maintained to the height of contour of the abutment *(top arrow)*.

arm then projects horizontally across the soft tissues adjacent to the abutment. The approach arm turns vertically to cross the gingival margin at 90 degrees and contacts the abutment at the height of contour. At this point, the clasp turns abruptly toward the prescribed undercut. The retentive component of the clasp then passes apical to the height of contour and engages the specified undercut. The retentive projection is gently curved and should point slightly toward the occlusal plane.

The mechanics of a modified T-clasp are nearly identical to those of a conventional T-clasp. As a result, modified T-clasps are often used in Kennedy Class I and Class II applications when retentive undercuts are located adjacent to the edentulous area(s).

Because the nonretentive projection is absent, the modified T-clasp provides improved esthetics in most applications. Therefore, modified T-clasps are often used when canines or premolars will serve as abutments.

*Y-clasp design.* From a practical perspective, a Y-clasp is equivalent to a T-clasp. A Y-clasp is formed when the approach arm terminates in the cervical third of the abutment, while the mesial and distal projections are positioned near the occlusal/incisal surface (see Fig 3-68).

As might be expected, the mechanics of a Y-clasp are similar to those of a T-clasp. On occasion, careful recontouring of the abutment surface will allow the Y-clasp to be converted to a standard T-clasp. This often provides an improved esthetic result.

*I-clasp design.* As with T- and Y-clasps, the I-clasp or I-bar derives its name from its shape (Fig 3-75;

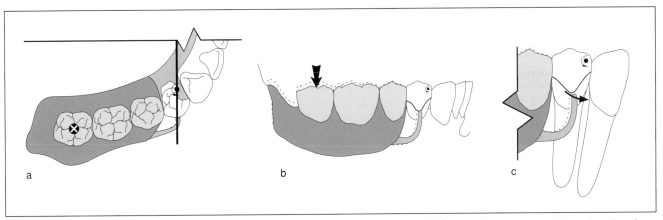

**Fig 3-77** A properly designed I-clasp direct retainer is placed on this mandibular first premolar abutment. Note that the clasp terminus is placed at the midfacial prominence of the abutment. *(a)* Upon loading, the extension base is displaced toward the underlying tissues, causing the removable partial denture to rotate around a fulcrum line passing through the distal rest on the first premolar. *(b)* As prosthesis rotation occurs, the retentive terminus of the I-clasp moves mesially, disengaging from the abutment. *(c)* Since the clasp disengages from the abutment surface, it induces no stress to the abutment, thus minimizing harmful force transference.

see also Fig 3-69). The approach arm typically originates from framework components in the edentulous area and projects horizontally across the soft tissues adjacent to the abutment. A gradual turn allows the approach arm to assume a vertical orientation and cross perpendicular to the free gingival margin. The clasp arm contacts the abutment surface over an area that extends from the measured undercut to the height of contour (Fig 3-76). Typically, the contact area between the clasp and the abutment is 2.0 to 3.0 mm in height and 1.5 to 2.0 mm in width. The approach arm has a half-round, cross-sectional geometry and is characterized by a gradual and uniform taper throughout its length.

Often, the I-clasp design is used in conjunction with a mesial rest. Upon loading, this rest serves as the center of rotation. As the posterior portion of the prosthesis moves toward the underlying soft tissues, the clasp terminus moves into an area of greater undercut (Fig 3-77). Hence, the retentive element disengages from the abutment, and torquing forces are minimized.

This design is commonly used in the treatment of Kennedy Class I and Class II partially edentulous arches. In these applications, proper placement of the clasp terminus is essential if the clasp is to release upon occlusal loading. Hence, the I-clasp

should be placed at or mesial to the midfacial prominence of the abutment (see Fig 3-77).

The I-clasp is an integral retentive component in two distinct design philosophies: the mesial rest/I-bar concept[14] and the RPI concept.[15] Of particular note is the latter, advanced by Dr A. J. Krol. His approach to prosthesis design provides a valid theoretical rationale for disengagement of the retentive clasp terminus during rotational movement of the removable partial denture. Widely accepted in the United States, this design philosophy calls for the use of a mesial rest, a distal guide plate, and an I-clasp retainer (mesial *r*est, distal *p*roximal guide plate, and *I*-clasp = RPI). This design philosophy is described in greater detail in chapter 8.

**Summary of retentive clasp assemblies** Selection of the most appropriate clasp assembly for a specific clinical situation must be based on a variety of factors. Prosthesis design should be kept as simple as the clinical situation permits. Unnecessarily complicated designs may be avoided by producing improved abutment contours. In many instances, this may be accomplished by carefully recontouring the surfaces of an abutment. In other instances, it may require the placement of one or more fixed restorations. Although the latter approach will result in added expense for the patient, the simplification in design can significantly improve the comfort, function, and longevity of the prosthesis.

Appropriate clasp selection is particularly important in Kennedy Class I and Class II applications. The application of forces must be carefully controlled to prevent the accelerated loss of removable partial denture abutments. If a mesiofacial undercut is available on the abutment tooth adjacent to a distal extension space, a combination clasp incorporating a wrought-wire retentive element should be used to dissipate functional stresses. If the retentive undercut is located on the distofacial or midfacial surface, an appropriate infrabulge clasp should be selected. If there are contraindications to the use of an infrabulge clasp, a reverse circlet clasp should be considered.

## ⌑ Indirect Retainers

A removable partial denture derives support from two main sources. Support may be available from periodontally sound natural teeth through properly constructed rests contacting well-prepared rest seats. In edentulous regions, the residual alveolar processes and associated soft tissues may provide support for well-adapted denture bases. Disparities in the support provided by natural teeth and soft tissues present distinct challenges in removable partial denture design.

A removable partial denture that is supported by healthy natural teeth (eg, Kennedy Class III and short-span Class IV applications) possesses adequate stability and retention to resist functional displacement. However, a removable partial denture that is not entirely bounded by natural teeth (eg, Kennedy Class I, Class II, and long-span Class IV applications) will move when a load is applied. A denture base that is supported at one end by a healthy natural abutment and at the other by movable soft tissues will rotate toward or away from the residual ridge when subjected to occlusal forces or the pull of sticky foods. The need to consider this movement has long been recognized. In 1880, F. H. Balkwill clearly described the rotational movement occurring within a prosthesis supported by natural teeth and soft tissues. In 1916, Prothero coined the term *fulcrum line* to identify the primary

axis of rotation.[4] Other potential axes, or fulcrum lines, clearly exist in removable partial denture applications and must be considered in the design and construction of such prostheses. Therefore, a discussion of terminology is in order.

The descriptive term *extension base* is frequently applied to a removable partial denture that extends from the natural abutment teeth onto the tissues of the residual ridge. Support for this type of prosthesis must be derived from the remaining teeth and the tissues underlying the denture bases. This is the case in Kennedy Class I, Class II, and long-span Class IV situations.

With regard to appropriate terminology, a Kennedy Class I partially edentulous condition may be restored with a *bilateral, distal extension removable partial denture*. A patient demonstrating a Kennedy Class II partially edentulous condition may receive a *unilateral, distal extension removable partial denture*. A patient displaying a Kennedy Class IV pattern of edentulism may be treated with a *mesial extension removable partial denture*. This nomenclature has found common use because it accurately describes the clinical and prosthodontic conditions at hand. Therefore, both Kennedy classification and extension base terminology are acceptable when used appropriately.

When an occlusal load is applied to a distal extension removable partial denture, the prosthesis rotates around a fulcrum line that passes through the most posterior rests—one on each side of the dental arch (Fig 3-78). Displacement of the prosthesis is limited by the hard and soft tissues of the residual ridge (Fig 3-79). Therefore, optimal resistance to displacement may be provided by broad and accurate adaptation of the denture base(s) to the supporting tissues. The chosen impression technique (eg, selective pressure or mucostatic) may exert a significant influence on the amount of denture base movement that results from functional loading.

Forces acting to dislodge the prosthesis in an occlusal direction also must be considered. Sticky foods or other substances may pull on the artificial teeth and move the extension base away from the underlying ridges. Active tissues such as the tongue and buccinator muscle also may displace the den-

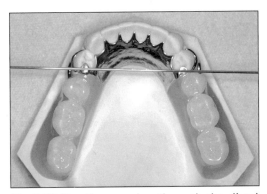

**Fig 3-78** The line passing through the distal rests on the mandibular first premolars designates the primary rotational fulcrum for this extension base removable partial denture. Application of an occlusal load to the denture teeth will result in rotational displacement of the prosthesis toward the underlying supporting tissues around the primary rotational fulcrum.

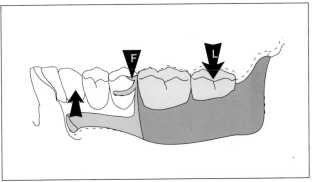

**Fig 3-79** Illustration of the fulcrum (F) established at the occlusal rest when a load (L) is applied to the extension base. Prosthesis rotation around this fulcrum causes the extension base to be displaced toward the underlying supporting tissues, while anterior aspects of the removable partial denture rotate in an occlusal direction *(arrow)*.

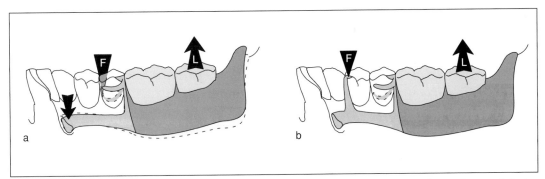

**Fig 3-80** *(a)* Illustration of the fulcrum (F) established at the retentive clasp terminus when a dislodging force (L) acts on the extension base. Rotation of the prosthesis causes the extension base to be displaced away from the supporting tissues, while the anterior portion of the prosthesis rotates in an apical direction. Rotation of the removable partial denture in this manner may result in unwanted prosthesis impingement into the soft tissues of the floor of the mouth. *(b)* This unwanted rotation may be effectively countered by placing a rest on the opposite side of the fulcrum from the extension base. In this scenario, impingement of the prosthesis into the floor of the mouth is negated as the fulcrum is transported to the anterior rest, also know as an indirect retainer.

ture base during speech, mastication, or swallowing. When a distal extension removable partial denture is subjected to such forces, the associated fulcrum line passes through the tips of the retentive clasps (Fig 3-80). Therefore, the practitioner must provide one or more components to limit such movement.

The framework component that resists rotational displacement of an extension base away from the supporting tissues is called an *indirect re-tainer*. When rotational forces are effectively counteracted by placement of indirect retainers, the removable partial denture is said to exhibit *indirect re-tention* (see Fig 3-80). All Kennedy Class I, Class II, and Class IV removable partial dentures require effective indirect retention.

To understand the importance of indirect retention, one must consider the effects of rotational movement. When the posterior portion of a Kennedy Class I or Class II removable partial den-

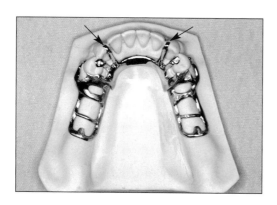

**Fig 3-81** The indirect retainers on the mandibular canines *(arrows)* provide additional support and rigidity to the lingual bar major connector.

ture is subjected to occlusally directed dislodging forces in the absence of properly designed indirect retention, two undesirable events ensue: *(1)* the denture base or denture bases move away from the supporting tissues, and *(2)* the anterior segment of the major connector impinges upon the underlying soft tissues (see Fig 3-80a). This results in transmission of potentially destructive forces to the hard and soft tissues of the dental arch. Consequently, these conditions must be avoided.

When well-designed indirect retention is included in Kennedy Class I and Class II applications, forces acting to displace the denture bases are negated. In this configuration, the rotational axis shifts from the retentive clasp tips to the indirect retainers (see Fig 3-80b). As long as the clasp assemblies adequately resist the vertical dislodging forces, the prosthesis remains in place. As dislodging forces are elevated beyond the retentive capacities of the clasp assemblies, the prosthesis moves away from the underlying tissues.

Although the concept of indirect retention was originally advanced by Dr W. E. Cummer as a means of resisting rotational displacement, properly designed indirect retainers often serve additional functions.[16] When in positive contact with a rest seat, an indirect retainer contributes to the overall support and stability of the removable partial denture. For a long-span lingual bar, properly constructed indirect retainers can provide additional support and rigidity to the major connector (Fig 3-81). In this application, effective indirect retention prevents traumatic contact with the underlying soft tissues during movement of the prosthesis.

## Factors determining effectiveness of indirect retainers

Indirect retention can only be achieved when one or more rigid indirect retainers are positioned in properly prepared rest seats. The relationship of an indirect retainer to its rest seat permits applied forces to be transmitted within the long axis of the abutment. As might be expected, additional factors influence the effectiveness of indirect retention. Each of these factors must be evaluated and understood within the three-dimensional context of partial denture movement.

Identification of the primary fulcrum line is extremely important in Kennedy Class I and Class II applications. As previously noted, the primary fulcrum line passes through the most posterior abutments (one on each side of the dental arch). To prevent displacement of an extension base away from the underlying residual ridge, one or more indirect retainers must be positioned on the opposite side of the fulcrum line (Fig 3-82).

The greater the distance between the fulcrum line and the indirect retainer, the more effective the direct retainer will be. Therefore, the position of the indirect retainer should be perpendicular to—and as far from—the primary fulcrum line as is practical (Fig 3-83). In certain instances, this location may be occupied by an edentulous space or a tooth that is unable to support an indirect retainer for periodontal reasons. Hence, it is often necessary to select a more suitable abutment. For practical purposes, indirect retainers should not

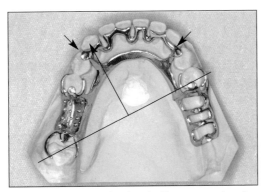

**Fig 3-82** When designing indirect retention for this removable partial denture framework, identification of the primary fulcrum line is necessary. The primary fulcrum line *(black line)* passes through the distal-most abutments on either side of the dental arch. Though inconvenient, a rest placed on the mesial aspect of the mandibular left canine *(long arrow)* would provide ideal indirect retention. Instead, rests located on the mesial occlusal surfaces of the first premolars *(short arrows)* provide adequate indirect retention.

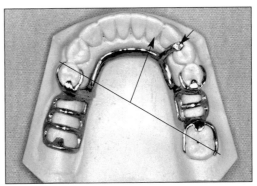

**Fig 3-83** The geometrically ideal position for indirect retention for this framework would be the mandibular right lateral incisor *(long arrow)*. This location is perpendicular to, and as far from, the primary fulcrum line as possible. However, since incisal rests are not practical, placing a rest on the right first premolar *(short arrow)* is a viable alternative that will provide adequate indirect retention.

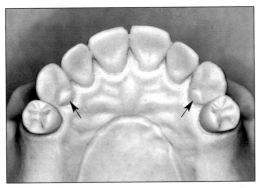

**Fig 3-84** Prepared cingulum rest seats on the maxillary canines *(arrows)* will function to support an anterior lingual plate.

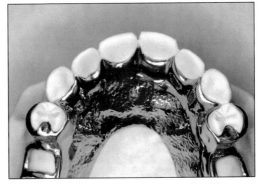

**Fig 3-85** The lingual plate on this maxillary removable partial denture framework is supported by properly designed cingulum rests on the canine teeth (see Fig 3-84).

be placed on maxillary or mandibular incisors. Canines and premolars are commonly used because of their increased periodontal support.

There is considerable confusion regarding the role of lingual plating in indirect retention. By definition, an indirect retainer is an occlusal, incisal, or cingulum rest that displays accurate and definitive contact with a properly designed, horizontally oriented rest seat. In contrast, the contact between a lingual plate and the associated anterior teeth occurs on inclined planes. Therefore, a lingual plate

does not serve as an indirect retainer. Nevertheless, if a lingual plate is adequately supported by properly designed rests at each end, the lingual plate may enhance the efficiency of the indirect retainers. In this configuration, the anterior teeth can partially offset dislodging forces on the denture base. The rests prevent apical migration of the lingual plate during functional loading and prevent orthodontic movement (ie, splaying) of the associated teeth (Figs 3-84 and 3-85).

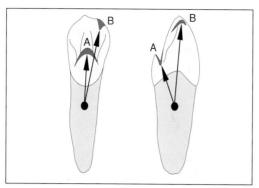

**Fig 3-86** When compared to a cingulum rest (A), the incisal rest (B) may deliver potentially harmful forces a greater distance from the abutment's center of rotation. Where practical, the cingulum rest is preferred over the incisal rest.

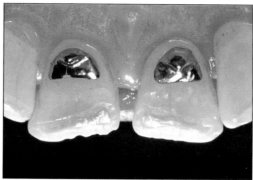

**Fig 3-87** In this situation, it was necessary to engage the maxillary central incisors with indirect retainers. Rather than penetrating the enamel with a conventional cingulum rest preparation or placing metal in esthetically unacceptable locations with an incisal rest, bonded rest seats were constructed. Conservative tooth preparation and enamel-metal bonding technology permitted reliable placement of these custom rest seats.

## Forms of indirect retainers

An indirect retainer is an auxiliary occlusal, cingulum, or incisal rest that contacts a properly designed rest seat when the removable partial denture is in place. In order to be effective, the indirect retainer must be rigid. If the indirect retainer is flexible, the prosthesis will not function as intended. In fact, potentially destructive forces may be amplified because of this lack of rigidity.

An occlusal rest is the preferred component for indirect retention. Because of its location and vertical orientation, an occlusal rest permits forces to be directed within the long axis of the corresponding abutment.

A cingulum rest also can be used as an effective indirect retainer. This rest generally is limited to maxillary canines. The normal morphology of this tooth lends itself to appropriate rest seat preparation with minimal recontouring. The practitioner must pay particular attention to the positions of opposing teeth and the locations of occlusal contacts. In addition, the practitioner must create adequate space for a properly designed rest seat and a sufficiently strong rest, but not at the expense of essential disclusive contacts.

An incisal rest also may provide indirect retention where other rests are contraindicated. This is particu-

larly true for maxillary and mandibular incisors, as well as mandibular canines. Because of the unfavorable lingual anatomy of these teeth, incisal rests may be the only acceptable option. Unfortunately, incisal rests are esthetically objectionable and exhibit long approach arms that may transfer harmful tipping forces to abutments (Fig 3-86).

If an incisor must be used, an incisal rest seat must be prepared. More effective indirect retention may be achieved by preparing the incisor to receive either a full coverage restoration or a cast metal rest seat that is bonded to the lingual surface of the tooth (Fig 3-87). The result should be a well-designed lingual rest seat that provides appropriate contours for the rest, contributes to optimal force distribution, and permits an effective means of indirect retention for the removable partial denture.

## ◲ Tooth Replacements

The prosthetic teeth of choice for removable partial dentures are commercially available, acrylic resin denture teeth (Fig 3-88). In most instances, the restoration of edentulous areas is accomplished by attaching such teeth to an acrylic resin denture base. Nevertheless, specific clinical conditions make the use of conventional denture teeth difficult, if not impossible. In

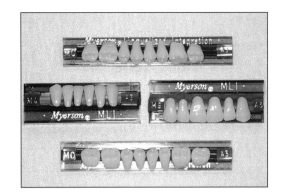

**Fig 3-88** Commercially available, acrylic resin denture teeth are most appropriate for removable partial dentures.

these situations, other forms of tooth replacement may provide more favorable results. Alternative methods of replacement include tube teeth, braided posts, reinforced acrylic pontics, and metal pontics. To choose the best method, the practitioner must carefully consider esthetic and functional requirements of the patient, the structural requirements of the proposed removable partial denture, and the materials to be used in prosthesis construction.

## Denture bases

Most denture bases are constructed using acrylic resins or cast metal alloys. The acrylic resins are typically heat-activated or chemically-activated polymethyl methacrylate resins. These resins are available in a variety of shades and may be used to establish the desired gingival colors and contours. Consequently, acrylic resin denture bases are preferred by most practitioners.

Denture bases also may be created using cobalt-chromium alloys, nickel-chromium alloys, Type IV gold alloys, titanium-aluminum-vanadium alloys, and commercially pure titanium. Advantages of metal denture bases include increased strength, improved adaptation to underlying tissues, improved hygiene, and enhanced thermal conductivity. The major drawbacks associated with metal denture bases involve the inability to reline or rebase poorly fitting areas. The use of metal-resin bonding systems has been suggested, but the clinical effectiveness of these procedures has not been well documented. Therefore, metal bases should be used primarily for residual ridges that are well healed and ideally contoured.

If a cast metal denture base is being considered, extreme care must be used during impression-making procedures. Overextension of metal borders may necessitate adjustment of the denture base alloy. These adjustment procedures are difficult and time consuming.

## Anterior tooth replacements

The replacement of anterior teeth, particularly single teeth, should normally be accomplished using fixed partial dentures or implant-supported restorations. However, there are instances in which the replacement of anterior teeth is best accomplished with a removable partial denture. Removable partial denture therapy should be considered in the following anterior applications:

1. In young patients, tooth preparation for a fixed restoration might compromise pulpal health. A removable partial denture can be used until more definitive therapy is possible.
2. For patients in poor general health, extended dental appointments may be contraindicated. Removable partial denture therapy often permits a reduction in "chair time."
3. Periodontal compromise of proposed abutments may contraindicate conventional fixed partial denture therapy. Removable partial denture therapy permits the distribution of forces throughout the dental arch, thereby creating a more favorable clinical situation.
4. The edentulous space may be too great for restoration with a fixed partial denture (Fig 3-89). Under such circumstances, a removable partial denture is indicated.
5. Severe resorption of the alveolar process may require the fabrication of excessively long, bulky, and

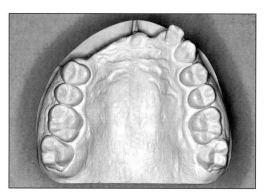

**Fig 3-89** Restoration of the missing maxillary teeth in this situation is best accomplished using a removable partial denture because of the severe destruction of the alveolar process, the need for esthetic lip support, the extensive span of the edentulous space, and the unfavorable nature of lateral incisors as fixed partial denture abutments.

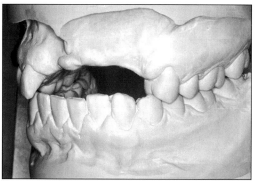

**Fig 3-90** The most predictable and convenient method to restore the missing soft and hard tissues of this edentulous alveolar process is with the denture base of a removable partial denture.

unhygienic pontics in a fixed partial denture (Fig 3-90). In such instances, a removable partial denture may provide improved esthetics and permit improved hygiene.

### Methods of anterior tooth replacement

There are two primary methods for replacing anterior teeth with removable partial dentures. Other methods exist, but should be considered modifications of these basic approaches:

1. Acrylic resin or porcelain teeth on an acrylic resin denture base
2. Reinforced acrylic pontics (RAPs)

Anterior tooth replacements are described in the following sections. Their advantages and limitations are presented.

**Anterior acrylic resin, composite resin, or porcelain teeth with acrylic resin denture bases** Today, commercially produced denture teeth are available in a seemingly limitless variety of shades, molds, and sizes. Although porcelain denture teeth are available, the overwhelming majority of prosthetic teeth are fabricated using acrylic resins and composite resins. Acrylic resin and composite resin teeth display wear characteristics that make them compatible with enamel and

dentin. In addition, these teeth can be reshaped with relative ease. Therefore, acrylic resin and composite resin teeth are preferred in most removable partial denture applications.

Unlike resin teeth, porcelain denture teeth produce significant wear of opposing enamel and dentin surfaces. Porcelain teeth also are difficult to adjust, and are susceptible to fracture. Consequently, the use of porcelain teeth in removable partial denture therapy is discouraged.

*Summary.* Following are the advantages of resin or porcelain teeth on acrylic resin denture bases:

- Most esthetic form of replacement because of wide variety of shades, molds, and sizes
- Acrylic resin denture base may be used to restore lost portions of alveolar process (through careful manipulation of denture base contour)
- Provides opportunity for conventional reline and rebase procedures

Following are the limitations of resin or porcelain teeth on acrylic resin denture bases:

- Does not work well for single-tooth replacement
- Resin denture base requires additional bulk for adequate strength

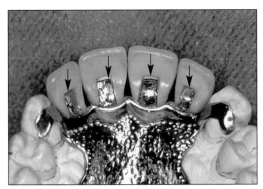

**Fig 3-91** The RAPs used on this removable partial denture will replace missing maxillary incisors. Note the metal struts that extend into the body of each denture tooth *(arrows)*. Once processed, acrylic resin will wrap around each strut, firmly attaching the denture teeth to the framework.

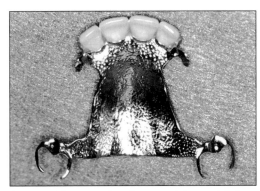

**Fig 3-92** The completed removable partial denture depicted in Fig 3-91. Processed acrylic resin completes the strong attachment of the denture teeth to the metal framework.

**Reinforced acrylic pontics** A reinforced acrylic pontic is an exceptionally strong and esthetic anterior tooth replacement. It consists of an acrylic resin denture tooth attached to a centrally located metal reinforcing strut that projects from the removable partial denture framework (Fig 3-91). Because the prosthetic tooth is primarily acrylic resin, the esthetics and wear characteristics of a reinforced acrylic pontic are considered favorable (Fig 3-92).

*Summary.* Following are the advantages of reinforced acrylic pontics:

- Exceptional strength and esthetics
- Can be designed so that occlusion is confined to the acrylic resin portion of the tooth
- Can be used in areas of restricted restorative space

Following are the limitations of reinforced acrylic pontics:

- Requires well-healed and favorably contoured residual edentulous ridge
- Little support can be gained from contact with the residual ridge
- Difficult to reline

## Posterior tooth replacements

### Methods of posterior tooth replacement

There are four primary methods for replacing posterior teeth with removable partial dentures. While other methods exist, they should be considered modifications of these basic methods:

1. Acrylic resin, composite resin, or porcelain teeth on an acrylic resin denture base
2. Tube teeth
3. Braided posts
4. Metal pontics

**Posterior acrylic resin, composite resin, or porcelain teeth on an acrylic resin denture base** The majority of missing posterior teeth are replaced using acrylic resin teeth on an acrylic resin denture base (Fig 3-93). Unfortunately, the occlusal surfaces of acrylic resin teeth tend to flatten with time and continued function. This results in decreased efficiency of the masticating surfaces, a gradual decrease in the occlusal vertical dimension, and an accompanying change in occlusal relationships (Fig 3-94). Patients with Kennedy Class I and Class II patterns of edentulism are particularly susceptible to these difficulties. Therefore, patients wearing distal extension prostheses must be maintained on a strict recall program to prevent the occurrence of such changes.

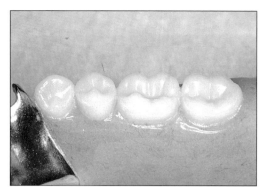

**Fig 3-93** Acrylic resin denture teeth are the most popular form of posterior tooth replacement used during the construction of removable partial dentures.

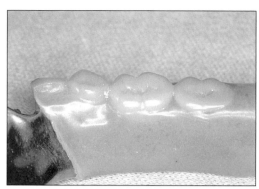

**Fig 3-94** Extended use of a removable partial denture frequently leads to wear of the acrylic resin denture teeth. Clinically, this may lead to decreased masticatory efficiency, decreased occlusal vertical dimension, and changes in occlusal relationships.

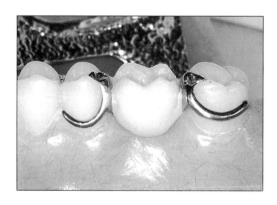

**Fig 3-95** This tube tooth was constructed to establish intimate contact between the gingival aspect of the denture tooth and the soft tissues of the edentulous ridge.

The use of porcelain denture teeth should be considered with great caution. As previously noted, porcelain denture teeth can produce significant wear of enamel and dentin surfaces. Porcelain denture teeth also may produce noticeable wear of feldspathic porcelains used in the fabrication of metal-ceramic restorations (eg, crowns and fixed partial dentures). Therefore, porcelain denture teeth should be used only when they will be opposed by a prosthesis with similar porcelain surfaces. Otherwise, the use of porcelain denture teeth should be discouraged.

**Posterior tube teeth** A tube tooth consists of a resin or porcelain denture tooth prepared by drilling a vertical channel from the ridge lap area toward the occlusal surface. An appropriately sized wax or plastic tube is placed in the channel, and the prosthetic tooth is properly positioned for waxing procedures. As the framework is waxed, the tube is attached to the wax pattern. The artificial tooth is then removed, leaving the wax or plastic tube in the desired position. Subsequently, the wax pattern is invested and cast. After the framework has been divested, finished, and polished, the prosthetic tooth is cemented onto the metal tube.

Tube teeth are frequently used for posterior tooth replacement and should be limited to the replacement of one to three missing teeth in Kennedy Class III partially edentulous applications (Fig 3-95). When constructed so that intimate contact is established between the gingival aspect of the tooth and the soft tissues of the edentulous ridge, the tube tooth displays excellent esthetics. Since there is no effective means of relining the prosthesis, tube teeth are seldom indicated for Kennedy Class I or Class II situations.

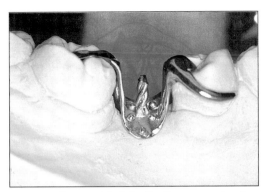

**Fig 3-96** The braided (helical) post projecting from the removable partial denture framework provides a reliable means of retaining the denture tooth to the framework.

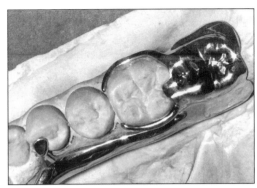

**Fig 3-97** A metal pontic was used on this removable partial denture because of severely restricted interarch space.

**Braided posts** From a mechanical perspective, a braided post is similar to a tube tooth. Both forms of tooth replacement are dependent upon a centrally located reinforcing strut. However, the methods used in strut construction are significantly different.

A braided post is created by twisting two small-diameter wax ropes around one another in a helical fashion. During the final stages of framework waxing procedures, the helical or "braided" ropes are attached at a prescribed position on the wax pattern. The framework is then cast and a metal reinforcing strut is produced (Fig 3-96). Subsequently, an acrylic resin denture tooth is fitted to the strut. This is accomplished by creating a slightly oversized channel that originates at the ridge lap portion of the tooth and projects occlusally. The acrylic resin tooth is then attached to the framework using heat-activated or chemically-activated resin.

A braided post permits the development of excellent esthetics. In addition, braided posts are easier to fabricate than are tube teeth. Consequently, braided posts are preferred by many practitioners.

**Posterior cast metal pontics** The use of cast metal pontics in removable partial denture applications is restricted to the replacement of posterior teeth (Fig 3-97). Such pontics are used where interarch space is extremely limited or where drifting of the remaining teeth has resulted in a space that is too narrow for placement of a denture tooth.

In most instances, a metal pontic is made from the same metal that forms the remainder of the partial denture framework. A veneer of acrylic resin or composite resin may be used to improve esthetics or to create an occlusal surface with wear characteristics similar to those of enamel or dentin. Gold alloy also may be used to create occlusal surfaces that are compatible with enamel or dentin. A variety of techniques for the creation of acrylic resin, composite resin, and gold alloy are available in the periodical literature.

## ⌷ References

1. Chayes HES. A system of movable-removable bridgework in conformity with the principle that "teeth move in function." Dent Rev 1917;31:85–123.

2. Roach FE. Conserving the natural teeth in supplying partial dentures. Dent Cosmos 1908;50:17–23.

3. Bonwill WGA. New methods of clasping artificial dentures to human teeth without injury versus immovable bridges. Dent Items Interest 1899;21:656–670.

4. Prothero JH. Prosthetic Dentistry, ed 2. Chicago: Medico-Dental, 1916:248, 250.

5. Kennedy E. Partial Denture Construction. Brooklyn: Dental Items of Interest, 1928:231–247.

6. DeVan MM. Preserving natural teeth through the use of clasps. J Prosthet Dent 1955;5:208–214.

7. Akers PE. Partial dentures. J Am Dent Assoc 1928;15:717–722.

8. Roach FE. Principles and essentials of bar clasp partial dentures. J Am Dent Assoc 1930;17:124–138.

9. Anusavice KJ. Phillip's Science of Dental Materials, ed 10. Philadelphia: Saunders, 1996:57, 237–271, 455–459, 631–654.

10. Stone ER. Tipping action of bar clasps. J Am Dent Assoc 1936;23:596–617.

11. Nesbitt NB. The cast clasp in removable bridge work. Dent Items Interest 1916;38:581–592.

12. Roach FE. The double-bow clasp. Dent Review 1913;27:1007–1013.

13. Applegate OC. Essentials of Removable Partial Denture Prosthesis, ed 3. Philadelphia: Saunders, 1965:177–178, 182–190.

14. Kratochvil F. Influence of occlusal rest position and clasp design on movement of abutment teeth. J Prosthet Dent 1963;13:114–124.

15. Krol AJ. RPI clasp retainer and its modifications. Dent Clinics North Am 1973;17:631–649.

16. Cummer WE. Partial denture service. In: Anthony LP (ed). The American Textbook of Prosthetic Dentistry in Contributions by Eminent Authorities, ed 7. Philadelphia: Lea & Febiger, 1942:753.

## ⌨ Bibliography

Anthony EP. Indirect retention in partial denture design. J Prosthet Dent 1966;16:1103–1110.

Applegate OC. The Partial Denture: Its Origin and Development [thesis]. Ann Arbor: Univ of Michigan School of Dentistry, 1937:43–44.

Applegate OC. Use of the paralleling surveyor in modern partial denture construction. J Am Dent Assoc 1940;27:1397–1407.

Asgar K, Peyton FA. Casting dental alloys to embedded wires. J Prosthet Dent 1965;15:312–321.

Avant WE. Factors that influence retention of removable partial dentures. J Prosthet Dent 1971;25:265–270.

Avant WE. Indirect retention in partial denture design. J Prosthet Dent 1966;16:1103–1110.

Bange AA, Phoenix RD, Duncan RC. Gold alloy cast to base metal removable partial denture frameworks. J Prosthet Dent 1994;72:137–140.

Bates JF. Cast clasps for partial dentures. Int Dent J 1963;13:610–614.

Bates JF. The mechanical properties of the cobalt-chromium alloys and their relation to partial denture design. Br Dent J 1965;119:389–396.

Beck HO. Alloys for removable partial dentures. Dent Clin North Am 1960;4:591–596.

Bezzon OL, Mattos MGC, Ribero RF. Surveying removable partial dentures: The importance of guiding planes and path of insertion for stability. J Prosthet Dent 1997;78:412–418.

Blatterfein L. Design and positional arrangement of clasps for partial dentures. N Y State Dent J 1952;22:305–306.

Blatterfein L. Study of partial denture clasping. J Am Dent Assoc 1951;43:169–185.

Blatterfein L. The use of the semiprecision rest in removable partial dentures. J Prosthet Dent 1969;22:307–332.

Breisach L. Esthetic attachments for removable partial dentures. J Prosthet Dent 1967;17:261–267.

Brudvik JS, Morris HF. Stress-relaxation testing. Part III: Influence of wire alloys, gauges, and lengths on clasp behavior. J Prosthet Dent 1981;46:374–379.

Brudvik JS, Wormley JH. Construction techniques for wrought wire retentive clasp arms as related to clasp flexibility. J Prosthet Dent 1973;30:769–774.

Brumfield RC. Tentative standard methods of testing precious metal dental materials. J Am Dent Assoc 1954;49:17–30.

Burns DR, Ward JE. A review of attachments for removable partial dentures: Part 1. Classification and selection. Int J Prosthodont 1990;3:98–102.

Calverely MJ, Cagna DR, Phoenix RD. Preferred design philosophies for distal extension RPDs in North American dental schools. J Dent Educ 1997;61:220.

Cecconi BT, Asgar K, Dootz E. The effect of partial denture clasp design on abutment tooth movement. J Prosthet Dent 1971;25:44–56.

Cecconi BT, Asgar K, Dootz E. Clasp assembly modifications and their effect on abutment tooth movement. J Prosthet Dent 1972;27:160–167.

Chayes HES. Bridgework conducive to health and the instrument for constructing it. Dent Items Interest 1939;37:267.

Chayes HES. Empiricism of bridgework. Dent Items Interest 1910;32:745.

Chayes HES. Movable-Removable Bridgework. New York: Chayes System Laboratories, 1922.

Chayes HES. Principles, functions and construction of saddles in bridge work. Dent Items Interest 1915;37:831.

Chick AO. Correct location of clasps and rests on dentures without stress-breakers. Br Dent J 1955;95:303–309.

Clayton JA, Jaslow C. A measurement of clasp forces on teeth. J Prosthet Dent 1971;25:21–43.

Colman AJ, Evans JH. Restoration of posterior edentulous areas when space precludes conventional treatment: A case report. Quintessence Int 1995;26:613–616.

Coy RE, Arnold PD. Survey and design of diagnostic casts for removable partial dentures. J Prosthet Dent 1974;32:103–106.

Craddock FW, Bottomleys GA. Second thoughts on clasping. Br Dent J 1954;46:134–137.

Cummer WE. Partial dentures. Dent Summary 1917;37:169–214.

Cummer WE. Partial dentures. In: Turner CR, Anthony LP (eds). The American Textbook of Prosthetic Dentistry in Contributions by Eminent Authorities, ed 5. Philadelphia: Lea & Febiger, 1928:324.

Cunningham DM. Comparison of base metal alloys and type IV gold alloys for removable partial denture frameworks. Dent Clin North Am 1973;17:719–722.

Donahue TJ. Factors that augment the role of direct retainers in mandibular distal-extension removable partial dentures. J Prosthet Dent 1988;60:696–699.

Firtell DN. Effect of clasp design upon retention of removable partial dentures. J Prosthet Dent 1968;20:43–52.

Fisher RL, Jaslow C. The efficacy of an indirect retainer. J Prosthet Dent 1975;34:24–30.

Frank RP, Brudvik JS, Nicholls JI. A comparison of the flexibility of wrought wire and cast circumferential clasps. J Prosthet Dent 1983;49:471–476.

Frank RP, Nicholls JI. An investigation of the indirect retainer. J Prosthet Dent 1977;38:494–506.

Garver DG. A new clasping system for unilateral distal-extension removable partial dentures. J Prosthet Dent 1978;39:268–273.

Gindea AE. A retentive device for removable dentures. J Prosthet Dent 1972;27:501–508.

Girardot RL. History and development of partial denture design. J Am Dent Assoc 1941;28:1399–1408.

Grasso JE. A new removable partial denture clasp concept. J Prosthet Dent 1980;43:618–621.

Grieder A, Cinotti WR. Periodontal Prosthesis, vol 2. St. Louis: Mosby, 1968:622.

Henrichsen S. Ball clasps for partial dentures. Dent Cosmos 1914;56:1194.

Jackley GA, Plummer KD. Bonding soft reline materials to base metals. J Prosthodont 1994;3:16–18.

Kabcenell JL. Effective clasping of removable partial dentures. J Prosthet Dent 1962;12:104–110.

Kotowicz WE, Fisher RL, Reed RA, Jaslow C. The combination clasp and the distal extension removable partial denture. Dent Clin North Am 1973;17:651–660.

Langer A. Combinations of diverse retainers in removable partial dentures. J Prosthet Dent 1978;40:378–384.

LaVere AM. Clasp retention: The effects of five variables. J Prosthodont 1993;2:126–131.

LaVere AM, Freda AL. A simplified procedure for survey and design of diagnostic casts. J Prosthet Dent 1977;37:680–683.

McCall JO. The periodontist looks at the clasp partial denture. J Am Dent Assoc 1951;43:439–443.

McCracken WL. Contemporary partial denture design. J Prosthet Dent 1958;8:71–84.

McGivney GP, Castleberry DJ. McCracken's Removable Partial Prosthodontics, ed 9. St. Louis: Mosby, 1995:255.

McKinnon KP. Indirect retention in partial denture construction. Dent J Aust 1955;27:221–225.

Miller EL, Grasso JE. Removable Partial Prosthodontics, ed 2. Baltimore: Williams & Wilkins, 1981:155.

Morris HF, Asgar K, Roberts EP, Brudvik JS. Stress relaxation testing. Part II: Comparison of bending profiles, microstructures, microhardnesses, and surface characteristics of several wrought wires. J Prosthet Dent 1981;46:256–262.

Morrison ML. Internal precision attachment retainers for partial dentures. J Am Dent Assoc 1962;64:209–215.

Nichols IG. Prosthetic Dentistry: An Encyclopedia of Full and Partial Denture Prosthesis. St. Louis: Mosby, 1930:599–600.

Preiskel HW. Precision Attachments in Prosthodontics: The Applications of Intracoronal and Extracoronal Attachments, vol 1. Chicago: Quintessence, 1984:139.

Rad MN, Yarmand MA. Design of a direct retainer for removable partial dentures. J Prosthet Dent 1974;31:457–459.

Renner RP. Semiprecision attachment-retained removable partial dentures. Quintessence Dent Technol 1994;17:137–144.

Rudd RW, Bange AA, Rudd KD, Montalvo R. Preparing teeth to receive a removable partial denture. J Prosthet Dent 1999;82:536–549.

Schneider R. Metals used to fabricate removable partial denture frameworks. J Dent Technol 1996;13:35–42.

Schneider RL. Significance of abutment tooth angle of gingival convergence on removable partial denture retention. J Prosthet Dent 1987;58:194–196.

Shohet H. Relative magnitudes of stress on abutment teeth with different retainers. J Prosthet Dent 1969;21:267–282.

Smith GP. Cast clasps: Their uses, advantages, and disadvantages. Am J Orthod Oral Surg 1947;33:479–483.

Stade EH, Stewart GP, Morris HF, Pesavento BA. Influence of fabrication technique on wrought wire clasp flexibility. J Prosthet Dent 1985;54:538–543.

Steffel VL. Planning removable partial dentures. J Prosthet Dent 1962;12:524–535.

Steffel VL. Simplified clasp partial denture designed for maximum function. J Am Dent Assoc 1945;32:1093–1100.

Stern WJ. Guiding planes in clasp reciprocation and retention. J Prosthet Dent 1975;34:408–414.

Stewart KL, Rudd KD. Stabilizing periodontally weakened teeth with removable partial dentures. J Prosthet Dent 1968;19:475–482.

Stobie JL. A Comparison of the Deflection Characteristics of Typical Removable Partial Denture Clasps [thesis]. Houston: Univ of Texas Dental Branch, 1969.

VandenBrink JP, Wolfaardt JF, Faulkner MG. A comparison of various removable partial denture clasp materials and fabrication procedures for placing clasps on canine and premolar teeth. J Prosthet Dent 1993;70:180–188.

Wakabayashi N, Mizutani H, Minoru A. All-cast-titanium removable partial denture for a patient with a severely reduced interarch distance: A case report. Quintessence Int 1997;28:173–176.

Warr JA. An analysis of clasp design in partial dentures. Phys Med Biol 1959;3:212–232.

Weinberg LA. Lateral force in relation to denture base and clasp design. J Prosthet Dent 1956;6:785–800.

Wiebelt FJ, Stratton RJ. Bracing and reciprocation in removable partial denture design. Quintessence Dent Technol 1985;9:15–17.

# Mechanical Principles Associated with Removable Partial Dentures

## ❑ Mechanics of Movement: Thinking Three-Dimensionally

To understand how intraoral forces act on a removable partial denture, the practitioner must begin with an understanding of basic mechanical concepts. Movement occurs when a resting object is acted upon by a sufficient force. In the human body, movement can occur in any of the three fundamental planes: horizontal, sagittal, or frontal. These planes are mutually perpendicular and therefore intersect one another at right angles. The intersection of any two planes forms a linear axis. Because there are three planes, there are also three axes. These are called the transverse axis, the vertical axis, and the sagittal axis (Fig 4-1). Rotational movement of an object around any one of the three axes can only occur within the plane that runs exactly perpendicular to that axis.

These same fundamental planes can be used to describe clinically relevant movement of removable partial dentures (Fig 4-2). Most movements of removable partial dentures do not occur within a single plane because the forces that cause them are a composite of forces from multiple planes. Fortunately, composite forces can be broken down into force vectors. This makes it possible to determine how much force, or what proportion of the total force, is occurring within any given plane.

Usually, a dominant force vector can be identified. This is the vector that causes the greatest concern in removable partial denture design (Fig 4-3). Consequently, design features are added to resist dominant forces.

During the design process, the practitioner must consider the ability of individual teeth to withstand forces. Fibers of the periodontal ligament are arranged to absorb axial forces (Fig 4-4). Unfortunately, these fibers do not offer similar protection when teeth are subjected to non-axial tipping or rotational forces. According to available information, the forces that teeth are best able to resist are those directed within their long axes. Experiments by Synge and Dyment in the 1930s produced conservative estimates that axial loading is tolerated over non-axial forces by a ratio of 17.5 to 1.[1] Consequently, non-axial forces of much smaller magnitude can be extremely destructive to the supporting structures of a tooth and should be avoided whenever possible.

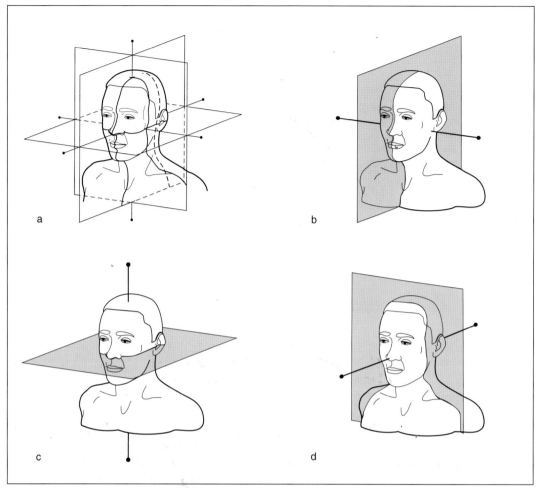

**Fig 4-1** *(a)* Three fundamental planes and three axes as related to the human head. *(b)* The first plane is a sagittal plane. Movement in this plane occurs relative to a mediolateral axis that is perpendicular to the sagittal plane. *(c)* A horizontal plane also exists. Movement in this plane occurs around a vertical axis that is perpendicular to the horizontal plane. *(d)* The final plane is a frontal plane. Movement in this plane occurs relative to an anterioposterior axis running perpendicular to the frontal plane.

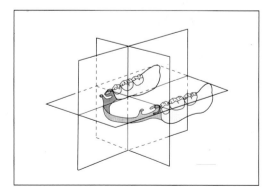

**Fig 4-2** Three fundamental planes can be used to describe potential movement of a removable partial denture. Prosthesis movement may occur in any one of these planes and around an axis (ie, fulcrum line) that is perpendicular to that plane.

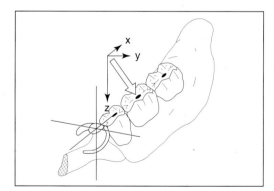

**Fig 4-3** The force acting on an object is usually a composite of forces in three dimensions. It may be broken down into its component force vectors in each of the three planes of space (x, y, and z). Note that force vector z is much greater than are vectors x or y. Vector z is the dominant direction of the applied force.

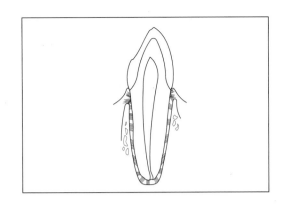

**Fig 4-4** Fibers of the periodontal ligament are arranged to resist vertical (ie, axial) forces more effectively than horizontal or torsional forces. The fibers act as a sling, countering vertical tooth displacement.

## ☐ Support and Force Distribution: Intact Versus Artificial Dentition

### Entirely tooth-supported prostheses

For purposes of discussion, consider a patient with intact dental arches in which teeth are well aligned and display optimal contact relationships. As the patient occludes, the teeth are subjected primarily to axial loading (Fig 4-5). Support is gained entirely from the periodontal ligaments of individual teeth. As might be expected, a similar situation occurs with a properly constructed fixed partial denture. Abutment teeth are rigidly connected and can provide optimal occlusal relationships in all functional movements (Fig 4-6).

Like a conventional fixed partial denture, a Class III removable partial denture is entirely tooth supported. As a result, forces are directed within the long axes of the abutments and are transmitted to the associated periodontal tissues (Fig 4-7). Compared with a fixed prosthesis, a removable prosthesis does not connect its abutments as rigidly to one another. Therefore, limited movement is possible, and this movement can result in non-axial loading of the abutment teeth during function. In most instances, off-axis loading in Class III applications is extremely limited.

### Combined tooth-tissue–supported prostheses

Classes I, II, and IV removable partial dentures introduce an important variable in the support of the prosthesis. They are not completely tooth supported but derive varying degrees of support from the tissues of the residual ridge. Utilizing the mathematical calculations of Synge and conservative estimates of tissue displacement, DeVan determined that the mucoperiosteum of the residual ridge offers only 0.4% of the support provided by a periodontal ligament.[2] In other words, soft tissues are 250 times more displaceable than are the adjacent teeth. This is particularly important when one considers the masticatory forces placed on an extension base during function.

Although initial masticatory forces may be oriented in the long axes of the abutments, differences in tooth and soft tissue support eventually result in non-axial loading. This occurs as the prosthesis pivots on the abutment closest to the extension base (Figs 4-8 and 4-9). The resultant forces can be extremely damaging to the abutments and must be controlled if clinical treatment is to be successful. Failure to consider these forces in the design of a removable partial denture can result in tooth mobility and restoration failure. Therefore, these forces must be controlled through optimal tissue health, maximum coverage of soft tissues, proper use of direct retainers, and placement of all components in their most advantageous positions.

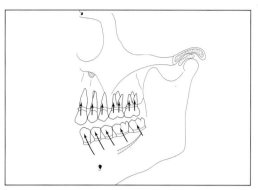

**Fig 4-5** Intact dental arches in which teeth are well aligned with optimal contact relationships experience mostly axial loading.

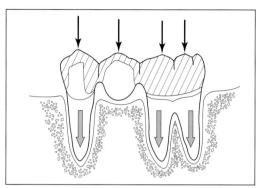

**Fig 4-6** Like the intact dentition, well-constructed fixed partial dentures are structurally able to resist both axial and non-axial loads. Support for the missing tooth is provided by the periodontal ligaments of the abutment teeth.

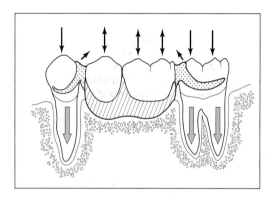

**Fig 4-7** Like a fixed partial denture, the tooth-supported, or Class III, removable partial denture derives support from abutments. Occlusal loading of the removable partial denture transmits stress down the long axes of the abutments *(shaded arrows)*. However, limited movement of the prosthesis, including a tendency to lift in function, is possible.

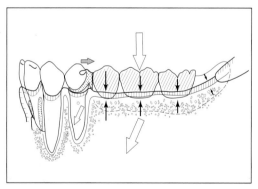

**Fig 4-8** Abutment tipping may occur when Class I removable partial dentures receive occlusal loads. The distal extension base supported by the underlying soft tissues is displaced more than is the abutment supported by periodontal ligament. The denture base rotates around an axis running through the rest adjacent to the edentulous space. This off-axis abutment loading may result in distal tipping.

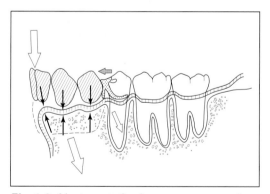

**Fig 4-9** Abutment tipping may occur when Class IV removable partial dentures receive occlusal loads. The anterior extension base supported by the underlying soft tissues is displaced more than is the abutment supported by periodontal ligament. The denture base rotates around an axis running through the rest adjacent to the edentulous space. This off-axis loading may result in mesial tipping.

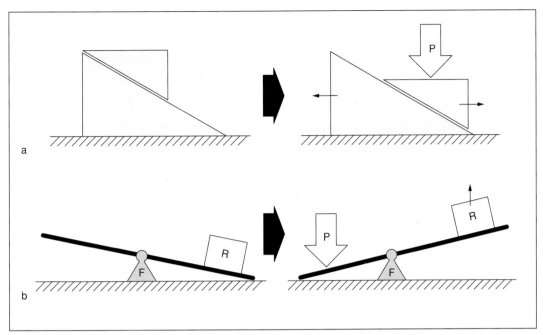

**Fig 4-10** During occlusal loading, a removable partial denture may transmit stresses to oral structures through the actions of two basic mechanical principles. *(a)* The inclined plane. In this system, two objects share an interface that forms an acute angle with the horizontal plane. Application of vertical power (P) causes the objects to move in opposite directions. *(b)* The lever. By definition, all levers consist of a fulcrum (F) about which the lever rotates, a power source (P) that mobilizes the lever to do work, and a resistance (R) to which the lever does work.

## ⌑ Lever and Inclined Plane Actions

The control of potentially damaging forces is the primary goal of removable partial denture design. When subjected to intraoral forces, a removable partial denture can perform the actions of two simple machines—the lever and the inclined plane (Fig 4-10).

A lever consists of a rigid bar, a fulcrum, an object to be moved, and an applied force. The efficiency of the system is dependent upon the arrangement of the fulcrum, the object, and the force in relation to the bar. There are three classes of levers: first, second, and third (Fig 4-11). A first-class lever has the potential to be very efficient, while a second-class lever is less efficient, and a third-class lever is the least efficient.

Figures 4-12 and 4-13 illustrate how the movement of a distal extension base may create a first-class lever. Movement of the extension base will cause the removable partial denture to rotate about the most distal abutment tooth. This creates a potentially damaging load on the teeth and soft tissues anterior to the distal abutment. A Class IV removable partial denture can

function in a similar manner, but it fulcrums about a mesial abutment.

As a rule, the longer the extension base, the greater the potential for damaging loads to be generated on the opposite side of the fulcrum line. This results in a greater need for design features that can minimize rotation. Most mesial extension bases are short, and functional loads are of a lesser magnitude. Consequently, the leverage-induced stresses are relatively limited. In contrast, distal extension bases generally are longer and are subjected to greater masticatory forces. Therefore, the practitioner must be certain to incorporate features that will halt rotation.

The distal extension partial denture presents the greatest potential for damaging loads because it rotates about three fulcrums (Figs 4-14 to 4-16). Movement usually takes place around all three fulcrums simultaneously. During the design process, the practitioner must consider these three fulcrums and the movement that may take place around them. Components of the prosthesis may then be positioned to counteract or prevent each of the rotations.

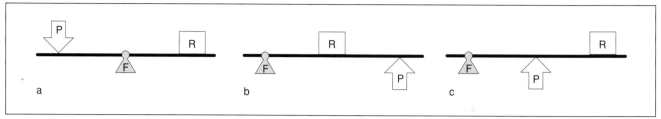

**Fig 4-11** *(a)* The most efficient lever, a first-class lever, positions the fulcrum (F) between the power source (P) and the resistance (R). *(b)* With a second-class lever, the power and fulcrum are on opposite ends of the lever and the resistance is in the middle. *(c)* The most inefficient lever is a third-class lever, for which the resistance is on one end, the fulcrum is on the other end, and power is applied in the middle.

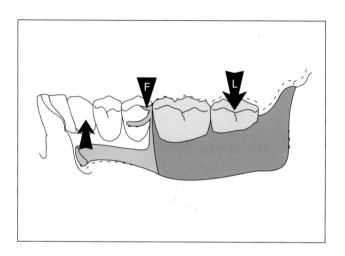

**Fig 4-12** When externally loaded, a distal extension removable partial denture may function as a first-class lever. A fulcrum (F) exists near the rest seat. The power that activates the lever results from occlusal loading (L) of the extension base. As the lever functions, aspects of the prosthesis anterior to the fulcrum will move in a superior direction *(arrow)*.

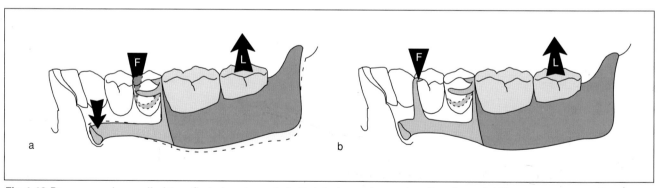

**Fig 4-13** Power may be applied to a first-class lever in both inferior and superior directions. *(a)* Circumstances tending to unseat the extension base provide superiorly directed power, or load (L), to the lever. Functioning through a fulcrum (F) near the terminus of the direct retainer, aspects of the denture anterior to the fulcrum move inferiorly *(arrow)*. *(b)* To resist this potentially damaging movement, appropriate design principles require an indirect retainer to be positioned anterior to the direct retainer. In this configuration, the indirect retainer serves as a fulcrum for the lever system, limiting inferior displacement of the lingual bar.

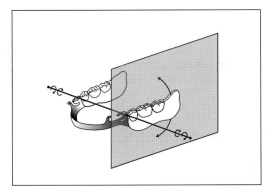

**Fig 4-14** A horizontal fulcrum line extends through the rests on the principal abutments. Rotational movement of the denture can occur around the fulcrum line in the sagittal plane. Denture movement occurs toward and away from the supporting ridge.

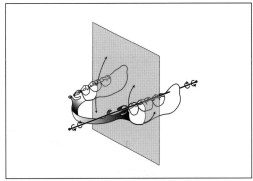

**Fig 4-15** A horizontal fulcrum line extends through the rest and along the edentulous ridge on one side of the arch. Rotational movement of the denture can occur around the fulcrum line in the frontal plane. Mediolateral rotational movement of the denture occurs relative to the edentulous alveolar process.

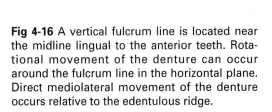

**Fig 4-16** A vertical fulcrum line is located near the midline lingual to the anterior teeth. Rotational movement of the denture can occur around the fulcrum line in the horizontal plane. Direct mediolateral movement of the denture occurs relative to the edentulous ridge.

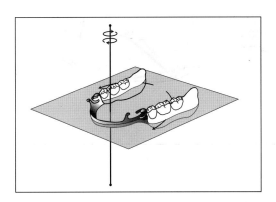

Components should not be added to the partial denture indiscreetly or by force of design habit. A practitioner who does not understand the biologic or physiologic requirements of a prosthesis will frequently design all partial dentures of a particular class in the same manner. This is one reason that removable partial dentures have not enjoyed overwhelming acceptance in the past. Only the practitioner who knows the health and condition of the oral tissues is qualified to design a removable prosthesis. To omit components because of a patient's objection to them or to make the prosthesis lighter or smaller is a disservice to the patient and compromises the basic philosophy of prosthodontics: preserving that which remains, rather than merely replacing that which has been lost.

## ❏ Forces Acting on the Removable Partial Denture

Removable partial dentures are subject to a composite of forces arising from three principal fulcrums. One fulcrum is on the horizontal plane that extends through two principal abutments, one on each side of the dental arch, and generally is termed the *principal fulcrum line* (see Fig 4-14). This fulcrum controls the rotational movement of the denture in the sagittal plane (ie, denture movement toward or away from the supporting ridge). Rotational movement around this fulcrum line is the greatest in magnitude, but is not necessarily the most damaging. The resultant force on the abutment teeth is usually mesio-apical or disto-apical,

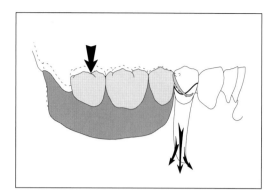

**Fig 4-17** Rotation of a Class I removable partial denture due to occlusal loading of the extension base occurs around a fulcrum located near the distal rest seat on the abutment. Stresses transferred to the abutment depend on a variety of factors, but are generally mesio-apical or disto-apical in direction.

with the greatest vector in the apical direction (Fig 4-17). As previously noted, the fibers of the periodontal ligaments are arranged so that axially aligned forces are resisted some 17 times greater than are non-axial loads. Therefore, horizontal or lateral forces of much less magnitude can be more destructive to the hard and soft tissues of the periodontium.

A second fulcrum line lies in the sagittal plane and extends through the occlusal rest on the terminal abutment and along the crest of the residual ridge on one side of the arch (see Fig 4-15). In a Class I situation, there would be two such lines, one on each side of the arch. This fulcrum line controls the rotational movements of the denture in the frontal plane (ie, a rocking movement over the crest of the ridge). This movement is easier to control than the first and usually not as great in magnitude. The resultant forces are more nearly horizontal and are not well resisted by the oral structures. Therefore, these forces can be moderately damaging and should be given thorough consideration in the design process.

The third fulcrum is located in the vicinity of the midline, just lingual to the anterior teeth (see Fig 4-16). This fulcrum line is oriented vertically and controls rotational movement in the horizontal plane (ie, the flat, arcuate movements of the prosthesis). Due to its orientation, the force resulting from this movement is almost entirely horizontal. Consequently, these forces can be extremely damaging and should receive significant attention during the design process.

Every effort must be made to control or minimize the rotational movements related to these three principal rotational axes. This requires careful thought and

meticulous planning throughout the design process. In turn, the chosen removable partial denture components must be properly constructed and positioned.

## ☐ Factors Influencing Magnitude of Stresses Transmitted to Abutment Teeth

### Length of edentulous span

The longer the edentulous span is, the longer the denture base will be, and the greater the leverage force transmitted to the abutment teeth will be. For each distal extension base, the fulcrum is located at or near the occlusal rest on the most posterior abutment tooth. During function, a load is applied to the artificial teeth, and the length of the lever arm (ie, denture base) determines how much force the associated abutments must withstand. Therefore, the practitioner must always be aware of the forces that are generated as a result of removable partial denture design. Although other factors such as the thickness of the mucosa and the total area of the residual ridge may affect clinical outcomes, the length of the edentulous span remains a factor that warrants particular attention.

When treatment is being planned, every effort should be made to retain an abutment posterior to the edentulous space. Preserving a posterior tooth to serve as vertical support, even as an overdenture abutment, results in improved patient service. Similarly, the placement of an endosseous dental implant can result in an equally valuable service.

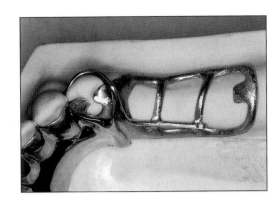

**Fig 4-18** A wrought-wire clasp arm direct retainer is located on the first premolar. This clasp provides optimal flexibility, shielding the abutment from harmful stress during prosthesis movement. Although stress transfer to the abutment is limited by this clasp design, stress transfer to the residual edentulous ridge is increased.

## Quality of ridge support

The form of the residual ridge can play a large part in distributing forces generated by the function of the partial denture. Large, well-formed ridges are capable of withstanding greater loads than are small, thin, or knife-edged ridges. Broad ridges with parallel sides permit the use of denture bases with longer vertical surfaces. These surfaces help stabilize the removable partial denture against lateral forces

The thickness and health of the mucoperiosteum also influence the loads transferred to abutment teeth. A healthy mucoperiosteum approximately 1 mm in thickness is capable of bearing a greater functional load than is thin, atrophic mucosa. Soft, flabby, displaceable tissue contributes little to the vertical support of the denture base. This type of tissue allows excessive movement of the denture base and permits forces to be transferred to the associated abutments.

## Clasp flexibility

In the discussion of components in chapter 3, it was noted that the more flexible the retentive arm of the clasp, the less load is transferred to the abutment. For this reason, the wrought-wire retentive clasp was recommended for chosen Class I and Class II applications. It was also noted that a flexible clasp arm offers less resistance to displacement in the horizontal plane, thus allowing the generation of more destructive, nonaxial loads (Fig 4-18). Therefore, as the flexibility of the clasp increases, the vertical and lateral stresses transmitted to the residual ridge are increased.

In practice, the dentist must decide which requires the most protection—an abutment or the associated residual ridge. If the periodontal condition of the abutment is good, a less flexible clasp, such as a vertical projection T- or modified T-clasp, may be indicated. A vertical projection clasp transfers a moderate percentage of an applied load to the abutment, and the remainder to the tissues of the residual ridge. If the periodontal support is questionable, a wrought-wire retentive clasp may be selected. This clasp places a smaller percentage of the load on the abutment, and a greater percentage on the residual ridge.

## Clasp design

A clasp that is designed to be passive when it is completely seated on the abutment tooth will exert less load on the tooth than will one that is not passive. As a result, the fit of a removable partial denture framework must be carefully refined to ensure that the prosthesis is completely seated. Only when the framework is completely seated will the retentive clasp arms be passive. If a clasp's retentive tip is designed and constructed to lie in a 0.010-inch undercut, but the framework is not completely seated, the retentive tip will not be passive. Instead, it will exert a continuous load on the abutment.

Refinement of the framework's fit is best accomplished by uniformly coating the tooth-contacting surfaces of the framework with a disclosing wax (Fig 4-19). As the framework is seated, wax is displaced. A tooth-to-metal binding will show through the wax. These areas are adjusted until the framework is completely seated and the clasp arms become passive. The

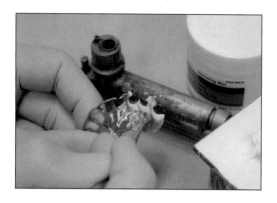

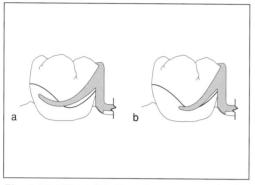

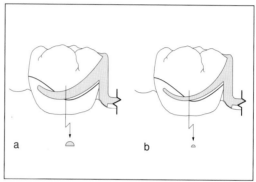

**Fig 4-19** The use of disclosing wax permits identification of areas requiring adjustment to optimize the fit of the framework.

**Fig 4-20** With all other factors equal, the greater the length of a clasp arm, the greater its flexibility. A long, gently curving clasp arm (a) has greater flexibility than a short, relatively straight clasp (b).

**Fig 4-21** Compared with a clasp fabricated with a gold-based alloy (a), a clasp arm constructed in chromium-based alloy (b) must be fabricated using a smaller cross-sectional diameter.

technique for fitting the framework is covered in detail in chapter 11.

A clasp should be designed so that during insertion or removal of the prosthesis, the reciprocal arm contacts the tooth before the retentive tip passes over the greatest bulge of the abutment. This will stabilize or neutralize the load to which the abutment is subjected as the retentive tip passes over the greatest bulge of the tooth.

## Length of clasp

As previously mentioned, the more flexible a clasp is, the less stress it will place on the corresponding abutment. Flexibility can be increased by lengthening the clasp. Doubling the length of a clasp will increase its flexibility fivefold. Clasp length may be increased by using a curved, rather than straight, course on an abutment tooth (Fig 4-20).

## Material used in clasp construction

A clasp constructed of a chromium-based alloy will normally exert a greater load on the abutment than will a gold-based alloy, all other factors being equal (eg, length, diameter). This is due to the greater rigidity of chromium-based alloys. To compensate for this difference in rigidity, clasp arms constructed using chromium-based alloys display smaller diameters compared with clasp arms constructed using gold-based alloys (Fig 4-21).

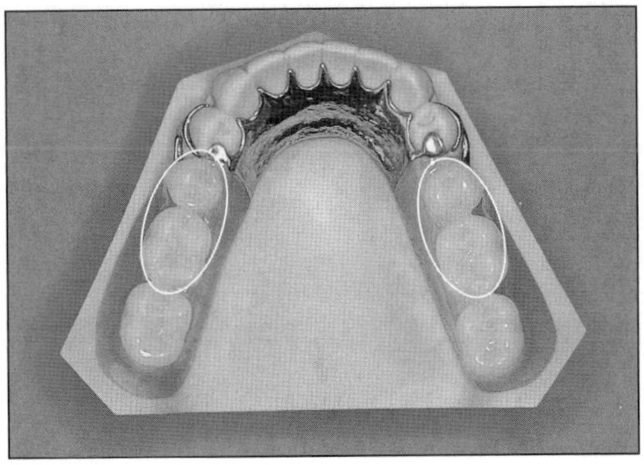

**Fig 4-22** Artificial teeth should be arranged so that masticatory forces are directed to the second premolar and first molar areas *(circled regions).*

## Surface characteristics of the abutment

The surface of a cast gold restoration offers more frictional resistance to clasp arm movement than does the enamel surface of a tooth. Therefore, an abutment restored with gold experiences greater stresses than does a tooth with intact enamel.

## Occlusal harmony

Many patients exhibit deflective occlusal contacts that generate horizontal force vectors. These vectors can be magnified by removable partial dentures and can be transmitted to the abutments and residual ridges. To prevent the transmission of destructive forces, the practitioner must be fully aware of occlusal conditions and of the mechanics of partial denture movement.

The opposing occlusion can play an important role in determining the load generated during closure. Some individuals with natural teeth can exert closing forces of 300 pounds per square inch. In contrast, many denture wearers may not be able to exceed 30 pounds per square inch. Therefore, a removable partial denture that opposes an intact dentition may be subjected to much greater loading than a removable partial denture opposed by a complete denture.

The area of the denture base against which the occlusal load is applied also influences the amount of load that is transferred to the abutment teeth and the residual ridge. If an extension base is loaded adjacent to the neighboring abutment, there will be minimal movement of the denture base. As loading moves farther from the abutment, movement of the denture base will be greater.

Ideally, the occlusal load should be applied in the center of the denture-bearing area, both anteroposteriorly and faciolingually. In most mouths, the second premolar and first molar regions represent the best areas for the application of the masticatory loads. Artificial teeth should be arranged so that the bulk of the masticatory forces are applied in these areas (Fig 4-22).

## Design Considerations: Controlling Stress

It is often argued that the theoretical aspects of partial denture design are of primary importance. In reality, clinical observation and experience must be used to balance what *should* happen with what *will* happen.

It has been stated that "No removable partial denture can be designed or constructed that will not be destructive in the mouth." This statement can be fully justified if all forces and movements are considered. There is no mechanism to counter all forces that may be applied to a removable partial denture. Nevertheless, a design philosophy that strives to control these forces within the physiologic tolerances of the teeth and supporting structures can be successful. Therefore, the design philosophy of this book is a combination of theoretical and clinical knowledge that a practitioner can learn and then use to achieve predictable results.

Past arguments about partial denture design philosophies have resulted in noticeable confusion.

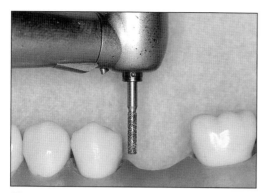

**Fig 4-23** A guiding plane is prepared on the distal surface of the second premolar using a cylindrical diamond bur.

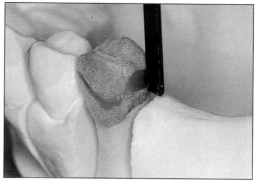

**Fig 4-24** A guiding plane is prepared on the distal surface of a wax pattern using a dental surveyor and a wax carving instrument. Careful execution of laboratory procedures will result in a surveyed crown that exhibits an accurate distal guiding plane.

As a result, many practitioners have abandoned their design responsibilities. If this textbook seems to oversimplify the design process, then it is done with the ultimate desire that the practitioner will accomplish the design based upon a thorough understanding of the anatomical, physiological, physical, and mechanical demands of removable partial denture service.

## Direct retention

The retentive clasp arm is the element of a removable partial denture that is responsible for transmitting most of the destructive forces to the abutments. Consequently, a removable partial denture should be designed to keep clasp retention at a minimum, and yet provide adequate retention to prevent dislodgment of the denture by unseating forces.

Other components of a removable partial denture may contribute to the retention of the prosthesis, thereby allowing a reduction in the amount of retention provided by clasps. Exploiting this retentive potential in widely separated areas of the mouth can result in reduced loads on the abutment teeth. As a result, the support and stability of the prosthesis also may be improved.

## Potential sources of additional retention

### Forces of adhesion and cohesion

For prosthetic purposes, adhesion may be defined as the attraction of saliva to the denture base and soft tissues, and cohesion may be defined as the attraction of saliva molecules for one another. Although it is impossible to develop a peripheral seal around the borders of a removable partial denture, adhesion and cohesion can still contribute to retention. To maximize this effect, each denture base must cover the maximum area of available support, and it must be accurately adapted to the underlying mucosa.

### Frictional control

A removable partial denture should be designed so that guiding planes are present on as many teeth as possible. Guiding planes are prepared surfaces that are parallel to each other and parallel to the path the denture takes as it is inserted and withdrawn from the mouth. These planes may be created on enamel surfaces (Fig 4-23) or on the surfaces of dental restorations (Fig 4-24). The frictional contact of the prosthesis against these parallel surfaces can contribute significantly to the retention of the removable partial denture.

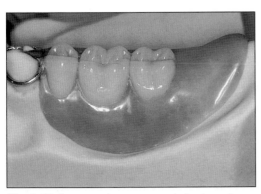

**Fig 4-25** A properly contoured denture base will contribute to retention and stability of the removable partial denture.

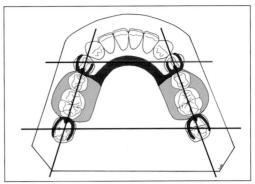

**Fig 4-26** Quadrilateral clasping requires direct retainers to be placed at both ends of the edentulous spaces in a Class III, Modification 1, partially edentulous arch. This design provides optimal retention and stability for the removable partial denture.

## Neuromuscular control

The innate ability of the patient to control the actions of the lips, cheeks, and tongue can be a major factor in the retention of a removable prosthesis. A patient who lacks the ability or coordination to control the movement of these structures may not be able to retain a prosthesis.

The design and contour of the denture base can greatly affect the patient's ability to retain a removable partial denture. Any overextension of the denture base can contribute to displacement of the prosthesis. As a result, clasping mechanisms will no longer be passive and will apply undesirable forces to the abutments. These forces may produce noticeable tooth movement and/or discomfort. Properly contoured denture bases prevent such difficulties and can enhance retention and stability of a removable partial denture (Fig 4-25).

## *Clasp position*

Most people who design removable partial dentures use too many retentive clasps. Often, the spatial distribution of retentive clasps is more important to retention than the number of clasps. The following guidelines should be followed when determining the appropriate placement of direct retainers.

## Quadrilateral configuration

The quadrilateral configuration is indicated for Class III arches, particularly when there is a modification space on the opposite side of the arch (Fig 4-26). A retentive clasp assembly should be positioned anterior and posterior to each edentulous space. This creates a stable mechanical situation in which leverage is effectively neutralized.

For a Class III arch in which no modification space exists, the goal should be to place two clasp assemblies adjacent to the edentulous space, and two clasp assemblies on the opposite side of the arch. The clasp assemblies on the intact side of the arch should be separated for additional mechanical stability. Consequently, one clasp assembly should be placed as far posteriorly as possible, and the other should be positioned as far anteriorly as space and esthetics will permit. This maintains the quadrilateral concept and represents an effective method of controlling loading.

## Tripodal configuration

Tripodal distribution is used primarily for Class II arches (Fig 4-27). One clasp assembly should be placed adjacent to the defining distal extension space. If there is a modification space on the contralateral side of the arch, the teeth anterior and posterior to the space should be clasped. If a modification space is not

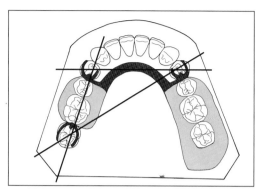

**Fig 4-27** For the Class II, Modification 1, partially edentulous arch, tripodal clasping is ideal. Direct retainers should be designed to engage abutments adjacent to both edentulous spaces.

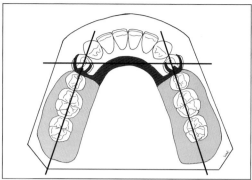

**Fig 4-28** For a Class I partially edentulous arch, bilateral clasping is indicated. Although this design does not permit optimal control of harmful forces, it is the best design for existing conditions.

present, one clasp should be positioned as far posteriorly as possible, and the other as far anteriorly as esthetics, space, and tooth contours will permit.

By creating a significant separation of the clasp assemblies on the dentate side, the practitioner can establish improved mechanical stability. Although the tripodal design is not as effective as the quadrilateral configuration, it is the most effective method for neutralizing leverage in a Class II situation.

### Bilateral configuration

Unfortunately, many removable partial dentures fall into the bilateral distal extension group (Class I arches) (Fig 4-28). In Class I applications, the most posterior tooth on each side of the arch should be clasped. This produces a bilateral configuration in which the clasps exert little or no neutralizing effects on leverage-induced stresses. Consequently, these stresses must be controlled by other means (eg, indirect retainers).

## *Clasp design*

### Cast circumferential clasp

The conventional cast circumferential clasp that originates from a disto-occlusal rest and engages a mesiofacial retentive undercut should not be used on a distal extension removable partial denture. The terminal third of this clasp reacts to movement of the denture base toward the tissue by placing a non-axial, tipping

force on the associated abutment (Fig 4-29). Long-term clinical observation indicates that this force is extremely destructive and must be avoided at all costs.

The reverse circlet clasp, a cast circumferential design that originates from a mesio-occlusal rest and engages a distofacial retentive undercut, may be used for distal extension applications. The mechanics of a reverse circlet clasp are very different from those of a conventional circumferential clasp (Fig 4-30). As an occlusal load is applied to the denture base, the retentive terminal of a reverse circlet clasp moves into a greater vertical undercut, but engages the abutment's mesiodistal height of contour. Consequently, a mesially directed force is imparted to the abutment. This mesially directed force may be well tolerated if sound proximal contact with the adjacent natural tooth (ie, buttressing) is present.

### Vertical projection clasp

A vertical projection T- or modified T-clasp may be used on an abutment adjacent to a distal extension edentulous space. Use of this clasp design is only appropriate when a retentive undercut is located on the distofacial surface of the abutment. It is not indicated when the tooth has only a mesiofacial undercut.

Upon loading of the extension base, a distal rest serves as a center of rotation. The tip of the retentive clasp moves apically and mesially. This minimizes potentially harmful torquing forces, while transmitting a relatively small, mesially directed force to the abut-

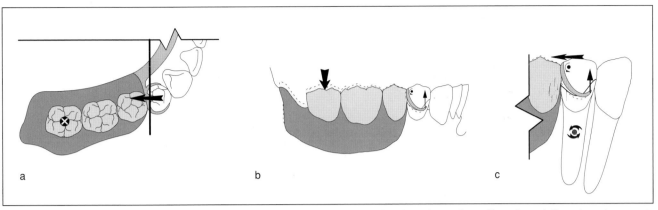

**Fig 4-29** *(a)* Use of a cast circumferential clasp arm to engage a mesiofacial undercut in a Class I partially edentulous arch should be avoided. *(b)* Occlusal loading of the extension base results in prosthesis rotation around the distal rest. *(c)* The proximal two thirds of the clasp arm moves anteriorly while the terminal one third of the clasp engages the abutment moving superiorly. Stress imparted to the abutment results in a tipping force that can be extremely destructive.

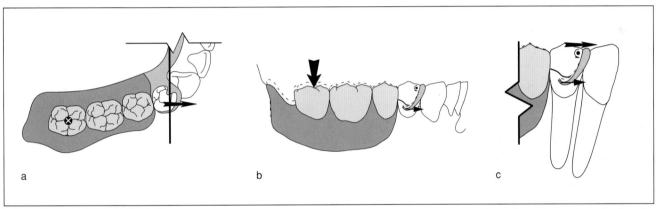

**Fig 4-30** *(a)* The reverse circlet clasp arm direct retainer engages a distofacial undercut in a Class I partially edentulous arch. *(b)* Occlusal loading of the extension base results in prosthesis rotation around a mesial rest seat. *(c)* As an occlusal load is applied to the denture base, the terminal one third of the clasp arm engages the abutment's mesiodistal height of contour. This imparts a mesially directed force on the abutment that is well tolerated if sound proximal contact with the adjacent natural tooth is present.

ment (Fig 4-31). The mesially directed force is well tolerated as a result of sound contact with the adjacent natural tooth (ie, buttressing).

Two design philosophies recommend elimination of the disto-occlusal rest when using a vertical projection I-clasp, or I-bar, in conjunction with a distal extension base. In these applications, a mesio-occlusal rest is substituted for the disto-occlusal rest. Adherents believe that a distal rotational axis passing through the disto-occlusal rest prevents release of the clasp assembly during occlusal loading. In contrast, a mesial rotational axis passing through the mesio-occlusal rest allows the clasp arm to disengage from the tooth surface by moving mesially and apically (Fig 4-32). By moving the occlusal rest mesially, the practitioner also alters the length of the lever arm (ie, the distance from the rest to the denture base). This yields an increasingly vertical movement of the denture base and results in force application that is better tolerated by the edentulous ridge.

The foregoing advantages must be weighed very carefully against a perceived disadvantage. If the rest adjacent to a distal extension base is omitted, displacement of the denture base will create space between the framework and the abutment surface (Fig 4-33). Food particles may collect in this area, preventing the pros-

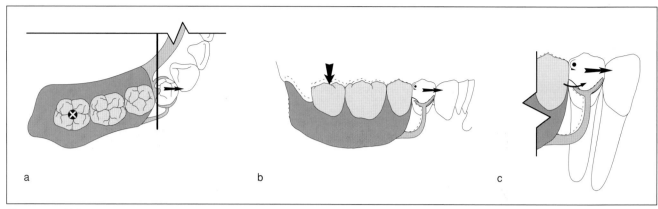

**Fig 4-31** *(a)* The vertical projection T-clasp engages a distofacial undercut in a Class I partially edentulous arch. *(b)* Occlusal loading of the extension base results in prosthesis rotation around a distal rest seat. *(c)* As the denture base is displaced toward the supporting tissues, the clasp terminus moves apically and mesially. This transmits a relatively small, mesially directed force to the abutment. This force is well tolerated because of contact with the adjacent natural tooth.

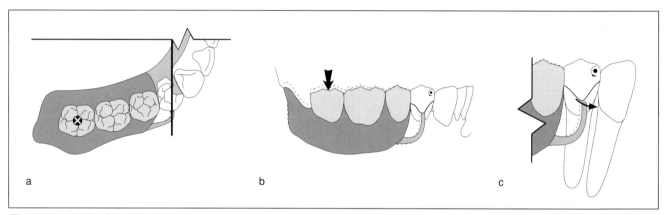

**Fig 4-32** *(a)* In the Class I arch, the vertical projection I-clasp engages a facial undercut at or mesial to the mesiodistal prominence of the abutment's facial surface. *(b)* Occlusal loading of the extension base results in prosthesis rotation around a mesial rest seat. *(c)* As the denture base moves toward the supporting tissues, the clasp terminus moves apically and mesially, disengaging the abutment. The theoretical mechanics of this design dramatically reduce stress transmission to the abutment.

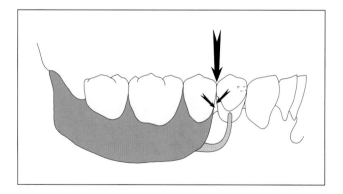

**Fig 4-33** Elimination of the rest from the distal surface of the abutment may permit impaction of food and debris between the abutment and the guide plate of the prosthesis *(arrows)*.

thesis from returning to its original position and transferring undesirable forces to the associated teeth and soft tissues. Food entrapment also may produce significant gingival irritation at the necks of the affected

teeth. While it may be argued that a properly prepared guiding plane will prevent food impaction, clinical experience indicates that impaction may be a problem.

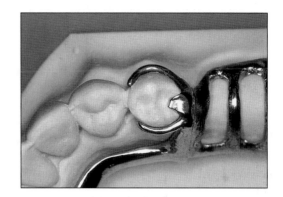

**Fig 4-34** The combination clasp on the second premolar consists of a flexible facial wrought-wire clasp, a lingual cast reciprocal clasp, a disto-occlusal rest, and a distal guide plate.

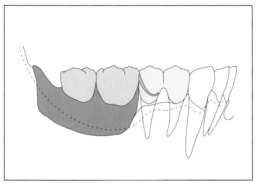

**Fig 4-35** The short, tapered root of the periodontally compromised first premolar (bone level represented by *broken line*) renders it a poor candidate for a removable partial denture abutment. By splinting the first and second premolars with a fixed partial denture, applied loads may be distributed between the two abutments, increasing their effectiveness.

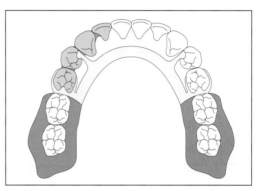

**Fig 4-36** Improved faciolingual stability can be achieved by extending the splint around the curve of the arch. Here, a fixed partial denture extending from the left second premolar to the left lateral incisor accomplishes this objective.

## Combination clasp

Often a tooth adjacent to a distal extension residual ridge presents with a mesiofacial undercut. Under these circumstances, a combination clasp can be employed to reduce the stresses transmitted to the abutment. A combination clasp consists of a cast reciprocal element and a wrought-wire retentive clasp (Fig 4-34). A wrought-wire clasp is more flexible than a conventional circumferential clasp by virtue of its cross-sectional shape and internal structure. The circular cross section of a wrought-wire clasp allows it to flex in any spatial plane, whereas a conventional circumferential clasp flexes primarily in one plane. Because of its omnidirectional flexure, a wrought-wire retentive arm can distribute stresses in multiple planes. A cast circumferential clasp would transfer most leverage-induced forces directly to the abutment. Consequently, a combination clasp is more "forgiving" than a cast circumferential clasp.

## *Splinting of abutment teeth*

A tooth with decreased periodontal support can sometimes be strengthened through the use of fixed splinting (Fig 4-35). Splinting two or more teeth actually increases the periodontal ligament area and distributes applied loads more effectively.

The use of fixed restorations often has the effect of stabilizing the abutment teeth in a mesiodistal direction. If one of the teeth included in the fixed splint is a canine, or if the splint extends anteriorly around the curve of the arch, the splinted teeth will be stabilized in a faciolingual direction as well (Fig 4-36).

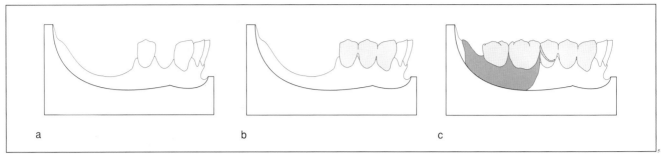

a        b        c

**Fig 4-37** *(a)* The lone standing second premolar is susceptible to excessive stress transfer from the removable partial denture. *(b)* A fixed partial denture extending from the second premolar to the canine will effectively stabilize the premolar abutment. *(c)* An improved prognosis can now be expected for the final restoration.

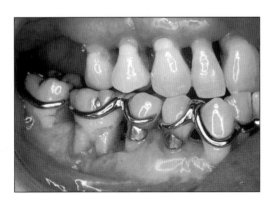

**Fig 4-38** This mandibular removable partial denture serves as a splint for the periodontally compromised teeth in the right posterior sextant. Multiple clasps, multiple rests, prepared guide planes, and a rigid major connector function to stabilize the mobile teeth.

Fixed splinting may be indicated when a loss of periodontal attachment has occurred. Nevertheless, it is seldom beneficial to splint an extremely weak abutment tooth to a strong tooth. The result is generally to weaken the strong abutment rather than strengthen the weak abutment.

Splinting is also indicated when the proposed abutment tooth has either a tapered root or short roots to the extent that there is not an acceptable amount of periodontal ligament attachment present. The joining of two such teeth by crowns will, in effect, produce an acceptable multirooted abutment tooth (see Fig 4-35).

One of the most important considerations for fixed splinting involves a lone-standing abutment adjacent to a distal extension space. Such a tooth is at risk because of the rotational forces it must withstand. In most instances, fixed splinting provides improved stabilization and a much better long-term prognosis (Fig 4-37).

Under some circumstances, splinting may be accomplished using a removable partial denture (Fig 4-38). This should not be attempted if fixed splinting is possible, because it is considered a compromised form of treatment. However, it is indicated when no other approach is feasible. The splinting consists of clasping more than one tooth on each side of the arch and using additional rests for increased support. It is not necessary for all clasps to be retentive. Prepared guiding planes may provide additional horizontal stability. Research indicates that rigid support of periodontally weakened teeth generally results in decreased mobility.

A principal advantage of splinting with a removable prosthesis is cross-arch stabilization. Teeth on both sides of the dental arch can provide resistance to horizontal forces. In most instances, this is accomplished by using well-adapted plating on the lingual surfaces of all remaining teeth.

Other forms of removable prostheses, such as the Swing-Lock partial denture, can be used to splint teeth effectively. Swing-Lock philosophy is presented in chapter 19.

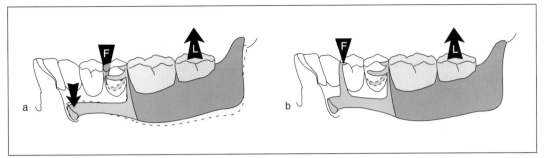

**Fig 4-39** *(a)* A dislodging force, or load (L), causes rotation of the prosthesis in which the extension base lifts away from the edentulous ridge, while anterior portions of the prosthesis rotate around the fulcrum (F) in an apical direction. Rotation of the prosthesis in this manner may result in unwanted impingement into the soft tissues of the floor of the mouth. *(b)* This rotation may be effectively countered by placing a rest on the opposite side of the previous fulcrum. This rest becomes the fulcrum and will limit impingement of the prosthesis into the floor of the mouth.

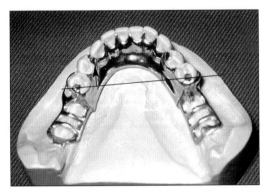

**Fig 4-40** For the Class I partially edentulous arch, indirect retainers *(arrows)* should be placed as far anterior to the fulcrum *(line)* as is practically possible. Here, mesio-occlusal rests on the first premolars serve as indirect retainers.

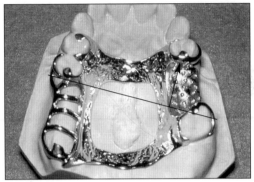

**Fig 4-41** The disto-occlusal rest on the left first premolar *(arrow)* is far enough anterior to the fulcrum *(line)* to function effectively as an indirect retainer.

## Indirect retention

An indirect retainer is a component that helps resist rotation and/or displacement of a removable partial denture. As a result, the indirect retainer is located on the side of the fulcrum line opposite the denture base (see chapter 3).

The indirect retainer is essential in the design of Class I and Class II removable partial dentures. Because of its position, the indirect retainer minimizes the rotation that occurs when a dislodging force is placed on a distal extension base (Fig 4-39). The indirect retainer also encourages vertical travel of the prosthesis when dislodging forces are applied. Hence, this component may reduce torquing forces at the associated abutment.

Because an indirect retainer is located at the end of a lever arm, it must be positioned in a definite rest seat. This allows forces to be directed within the long axis of the abutment.

As might be expected, the need for indirect retainers varies with each type of removable partial denture. Indirect retention must always be used in a Class I arch. The indirect retainer or retainers must be positioned as far anterior to the fulcrum line as possible (Fig 4-40).

Although indirect retention is not as critical in a Class II arch as in a Class I arch, it is still required. If there is a modification space on the tooth-supported side of the arch, abutment teeth on both sides of the space should be rested. The fulcrum line will run through the most posterior abutment on the tooth-supported side and the terminal abutment on the distal extension side (Fig 4-41). The most anterior abutment on the tooth-supported side, with its rest and clasp assembly, may be located far enough anterior to

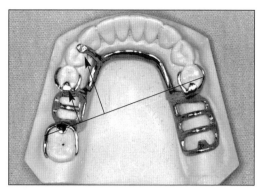

**Fig 4-42** The disto-occlusal rest on the left second premolar *(short arrow)* is too close to effectively serve as an indirect retainer. Therefore, the design of this framework includes a mesio-occlusal rest on the left first premolar *(long arrow)*. This rest is far enough anterior to the fulcrum *(line)* to provide effective indirect retention.

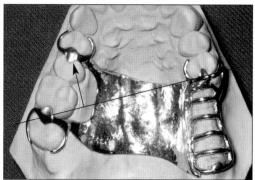

**Fig 4-43** This Class II removable partial denture framework employs an embrasure rest between the left first and second premolars *(arrow)* as an indirect retainer. This rest is far enough anterior to the fulcrum *(line)* to serve as an effective indirect retainer.

the fulcrum line to serve as the indirect retainer. However, a definite rest seat positioned farther anteriorly may increase the effectiveness of indirect retention (Fig 4-42).

If there is no modification space on the tooth-supported side of the arch, the practitioner should identify the most posterior tooth with favorable contours for clasping (Fig 4-43). This places the fulcrum line in a posterior position and allows the indirect retainer to be positioned farther from this axis of rotation. To develop a desirable clasping configuration, a third abutment should be located on the tooth-supported side as far anteriorly as is practical. The chosen abutment must display suitable contours for clasping, and the resultant clasp assembly should not interfere with esthetics. This clasp assembly may serve as the indirect retainer if it is located far enough anterior to the fulcrum line.

For a Class III arch, indirect retention is not ordinarily required because there is no extension base with which to create a lever arm.

In certain Kennedy Class III applications, the tooth posterior to the edentulous space does not display suitable contours for partial denture retention. Clinical findings also may contraindicate the placement of a surveyed restoration to improve tooth contours. If clinical evidence indicates that the abutment can provide support and stability for a removable partial denture, the practitioner may choose to place a nonretentive clasp assembly on the tooth. This assembly can greatly enhance support and stability of the removable partial denture, but will change the mechanics of the prosthesis. Upon the application of a seating force, the removable partial denture will function as an entirely tooth-supported Kennedy Class III prosthesis. In contrast, a force that tends to unseat the denture base will cause the removable partial denture to act as a Kennedy Class II prosthesis. Under these circumstances, clasping may be consistent with that of a conventional Class III prosthesis. Nevertheless, the practitioner must incorporate appropriate indirect retention in the framework design to account for the rotational movement that will occur when an unseating force is applied to the denture base.

A similar situation may occur in a Kennedy Class II arch with a modification on the opposite side of the arch (Fig 4-44). In this instance, placement of a nonretentive clasp assembly distal to the modification space will cause the prostheses to function as a Class I prosthesis when an unseating force is applied. Hence, the practitioner must incorporate appropriate indirect retention in the prosthesis design to minimize detrimental rotation.

The consideration for a Class IV arch is the reverse of that for Class I and Class II arches. Since the extension base for a Class IV arch is anterior to the fulcrum

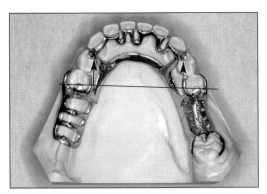

**Fig 4-44** A usable undercut was not available on the right third molar, resulting in a nonretentive clasp assembly for this abutment. This prosthesis will function like a Class I removable partial denture as forces act to lift the denture bases away from the edentulous ridges. Therefore, additional indirect retainers must be added. Mesio-occlusal rests on the right and left first premolars *(arrows)* will serve this function.

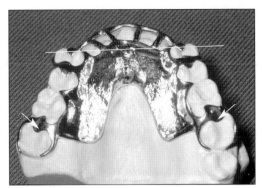

**Fig 4-45** Forces acting to move the denture base away from the edentulous ridge in a Class IV removable partial denture must be resisted by indirect retainers positioned posterior to the fulcrum *(line)*. Embrasure rests *(arrows)* provide effective indirect retention for this framework.

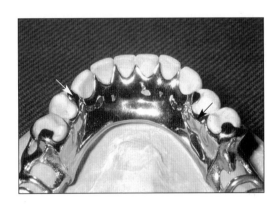

**Fig 4-46** Mesio-occlusal rests on the first premolars *(arrows)* serve to support this long lingual plate major connector.

line, indirect retention must be located as far posteriorly as possible (Fig 4-45). Consequently, occlusal rests and clasp assemblies must be positioned on posterior teeth that display favorable contours for direct clasping and support.

## Auxiliary rests

Auxiliary rests may be needed to provide additional vertical support for lingual plate major connectors, long lingual bar major connectors, and large palatal major connectors. Auxiliary rests must always accompany lingual plating of the anterior teeth and must be located no farther distal than the mesial fossae of the first premolars (Fig 4-46).

## Occlusion

A smoothly functioning occlusion that is in harmony with the movements of both the temporomandibular joints and the neuromusculature will minimize the load transferred to the teeth and soft tissues.

Neither the metal of the framework nor the artificial teeth of the partial denture should receive the initial occlusal contact as the jaws come together. All components of a removable partial denture must be coordinated with mandibular movements and the guiding influences of the remaining natural teeth. Furthermore, the contacts of the remaining natural teeth must be the same whether the removable partial denture is in the mouth or not.

The occlusal surfaces of the artificial teeth can transmit varying amounts of force to the supporting structures. The number of teeth being replaced may be reduced to decrease the amount of load transferred to the residual ridge.

Artificial posterior teeth should possess sharp cutting surfaces to be as efficient as possible and to avoid the need for excessive forces in mastication. Despite the need for sharp cutting surfaces, steep cuspal inclines on the artificial teeth should be avoided because they tend to permit the development of horizontal forces that can produce torsional stresses on the abutment teeth.

## Denture bases

Each denture base should be designed to cover as extensive an area of supporting tissue as possible. The stress created by the partial denture in function will thus be distributed over a larger area, so no single area will be subjected to stress beyond its physiologic limits.

Denture base flanges should be made as long as possible to help stabilize the denture against horizontal movements.

A mandibular distal extension denture base must always extend onto the retromolar pad area of the mandible, while a maxillary distal extension denture base must always cover the tuberosity. Both structures are capable of bearing more load than is the alveolar ridge anterior to them.

Despite the desire for extensive coverage, care must be taken to avoid overextension of denture bases. Interference with the functional movements of the surrounding soft tissues will produce displacement or "lifting" of the denture bases. As a result of this movement, undesirable forces will be applied to the abutments.

The more accurate the adaptation of the denture base to the residual ridge, the better the retention will be. This is partially due to the forces of adhesion and cohesion. The denture base also may engage small tissue undercuts and thereby contribute to retention of the prosthesis. In most instances, these contributions are relatively small.

The type of impression used to record the tissues of the residual ridge will influence the amount of stress the residual ridge can effectively withstand. The mucosa of the residual ridge is displaceable to varying degrees, and it can be recorded with a variety of impression materials and techniques. Clinical procedures for accurately recording the functional form of the residual ridge are presented in chapter 12.

The external or polished surfaces of the denture base also must be contoured properly to assist in retention of the prosthesis. If these surfaces are properly contoured, movement of the partial denture will be reduced and prosthetic service will be improved.

## Major connectors

In the mandibular arch, a lingual plate major connector that is properly supported by rests can aid in the distribution of functional stresses to the remaining teeth (Fig 4-47). The lingual plate major connector is particularly effective in supporting periodontally weakened anterior teeth.

The geometry of a lingual plate also adds rigidity to the major connector by positioning the metal in multiple planes. The added rigidity contributes to the effectiveness of cross-arch stabilization. Loads generated on one side of the arch are transmitted through the major connector to the teeth on the opposite side, thus reducing the stresses developed within any single portion of the arch.

In the maxillary arch, a palatal major connector that contacts several of the remaining natural teeth via lingual plating can distribute applied loads over a large area (Fig 4-48). The major connector must be rigid, and it must receive vertical support from rests on several teeth.

The hard palate often provides a valuable area for support. A maxillary major connector that employs maximum coverage of this area can contribute greatly to the support, stability, and retention of the prosthesis. This substantially reduces the stresses transferred to the abutments.

## Minor connectors

The most intimate contact between an abutment and a removable partial denture occurs at the interface between a guiding plane and the corresponding minor connector (ie, proximal plate). This enamel-to-metal contact serves two major purposes. First, it provides a

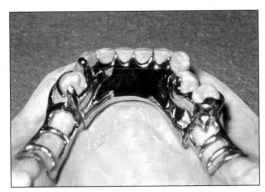

Fig 4-47 This properly designed and sufficiently rigid lingual plate major connector will effectively distribute stresses throughout the mandibular arch.

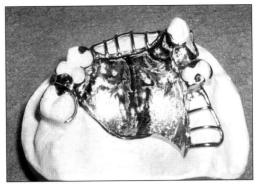

Fig 4-48 The combination of broad palatal coverage and lingual plating will effectively distribute applied loads throughout the maxillary arch.

distinct path of insertion and removal, thereby helping to retain the prosthesis. Second, it offers improved stability to the prosthesis by providing increased resistance to horizontally directed forces.

Because lateral forces are the most destructive, their control is essential. If guiding planes on additional abutment teeth are incorporated, the force that must be resisted by each tooth can be minimized. In this way, the physiologic limit of any single tooth will not be exceeded.

## Rests and rest seats

Properly prepared rest seats help to control stresses by directing forces within the long axes of the abutments. As previously noted, periodontal ligaments are capable of withstanding vertical forces, but are susceptible to damage when subjected to horizontal or torsional forces.

One of the most critical requirements of a rest seat is that the floor of the preparation must form an angle of less than 90 degrees with the proposed path of insertion (defined by the guiding plane). This permits the rest to grasp the tooth securely and prevent its migration. If the enclosed angle formed by the base of the rest seat and the established guiding plane is greater than 90 degrees, an inclined plane action may be established and tooth migration may occur.

Occlusal rest seats must present gently rounded contours. As forces are applied to the partial denture, the rest must be free to move within the rest seat. This

movement of the rest within the rest seat is similar to a ball-and-socket joint and permits the release of stresses that would otherwise be transferred to the abutment. While cingulum rest seats and incisal rest seats display geometries that are very different from occlusal rest seats and from one another, the importance of stress release remains critical. Therefore, the practitioner must ensure that all rest seats are properly prepared and that the corresponding rests are properly fitted.

The number of abutment teeth influences the amount of force that each tooth must withstand. Therefore, as the number of abutments is increased, the amount of stress that must be borne by any single abutment is decreased.

## References

1. Synge JL, Dyment ML. The elasticity of the periodontal membrane. Oral Health 1935;25:105–109.
2. DeVan MM. The prosthetic problem—Its formulation and suggestions for its solution. J Prosthet Dent 1956;6: 291–301.

## Bibliography

Applegate OC. Keeping the partial denture in harmony with biologic limitations. J Am Dent Assoc 1951;43:409–419.

Applegate OC. Stresses induced by a partial denture upon its supporting structures and practical methods of control. Proc D Centenary 1940:308–319.

Angsberger RH. Abutment stabilization through endosseous and cross-arch splinting. J Prosthet Dent 1971;26:406–413.

Avant WE. Factors that influence retention of removable partial dentures. J Prosthet Dent 1971;25:265–269.

Aviv I, Ben-Ur Z, Cardash HS. An analysis of rotational movement of asymmetrical distal-extension removable partial dentures. J Prosthet Dent 1989;61:211–214.

Craig RG, Farah JW. Stresses from loading distal-extension removable partial dentures. J Prosthet Dent 1978;39:274–277.

El Chaukawi HG, Goodkind RJ, DeLong R, Douglas WH. The effect of the resilient-layer distal-extension partial denture on movement of the abutment teeth; a new methodology. J Prosthet Dent 1988;60:622–629.

Frechette AR. Partial denture planning with special reference to stress distribution. J Ontario Dent Assoc 1953;30:318–329.

Friedman J. Abutment sites and spaces in partial denture case analysis. J Prosthet Dent 1954;4:803–812.

Granger ER. Mechanical principles applied to partial denture construction. J Am Dent Assoc 1941;28:1943–1951.

Hekneby M. Model experiments on the transmission of forces from a lower free end partial denture to the supporting teeth [in Danish]. Tandlaegebladet 1967;71:1097–1119.

Henderson D, Steward TE. Design and force distribution with removable partial dentures. J Prosthet Dent 1976;17:350–364.

Hughes GA. Review of the basic principles of removable partial denture prosthesis. Fortn Rev Chic Dent Soc 1947;13:9–13.

Mahler DB, Terkla IG. Analysis of stress in dental structures. Dent Clin North Am 1958;2:789–798.

McLean DW. Fundamental principles of partial denture construction. J Tenn Dent Assoc 1939;19:108–118.

Schuyler CH. The partial denture as a means of stabilizing abutment teeth. J Am Dent Assoc 1941;28:1121–1125.

Weinberg LA. Lateral force in relation to the denture base and clasp design. J Prosthet Dent 1956;6:785–800.

White JT. Visualization of stress and strain related to removable partial denture abutments. J Prosthet Dent 1978;40:143–151.

# The First Diagnostic Appointment

## ☐ Importance of the Diagnostic Phase of Treatment

Many failures in removable partial denture treatment can be traced to inadequate diagnosis and incomplete treatment planning. Therefore, a thorough, properly sequenced treatment plan is essential to successful removable partial denture therapy. The formulation of an appropriate treatment plan requires careful evaluation of all pertinent diagnostic data. Information must be obtained from patient interviews, radiographic evaluation, oral examination, diagnostic mounting of casts, preliminary survey and design procedures, and appropriate consultations with medical and dental specialists. Too often, the design of a removable partial denture is determined after all other phases of patient treatment have been completed. This approach generally results in failure. Decisions regarding teeth to be retained, surgical procedures to be employed, and restorations to be placed must be made with the ultimate design of the prosthesis in mind. Hence, survey and design procedures must be considered key elements in the diagnostic phase of treatment.

## ☐ Organizing the Diagnostic Examination

The examination can be completed most effectively and expeditiously if two appointments are used. During the first appointment, a thorough health history should be completed and reviewed. A preliminary examination of the oral cavity should be performed to identify conditions requiring immediate attention, and a dental prophylaxis and radiographic survey should be completed. Finally, accurate maxillary and mandibular impressions should be made, and diagnostic casts should be generated.

During the second appointment, facebow and jaw relation records should be made. Using these records, diagnostic casts should be mounted in an appropriate dental articulator. In addition, a definitive oral examination should be completed. Radiographic evaluation should be correlated with clinical findings, and arrangements for consultation should be made. Procedures for the second diagnostic appointment are described in chapter 6.

When all relevant information has been gathered, the practitioner should perform survey and design procedures. In turn, a properly sequenced treatment plan should be formulated and presented to the patient.

## ▢ Health Questionnaire

The purpose of a health questionnaire is to provide information about a patient's well-being and to highlight potential problems. Therefore, a health questionnaire should provide information regarding local and systemic conditions that may affect the patient's treatment. Any positive responses or questionable answers should be explored during the patient interview.

Evaluation of a patient's blood pressure is an important part of the health evaluation process. It has been estimated that more than 20 million Americans exhibit hypertension.[1,2] Of that number, approximately one half have been diagnosed and one fourth are receiving adequate therapy.[3] These facts should motivate health professionals to screen all patients for hypertension. Any patient with systolic pressure exceeding 130 mm Hg or diastolic pressure exceeding 90 mm Hg should be considered to have a potentially serious medical condition for which medical consultation is indicated.

## ▢ Patient Interview

The next step in the examination procedure is the patient interview. During this phase of the diagnostic process, the practitioner should establish rapport with the patient, gain insight into the psychologic makeup of the patient, explore physical problems that may affect the treatment, and determine the patient's expectations for restorative therapy.

### Establishing rapport

Dr Carl Boucher put the initial patient contact into proper perspective when he said, "The first five minutes spent with a patient represent the most important period of dentist-patient interaction. Patients should feel that the dentist is genuinely interested in them and in helping to solve their dental problems."[4] Practitioners must not overlook the importance of these interactions because they represent the groundwork for future

dental treatment. In addition, these early interactions provide essential information regarding patient attitudes and expectations.

In 1961, Dr M. M. DeVan stated, "We should meet the mind of the patient before we meet the mouth of the patient."[5] DeVan's statement underscores the importance of effective communication between patient and practitioner. It is essential that a practitioner understand the patient's needs, desires, and expectations before initiating treatment. The patient's attitudes and opinions relative to the dentist and dentistry can greatly influence the success or failure of treatment. Many clinically acceptable prostheses have been discarded because patients were not mentally prepared to receive them.

### Gaining insight into a patient's psychological makeup

A patient's psychological makeup is an important factor in dental treatment. Psychological makeup will influence the difficulty of clinical treatment, as well as the success or failure of treatment outcomes.

In 1950, Dr M. M. House classified patients into four major categories based upon psychological characteristics: philosophical, exacting, hysterical, and indifferent.[6] Philosophical patients are the easiest to treat. They are mentally well adjusted and easygoing. They accept responsibility for having lost their teeth, and they recognize the need for prosthetic replacement. Furthermore, these patients understand that they have a role in maintaining their dental health. These individuals adjust to any prosthesis that is reasonably well designed and constructed, and usually do not present problems for the dentist.

Exacting patients are precise in everything they do. They are immaculate in dress and appearance. Their nature is to be satisfied only by perfection. They may demand that the dentist explain every step of the treatment in detail. These patients should not be promised that they will be able to wear a prosthesis without any inconvenience, because they will expect the dentist to live up to such promises. Potential problems and inconveniences should be explained in detail before treatment is initiated. A logical explanation may be perceived as an excuse if given after a problem has arisen. Additional appointment time should be scheduled for exacting patients because they demand undivided attention, effort, and patience. These patients have high expectations and are difficult to treat. Yet, when satisfied, these patients become enthusiastic supporters of the dentist and valuable assets to the dental practice.

A hysterical patient must be recognized before treatment is initiated to avoid a highly unpleasant experience for both patient and dentist. Hysterical patients may be extremely apprehensive about undergoing dental treatment. They also tend to complain without justification. Many are convinced they will never be able to wear dental prostheses. Hysterical patients do not accept responsibility for any of their dental problems. Patients who have debilitating systemic or psychiatric disorders are often included in this category. They must be advised that their dental problems may be related to systemic or psychiatric conditions. Adjunctive medical and psychiatric therapies may be useful in the treatment of hysterical patients. Unless the attitudes of such patients are changed, the probability of successful dental treatment is minimal.

Indifferent patients also present significant problems for dental practitioners. Indifferent patients are characterized by lack of motivation or concern about existing oral conditions. These patients tend to ignore instructions and to be uncooperative throughout treatment. They may exhibit little concern about appearance and function of the remaining teeth. Unless these patients can be taught to appreciate the importance of replacing missing teeth and maintaining oral health, the prognosis for dental treatment is poor.

## Evaluating the effects of physical problems on dental treatment

Another objective of the patient interview is to evaluate physical problems that may affect the patient's treatment. Positive responses on the health questionnaire must be explored in detail. The symptoms and manifestations of disease should be reviewed and carefully evaluated to determine potential effects upon dental treatment. There are too many systemic disturbances to rely on memory alone. Therefore, the practitioner should consult current reference materials during this process. When any doubt exists, the most prudent action is to seek medical consultation before dental treatment is initiated. Knowing that the patient has a systemic disturbance is not enough. The dentist must understand how the disease may affect treatment of the patient. Following are some systemic disturbances that can exert significant effects on dental treatment.

### Diabetes

Uncontrolled diabetes is frequently accompanied by multiple small oral abscesses and poor tissue tone. The disease should be brought under control before prosthodontic treatment is initiated. The decreased resistance to infection exhibited by diabetic patients necessitates special care during treatment and follow-up. Diabetic patients often display reduced salivary output. This significantly reduces a patient's ability to wear a prosthesis and increases the likelihood of dental caries.

### Arthritis

Arthritic changes in the temporomandibular joint of a patient may produce changes in occlusion. Arthritic changes also may create difficulties in the determination and recording of jaw relations.

### Paget disease

Patients with Paget disease may show enlargement of the maxillary tuberosities. This can cause changes in the fit and occlusion of prostheses. A frequent recall program should be instituted for patients with Paget disease.

### Acromegaly

A patient with acromegaly may have enlargement of the mandible. Consequently, patients with acromegaly should be examined frequently to evaluate the fit and function of removable prostheses.

### Parkinson disease

Parkinson disease is characterized by rhythmic contractions of the musculature, including the muscles of mastication. The symptoms are sometimes so severe that it is impossible for a patient to insert and remove a removable partial denture, let alone practice the oral hygiene procedures necessary for the maintenance of oral health. Impression procedures also may be compromised by the presence of excessive quantities of saliva.

## Pemphigus vulgaris

Pemphigus vulgaris is a disease that usually begins with formation of bullae in the oral cavity with gradual extension to the skin. Before 1959, the disease was usually fatal; however, current treatment regimens have resulted in a good prognosis. In the acute phase, oral discomfort and dryness of the mouth are common symptoms. These symptoms may be erroneously linked to the presence of a removable prosthesis. Consequently, patients have been known to go from dentist to dentist for the relief of pain, or the fabrication of new prostheses. When the disease is controlled with appropriate medications, patients can wear prostheses successfully. However, care must be taken to establish smooth, polished borders in the finished prostheses. Greater than normal postinsertion care also can be anticipated.

## Epilepsy

Epileptic patients present special problems in treatment planning and restorative therapy. A grand mal seizure may result in fracture and aspiration of a prosthesis, and possibly the loss of additional teeth. Therefore, consultation with the patient's physician should be carried out before treatment is initiated. The construction of removable partial dentures is usually contraindicated if the patient has frequent, severe seizures that occur with little or no warning. However, if the seizures are well controlled, or if the patient has adequate premonition to permit removal of prostheses, a removable partial denture may be indicated.

All materials used in the construction of a prosthesis for an epileptic patient must be radiopaque so that any part of the prosthesis that is swallowed or aspirated during a seizure can be located radiographically. If the patient's medication includes phenytoin, one must take particular care to ensure that the removable partial denture does not irritate the gingival tissues. Otherwise, gingival hypertrophy may result.

## Cardiovascular disease

Patients with the following cardiovascular conditions require medical consultation before the initiation of dental procedures:

- Acute or recent myocardial infarction
- Unstable or recent onset of angina pectoris
- Congestive heart failure
- Uncontrolled arrhythmia
- Uncontrolled hypertension

Several other cardiovascular conditions also may warrant medical consultation. Prophylactic antibiotic therapy is always recommended if surgical procedures are to be accomplished for patients with a congenital or rheumatic valvular heart disease, cardiac murmurs, or repaired coarctation of the aorta. There is conflicting evidence regarding the need for prophylactic medication when lesser degrees of tissue trauma are anticipated, such as the placement of restorations and the making of impressions. In addition, many physicians do not recommend antibiotic prophylaxis for patients with a history of rheumatic fever if there has not been cardiac involvement. Because a patient's knowledge of the condition may not be completely accurate, the most prudent procedure for the dentist is to request a medical consultation with the patient's physician.

## Cancer

Due to its many forms, cancer may affect removable partial denture therapy in numerous ways. The treatment of cancerous lesions with ionizing radiation and chemotherapy also may impact removable partial denture therapy. Oral complications are a common side effect of radiation and chemotherapy for malignancies in areas other than the head and neck. The most common oral complications are mucosal irritations, xerostomia, bacterial infections, and fungal infections. These conditions may complicate the construction and wear of removable partial dentures. An investigation conducted by Sonis and colleagues in 1978 indicated that 40% of all patients treated with chemotherapy and radiotherapy for malignancies remote from the oral cavity developed some form of oral complication.[7] The incidence varied with the type of malignancy: Hodgkin disease, 100%; leukemia, 66.7%; mesenchymal cancer, 37.5%; gynecologic cancer, 33.3%; non-Hodgkin lymphoma, 33.3%; adeno-carcinoma of bowel, 20%; and breast cancer, 11.5%.

## Transmissible diseases

Hepatitis, tuberculosis, influenza, human immuno-deficiency virus (HIV), and other transmissible diseases pose a particular hazard for patients, dental auxiliaries, and dentists. These diseases may be transmitted by contact with contaminated blood, saliva, aerosols, and instruments. Additional hazards exist during the prosthodontic phases of treatment. Impression trays and materials may be contaminated when impressions are made. If impressions are not properly disinfected, the resultant casts also may permit the transmission of disease. Contaminated polishing wheels, pumice, pumice pans, and prostheses may cause aerosol contamination of the laboratory and the dental office. Hence, it is imperative that dental personnel take precautions to prevent contamination and disease transmission.

## Evaluating the effects of drugs on treatment

No dentist or physician can be expected to remember the effects, side effects, and interactions of all drugs. However, each dentist is responsible for determining which medications a patient is taking and for using current reference information to determine what effects these medications may have on dental treatment.

Increasing age usually is accompanied by an increase in (1) the need for some type of prosthodontic treatment and (2) the use of prescription and non-prescription drugs. The proportion of persons on some type of medication is 1 in 4 for teenagers, 1 in 3 for young adults, 1 in 2 for persons in their 40s, and 2 in 3 for persons aged 50 and older.[8] Therefore, at least half of the patients requiring prosthodontic treatment are likely to be taking one or more drugs that could affect dental treatment. Following are some of the frequently prescribed drugs that can affect treatment.

## Anticoagulants

Postsurgical bleeding may be a problem for patients receiving anticoagulants. This is particularly true for patients undergoing extractions, osseous recontouring, or soft tissue surgeries. These patients should be referred to qualified oral surgeons or periodontists for management of the surgical phases of treatment.

## Antihypertensive agents

The most significant side effect of antihypertensive drugs is orthostatic hypotension, which may result in syncope when a patient suddenly assumes an upright position. As a result, care must be taken when the patient rises from the dental chair. The patient should be questioned about feeling dizzy or weak. If symptoms persist, the patient should not be allowed to leave the office unaccompanied. Treatment for hypertension also may include prescription of a diuretic agent. This may contribute to a decrease in saliva and an associated dry mouth.

## Endocrine therapy

A patient undergoing endocrine therapy may experience severe oral discomfort related to dry mouth (ie, xerostomia). If the patient is wearing a prosthesis, it could be mistakenly blamed for causing the discomfort.

## Saliva-inhibiting drugs

Methantheline (Banthine, Searle, San Juan, Puerto Rico), atropine, and their derivatives are sometimes used to control excessive salivary secretion. These drugs are particularly useful when a practitioner is making impressions. Saliva-inhibiting drugs are contraindicated in patients with cardiac disease because of their vagolytic effects. These drugs also should be avoided in patients with prostatic hypertrophy and glaucoma. Salivary flow should be controlled by mechanical means in these patients.

## Ascertaining a patient's expectations of treatment

An important objective of the interview is to ascertain a patient's expectations of dental treatment. In turn, the practitioner should determine whether these expectations are realistic in the light of the patient's oral and physical conditions. Any removable partial denture will complicate oral hygiene procedures, occupy space in the oral cavity, and require a learning and adaptation period. If a patient cannot tolerate these inconveniences, the chances for successful treatment are extremely limited. If the patient's expectations cannot be changed through explanation and education, treatment should not be undertaken.

## Obstacles to a successful interview

Several obstacles must be overcome during the interview process if a dentist is to provide appropriate treatment. The first obstacle is a lack of attention. Too often the dentist is lecturing rather than listening. Certainly patient education is an important part of dental treatment, but the patient interview is not the appropriate time for patient education. Valuable information may be gained from patients by simply allowing them to talk. Their opinions regarding previous dental care and current oral conditions may be determined by asking a few general questions. Patient desires, needs, and expectations also may be clarified during this portion of the interview.

In many instances, the dentist is inattentive when observation and interpretation of the patient's actions are required. The patient's body language and things that are left unsaid may be more indicative than the words being used. Simple actions such as smiling with a closed mouth or placing the hand in front of the mouth during speech may indicate the patient's true feelings about the appearance of his or her teeth (Fig 5-1). Middle-aged patients may say that obtaining good function and comfort is all they expect from a partial denture, while their immaculate dress, mannerisms, or excessive use of cosmetics may communicate that appearance is of critical importance. The dentist should be aware of such behavior before beginning treatment.

Another obstacle to a successful interview may be the dentist's choice of words. Professional terms such as *esthetics, centric relation, vertical dimension, stability, hypertrophy,* and *edema* may be misinterpreted or completely misunderstood by the patient. Patience, clarity of speech, and the use of understandable terms are essential throughout dental treatment.

Patients may be reluctant to provide information that they believe is irrelevant to dental treatment. Information about systemic problems or drug usage may be particularly difficult to obtain. The dentist must explain the importance of this information and be relentless in obtaining a current and thorough history.

## Keys to a successful interview

### Dentist's attitude and behavior

A dentist's attitude and behavior during the interview have a great impact on its ultimate success or failure. A patient who perceives the dentist as caring, understanding, and respectful is more likely to be honest and cooperative. The dentist can communicate concern for the patient by employing the following behaviors:

1. The dentist should face the patient, preferably at the same level, and should appear relaxed and unhurried (Fig 5-2).
2. The dentist should make eye contact with the patient, looking directly at the patient and displaying complete attention rather than studying radiographs or writing (see Fig 5-2).
3. The dentist should employ appropriate head nodding, verbal following, and verbal reflection. In verbal following the dentist makes a short comment such as "I see," "I understand," or "That is unusual," to indicate attention to what is being said and to encourage the patient to continue to provide information. Verbal reflection involves paraphrasing what the patient has said to ensure that the intended meaning has been understood.

### Phrasing of questions

The phrasing of questions is very important to the success of a patient interview. When general information is sought, the question should be phrased so that a simple *yes* or *no* will not suffice as an answer. For example, questions such as, "Are you frightened or nervous about visiting the dentist?" limit responses to *yes* or *no*. On the other hand, open-ended statements such as, "Tell me about your feelings when you have to go to the dentist," require the patient to provide more information and thereby permit a more accurate assessment of the patient's opinions and experiences.

## Structure of the interview

### Dental history

Valuable information can be obtained by reviewing the patient's dental history. It is important to find out why teeth were extracted. A question such as, "Have you had any of your permanent teeth removed?" followed

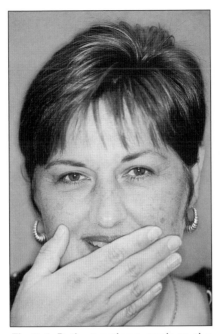

**Fig 5-1** Patient actions, such as the placement of a hand over the mouth, may indicate concern about appearance of teeth.

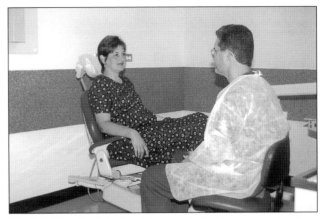

**Fig 5-2** The dentist should be seated at the same level as the patient. The dentist should face the patient and appear relaxed and unhurried.

by, "Why were these teeth removed?" can provide valuable information for treatment planning. If the teeth were lost as a result of caries, special emphasis should be placed on improving the patient's oral hygiene. If the teeth were lost as a result of periodontal disease, every effort should be made to limit its progression.

If the patient has an existing removable partial denture, the dentist should gather information regarding patient satisfaction. A patient who has had favorable experiences with an existing removable partial denture probably will have favorable experiences with future removable partial dentures. The patient should be asked, "What do you like best about your existing removable partial denture?" These features should be incorporated into the new prosthesis. The patient also should be asked, "What do you like least about your existing removable partial denture?" If possible, these features should be modified to permit improved removable partial denture service.

If several prostheses have been constructed over a relatively short time, the patient may have complaints that are unjustified. The existing prostheses should be evaluated to determine their suitability. In addition, the patient should be asked, "Why were you dissatisfied with the partial dentures?" If the dentist believes

that the complaints are justified, patient treatment may be undertaken. If the complaints appear unjustified, the realities of removable partial denture service should be explained to the patient. Subsequently, the dentist should decide whether to undertake dental treatment.

### Diet

The patient's diet should be evaluated. If cough drops, breath mints, soft drinks, hard candy, coffee with sugar, or other sugar-containing products are used on a regular basis, a change must be effected. The problems caused by sugars are compounded by the wearing of a removable partial denture because the prosthesis shields the microorganisms from the cleansing and buffering action of the patient's saliva.

### Habits

Oral habits should be evaluated to determine whether they will affect the prognosis of restorative treatment.

**Bruxism and clenching** Bruxism and clenching may exert significant effects on the prognosis of removable partial denture therapy (Fig 5-3). If either habit persists following treatment, it may result in unfavorable

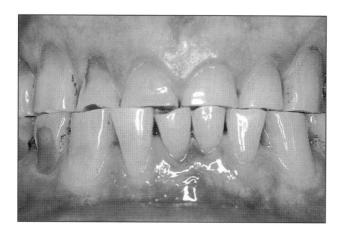

**Fig 5-3** Bruxism and clenching may cause significant loss of tooth structure and complicate therapy.

loading of the prosthesis and lead to the early loss of abutments. Bruxism is often initiated by interceptive occlusal contacts (ie, occlusal prematurities). The occlusion should be analyzed to determine whether correction is indicated. If efforts to eliminate the bruxism are unsuccessful, the patient should wear an occlusal device or night guard to help protect the remaining teeth. Some patients who clench their teeth to relieve tension have such an ingrained clenching habit that they do not realize that an interocclusal space is normal. Patient education and special jaw exercises may be instrumental in eliminating these habits.

**Tongue thrusting** If a tongue-thrust habit has been a contributing factor in tooth loss, continuation of the habit could place harmful stresses on partial denture abutments. If possible, the habit should be eliminated before a prosthesis is constructed. If the habit cannot be eliminated, the removable partial denture should be designed to distribute the forces to as many teeth and supporting structures as possible.

### Expectations of treatment

Some indication of the patient's expectations may have been gained when the dental history was reviewed. Further questioning may provide additional insights. The dentist may pose questions such as, "What do you expect from having a partial denture made?" or "What things would you like to have changed if a new partial denture is made?" If the patient has unrealistic expectations (eg, a removable partial denture without a major connector crossing the palate), the

treatment plan should be altered or patient expectations should be changed through education. If neither can be accomplished, it would be inappropriate to treat the patient.

### Questions from the patient

Asking whether the patient has specific questions or concerns is a good way to conclude the interview. In addition, it allows the patient to open new subject areas and to provide additional information.

## Observing the patient's physical characteristics

During the interview, it is important to note any relevant physical characteristics displayed by the patient. For example, if a patient exhibits a speech problem, it is important that the problem be recognized before construction of a removable partial denture. Otherwise, this problem may be attributed to the prosthesis.

Neuromuscular deficits and neuromotor damage also should be noted. A patient with poor neuromuscular coordination may require additional time to adapt to a removable partial denture. A patient who has suffered a stroke or other neuromotor damage is likely to have difficulty placing and removing a removable partial denture. Patients with such deficits also may have difficulty maintaining adequate levels of hygiene of the oral cavity and the prosthesis.

The length and the mobility of a patient's lips are also important characteristics that should be carefully examined. Patients with short or highly mobile lips

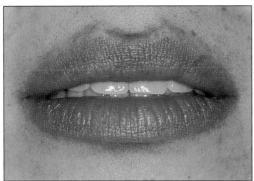

**Fig 5-4** The patient's upper lip should be evaluated to determine its resting length.

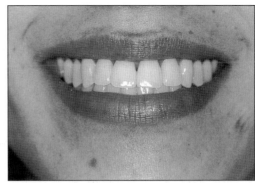

**Fig 5-5** The patient's upper lip also should be evaluated when the patient smiles. This will provide important information regarding the mobility of the patient's upper lip.

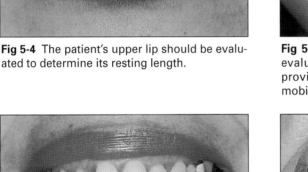

**Fig 5-6** A patient with a short or highly mobile upper lip is likely to expose the marginal gingivae upon smiling. Additional effort is required to ensure that a prosthesis will harmonize with the patient's existing gingival contours and coloration.

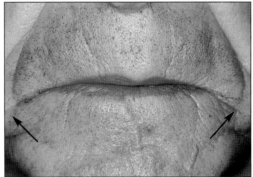

**Fig 5-7** Folding or creasing at the commissures *(arrows)* often indicates a decrease in the patient's occlusal vertical dimension.

present significant challenges in the construction of esthetically pleasing removable partial dentures (Figs 5-4 to 5-6). Esthetics may be compromised if the clasp arms, denture borders, or other components are visible when the patient smiles or speaks.

Facial changes that indicate a decrease in occlusal vertical dimension should be evaluated and treated with great care (Fig 5-7). Treatment should be preceded by placement of an occlusal device and determination of an acceptable occlusal vertical dimension. Failure to identify the correct occlusal vertical dimension may result in the fabrication of prostheses that are woefully inadequate. These prostheses may cause intrusion or migration of the remaining teeth, resulting in failure of the restorative effort. The importance of appropriate maxillomandibular relationships is discussed in chapter 13.

## ⊟ Infection Control in Clinical Prosthodontics

During the past 15 years, infection control has assumed an increasingly prominent role in the health care sciences. The accumulation and dissemination of scientific information has placed the topic in front of health care workers and the general public alike. As a result, numerous infection control procedures have been instituted. These procedures and policies continue to evolve as additional information is provided. Because of the rapid nature of these changes, it would be impossible for the authors to provide a complete list of current infection control recommendations. Therefore, the following sections provide only broad guidelines for infection control. For more specific information, reference to documents published by the

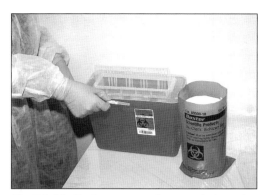

**Fig 5-8** Medical waste products and sharp instruments must be placed in appropriate containers. Disposal of these items must conform with EPA guidelines.

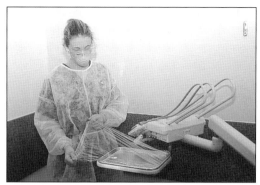

**Fig 5-9** Operatory surfaces should be covered using impermeable barriers such as plastic wrap. Note that the operator is wearing the appropriate personal protective equipment: disposable mask, gown, and gloves and protective eyewear.

American Dental Association (ADA), the Occupational Safety and Health Administration (OSHA), and similar organizations is recommended.

### Personal protective equipment

The most important measure to minimize disease transmission between patients and dental care providers is the routine use of gloves. All personnel having direct patient contact should wear disposable gloves. In most instances, latex gloves are preferred because of their tactile characteristics, availability, and minimal cost. For persons with latex allergies, a variety of nonlatex gloves are available.

Disposable masks, gowns, and gloves and protective eyewear should be worn during clinical appointments. This is particularly important when aerosols will be generated. In addition, all medical waste products must be disposed of as mandated by the Environmental Protection Agency (EPA) (Fig 5-8). These products include sharps (ie, needles, blades, broken glass), human tissues removed during surgery, and blood-soaked materials. State regulations involving disposal of these materials may vary and should be consulted before any action is taken.

### Surface coverage

Disease-causing microorganisms may be transferred from infected patients to environmental surfaces and these microorgansims may remain viable for prolonged periods (hours to days). Contact with contaminated surfaces may result in disease transmission. Therefore, preventive measures must be taken to control or block cross-infection in clinical settings.

The most practical and effective method of managing operatory surface contamination is the use of impermeable barriers (eg, plastic wrap) to shield surfaces from direct or indirect exposure (Fig 5-9). Plastic wrap can be used on light handles, controls, chair switches, evacuator controls, air-water syringes, saliva ejectors, bracket tables, soap dispensers, and other areas at the operator's discretion. Surface covers must be changed between patients to minimize the probability of disease transmission.

### Chemical cleaning and disinfection

Chemical cleaning and disinfection is necessary for those surfaces that cannot be covered but may become contaminated during patient treatment. A number of disinfectants are available at this time. Practitioners are referred to infection control guidelines for prescribed applications.

### Instrument sterilization

All instruments that can withstand heat sterilization must be thoroughly cleaned and heat sterilized between uses. Chemical disinfection of these items is un-

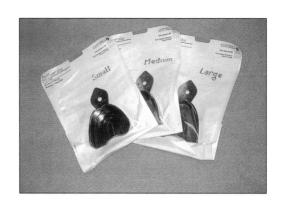

**Fig 5-10** Metal impression trays should be sterilized and stored in unopened bags.

acceptable. Instruments to be heat sterilized should cleaned by scrubbing with hot water and soap or by using an ultrasonic cleaner with an appropriate cleaning solution. Instruments should then be dried, wrapped, packaged, and heat sterilized. Reusable items that cannot be heat sterilized must be cleaned and treated with ethylene oxide or an EPA-registered chemical sterilant. The practitioner should ensure that manufacturers' recommendations are strictly followed.

## Prosthodontic clinical protocol

### Impression trays

Cleaning, sterilization, and storage of stock impression trays minimizes potential health hazards. Metal trays should be cleaned immediately after separating the impressions and casts. Trays should be soaked in a detergent solution and wiped with alcohol sponges to remove adhesives, deposits, and stains. Trays should then be placed in appropriate bags and sterilized. Following sterilization, trays should be stored in the unopened bags (Fig 5-10).

### Instruments, articulators, custom trays

All instruments, including laboratory knives, wax spatulas, acrylic burs, and wax carvers should be cleaned and sterilized following each use. Custom impression trays, record bases, and occlusion rims must be disinfected after construction. A 2-minute application of an approved sodium hypochlorite solution may be used to disinfect these items.

### Disinfecting impressions

Alginate impressions should be rinsed thoroughly in running tap water to remove all traces of saliva and sprayed with an appropriate sodium hypochlorite solution. Impressions should be loosely wrapped in plastic and set aside for not less than 2 minutes. Casts should be poured not more than 12 minutes after removal of an alginate impression from the mouth. Other impressions such as polysulfide, polyvinyl siloxane, polyether, and zinc oxide–eugenol should be disinfected as described for alginate impressions. The prescribed times for pouring casts are material specific.

### Denture asepsis

New removable partial dentures should be washed thoroughly with a brush and germicidal soap, then rinsed using clean tap water. Individual prostheses should be sprayed with a dilute sodium hypochlorite solution and allowed to stand undisturbed for 2 minutes. At the end of this period, prostheses should be rinsed in tap water once again. Prostheses then should be sealed in watertight bags containing clean tap water. Shortly before insertion, prostheses should be removed from the sealed bags and again sprayed with a dilute sodium hypochlorite solution and allowed to stand for 2 minutes. Finally, prostheses should be thoroughly rinsed in tap water to remove any remaining sodium hypochlorite solution from the exposed surfaces. Removable partial dentures should not be immersed in concentrated sodium hypochlorite solutions, nor should they be exposed to dilute sodium hypochlorite solutions for prolonged periods. Most alloys used in removable partial denture construction will become pitted and/or discolored if these recommendations are not followed.

Prostheses that have been worn by the patient should be disinfected prior to modification. These prostheses should be disinfected in the same manner as new prostheses. Following modification, removable partial dentures should be disinfected again. At this stage, prostheses should be rinsed in cool running water and evaluated clinically.

# ▢ Initial Examination

## Detection of problems requiring immediate attention

A preliminary examination must be performed during the first appointment to identify problems requiring immediate attention. Extensive carious lesions may require excavation to determine whether there is pulpal involvement. Provisional restorations may be required to relieve discomfort or restore tooth contours. Oral conditions caused by ill-fitting removable partial dentures also may require immediate attention. Adjustment or temporary relining of existing prostheses should be accomplished to eliminate patient discomfort and allow recovery of the damaged tissues.

## Evaluation of oral hygiene

Evaluation of a patient's oral hygiene is essential for appropriate treatment planning. Inadequate oral hygiene must be recognized early in the diagnostic procedure to allow initiation of an effective oral hygiene program. Having witnessed the decline of a beautifully restored mouth, one realizes the true value of oral hygiene instruction and patient education. It is important to remember that the ultimate success of dental treatment relies on the home care of the patient as well as the technical procedures performed by the dentist.

It is the dentist's responsibility to explain

1. The signs and symptoms of dental disease
2. The materials and techniques for proper home care
3. The patient's responsibilities in preventing further dental disease

Only after patients have acknowledged their responsibilities and demonstrated their motivation and ability to maintain good oral hygiene should extensive restorative therapy be initiated.

## Evaluation of caries susceptibility

The presence of a large number of restored teeth, signs of recurrent caries, and evidence of decalcification indicate that the patient is susceptible to caries. Unless an exceptional level of plaque control can be achieved, the prognosis for treatment will be poor. Hence, the placement of crowns, fixed partial dentures, and removable partial dentures should not be considered until the patient demonstrates acceptable, sustained oral hygiene practices. If this is not accomplished, it is likely that the completed restorations will fail as a result of continued caries progression.

## Oral prophylaxis

Scaling and oral prophylaxis should be performed if necessary. The definitive intraoral examination, diagnostic impressions, and diagnostic casts will be more accurate if the teeth are clean.

## Radiographs

A complete series of periapical and bite-wing radiographs is an indispensable part of the dental examination for a prospective removable partial denture patient (Fig 5-11). Periapical radiographs are essential for determining the crown-to-root ratios of remaining teeth and the condition of the associated periodontal tissues. Bite-wing radiographs are helpful in identifying interproximal caries on the remaining teeth. A panoramic radiograph is ideal for screening for pathologic conditions, but is not adequate for the definitive examination of a removable partial denture patient (Fig 5-12). Evaluation of radiographs is described in chapter 6.

## Diagnostic impressions and casts

A dental examination for a partially edentulous patient must be considered incomplete unless it includes the evaluation of accurate diagnostic casts (Fig 5-13). Diagnostic casts permit analysis of hard and soft tissue contours. These casts provide valuable information about the space that a removable partial denture may occupy. They permit evaluation of existing tooth contours and may indicate the need for fixed restorations on one or more remaining teeth. In addition, di-

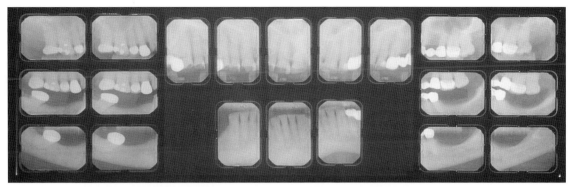

**Fig 5-11** A complete series of bite-wing and periapical radiographs should be made for any prospective removable partial denture patient.

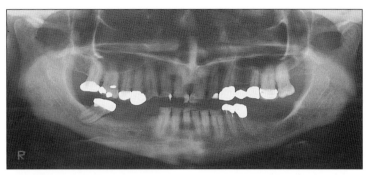

**Fig 5-12** A panoramic radiograph may be a useful adjunct during the examination process.

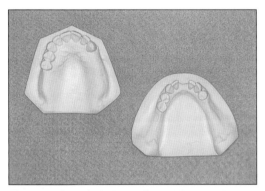

**Fig 5-13** Occlusal view of maxillary and mandibular casts. Accurate diagnostic casts are an essential part of the dental examination for a partially edentulous patient.

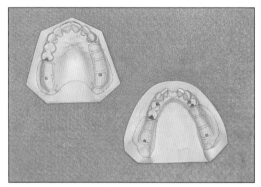

**Fig 5-14** Occlusal view of casts after designs have been drawn. These designs serve as blueprints for tooth modification and prosthesis construction.

agnostic casts sometimes indicate the need for surgical correction of exostoses, prominent frena, and soft tissue undercuts.

During the treatment-planning process, diagnostic casts are surveyed. Proposed designs are drawn directly on the diagnostic casts (Fig 5-14). Individual casts then serve as blueprints for the placement of restorations, the recontouring of teeth, and the preparation of rest seats. These casts also may be helpful

during treatment-planning presentations. Patients are more likely to approve a treatment plan if they can visualize existing problems than they are if they must rely upon a verbal description.

Diagnostic mounting of the casts on a suitable articulator also should be accomplished. This process permits assessment of the occlusion and the available restorative space. Because the casts are normally mounted and evaluated during the second diagnostic appointment, these procedures are discussed in chapter 6. The procedures for making diagnostic impressions and casts are presented in the following sections.

## Physical properties and working characteristics of alginate impression material

Irreversible hydrocolloid impression material, commonly known as alginate, is the material of choice for diagnostic impressions. Because of its accuracy and handling characteristics, alginate impression material is suitable for making diagnostic and final impressions for removable partial dentures. Alginate is easy to use and is relatively inexpensive. However, it is one of the most abused impression materials in dentistry. Knowledge of the physical properties and working characteristics of irreversible hydrocolloid is essential if the material is to be used successfully.

Alginate impression material is supplied in powdered form. Water is mixed with the powder to form a viscous sol, which yields an elastic gel through a series of chemical reactions.

Alginate powder is available in bulk containers and in pre-weighed packets (Fig 5-15). Although convenient, individual packets are more expensive than equal volumes of bulk alginate.

While irreversible hydrocolloid is not usually considered to have a shelf life, the method of storage is very important. Alginate deteriorates rapidly when subjected to elevated temperatures and high humidity. Alginate stored at 65°C (149°F) for 1 month has been shown to be unsuitable for use. Evidence of deterioration has even been shown after storage at 54°C (129°F).[9] This deterioration is thought to be caused by depolymerization of the alginate constituent. Once a container of alginate is opened, the material can show measurable deterioration within 3 days. Repeated opening of the container and exposure of its contents to humidity contribute to rapid deterioration of the powder. Alginate that has deteriorated because of heat or moisture will become thin during mixing, exhibit erratic setting times, have reduced strength, and display high degrees of permanent deformation within the impression. Alginate also can be contaminated by gypsum. Small amounts of dental stone left in a mixing bowl or on a spatula can contaminate alginate and accelerate its set. Therefore, it is essential that mixing bowls used for alginate impression materials be free of gypsum products.

The water-powder ratio has a significant effect on the working characteristics of alginate impression material. This is particularly important when alginate is used for making impressions of the dental arches. Changes in the water-powder ratio will affect the consistency and setting time of the mixed material as well as the strength and quality of the impression. An extremely thick mix will not record fine detail. A thin mix will flow out of the impression tray and away from the tissues. Furthermore, a thin mix of alginate will tear upon removal from the mouth and will result in an unacceptable impression. However, despite changes in consistency and setting time, the accuracy of irreversible hydrocolloid is not affected by changes in the water-powder ratio. Extremely thin mixes of alginate may be used for duplicating casts with no loss of accuracy. Ideally, a dentist should work with a predetermined amount of powder for every impression. The amount of water may be adjusted to obtain subtle variations in consistency of the impression material.

Measurement of alginate powder may be accomplished by volume or by weight. Volumetric measurement is performed using a scoop provided by the manufacturer. This method is inaccurate because alginate powder may be loosely or tightly packed into the scoop. The amount of powder per scoop is dependent upon whether the material in the container was "fluffed" or compacted at the time of measurement and whether excess powder was pressed into the scoop or simply scraped off the top. Inconsistencies in measurement produce significant variations in water-powder ratios. These variations often result in unpredictable handling properties.

Weight measurement of alginate powder is more accurate and more consistent than volumetric measurement and therefore is the preferred method for dividing and dispensing alginate powder. As was mentioned previously, manufacturers sell alginate powder in pre-weighed foil packets; however, purchasing the material in bulk is more economical. As a result, many practitioners choose to buy the material in bulk and weigh it prior to clinical use.

Once a canister of alginate powder is opened, its entire contents should be accurately weighed into 28-g increments (the amount needed for most impressions)

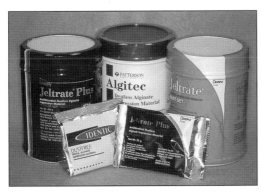

**Fig 5-15** Alginate impression powders are available in bulk containers and pre-weighed packets.

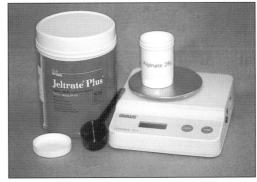

**Fig 5-16** Bulk materials should be accurately weighed using an appropriate scale. Alginate powders should be stored in properly labeled, moisture-proof containers.

and placed in properly labeled, moisture-tight containers (Fig 5-16). When the material is needed, 68 to 72 mL of water is accurately measured and mixed with the powder. This range permits variation of the water-powder ratio to satisfy the requirements of the patient being treated. It is important to note that some water supplies contain large amounts of minerals that can adversely affect the accuracy and the setting time of alginate impression materials. If the practitioner is concerned about the mineral content of the local water supply, distilled or demineralized water should be used.

The setting time of alginate is determined by the manufacturer. Both fast- and regular-set materials are available. The dentist can alter the setting time somewhat by varying the temperature of the water used. Most manufacturers recommend the use of 22°C (72°F) water. Cooler water will provide more working time, whereas slightly warmer water will hasten the set of the impression material. Some brands of alginate exhibit greater sensitivity to temperature change than others. Certain products have shown as much as a 20-second change in gelation time for each 1°C change in the temperature of the water.[9] Refrigeration of the mixing bowl and water can greatly increase the working time. The refrigeration of pre-packaged and pre-weighed powder is not recommended since condensation may affect the accuracy and working properties of the material.

### Storage of alginate impressions

A definite disadvantage of alginate impressions is that they cannot be stored for an appreciable length of time. Measurable distortion occurs if a cast is not poured within 12 minutes of impression removal.[10-14] The primary mechanisms of distortion are evaporation and absorption of liquids.

Evaporation of water results in shrinkage of alginate impression material. This produces distortion of alginate impressions and inaccuracy of associated casts. Therefore, alginate impressions should not be exposed to the atmosphere for more than 12 minutes. Even at 100% humidity, water is eliminated from alginate impression material through a process called *syneresis*. As the moisture content of the material changes, shrinkage of the impression occurs.

In addition to losing water, alginate impression materials also may absorb liquids. This process of absorption, termed *imbibition*, results in localized expansion of the completed impression. This causes distortion of the impression and leads to inaccuracies in the corresponding cast. As a result, an alginate impression should never be wrapped in wet paper towels or immersed in a liquid.

### Sticking of alginate

A potential problem in using irreversible hydrocolloid is the tendency for this material to stick to the teeth (Fig 5-17). Sticking occurs when alginate radicals within the impression material form chemical bonds with hydroxyapatite crystals of the enamel. As the impression is removed, tearing of the alginate occurs. This produces surface inaccuracies in the impression and the resultant cast (Fig 5-18).

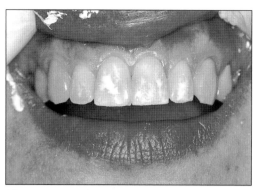

**Fig 5-17** Under certain conditions, alginate impression materials may stick to the teeth.

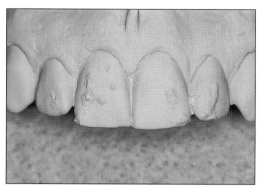

**Fig 5-18** Sticking of alginate results in an inaccurate dental cast.

Sticking generally occurs on the facial surfaces of the teeth and also may occur on the cusp tips. As a result, the practitioner should examine these surfaces immediately after removing an alginate impression. If sticking occurs, alginate should be removed from the teeth with appropriate instruments. The practioner should also thoroughly examine each impression immediately after its removal. If sticking has occurred, the facial surfaces of the impression will present characteristic roughened or scaly surfaces.

Three factors contribute to sticking. First, many dentists polish the teeth following mouth preparation for removable partial dentures. If impressions are made after thorough polishing of the teeth, sticking is more likely to occur. Therefore, only light cleaning of the teeth should be accomplished immediately before impressions are made. If thorough cleaning is necessary, impression procedures should be deferred to a subsequent appointment.

Second, there is a greater tendency for alginate to stick if the teeth are dry. Adequate moisture control can be accomplished by packing the mouth with gauze pads before making an impression. Gauze pads must be gently removed before the impression material is placed in the oral cavity. Drying with compressed air is contraindicated, because this minimizes the moisture content of tooth surfaces and contributes to the sticking of alginate.

Third, there is a greater tendency for sticking to occur if repeated impressions are made. The film that protects enamel from the sticking of alginate is lost during repeated attempts to make a satisfactory impression. Once sticking occurs, it becomes more severe with each subsequent impression. Therefore, a good impression technique should be used so that several attempts are not necessary. If sticking does occur, the practitioner should delay impression procedures until a subsequent appointment or take measures to prevent the alginate from sticking. A common preventive measure is to use a prophylaxis paste to which silicone ointment has been added. This produces a thin film of silicone that prevents sticking of the alginate impression material. An alternative method is to wipe small amounts of silicone ointment onto the vulnerable areas of the teeth. When using this technique, the practitioner must ensure that excess silicone is removed or it will make the impressions inaccurate. Alternatively, the dentist may have the patient suck on sour candy, chew sour gum, or swish whole milk. These procedures accelerate the production of a protective film over the teeth and minimize sticking of alginate. However, for some patients none of these measures will be effective. In these instances, impression procedures should be delayed for at least 24 hours.

### Position of patient and dentist during impression-making procedures

The position of the patient and the dentist can have a significant impact upon impression-making procedures. Experience suggests the patient should be seated upright and the dentist should be standing during these procedures. This enhances patient comfort

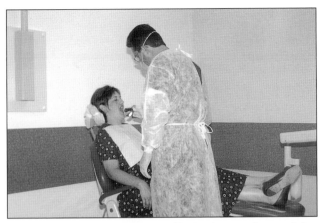

Fig 5-19 When making a mandibular impression, a right-handed operator should stand to the right and in front of the patient. Note that the patient is positioned so the mandibular arch is parallel to the floor.

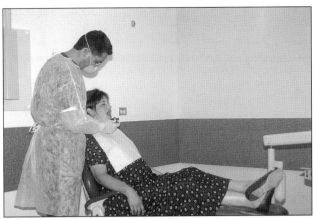

Fig 5-20 When making a maxillary impression, a right-handed operator should stand to the right of and behind the patient.

and provides the dentist with appropriate access, control, and field of vision.

The patient should be positioned so the occlusal plane is parallel to the floor when the patient's mouth is open. This differs slightly for maxillary and mandibular arches; therefore, some adjustment of the chair is necessary between impressions. The height of the chair should be adjusted so the patient's mouth is at the same level as the dentist's elbow. This permits increased operator comfort during impression procedures.

When making a mandibular impression, a right-handed dentist should stand to the right and in front of the patient (Fig 5-19). This permits the dentist to hold the impression tray in the right hand while manipulating the right corner of the patient's mouth with the left hand. When making a maxillary impression, a right-handed dentist should stand to the right of and behind the patient. This permits the dentist's left arm and hand to encircle the patient's head and manipulate the left corner of the mouth (Fig 5-20).

## Impression trays

Stock impression trays for dentate and partially edentulous dental arches are of four basic types: nonperforated metal trays, perforated metal trays, nonperforated plastic trays, and perforated plastic trays (Fig 5-21). Nonperforated metal trays are the trays of choice for removable partial denture applications.

These trays are rigid and properly confine alginate impression materials, making it easier for the operator to obtain properly extended impressions. Although perforated trays are rigid, they do not confine the impression materials as well as nonperforated trays and may result in impressions that are underextended and incomplete. The use of plastic trays, which are generally too flexible to ensure the accuracy of alginate impressions and the associated casts, should be avoided.

Checking maxillary tray for correct size The width of the dental arch is the most important factor in determining tray size. Ideally, there should be a clearance of 5 to 7 mm between the inner flanges of the tray and the facial surfaces of the remaining teeth and soft tissues (Fig 5-22).

When checking the size of a maxillary impression tray, the operator should stand to the right of and behind the patient. The operator's left arm should extend behind the patient's head, and the left hand should be used to manipulate the left corner of the patient's mouth. The impression tray should be held in the right hand with the thumb on top of the handle and the index and middle fingers under the handle. The right posterior flange of the tray should be used to engage the right corner of the mouth. The impression tray should be rotated into the mouth while the dentist manipulates the left corner of the mouth with the left

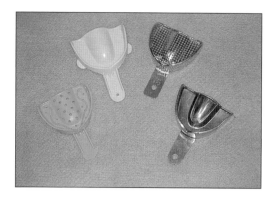

**Fig 5-21** Stock impression trays may be made from plastic or metal, and may be perforated or nonperforated. Nonperforated metal trays are recommended for removable partial denture applications.

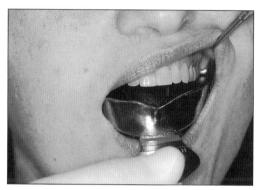

**Fig 5-22** There should be 5 to 7 mm of space between the internal surfaces of the tray and the facial surfaces of the teeth and soft tissues.

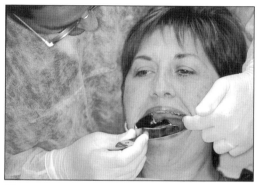

**Fig 5-23** When placing a maxillary tray, the dentist should use the left hand to manipulate the left corner of the mouth. The right posterior flange of the tray should be used to manipulate the right corner of the mouth.

hand (Fig 5-23). At this stage, the operator should visually assess the relationship between the tray and the facial surfaces of the teeth. As previously noted, a clearance of 5 to 7 mm should be present. This space is necessary to ensure the impression material will be thick enough to spring over the undercuts. Too large a tray may be difficult to insert because of interference with the coronoid processes of the mandible.

Frequently, a tray that displays the proper width is not long enough to cover the desired impression area. In other instances, more than 5 to 7 mm is present between the tray and the palatal tissues. If a maxillary impression is attempted in such an instance, the alginate impression material may sag before gelation is complete, resulting in an impression that appears to be accurate but is not. Improperly fitting trays should always be modified before making alginate impressions. The length of the tray and excessive palatal space can be corrected easily through the use of modeling plastic.

**Checking mandibular tray for correct size** A mandibular tray should provide 5 to 7 mm of space both facial and lingual to the remaining teeth and residual ridge. If a tray extends too far lingually, there is a tendency to trap the tongue or the floor of the mouth. The problem should be corrected by selecting a tray of a different size or by bending the lingual flanges of the tray to provide the required clearance.

When evaluating the size of a mandibular tray, a right-handed dentist should be positioned to the right and in front of the patient. The patient's mandibular occlusal plane should be at the level of the dentist's elbow. The impression tray should be held in the right hand, and the left thumb and index finger should be used to manipulate the right corner of the patient's mouth. The left posterior flange of the tray should engage the left corner of the mouth. As the right flange of the tray is rotated toward the mouth, the left thumb and index finger should be used to manipulate the right corner of the mouth. As the tray is rotated into position, the patient should be instructed to gently raise the tongue. This will ensure that the tongue is not trapped beneath the tray. Upon passing the corner of the mouth, the tray should be straightened and positioned over the teeth. The patient should then be instructed to rest the tip of the tongue on the anterior section of the tray. By depressing the lower lip, the dentist can easily see the buccal and lingual clearance between the teeth and the tray.

### Customizing a stock impression tray

Frequently, a stock impression tray does not fit the associated dental arch. In such instances, the fit of the impression tray can be improved using modeling plastic (Figs 5-24 to 5-30). The modeling plastic should be softened in a water bath at 60°C (140°F), kneaded, adapted to the tray, and formed to the general contours of the impression area. At this stage, the modeling plastic should be tempered in the water bath and seated in the mouth. The tray should be seated and removed several times while the modeling plastic is in a softened state. This is done to ensure that the tray does not become locked into hard and soft tissue undercuts. Following manipulation, the tray should be removed from the oral cavity and chilled in ice water. Subsequently, the modeling plastic should be trimmed with a sharp knife to provide 5 to 7 mm of clearance. Alginate adhesive should then be applied to the modeling plastic and the inner surface of the tray.

### Control of gagging

A relatively small percentage of patients experience difficulties, which generally involve gagging, during impression procedures. Before initiating impression procedures, the dentist should ask whether the patient has had impressions made in the past. If this is the patient's first experience, a brief description of the procedures should be given. The dentist should appear relaxed, and the explanation should be delivered in a smooth, even tone. The impression material may be described as a thick cream that sets to a rubber consistency in about 2 minutes. After describing the impression procedure, the dentist should then proceed in a confident manner. Dentists usually encounter problems with gagging when they are in the early stages of clinical practice and approach impression making in a nervous or anxious manner. Under no circumstances should the dentist bring up the subject of gagging, since this may cause the patient to become nervous or hesitant; it should only be addressed if the patient reports past difficulties with gagging during impression making.

The dentist should employ the following procedures to minimize or prevent gagging.

1. The patient should be seated in an upright position with the occlusal plane parallel with the floor.
2. When indicated, the maxillary tray should be modified using modeling plastic. A narrow band of unrelieved modeling plastic should be maintained at the posterior border of the impression area. This band of modeling plastic should prevent alginate from running posteriorly as the tray is inserted.
3. The patient should be directed to use an astringent mouthwash and cold water rinse just before the impression is made. The use of an anesthetic spray is usually contraindicated. Anesthetic spray will cause numbness of the tongue and soft palate and may contribute to gagging.
4. The impression tray should not be overfilled with impression material.
5. The posterior portion of the impression tray should be seated first. Then, the anterior portion of the tray should be rotated into position. This permits excess impression material to be displaced in an anterior direction—away from the soft palate and airway.
6. The patient should be instructed to keep the eyes open during the impression procedure. This encourages the patient to focus upon the surroundings rather than the impression procedure. It may be helpful to have the patient focus on a small object.
7. The patient should be directed to breathe through the nose. The dentist should encourage slow, deep breaths.
8. All instructions should be given in a calm, firm manner.

It is important to recognize that most gagging problems are psychological rather than physical. Confidence in the dentist will help eliminate many of these problems. However, a very small percentage of patients have a true, uncontrollable gag reflex. In these patients, the simple procedure of introducing an empty tray into the mouth may initiate severe gagging. Therefore, additional measures may be necessary to

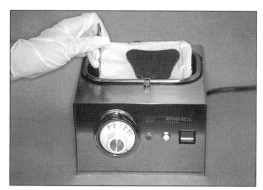

**Fig 5-24** Modeling plastic is softened in a water bath at 60°C (140°F).

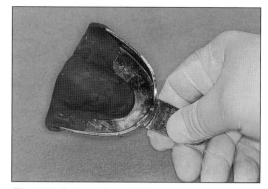

**Fig 5-25** Softened modeling plastic is carefully adapted to the impression tray.

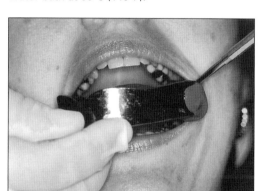

**Fig 5-26** The impression tray is properly seated in the oral cavity.

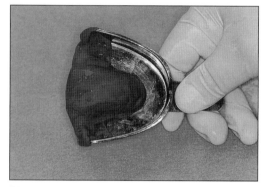

**Fig 5-27** Upon removal from the mouth, the modeling plastic is inspected for evidence of accurate adaptation.

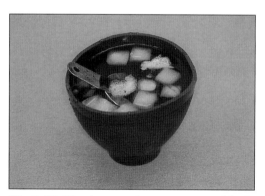

**Fig 5-28** The impression tray assembly is chilled in ice water to facilitate trimming of the modeling plastic.

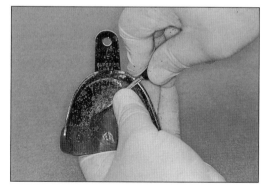

**Fig 5-29** The modeling plastic is trimmed to permit 5 to 7 mm of clearance.

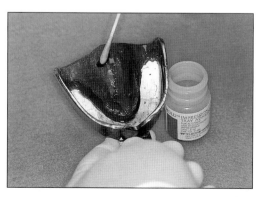

**Fig 5-30** Alginate adhesive is applied to the modeling plastic and inner surfaces of the tray.

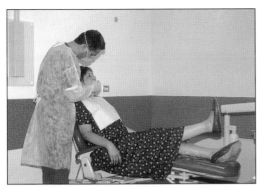

**Fig 5-31** The "leg lift" technique may be used to minimize gagging during impression procedures.

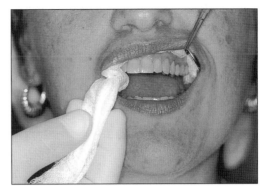

**Fig 5-32** Gauze is placed in the oral cavity to facilitate moisture control.

complete the impression process. The following procedures will allow a dentist to make impressions for almost any patient who is physically and psychologically able to follow instructions.

1. The patient should be instructed to take a deep breath and hold it while the dentist checks the size and adaptation of the tray. Most patients will not gag while holding their breath. As a result, the dentist can complete short procedures without the danger of the patient gagging.
2. The patient should be directed to rinse the mouth with astringent mouthwash and then with cold water. This combination will minimize the flow of saliva during impression procedures and will decrease the likelihood of gagging.
3. A fast-setting alginate should be used to hasten the set of the impression material. Slightly warmer water also may be used to shorten the gelation period.
4. The "leg-lift" technique may be used during the impression procedure. The patient should be directed to lift one leg off the dental chair and to keep it raised at all times (Fig 5-31). As fatigue sets in, it will usually be necessary to firmly command the patient to keep the leg lifted. The mixing of alginate should not be initiated until the patient appears to be tiring. When fatigue is noticeable, the alginate should be mixed and the impression made. The dentist should ensure that the patient's leg remains raised throughout the procedure. The leg-lift procedure is intended to distract the patient by focusing attention on another process. Its success is proba-

bly based on a combination of distraction, muscular fatigue, and anger directed at the dentist. However, once the patient understands that an impression can be made with little or no discomfort, additional procedures may be accomplished with a reduced tendency toward gagging.

### Control of saliva

As was mentioned earlier, alginate has a tendency to stick to teeth if the teeth are too dry. In contrast, excessive amounts of saliva can displace alginate impression material and contribute to an inaccurate impression. In most cases, saliva can be controlled by having the patient rinse the mouth with an astringent mouthwash and then with cold water. Subsequently, the patient's mouth should be packed with 4 × 4–inch gauze that has been unfolded to form an absorptive strip (Fig 5-32). In the maxillary arch, one gauze strip should extend from the posterior portion of the right buccal vestibule to the posterior portion of the left buccal vestibule. The patient should be instructed to hold a second strip against the tissues of the palate. In the mandibular arch, one gauze strip should extend from the right buccal vestibule to the left buccal vestibule. A second gauze strip should be positioned in the lingual sulcus by having the patient raise the tongue, placing the gauze, and then having the patient relax the tongue. The gauze should be gently removed immediately before the impression is made.

Some patients secrete excessive amounts of thick mucinous saliva from the palatal salivary glands. This saliva displaces the alginate and results in inaccurate

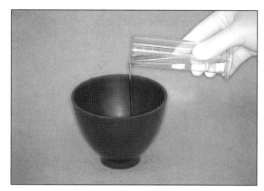

**Fig 5-33** Water is precisely measured and placed into a clean mixing bowl.

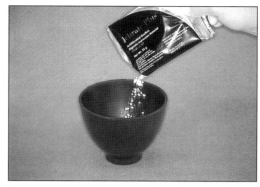

**Fig 5-34** At this stage, alginate powder is sifted into the water.

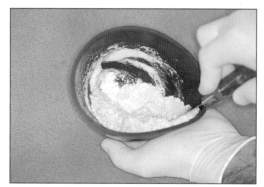

**Fig 5-35** A broad-bladed spatula is used to incorporate the alginate powder into the water.

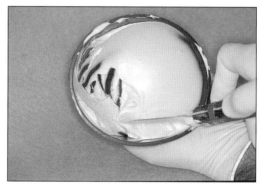

**Fig 5-36** During the mixing process, alginate impression material is pressed against the side of the bowl to minimize air entrapment.

impressions. These patients should be instructed to rinse with an astringent mouthwash. In turn, gauze sponges dampened in warm water should be used to place pressure over the posterior palate, causing the palatal glands to empty. Patients should then be directed to rinse the mouth with ice water. At this point maxillary impressions can be made.

In rare instances, a patient will secrete so much saliva that it becomes extremely difficult to make accurate impressions. The use of an antisialagogue in combination with mouth rinses and gauze packs may be used to control salivary flow in such instances. A 15-mg propantheline bromide tablet taken 30 minutes before the impression appointment may be indicated in certain instances. However, antisialagogues should not be prescribed in the presence of medical contraindications such as glaucoma, prostatic hypertrophy, or cardiac conditions in which any increase in the heart rate is to be avoided.

## Mixing alginate impression material

Alginate may be mixed by hand spatulation, mechanical spatulation, or mechanical spatulation under vacuum. The objective is a smooth, bubble-free mix of alginate. In hand spatulation, a measured amount of distilled water at approximately 22°C (72°F) should be placed into a rubber mixing bowl (Fig 5-33). Subsequently, pre-weighed alginate powder should be sifted from its container into the water (Fig 5-34). Mixing should begin slowly using a stiff, broad-bladed spatula (Fig 5-35). When all of the powder has been thoroughly wetted, the speed of spatulation should be increased. During this process, the spatula should be used to press the alginate impression material against the sides of the bowl (Fig 5-36). This ensures that the material is completely mixed and minimizes air entrapment. Spatulation should continue for a minimum of 45 seconds. Insufficient spatulation can result in failure of the ingredients to dissolve sufficiently. In turn, the change from

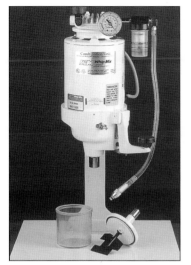

**Fig 5-37** Vacuum spatulation is performed using a specially designed mixing apparatus consisting of a rotary mixing device, a vacuum pump, and the associated mixing bowl.

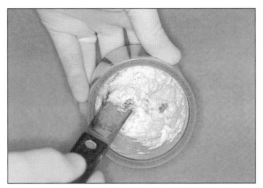

**Fig 5-38** A broad-bladed spatula is used to incorporate the alginate powder into the water.

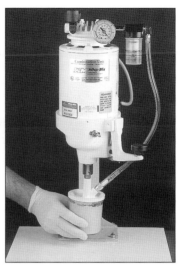

**Fig 5-39** The mixing bowl is properly assembled, the vacuum tubing is attached, and the alginate impression material is spatulated for 15 seconds.

a sol to a gel may not occur uniformly throughout the mass of alginate, resulting in a significant reduction in the strength of the material. An incompletely spatulated mix will appear lumpy and granular and will exhibit numerous areas of trapped air. Complete spatulation will result in a smooth, creamy mixture.

The most consistent method for making a smooth, bubble-free mix is mechanical spatulation under vacuum (Fig 5-37). When using this method, a prescribed amount of water should be added to a mechanical mixing bowl. Pre-weighed alginate should be sifted into the water and thoroughly incorporated by hand spatulation (Fig 5-38). The lid of the mixing bowl should be properly positioned and the vacuum apparatus should be activated. The impression material should be mechanically spatulated under 20 lbs of vacuum for 15 seconds (Fig 5-39). Shorter spatulation may result in incomplete mixing of the impression material. Longer spatulation may result in a greatly reduced setting time of the alginate material and could affect the strength of the gel.

### Loading the impression tray

Small increments of the impression material should be placed in the tray and forced under the rim (Fig

5-40). Placing too large a portion of alginate at one time increases the probability of trapping air. Impression material should be added until it is level with the flanges of the tray. Overfilling should be avoided. A moderate amount of impression material (approximately 20 cm$^3$) should be placed into a large-diameter syringe using a spatula (Fig 5-41). At this stage, the plunger should be replaced and the impression should be made.

### Making impressions

The mandibular impression should be made first because it usually entails less patient discomfort, and patient confidence is increased when an impression has been successfully completed. While holding the tray with the left hand, the dentist should use the right hand to remove gauze pads from the patient's mouth. The syringe should be used to introduce impression material into the facial and lingual vestibules (Fig 5-42). Additional material should be placed on the occlusal surfaces of the teeth. The index finger of the right hand should be used to force this material into the interproximal spaces and occlusal depressions. Immediately thereafter, the filled impression tray should be placed into the oral cavity and properly

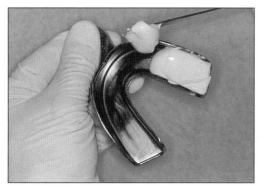

**Fig 5-40** The tray is loaded by placing small increments of alginate impression material under the rim. Impression material is loaded until it is level with the flanges of the tray.

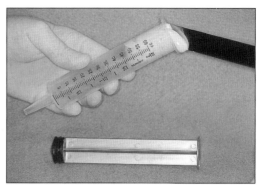

**Fig 5-41** Alginate impression material is loaded into a large-diameter syringe.

seated (Fig 5-43). The lips and cheeks should be pulled apically and then outward at a 45-degree angle to properly form the peripheries of the impression.

It is essential that the dentist maintain the position of the tray during the entire gelation period. This can be accomplished most effectively by placing the forefinger of each hand on top of the tray in the premolar area, and by placing the thumbs under the patient's chin (Fig 5-44). The dentist should maintain an even amount of pressure on the tray even if the patient opens or closes the mouth. Any movement of the tray during the gelation period will result in an inaccurate impression. Therefore, allowing the patient or the assistant to hold the tray should be avoided. Gelation of the alginate impression material should be complete within 2 to 3 minutes.

Following completion of the setting process, the impression should be removed and inspected. An impression should be repeated if voids are present in critical areas. See the following sections for additional details on the removal and inspection of the impression.

When making the maxillary impression, the dentist should be positioned to the right of and behind the patient. The patient should be instructed to rinse with an astringent mouthwash followed by cold water. Gauze pads should be used for moisture control. A large-diameter syringe should be used to place alginate impression material into the vestibules and onto the occlusal surfaces of the teeth. In addition, a moderate amount of impression material should be applied to the palate (Fig 5-45). Failure to accomplish this step may result in an impression with a large void

in the palatal area. When the material has been applied to the desired surfaces, it should be wiped into the interproximal spaces and occlusal depressions.

The loaded maxillary tray should be grasped with the thumb and forefinger of the right hand. As the right posterior flange of the impression tray engages the right corner of the mouth, the dentist's left hand should be used to retract the left corner of the mouth. Once the tray is in the mouth, the thumb and forefinger of the left hand should be used to raise the upper lip. This permits the dentist to see the relationship between the labial flange of the tray and the facial surfaces of the teeth or residual ridge.

Care should be taken to ensure that the tray is properly aligned during the insertion process. This can be evaluated by looking at the patient's head from above and behind, and by observing the position of the tray handle. The handle should protrude from the center of the mouth and should be oriented parallel to the sagittal plane (Fig 5-46). After the proper orientation has been verified, the tray should be seated. During this process, the cheeks should be lifted upward and outward to prevent the buccal tissues from being trapped by the flanges of the tray. The upper lip also should be lifted upward and outward to allow good visibility and to avoid trapping the lip between the flange of the tray and the anterior teeth. The tray must not be overseated. Overseating produces contact between the internal surfaces of the tray and the occlusal or incisal edges of the teeth, thereby producing an inaccurate impression. The tray should be stabilized throughout the set of the impression material by maintaining light

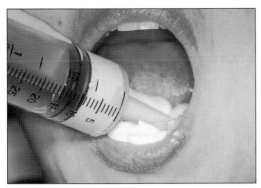

**Fig 5-42** The syringe is used to introduce impression material into the mandibular vestibules and lingual sulci.

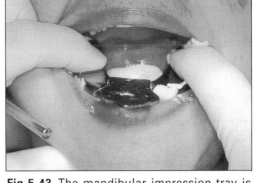

**Fig 5-43** The mandibular impression tray is properly seated.

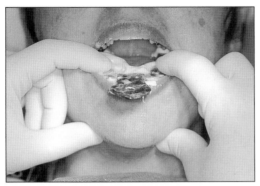

**Fig 5-44** The impression tray is supported throughout the gelation process.

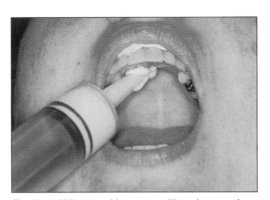

**Fig 5-45** When making a maxillary impression, a moderate amount of alginate impression material should be applied to the palate.

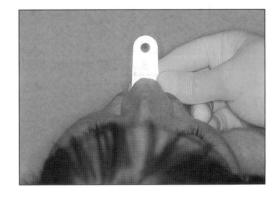

**Fig 5-46** When viewed from above and behind the patient, the handle of the impression tray is oriented parallel to the sagittal axis.

pressure over the premolar areas on both sides of the arch. The alginate impression material should set within 2 to 3 minutes.

Following completion of the gelation process, the impression should be removed and inspected. If voids are present in critical areas, the impression procedure should be repeated. Removal and inspection of the impression are discussed in greater detail in the following sections.

### Removal of impression from the mouth

Clinically, the initial set of alginate is determined by a loss of surface tackiness. An alginate impression should be left in the mouth for an additional 2 to 3 minutes after this initial set to permit the development of additional strength. Early removal of an alginate impression may lead to unnecessary tearing of the impression material. It is important to note that the gel strength doubles during the first 4 minutes after initial

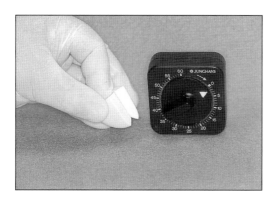

**Fig 5-47** A small mound of the original mix of alginate that has been set aside fractures cleanly upon bending, indicating that the alginate impression material may be removed from the mouth.

gelation. Beyond 4 minutes, no further strengthening occurs. In fact, impressions left in the mouth for 5 or more minutes exhibit noticeable distortion. There are two reliable methods of determining the correct time for removal of an alginate impression:

1. A timer can be used to measure the 2- to 3-minute period after initial gelation.
2. A small mound of the original mix of alginate can be placed on a glass or metal surface. When this alginate will fracture cleanly with finger pressure, the impression is ready to be removed from the mouth (Fig 5-47).

The physical strength of alginate gel is such that a sudden force is more successfully resisted than a slow, sustained force. The material also displays improved elastic recovery when an impression is rapidly removed. Therefore, alginate impressions should be removed from the mouth with a rapid, sustained tug. This results in a more accurate impression and cast.

The following technique makes it possible to remove an impression without significant distortion of the alginate: The lips and cheeks should be retracted to partially break the seal and facilitate impression removal. For a maxillary impression, the right thumb should be placed on top of the tray handle. The middle and index fingers should be placed on the underside of the handle and should extend onto the palatal segment of the tray. This prevents the tray from striking the mandibular teeth and tissues during tray removal. At this point, the impression should be removed with a rapid tug directed parallel to the long axes of the teeth. For a mandibular impression, the right thumb should be placed on the underside of the tray handle. The

middle and index fingers should extend onto the upper surface of the tray to prevent damage to the opposing teeth. The mandibular impression also should be removed with a rapid tug directed parallel to the long axes of the teeth. Rocking or slowly teasing the impression from the mouth will result in irreversible distortion of the impression material and should be avoided.

### Inspecting the impression

Following removal from the mouth, the impression should be inspected using a good light source and magnification (Figs 5-48 and 5-49). An impression should be repeated if there are any doubts regarding its accuracy. The practitioner should be aware of problems that occur consistently so that steps may be taken to address these deficiencies. Common problems include layering of the impression material, improper positioning of the tray, and entrapment of the tongue or other tissues by the flanges of the impression tray.

Layering is caused by the premature gelation of the syringe material. Alginate applied with the syringe should be 3 to 4 mm thick. If the impression material is too thin, the heat of the oral cavity may cause the material to set before the tray can be seated. This produces a distinct border between the syringe material and the tray material, and results in a layered impression.

Improper tray placement is caused by poor visibility. During insertion of the impression tray, the left hand should be used to manipulate one corner of the patient's mouth, while the posterior flange of the impression tray should be used to control the opposite corner of the mouth. The fingers should be used to manipulate the lip and provide optimum visibility during the seating process. The tray should be carefully seated

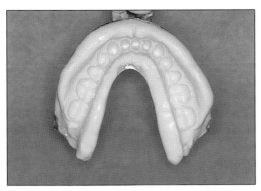

**Fig 5-48** Upon removal of the tray from the mouth, the mandibular impression is thoroughly inspected.

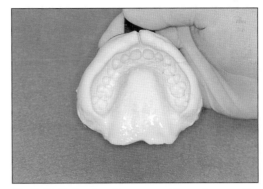

**Fig 5-49** Following its removal from the mouth, the maxillary impression is inspected.

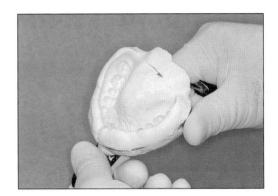

**Fig 5-50** Unsupported alginate material is removed from the impression.

so its flanges are apical to the gingival margins of the teeth. Overseating may cause the cusps of the teeth to contact the tray and result in an inaccurate impression. In addition, great care must be exercised when seating the tray in a patient with tori or other exostoses since contact with the overlying soft tissues may cause significant discomfort.

Entrapment of the tongue and other soft tissues also should be avoided. Upon seating of the mandibular impression tray, the patient should be asked to raise, protrude, and then relax the tongue. By raising and protruding the tongue, the patient prevents its confinement by the lingual flanges of the tray. With the subsequent relaxation of the tongue, the form of the lingual vestibule may be recorded.

Following are other common reasons for rejecting an impression:

1. Inadequate extension of the impression
2. Voids in critical areas
3. Tearing in critical areas
4. Alginate sticking to the teeth

5. Alginate separated from the underlying impression tray (Although it appears the alginate can be pushed back into contact with the tray, this will result in an inaccurate impression and an inaccurate cast.)
6. Rough or granular impression with poor tissue detail (This indicates inadequate spatulation, delayed insertion, or premature removal.)

A review of causes and solutions for common problems associated with making diagnostic alginate impressions is presented in Table 5-1 at the end of the chapter.

If the impression is acceptable, unsupported alginate material is removed (Fig 5-50).

### Cleaning the impression
Failure to remove saliva from the impression will result in an inaccurate cast. Therefore, saliva should be carefully removed from the impression surface before the associated cast is poured. Most patients have thin, serous saliva. This type of saliva can be removed by briefly holding the impression under a gentle stream of

153

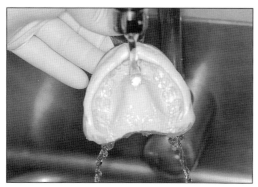

**Fig 5-51** Each impression is cleaned to remove saliva and unwanted oral fluids.

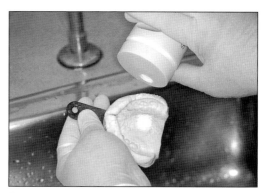

**Fig 5-52** A thin layer of dental stone is sprinkled on the surface of the impression. This stone serves as a disclosing agent for adherent saliva.

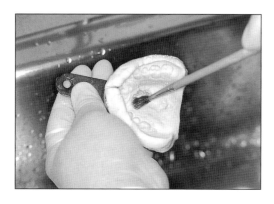

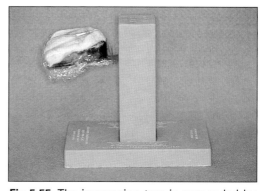

**Fig 5-53** Adherent saliva is removed using a wet camel-hair brush and light pressure.

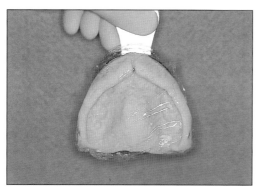

**Fig 5-54** The impression is sprayed with an appropriate disinfectant and lightly covered with plastic wrap.

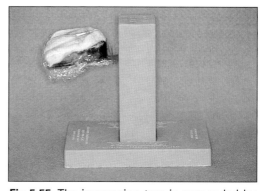

**Fig 5-55** The impression tray is suspended by its handle.

cool tap water (Fig 5-51). If running tap water is not effective, the saliva can be removed using a soft camel-hair brush and a mild detergent.

On the other hand, some patients have thick, ropy saliva that is difficult to remove. Therefore, it is recommended that a thin layer of dental stone be sprinkled on the surface of the impression (Fig 5-52). The stone adheres to the saliva and acts as a disclosing agent.

When the impression is placed under running tap water, the saliva can be removed by light brushing with a wet camel-hair brush (Fig 5-53). All traces of saliva should be removed before proceeding.

### Disinfecting the impression

Following the cleaning process, each impression should be sprayed with an appropriate disinfectant.

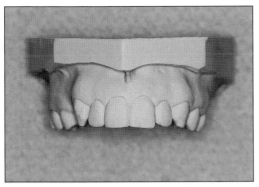

**Fig 5-56** Cast with a dense, abrasion-resistant surface.

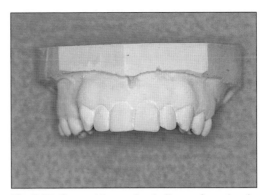

**Fig 5-57** Cast with a soft, chalky surface that is easily abraded.

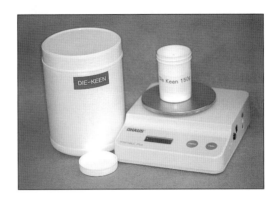

**Fig 5-58** Gypsum products should be proportioned by weight and stored in properly labeled, moisture-proof containers.

The impression should be loosely covered with plastic wrap and set aside for an appropriate period (Fig 5-54). This period may vary from 2 to 10 minutes depending on the disinfectant. At this time, care must be taken not to place pressure on the peripheries of the impression. Such pressure can lead to distortion of the alginate impression material. The tray should be suspended by its handle in a tray holder (Fig 5-55) or a slightly open drawer; placing the tray on a table may cause distortion of the alginate. It is also important to note that the use of compressed air to remove the disinfectant may cause dehydration of the impression surface, resulting in distortion of the impression and associated cast, and therefore should be avoided.

### Importance of water-powder ratio in making the cast

A cast with a dense, abrasion-resistant surface is essential in all phases of removable partial denture design and construction (Figs 5-56 and 5-57). The surface hardness of a stone cast is directly related to its com-

pressive strength, and the compressive strength of a stone cast is directly affected by the water-powder ratio used in making the cast.

All gypsum products, whether dental plaster or dental stone, require only 18.61 mL of water to react with 100 g of powder to form calcium sulfate dihydrate.[15] All remaining water occupies space in the cast, thereby reducing the compressive strength. Seemingly small volumes of water can exert significant effects upon the compressive strengths of dental casts. For example, if 30 rather than 27 mL of water is mixed with 100 g of Type III dental stone, the compressive strength will be reduced from 4,500 to 3,000 psi. As a result, manufacturers' recommendations for water-powder ratios should be strictly observed.

To ensure consistent water-powder ratios, all gypsum products should be measured by weight rather than by volume. Gypsum powder should be weighed in amounts suitable for pouring single impressions and stored in properly labeled, moisture-proof containers such as ointment jars (Fig 5-58). Usually 150 g is adequate for a single pour. This procedure will en-

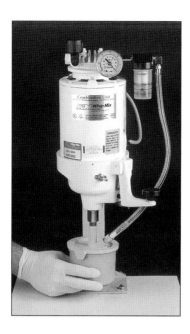

**Fig 5-59** Dental stone is mechanically spatulated under vacuum for 15 to 20 seconds.

sure a correct water-powder ratio, prevent deterioration, reduce waste, and promote efficiency.

Gypsum products should not be stored in open containers, where air exposure will cause the hemihydrate to absorb moisture from the air. Moisture contamination will cause the formation of calcium sulfate dihydrate crystals within the powder. This may accelerate or retard the setting of dental stone depending upon the severity of moisture contamination. Moisture contamination will reduce both the compressive strength and the surface hardness of the resultant casts.

### Mixing dental stone
The objective in mixing dental stone is to make a homogenous, bubble-free mix that will produce a dense, accurate cast. Water should be carefully measured and poured into a mixing bowl. Pre-weighed powder should be slowly sifted into the water to avoid air entrapment. The powder should be slowly incorporated into the water using a broad, stiff-bladed spatula. Care should be taken to avoid a whipping action, which would incorporate air into the mixture. Mixing should continue until a smooth consistency is achieved; 60 to 90 seconds usually is adequate. Prolonged spatulation, which can break up the crystals of gypsum that have formed and weaken the final cast, should be avoided. When possible, mechanical spatulation under vacuum should be used instead of hand mixing; mixing time

should then be reduced to 15 to 20 seconds (Fig 5-59). This process will provide reduced porosity in a mix of dental stone. After the mixing is complete, light vibration should be used to eliminate air inclusions.

### Pouring the cast
An acceptable impression can be ruined during pouring and trimming procedures. Therefore, the techniques for pouring and trimming diagnostic casts should be as exacting as those used for making master casts. A minimal expansion dental stone (ADA Type III or IV) should be used for diagnostic and master casts. Minimal expansion dental stones exhibit exceptional accuracy, surface detail, and abrasion resistance, and are therefore ideal for removable partial denture applications.

**Two-stage pour technique** Alginate impressions cannot be boxed and poured like complete denture impressions. Therefore, a two-stage technique should be employed for all casts used in the design and fabrication of removable partial dentures. The two-stage technique produces casts in which the teeth and soft tissue areas are the densest and most abrasion-resistant parts.

When a fresh mix of dental stone is tapped or vibrated, water immediately rises to the surface. If an impression is filled with dental stone and inverted so the teeth and residual ridges are facing upward, a similar process occurs. Manipulation, movement, or vi-

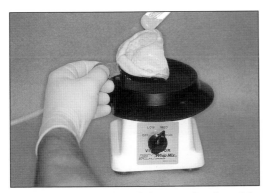

**Fig 5-60** The handle of the tray is placed in contact with a properly adjusted vibrator. Increments of stone are introduced and the impression is carefully filled.

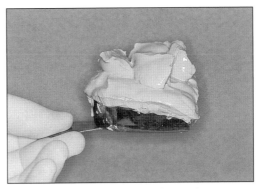

**Fig 5-61** Irregular mounds of dental stone are added to the exposed surface of the initial pour.

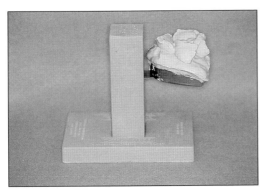

**Fig 5-62** The impression tray is suspended by its handle until the stone has reached its initial set.

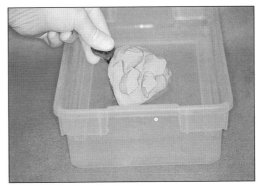

**Fig 5-63** The impression-cast assembly is placed in a container of clear slurry water for 4 to 5 minutes.

bration of the freshly mixed stone produces movement of water toward the surface of the impression. Therefore, the stone that makes up the teeth and residual ridges contains more water than do other portions of the cast. The surface of the resultant cast is weak and may be abraded easily. For these reasons, a single-stage or inversion technique should be avoided.

Pouring should be initiated within 12 minutes of impression removal. In the two-stage technique, an initial mix of stone is used to fill the impression. A small amount of stone should be added to one of the posterior extensions of the impression. The handle of the tray should be placed against a vibrator, and the impression tray should be tipped to permit a controlled flow of dental stone (Fig 5-60). The flow of the stone should be slow enough that it can be observed filling each individual tooth impression. Rapid flow or excessive vibration can cause air to be trapped at the impression-cast interface. Small increments of stone should be added

to the posterior extension of the impression until all borders are covered by 6 to 8 mm of stone. Stone should not be permitted to flow onto the sides of the impression tray because this will lock the cast onto the tray. The exposed surface of the poured stone should be left rough. Irregular mounds of stone should be added to this surface to provide locking undercuts for the second pour (Fig 5-61).

The tray should be suspended by the handle until the stone has reached its initial set (Fig 5-62). This should occur in 12 to 15 minutes. If any movement or vibration occurs during this period, water will rise toward the free surface of the dental stone, causing the stone in the anatomic portions of the cast to become more dense.

After the initial set, the impression-cast assembly should be placed in a bowl of clear slurry water for 4 to 5 minutes to thoroughly wet the first pour of dental stone (Fig 5-63). Clear slurry is a supersaturated solu-

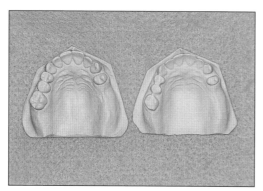

**Fig 5-64** Identical casts were stored in clear slurry water *(left)* and tap water *(right)* for 14 days. Notice the dissolution of the cast that was stored in tap water.

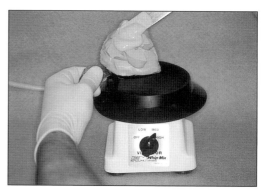

**Fig 5-65** A fresh mix of dental stone is prepared and vibrated onto the retentive nodules.

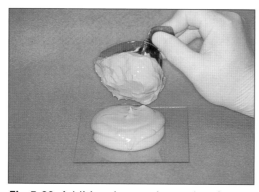

**Fig 5-66** Additional stone is used to form a patty. The impression is inverted and placed on the stone patty.

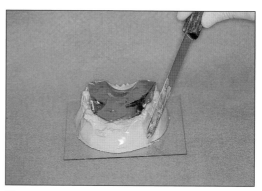

**Fig 5-67** A spatula is used to shape the base of the cast.

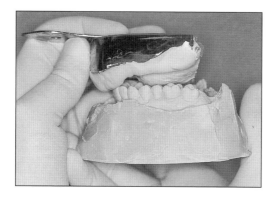

**Fig 5-68** The impression and cast are separated 45 to 60 minutes after initiation of the first pour.

tion of calcium sulfate made by placing chips of dental stone in water for 48 hours. Because it is a saturated solution, clear slurry permits wetting of the first pour without dissolution of the stone. A cast should never be soaked in tap or distilled water because dental stone is soluble in these liquids. If a stone cast is immersed in running water, its linear dimensions may decrease approximately 0.1% for every 20 minutes of exposure (Fig 5-64).

After the first pour has soaked for 5 minutes, a second mix of dental stone is prepared as described earlier. Some of the freshly mixed stone should be vibrated onto the roughened surface of the first mix (Fig 5-65). The remaining stone should be used to form a

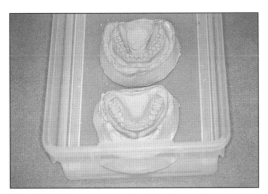

Fig 5-69 Casts are soaked in clear slurry water before grinding procedures are undertaken.

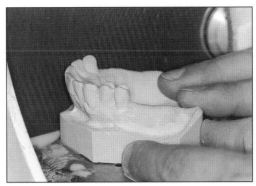

Fig 5-70 If a cast is not soaked, grinding residue will stick to the surface of the cast and compromise its accuracy.

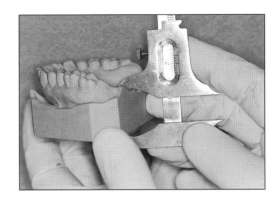

Fig 5-71 The base of the maxillary cast is trimmed until it is 10 to 13 mm at its thinnest point.

patty, and the impression should be inverted and placed onto this patty of stone (Fig 5-66). A spatula or similar instrument should be used to shape the base of the cast (Fig 5-67). In the case of a mandibular impression, the tongue space should be smoothed. Special care should be taken to avoid locking the stone onto the impression tray.

Between 45 and 60 minutes after the first pour, the cast and impression should be separated (Fig 5-68). An alginate impression should not be allowed to remain in contact with the associated cast for more than 60 minutes. Extended contact between alginate and dental stone will result in etching of the cast surface.

### Trimming the cast

Each dental cast should be soaked in clear slurry water (Fig 5-69) to facilitate grinding procedures and to prevent stone residue from sticking to the surface of the cast. A dry cast placed on a cast trimmer acts like a blotter or sponge. Grinding residue from the cast trim-

mer is absorbed onto the surface of the cast and is impossible to remove (Fig 5-70). Attempts to eliminate the residue with a brush will cause damage to the surface of the cast. The most effective way to avoid this problem is to wet the cast thoroughly before shaping it on the cast trimmer. The practitioner also must ensure that an adequate stream of water is flowing through the cast trimmer during the grinding process. In addition, a pan of clear slurry water should be positioned next to the cast trimmer so grinding residue may be rinsed from the cast periodically.

The base of the cast should be trimmed so that the occlusal surfaces of the teeth are parallel to the base. The base should be trimmed until it is 10 to 13 mm thick at its thinnest point, usually the center of the hard palate for a maxillary cast and the depth of the lingual sulcus for a mandibular cast (Fig 5-71).

The posterior border of the cast should be trimmed to form an angle of 90 degrees with the base. When viewed from an occlusal perspective, the poste-

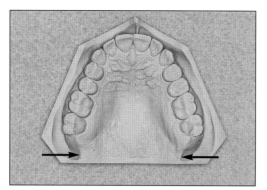

**Fig 5-72** Important structures such as the hamular notches *(arrows)* and tuberosities of the maxillary cast have remained intact.

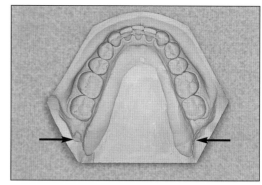

**Fig 5-73** The retromolar pads *(arrows)* have been preserved on the completed mandibular cast.

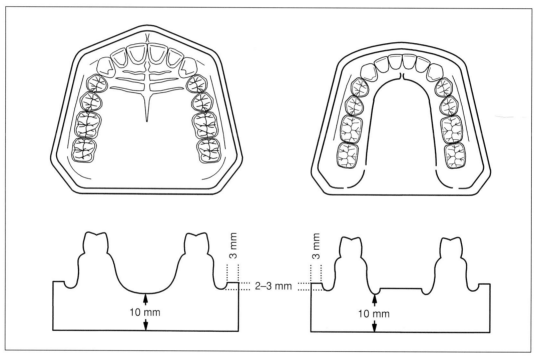

**Fig 5-74** Specifications for trimming maxillary *(left)* and mandibular *(right)* casts.

rior surface should be perpendicular to the midline of the palate. Care should be taken to preserve essential landmarks such as the hamular notches and tuberosities of a maxillary cast and the retromolar pads of a mandibular cast (Figs 5-72 and 5-73).

The sides of the cast should be trimmed at 90 degrees to the base (Fig 5-74). Care should be taken to avoid overtrimming the lateral aspects of a cast, which could eliminate the vestibular and buccal shelf areas. A land area of 2 to 3 mm should be maintained around the entire cast. The sides of the cast should be joined to the posterior surface by trimming just posterior to the hamular notches or retromolar pads (see Fig 5-74). As mentioned earlier, overtrimming these areas must be avoided. The hamular notches and retromolar pads are essential landmarks that must be preserved.

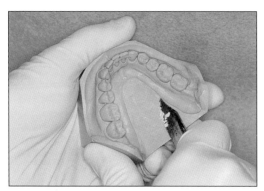

**Fig 5-75** The tongue space of the mandibular cast is trimmed flat. The integrity of the lingual sulcus is maintained.

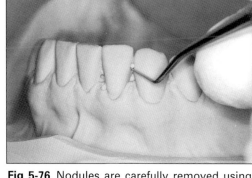

**Fig 5-76** Nodules are carefully removed using a fine, pointed instrument.

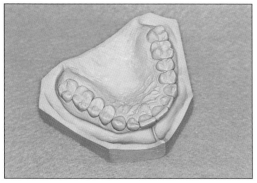

**Fig 5-77** An accurate and properly trimmed maxillary cast.

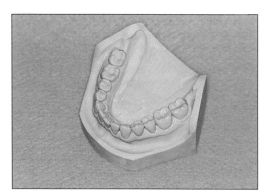

**Fig 5-78** An accurate and properly trimmed mandibular cast.

The anterior borders of maxillary and mandibular casts should be trimmed differently (see Fig 5-74). The anterior border of a maxillary cast should be angular, originating from the canine area on each side and extending to a point anterior to the central incisors. The anterior border of a mandibular cast should be gently curved, originating from the canine area on one side of the arch extending to the opposite canine area. The curve should follow the form of the arch. In both instances, care should be taken to avoid damage to the teeth and vestibular areas.

The tongue space should be trimmed flat, while maintaining the integrity of the lingual frenum and the lingual sulcus (Fig 5-75). Nodules of stone caused by voids in the impression should be carefully removed from noncritical areas (Fig 5-76). After thoroughly soaking the cast in clear slurry water, voids in the base and other noncritical areas of the cast should be filled with a thin mix of stone. Accurate, properly trimmed casts are essential in a wide variety of dental procedures. As a result, care must be taken to ensure that impressions and casts accurately represent the hard and soft tissue contours of the oral cavity (Figs 5-77 and 5-78).

### Causes of surface roughness on dental casts

There are several potential causes of surface roughness on dental casts. Perhaps the most common cause of surface roughness is adherence of alginate impression material to the enamel. This produces localized tearing of the impression material and results in noticeable surface irregularities on cast surfaces. If surface roughness is a consistent problem, one should suspect incompatibility between the alginate and the stone used for pouring the cast. Changing the brand of either the alginate or stone may correct the problem.

Surface roughness also may be caused by saliva or other fluids on the surface of an impression. Unwanted liquids should be eliminated from an impression by blotting with a dry tissue. As mentioned earlier, compressed air should not be used because it may cause dehydration and distortion of the impression material. Other possible causes of irregular surfaces on a cast include insufficient spatulation of the alginate, premature removal of an impression from the mouth, insufficient spatulation of dental stone, the use of contaminated stone, or the use of a single-pour technique.

It is also important to remember that an alginate impression should be removed from the cast 45 to 60 minutes after completion of the first pour. Leaving the impression in contact with the cast for an extended period may cause etching of the cast surface. This produces a soft, chalky surface. There is also danger that the cast will be abraded as the alginate shrinks and hardens.

A summary of the causes and solutions for common problems associated with diagnostic casts is presented in Table 5-2 at the end of the chapter.

## Length of appointment

Most practicing dentists will use auxiliary personnel to assist in completion of the health questionnaire, to record the blood pressure, to perform oral prophylaxis, and to make and develop radiographs. The patient interview, preliminary examination, and diagnostic impression procedures can easily be completed in a 1-hour appointment if the procedures are efficiently organized. Dental students, who will likely be completing all the steps themselves will probably require 3 to 4 hours to complete the first diagnostic appointment.

**Table 5-1** Causes and solutions for common problems associated with making diagnostic alginate impressions

| Problem | Probable cause | Solution |
|---|---|---|
| 1. Alginate sticks to teeth | Teeth too clean from overly vigorous pumicing | Pumice lightly; delay impression making until after thorough prophylaxis; use silicone as protective coating for teeth |
| | Teeth too dry | Avoid air drying of teeth; isolate arch with gauze packs |
| | Loss of protective film from teeth due to repeated impressions | Use good technique so repeated impressions not necessary; delay impression until another day |
| | Any of the above | Use silicone protective film; have patient suck on sour (citrus) candy or swish with whole milk |
| 2. Voids in impression | Poor mix of alginate | Spatulate for 45 to 60 seconds by hand or 15 seconds mechanically; wipe alginate along side of bowl during spatulation; use mechanical spatulation under vacuum |
| | Alginate did not flow to all areas | Wipe alginate on teeth, on palate, and into vestibular areas after mouth has been isolated with gauze packs; avoid mix that is too thick or too thin by using correct water-powder ratio; measure alginate by weight, not volume; avoid deterioration of alginate by heat or moisture contamination |
| 3. Peripheral underextension | Alginate did not flow into peripheral areas or poor mix of alginate | See No. 2 |
| | Tray too small, so material not carried into vestibule | Use tray with 5- to 7-mm clearance |
| | Tray incorrectly seated | Center tray with handle pointing straight out of mouth; retract lips with fingers so correct position of tray can be seen; seat tray so borders go below gingival marginal areas; avoid overly large trays, which will interfere with coronoid processes of mandible |
| | Cheeks, lips, or floor of mouth trapped under tray | Pull out cheeks; retract lips; have patient protrude tongue before final seating of tray |
| 4. Alginate tears when impression removed | Mix of alginate is too thin or too thick | Use water-powder ratio recommended by manufacturer; measure alginate by weight instead of volume; avoid deterioration of alginate by heat or moisture |
| | Impression removed from mouth too soon | Keep impression in mouth 2 to 3 min after it loses its tackiness |
| | Inadequate bulk of alginate | Select tray with 5- to 7-mm clearance; center tray properly; relieve modeling plastic used to modify tray |
| | Use of deteriorated alginate | Store bulk alginate in airtight containers at room temperature |
| | Prolonged or insufficient spatulation | Spatulate for 45 to 60 seconds by hand or 15 seconds mechanically |
| | Improper removal from mouth | Avoid rocking or teasing out of impression; remove with snap, applying force along long axes of teeth |

**Table 5-1 (cont)** Causes and solutions for common problems associated with making diagnostic alginate impressions

| Problem | Probable cause | Solution |
|---|---|---|
| 5. Lack of detail or grainy appearance | Prolonged or insufficient spatulation | Spatulate for 45 to 60 seconds by hand or 15 seconds mechanically |
| | Insufficient flow of material | Use tray that confines alginate; use correct water-powder ratio to avoid a mix that is too thin or too thick; measure by weight; avoid deterioration of alginate by heat or moisture |
| | Impression removed from mouth too soon | Hold steady in mouth for 2 to 3 min after tackiness is gone from alginate surface |
| 6. Alginate sets before tray completely seated | Mixing water too warm | Use water temperature of 22°C (72°F), or lower if more working time required |
| | Particles of dental stone (calcium sulfate) in mixing bowl | Use different mixing bowls and spatulas for alginate and stone |
| | Prolonged spatulation of alginate | Spatulate for 45 to 60 seconds by hand or 15 seconds mechanically |
| | Use of deteriorated alginate | Store at room temperature; avoid moisture contamination by measuring and sealing all contents of bulk containers of alginate |
| | Layer of material painted in mouth too thin | Wipe larger amounts onto teeth and into vestibules; introduce tray immediately by having tray filled before painting in mouth |
| | Fast-set alginate used | Use regular-set alginate |
| 7. Patient gags when tray is fit or impression made | Patient is fearful and lacks confidence in dentist | Proceed with confident, well-organized manner; use simple explanations; avoid talk about gagging |
| | Alginate flowing out of tray and into patient's throat | Seat patient upright with occlusal plane parallel with floor; correct maxillary tray with modeling plastic; avoid overfilling of tray |
| | Patient tense | Instruct patient to keep eyes open and focused on a small object; instruct patient to breathe through nose at normal rate |
| | Palate numb because of use of topical anesthetic | Avoid topical anesthetics; use astringent mouthwash and cold water rinses instead |
| | Patient has severe gag reflex | Ask patient to hold breath while tray is fit or corrected; use the "leg-lift" procedure; use fast-set alginate or accelerate the set of alginate by using warmer water |
| 8. Alginate displaced by saliva in palate | Mucinous saliva not removed from palate | Have patient use astringent mouthwash and cold water rinse; wipe and isolate palate with 2 × 2–inch gauze |
| | Excessive secretion by palatal mucous glands | Use warm gauze pads to milk palatal glands, followed by cold pads to constrict gland openings |
| | Patient produces copious amounts of saliva | Premedicate with 15 mg of propantheline bromide (Pro-Banthine, Searle, San Juan, Puerto Rico) 30 min before procedure if no contraindications |
| 9. Alginate pulled away from tray | Alginate not forced under rim lock | Use small increments and force alginate into rim lock areas |
| | Alginate does not stick to modeling plastic | Use alginate to coat entire inner surfaces of tray and modeling plastic |
| | Alginate stuck to teeth | See No. 1 |

**Table 5-2** Causes and solutions for common problems associated with casts made from alginate impressions

| Problem | Probable cause | Solution |
|---|---|---|
| 1. Cast has rough surface | Incompatibility between alginate and dental stone | Change brand of alginate or stone to obtain compatible combination |
| | Insufficient spatulation of stone | Spatulate until smooth homogenous mix is attained (60 to 90 seconds by hand or 15 to 20 seconds by mechanical spatulation under vacuum) |
| | Sticking of alginate to teeth | See No. 1 in Table 5-1 |
| | Saliva retained on impression | Rinse in running water until alginate has rough feel; use soap suds and camel-hair brush to remove saliva; use dry dental stone as a disclosing agent and remove saliva with camel-hair brush and running water |
| | Water left on impression | Blot water with dry tissue paper; avoid use of compressed air |
| | Poor mix of alginate; insufficient spatulation | Spatulate for 45 to 60 seconds by hand or 15 seconds mechanically |
| | Use of single-pour technique; water rose to tissue/tooth surface of impression | Use two-stage pour technique |
| 2. Surface of cast has chalky appearance | Incompatible alginate-stone combination | Change brand of alginate or stone to obtain compatible combination |
| | Film of stone slurry on cast after dry cast trimmed on model trimmer | Thoroughly soak cast in clear slurry water before trimming; rinse periodically in clear slurry water while trimming |
| | Impression left in contact with cast for prolonged period | Separate impression from cast 45 to 60 min after first pour |
| 3. Cast has a soft surface | Too much water in mix of stone | Use acceptable water-powder ratio; measure stone by weight instead of volume |
| | Use of inverted single-stage pour technique; water rose to tissue/tooth surface of impression | Use two-stage pour technique |
| | Use of moisture-contaminated stone | Premeasure stone and store in airtight container; avoid use of open bins for stone storage |
| | Water or stone powder added to improper water-powder ratio mix after mixing has been started | Measure correct amount of water and weigh correct amount of stone for acceptable water-powder ratio |
| | Stone spatulated too long | Spatulate for 60 to 90 seconds by hand or 15 to 20 seconds mechanically |
| 4. Cast breaks when impression separated from cast | Premature removal of impression from cast | Separate cast from impression 45 to 60 min after first pour |
| | Too much water in mix of stone | Measure water and weigh powder for correct water-powder ratio |
| | Use of single-stage pour technique | Use two-stage pour technique |
| | Water left in tooth impression | Blot all water with dry tissue paper |
| | Low compressive strength of dental stone because of moisture-contaminated stone, adding powder or water while mixing stone, or prolonged spatulation | Store stone correctly; measure water and weigh powder before mixing; spatulate for 60 to 90 seconds by hand or 15 to 20 seconds mechanically |
| | Alginate impression left in contact with cast overnight | Separate impression from cast 45 to 60 min after first pour |

**Table 5-2 (cont)** Causes and solutions for common problems associated with casts made from alginate impressions

| Problem | Probable cause | Solution |
|---|---|---|
| 5. Separation of cast between first and second pours of stone | Failure to leave surface of first pour with mechanical retention for second pour | Leave surface of first pour rough; add small irregular mounds of stone to soft surface of first pour |
| | Failure to thoroughly wet first pour before adding second pour | After initial set of first pour, soak cast and impression in clear slurry water for 5 min |
| 6. Voids in surface of cast | Air trapped in mix of stone because of inadequate or improper mixing | Sift powder into water to avoid air entrapment; hand spatulate 60 to 90 seconds, avoiding any whipping action, or mechanically mix stone under vacuum for 15 to 20 seconds; lightly vibrate mix until no more air bubbles come to surface |
| | Cast poured too rapidly and air trapped on surface of impression | Add small increments of stone to the same posterior extension of impression with light vibration and allow stone to flow slowly to fill all areas of impression |
| | Overvibration during pouring | Use light vibration only; flowing stone should not bounce |
| 7. Underextension of cast | Cast overtrimmed; hamular notch, retromolar pad, or vestibular areas obliterated | Take care in trimming of casts on model trimmer to avoid removal of critical areas |
| | First pour of alginate did not cover all peripheral areas of impression | Fill impression completely and cover all peripheral border areas with 5 to 6 mm of stone during first stage of pour |
| | Peripheral underextension of alginate impression | See No. 3 in Table 5-1 |
| 8. Erratic setting time of stone | Contamination of stone by heat or moisture | Pre-weigh and store stone in airtight containers |
| 9. Cast is inaccurate; not a true reproduction of the anatomy of the mouth | Loss of moisture content of impression because of syneresis, resulting in release of strains | Pour cast within 12 min after removal of impression from mouth; avoid excessive drying of impression |
| | Release of strains and swelling due to water | Do not store impression in water or other solutions; do not wrap impression in wet paper towel |
| | Strains or distortion in impression caused by its movement during gelation | Maintain impression in position until it is ready for removal; do not have assistant or patient hold impression |
| | Impression removed before gelation complete | Maintain impression in position for 2 to 3 min after alginate has lost its tackiness |
| | Strains induced in impression during its removal from mouth | Remove impression with a snap, applying force directly along long axes of teeth |
| | Use of nonrigid impression tray | Avoid use of trays that lack rigidity |
| | Use of inaccurate impression | See Table 5-1 |
| | Surface of cast lost by washing or soaking cast in tap water | Use clear slurry water whenever cast needs to be soaked or washed |
| | Teeth contacted tray during making of impression, allowing stone to flow between impression and tray | Retract lips for good visibility when seating tray; seat tray slightly beyond the landmark of the gingival margins |
| | Alginate displaced or strains induced by setting tray on bench top | Suspend tray by its handle in a tray holder or a slightly opened drawer |
| | Distortion in palate due to failure to correct tray | Correct palatal area of maxillary tray with modeling plastic; after modeling plastic chilled, trim to provide 5- to 7-mm clearance for alginate |

## ⊔ References

1. The sixth report of the Joint National Committee on prevention, detection, evaluation, and treatment of high blood pressure. Arch Intern Med 1997;157:2413–2446.

2. Little JW. The impact on dentistry of recent advances in the management of hypertension. Oral Surg Oral Med Oral Pathol Oral Radiol Endod 2000;90:591–599.

3. McInnes GT. Integrated approaches to management of hypertension: Promoting treatment acceptance. Am Heart J 1999:138:252–255.

4. Boucher CO (ed). Swenson's Complete Dentures, ed 6. St. Louis: Mosby, 1970.

5. DeVan MM. The transition from natural to artificial teeth. J Prosthet Dent 1961;11:677–688.

6. House MM. Full denture technique. Prepared from the notes of Study Club #1 by Conley FJ, Dunn AL, Quesnall AJ, Rogers RM. September 1950.

7. Sonis ST. Sonis AL, Lieberman A. Oral complications in patients receiving treatment for malignancies other than of the head and neck. J Am Dent Assoc 1978;97:468–472.

8. Kaufman DW, Kelly JP, Rosenberg L, Anderson TE, Mitchell AA. Recent patterns of medication use in the ambulatory adult population of the United States: The Slone survey. JAMA 2002;287:337–344.

9. Anusavice KJ (ed). Phillips' Science of Dental Materials, ed 10. Philadelphia: Saunders, 1996.

10. Combe EC, Burke FJT, Douglas WH. Dental Biomaterials. Boston: Kluwer, 1999:294.

11. Miller MW. Syneresis in alginate impression materials. Br Dent J 1975;139:425–430.

12. Osborne J, Lammie GA. The manipulation of alginate impression material. Br Dent J 1954;96:51–58.

13. Rudd KD, Morrow RM, Rhodes JE. Dental Laboratory Procedures. Vol 3: Removable partial dentures. St. Louis: Mosby, 1986:6.

14. Skinner EW, Carlisle FB. The use of alginate impression materials in the Sears' hydrocolloid impression technique. J Prosthet Dent 1956;6:405–411.

15. Craig RG, Powers JM (eds). Restorative Dental Materials, ed 11. St. Louis: Mosby, 2002.

## ⊔ Bibliography

Anderson JN. Flow and elasticity in alginates. Dent Prog 1970;1:63–70.

Ayers HD Jr, Phillips RW, Dell A, Henry RW. Detail duplication test used to evaluate elastic impression materials. J Prosthet Dent 1960;10:374–380.

Bergman B, Ericson G. Cross-sectional study of the periodontal status of removable partial denture patients. J Prosthet Dent 1989;61:208–210.

Beumer J III, Curtis TA, Morrish RB Jr. Radiation complications in edentulous patients. J Prosthet Dent 1976;36:193–203.

Chandler JA, Brudvik JS. Clinical evaluation of patients eight to nine years after placement of removable partial dentures. J Prosthet Dent 1984;58:736–743.

Dao N, Caputo AA, Lucatorto FM, Matyas J. Effects of disinfectants on dimensional accuracy of impression materials. J Prosthet Dent 1990;64:25–31.

Deneen LJ, Heid DW, Smith AA. Effective interpersonal and management skills in dentistry. J Am Dent Assoc 1973;87:878–880.

Drennon DG, Johnson GH, Powell GL. The accuracy and efficacy of disinfection by spray atomization on elastomeric impressions. J Prosthet Dent 1989;62:468–475.

Fleece L, Linton P, Dudley B. Rapid elimination of a hyperactive gag reflex. J Prosthet Dent 1988;60:415–417.

Gordon GE, Johnson GH, Drennon DG. The effect of tray selection on the accuracy of elastomeric impression materials. J Prosthet Dent 1990;63:12–15.

Harris WT Jr. Water temperature and accuracy of alginate impressions. J Prosthet Dent 1969;21:613–617.

Herrera SP, Merchant VA. Disinfection of alginate, polysulfide, vinyl polysiloxane and polyether dental impressions. J Dent Res 1985;64:194.

House MM. Full denture technique. Notes of House Study Club No. 1, 1960.

House MM. An outline for examination of mouth condition. Dominion Dent J 1921;33:97–100.

Kaiser DA, Nicholls JI. A study of distortion and surface hardness of improved artificial stone casts. J Prosthet Dent 1976;36:373–381.

Katberg JW. Cross-contamination via the prosthodontic laboratory. J Prosthet Dent 1974;32:412–419.

Krol AJ. A new approach to the gagging problem. J Prosthet Dent 1963;13:611–616.

Look JO, Clay DJ, Gong G, Messer HH. Preliminary results from disinfection of irreversible hydrocolloid impressions. J Prosthet Dent 1990;63:701–707.

Merchant HW, Carr AA. Blood pressure measurement: Problems and solutions. J Am Dent Assoc 1977;95:98–102.

Morrow RM, Brown CE Jr, Stansbury BE, DeLorimier JA, Powell JM, Rudd KD. Compatibility of alginate impression materials and dental stones. J Prosthet Dent 1971;25:556–566.

Nassif J. A self administered questionnaire—An aid in managing complete denture patients. J Prosthet Dent 1978;40:363–366.

Phillips RW, Price RR, Renking RH. The use of alginate for indirect restorations. J Am Dent Assoc 1953;46:393–403.

Phoenix RD. Department of Prosthodontics Junior Complete Denture Clinical Manual. San Antonio: Univ of Texas Health Science Center at San Antonio Dental School, 2000.

Pierce LH, Goodkind RJ. A status report of possible risks of base metal alloys and their components. J Prosthet Dent 1989;62:234–238.

Plainfield S. Communication distortion. The language of patients and practitioners of dentistry. J Prosthet Dent 1969;22:11–19.

Rahn AO, Matalon V, Drane JB. Prosthetic evaluation of patients who have received irradiation to the head and neck regions. J Prosthet Dent 1968;19:174–178.

Rowe AH, Forrest JO. Dental impressions: The probability of contamination and a method of disinfection. Br Dent J 1978;145:184–186.

Rudd KD, Morrow RM. Premedication: An aid in obtaining accurate complete denture impressions. J Prosthet Dent 1967;18:86–89.

Rudd KD, Morrow RM, Bange AA. Accurate casts. J Prosthet Dent 1969;21:545–554.

Rudd KD, Morrow RM, Brown CE Jr, Powell JM, Rahe AJ. Comparison of effects of tap water and slurry water on gypsum casts. J Prosthet Dent 1970;24:563–570.

Rudd KD, Morrow RM, Strunk RR. Accurate alginate impressions. J Prosthet Dent 1969;22:294–300.

Sauser CW. Pretreatment evaluation of partially edentulous patients. J Prosthet Dent 1961;11:886–893.

Schelb E, Cavazos E, Kaiser DA, Troendle K. Compatibility of Type IV dental stones with polyether impression material. J Prosthet Dent 1988;60:540–544.

Schutt RW. Bactericidal effect of a disinfectant dental stone on irreversible hydrocolloid impressions and stone casts. J Prosthet Dent 1989;62:605–606.

Tolentino AT. Prosthetic management of patients with pemphigus vulgaris. J Prosthet Dent 1977;38:254–260.

# The Second Diagnostic Appointment

The second diagnostic appointment should be used to complete the collection and evaluation of diagnostic data. A definitive oral examination is essential. The patient's occlusion should be evaluated. Radiograph findings should be correlated with the clinical findings. Medical and dental consultations should be requested if necessary.

## ❏ Mounted Diagnostic Casts

Mounted diagnostic casts are fundamental diagnostic aids in dentistry (Fig 6-1). Therefore, mounting procedures should be accomplished with great care. Accurately mounted diagnostic casts may be used in the following ways:

1. Accurately mounted diagnostic casts supplement examination of the oral cavity. Malpositioned teeth, low-hanging tuberosities, compromised interarch space, and defective restorations are readily apparent when accurate casts are correctly mounted on a suitable articulator.

2. Accurately mounted casts permit detailed analysis of a patient's occlusion. Mounted casts permit improved visual access, unimpeded by the patient's lips, cheeks, and tongue. Therefore, the dentist may evaluate occlusal relationships from facial and lingual perspectives. The resultant information may be essential in treatment planning and prosthesis design.

3. Mounted casts are helpful in patient education. By viewing accurately mounted casts, patients may gain an improved understanding of existing oral conditions, proposed treatment regimens, and potential difficulties.

4. Accurately mounted casts provide a record of the patient's condition before treatment. This record can be of great value if a conflict should arise during the course of treatment.

The primary objective of a diagnostic mounting procedure is to properly position the diagnostic casts on a dental articulator. To accomplish this objective, the casts must be properly related to one another, and to the opening/closing axis of the articulator. For purposes of discussion, a diagnostic mounting procedure

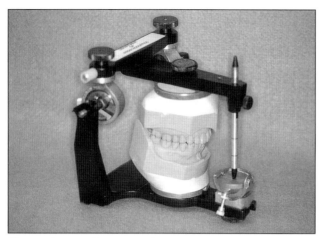

**Fig 6-1** Accurately mounted diagnostic casts are an essential part of diagnosis and treatment planning.

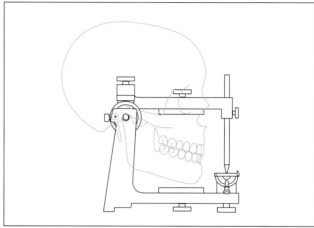

**Fig 6-2** The three-dimensional relationship between a patient's maxillary arch and the mandibular condyles must be simulated in the diagnostic mounting. A facebow is used to record this relationship and transfer it to an articulator.

may be divided into three distinct phases. These phases may be described as follows:

1. Orientation of the maxillary cast to the condylar elements of an articulator by means of a facebow transfer.
2. Orientation of the mandibular cast to the maxillary cast at the patient's centric jaw relation by means of an accurate centric relation record.
3. Verification of these relationships by means of additional centric relation records and comparison of occlusal contacts on the articulator with those in the mouth.

## Facebow transfer

The first step in a diagnostic mounting procedure involves mounting the maxillary cast on a semiadjustable articulator. The three-dimensional relationship between the patient's maxillary arch and mandibular condyles must be simulated in the diagnostic mounting. To accomplish this, the maxillary cast must be related to the condylar elements of the articulator exactly as the maxillary arch is related to the patient's condyles (Fig 6-2). A facebow transfer provides this orientation.

There are numerous facebows available to the clinician. It is necessary to select a facebow that is compatible with the articulator that is to be used. For purposes of explanation, a Hanau Spring-Bow and a

Hanau Wide-Vue articulator (Waterpik, Fort Collins, CO) will be described.

### Equipment and supplies for facebow transfer

The following equipment and supplies are needed for a facebow transfer:

1. Accurate maxillary cast
2. Semiadjustable articulator
3. Facebow and bite fork compatible with the chosen articulator
4. Red cake modeling plastic
5. Bunsen burner
6. Millimeter ruler and marking pencil
7. Dental stone, mixing bowl, and spatula
8. Stone-separating medium (Super-Sep, Kerr, Romulus, MI)

### True hinge axis

The most accurate method for making a facebow transfer is to determine the patient's true hinge axis and to use this axis in positioning the facebow. However, locating a patient's true hinge axis is time consuming and often unnecessary.

Arbitrary hinge axis points may be located using various methods. These points have proven acceptable in more than 90% of patients. Consequently, most facebow procedures are based upon arbitrary axis points.

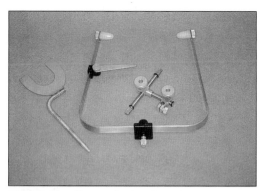

**Fig 6-3** The Hanau Spring-Bow is an arbitrary facebow. Like many arbitrary facebows, the Spring-Bow is placed into the patient's ears.

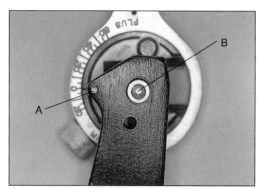

**Fig 6-4** The chosen articulator should include orientation pins (A), which facilitate placement of the facebow. These pins relate the facebow to the opening and closing axis of the articulator (B).

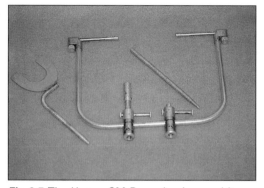

**Fig 6-5** The Hanau SM Bow also is an arbitrary facebow. When using this facebow, the posterior styli are placed against prescribed points on the patient's skin.

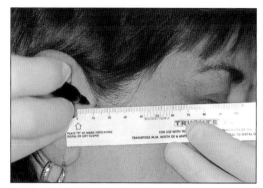

**Fig 6-6** Beyron's point is located 13 mm anterior to the margin of the tragus on an imaginary line connecting the tragus and the outer canthus of the eye. This point should be marked to permit ease of identification.

## Arbitrary hinge axis

The selection of arbitrary hinge axis points is dependent upon the type of facebow and articulator being used. Many facebows such as the Hanau Spring-Bow are placed into the patient's ears, much like a stethoscope (Fig 6-3). These "ear-type" facebows record the positions of the external auditory openings. Because the external auditory openings are superior and posterior to a patient's true hinge axis, some correction is necessary. This correction is accomplished when the facebow is transferred to a corresponding articulator (Fig 6-4). The distance and direction of this correction is determined by the manufacturer and is based upon anatomic averages. The result is an estimated or "arbitrary" hinge axis.

Other facebows such as the Hanau SM (Fig 6-5) require that the styli be placed at prescribed points on the face. Several arbitrary axis points have been described. One of the most commonly used points is Beyron's point. To locate Beyron's point, the operator must establish an imaginary line connecting the posterior margin of the tragus with the outer canthus of the eye. Using this line as a reference, the operator identifies and marks a point 13 mm anterior to the margin of the tragus. The same procedure is accomplished on the opposite side of the patient's face (Fig 6-6). Subsequently, the facebow is placed and the styli are positioned over the predetermined marks. The styli establish an arbitrary hinge axis that can be transferred to an articulator.

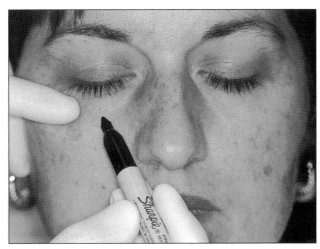

Fig 6-7 The infraorbital notch serves as an anterior point of reference when using a Hanau facebow. The infraorbital notch also should be marked for ease of identification.

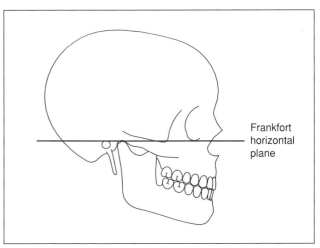

Fig 6-8 The plane established by the external auditory openings and the infraborbital notch is approximately parallel to the Frankfort horizontal plane.

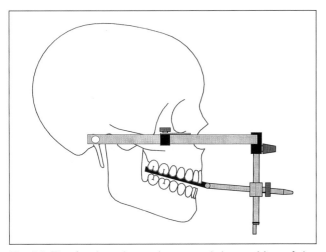

Fig 6-9 The facebow is used to record the position of the maxillary arch relative to the mandibular condyles.

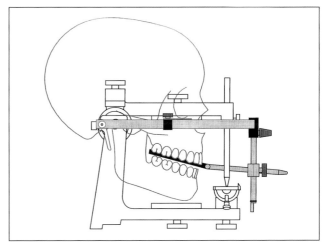

Fig 6-10 The spatial information recorded in Fig 6-9 then is transferred to an appropriate articulator. This permits proper orientation of the maxillary cast on the articulator.

### Anterior or third point of reference

An anterior or third point of reference is recommended for positioning a facebow on a patient's face. Different articulator and facebow combinations require different anterior points of reference, so it is important to follow the manufacturer's recommendations. As an example, the infraorbital notch is selected when a Hanau facebow is used (Fig 6-7). The plane established by the external auditory openings and the infraorbital notch is approximately parallel to the Frankfort horizontal plane (Fig 6-8). This allows the dentist to record the orientation of the maxillary arch using the Frankfort horizontal as a reference. When the facebow is transferred to the articulator, the Frankfort horizontal may be reestablished in relation to the upper member of the articulator (Figs 6-9 and 6-10). This permits proper orientation of the maxillary cast on the articulator. Proper orientation of the maxillary cast is essential in occlusal analysis, tooth arrangement, and esthetic evaluation. Therefore, the use of an anterior point of reference is strongly recommended.

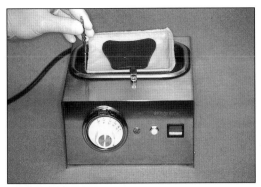

**Fig 6-11** Red cake modeling plastic is heated in a water bath maintained at 60°C (140°F).

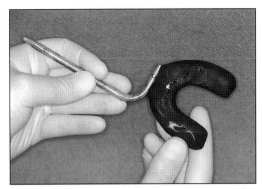

**Fig 6-12** When heated, red cake modeling plastic is adapted to a bite fork.

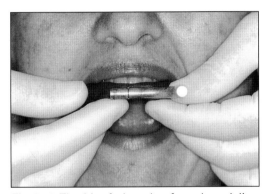

**Fig 6-13** The bite fork and softened modeling plastic are positioned over the maxillary teeth and gentle pressure is applied.

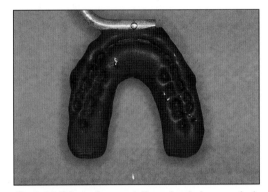

**Fig 6-14** When the modeling plastic has cooled, the bite fork is removed from the mouth. Indentations produced by the maxillary incisal and occlusal surfaces should be evident in the modeling plastic.

### Technique

The technical steps involved in making a facebow transfer vary somewhat depending on the facebow and articulator being used. However, the following steps apply for all facebow procedures:

1. Preparation of bite fork
2. Orientation of facebow to bite fork and reference points
3. Orientation of facebow to articulator
4. Attachment of maxillary cast to articulator

**Preparation of bite fork** A cake of red modeling plastic should be softened in a water bath at 60°C (140°F) and adapted to both sides of a bite fork (Figs 6-11 and 6-12). While the modeling plastic is still soft, the bite fork should be properly positioned in the mouth (Fig 6-13). The dentist should apply gentle pressure to en-

sure that the surfaces of the maxillary teeth are accurately recorded. The patient should then be directed to close lightly into the modeling plastic on the underside of the bite fork. The dentist should maintain the position of the bite fork until the modeling plastic has cooled.

When the modeling plastic has cooled, the bite fork should be removed from the mouth and inspected. Indentations produced by the incisal and occlusal surfaces should be evident in the modeling plastic (Fig 6-14). In addition, there should be no "show-through" of the underlying bite fork. If these conditions have been met, the modeling plastic should be chilled in ice water and trimmed so that only the indentations of the cusp tips remain (Fig 6-15).

If the remaining maxillary teeth are not widely distributed, stability of the modeling plastic record may be adversely affected. To address this problem, an accu-

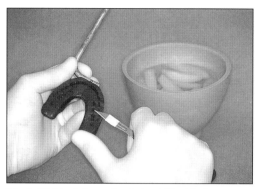

**Fig 6-15** Modeling plastic is chilled in ice water and properly trimmed.

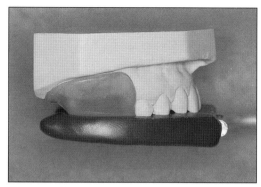

**Fig 6-16** If distribution of the remaining teeth will not permit accurate orientation of the associated dental cast, a well-adapted record base should be used. The record base provides increased contact with facebow assembly and permits a more accurate articulator mounting.

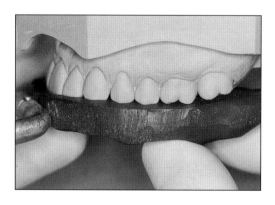

**Fig 6-17** The maxillary cast is placed into the modeling plastic record to verify accurate fit and stability.

rately fitting acrylic resin baseplate and wax occlusion rim should be fabricated on the maxillary cast. The baseplate and occlusion rim should be used to provide additional contact with the modeling plastic record (Fig 6-16) and improve accuracy of the facebow transfer.

After the record has been inspected and trimmed, the maxillary cast should be seated in the record to verify fit and stability (Fig 6-17). Before the cast is placed into the record, the maxillary cast should once again be inspected for inaccuracies. All nodules on the occlusal surfaces of the stone teeth should be removed. Subsequently, the maxillary cast should be placed into the imprints on the superior surface of the modeling plastic record. If the accuracy of the record is doubtful (eg, if the cast rocks or is not completely seated), the cuspal imprints may be corrected by gently heating the surface of the modeling plastic and repositioning the bite fork in the mouth. If the cast does not fit the mod-

eling plastic record following this process, inaccuracy of the maxillary cast should be suspected. The dentist must ensure the accuracy of the master cast and the modeling plastic record before proceeding.

**Orientation of facebow to bite fork and reference points** The bite fork and modeling plastic registration should be firmly seated on the patient's maxillary teeth. The patient should be directed to close into the indentations made by the mandibular teeth. In this manner, the patient can maintain the position of the bite fork with occlusal pressure. This frees the dentist's hands and facilitates placement of the facebow.

The following description relates to use of a Hanau Spring-Bow and a Hanau Wide-Vue articulator. If other combinations of facebows and articulators are used, appropriate departures from this description will be necessary.

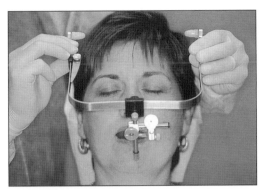

Fig 6-18 The bite fork is properly positioned on the patient's teeth; then the facebow is guided onto the stem of the bite fork.

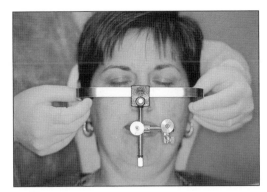

Fig 6-19 The earpieces of the facebow are gently guided into the external auditory openings.

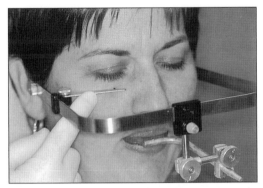

Fig 6-20 The orbital pointer is positioned to the level of the infraorbital notch.

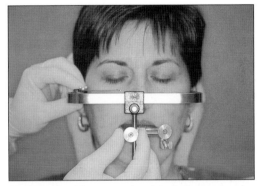

Fig 6-21 At this stage, the thumbscrews on the facebow are tightened. These screws maintain the spatial relationships between the facebow and the bite fork.

The Spring-Bow is an "ear-type" facebow. It is based upon anatomic averages and may be described as an arbitrary facebow. The styli of ear-type facebows are positioned in the external auditory openings. As a result, ear-type facebows are very convenient and are commonly used.

Clinically, a Spring-Bow should be guided onto the stem of the bite fork where it protrudes from the patient's mouth (Fig 6-18). The bow should then be stretched open and swung downward so the earpieces enter the external auditory openings on each side of the patient's face (Fig 6-19). The orbital indicator should be released and carefully rotated toward the patient until its tip approximates the infraorbital notch on the patient's right side (Fig 6-20). The bow should be raised or lowered to permit alignment of the orbital indicator with the lower border of the orbit (ie, orbitale). In this manner, the earpieces and orbital in-

dicator record the Frankfort horizontal plane. When this process has been completed, the three thumbscrews on the facebow should be tightened in proper sequence (Fig 6-21).

**Orientation of facebow to the articulator** The Hanau Wide-Vue is a semiadjustable articulator with a fixed intercondylar width. This type of instrument is adequate for most diagnostic procedures.

The following steps should be used in preparing the articulator and orienting the facebow to the articulator.

1. The articulator should be cleaned and properly adjusted. The condylar guidance should be set at 30 degrees, the lateral or Bennett guide at 15 degrees, and the incisal table at 0 degrees. The condylar balls should be locked in the rearmost position (Fig 6-22).

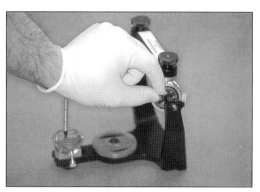

**Fig 6-22** An appropriate articulator is adjusted to receive the facebow. Condylar locking mechanisms are tightened.

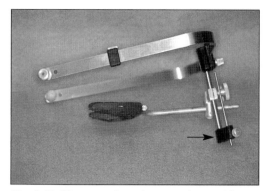

**Fig 6-23** The anterior elevator *(arrow)* is attached to the transfer rod.

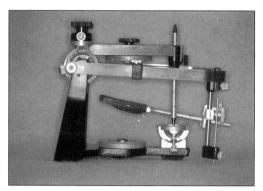

**Fig 6-24** The facebow is properly positioned on the articulator.

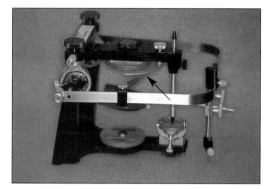

**Fig 6-25** The facebow is adjusted to the proper vertical position. The anterior elevator is adjusted to maintain this vertical position. *Arrow* indicates contact of orbital indicator with the orbital plane device.

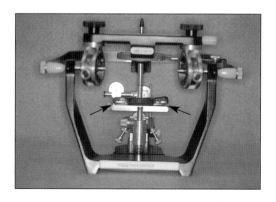

**Fig 6-26** The cast support is attached to the lower member of the articulator and adjusted to stabilize the bite fork. *Arrows* denote the bite fork resting lightly on the cast support.

2. The anterior elevator should be attached to the transfer rod. The elevating pin should be adjusted to its uppermost position and secured with the thumbscrew (Fig 6-23).
3. The Spring-Bow should be stretched open and the earpieces should be positioned on the auditory pins on the lateral aspects of the articulator. At this

stage, the anterior portion of the Spring-Bow should rest on the elevating pin (Fig 6-24).
4. The orbital plane device should be attached to the undersurface of the articulator's upper member. The anterior portion of the facebow should be raised or lowered until the superior surface of the orbital indicator contacts the undersurface of the orbital plane

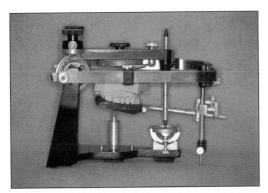

**Fig 6-27** The base of the maxillary cast is indexed, treated with an appropriate separating medium, and properly related to the indentations in the modeling plastic.

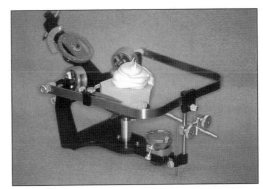

**Fig 6-28** A mixture of low-expansion dental stone is prepared and placed on the base of the cast.

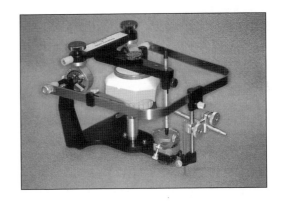

**Fig 6-29** The articulator is returned to a closed position. The mounting stone is shaped and smoothed.

device. The elevating pin should then be adjusted to maintain this vertical position (Fig 6-25).

5. The cast support should be attached to the lower member of the articulator and should be adjusted to stabilize the bite fork during mounting procedures (Fig 6-26).

**Attachment of maxillary cast to articulator** Following are the steps involved in attaching the maxillary cast to the articulator.

1. The base of the maxillary cast should be indexed, and an appropriate separating medium should be applied to the indices. At this stage, the maxillary cast should be properly seated in the modeling plastic record (Fig 6-27).
2. A mix of low-expansion dental stone should be prepared according to the manufacturer's directions. The upper member of the articulator should be raised to an open position, and the freshly prepared dental stone should be placed on the base of

the cast (Fig 6-28). This stone should extend superiorly so it will engage the upper mounting ring when the articulator is closed. The upper member of the articulator should be returned to the closed position. The dentist should ensure that the incisal pin is in contact with the incisal table. The dental stone should be contoured to engage the openings in the mounting ring. External contours should be smooth (Fig 6-29).

## *Centric relation record*

Centric relation is the physiologic relationship of the mandible to the maxilla when both condyles are properly related to their articular discs, and the condyle-disc assemblies are stabilized against the posterior slopes of the articular eminences. Hence, it is a bone-to-bone relationship of the mandible to the maxilla and is independent of tooth contact. This relationship is fundamental to any diagnostic evaluation of a patient's occlusion.

More than 90% of patients do not routinely close their jaws at the centric relation position. This occurs generally because the final stage of closure is guided by the occlusal and incisal surfaces of the remaining teeth. During this process, the teeth are directed toward a position of maximum contact termed *maximal intercuspal position*. To accommodate this position, one or both condyles may be forced to move anteriorly or anteriorly and laterally. When this occurs, maximal intercuspal position and centric relation do not coincide.

In spite of this phenomenon, diagnostic casts should be mounted at the patient's centric relation position for several reasons. From a muscular standpoint, centric relation is an extremely desirable position. The muscles associated with the articular disc and head of the condyle are in a relaxed state when the mandible assumes its centric relation position. Hence, there is a decreased likelihood of muscular fatigue and symptoms of temporomandibular dysfunction. In addition, centric relation is one of the few maxillomandibular relationships that can be repeatedly achieved. This permits fabrication of multiple records and verification of diagnostic mountings on a dental articulator.

Wear facets that are invariably present between centric relation and maximal intercuspal position attest to the fact that all patients close at centric relation at least part of the time. Interferences between centric relation and maximal intercuspal position are the most common causes of bruxism, accelerated wear, and temporomandibular dysfunction. These interferences are present to a much greater degree in partially edentulous patients because of tipping, drifting, and extrusion of teeth, which commonly occur when continuity of a dental arch is lost.

The decision whether to construct the prosthesis at centric relation or maximal intercuspal position must be made following consideration of all diagnostic data. With the exception of a small percentage of patients whose centric relation and maximal intercuspal positions coincide, a patient must be assisted or guided when the centric relation is recorded. To ensure consistency in achieving this position, the muscles controlling the movements of the mandible must be relaxed. Because patients exhibit varying degrees of muscle relaxation, the difficulty encountered will vary considerably from patient to patient. The determina-

tion of centric relation is difficult if there is splinting of the muscles associated with pain, hypertonicity of the muscles associated with occlusal interferences, or an appreciable degree of muscular tension.

Accurate recording of centric relation is impossible if the patient is suffering from acute temporomandibular joint or muscle disturbances. In most instances, the use of an occlusal device (ie, orthosis) is indicated to aid in the relief of the symptoms of these disturbances before an attempt is made to record centric relation.

Ramfjord and Ash have stated that the following three factors must be controlled in order to succeed in determining centric relation: (1) emotional stress; (2) pain in the temporomandibular joints or the musculature concerned with mandibular movement; and (3) "muscle memory," or the proprioceptive reflex resulting from occlusal interferences.[1] Because patients exhibit varying degrees of muscular and emotional relaxation, each practitioner should be familiar with more than one method for determining centric relation.

## Recommended method for determining centric relation

The following method should be attempted initially because it is designed to control the three factors described in the preceding section.

1. The patient should be comfortably seated in the dental chair. The backrest should be tilted to about 60 degrees to promote patient comfort and facilitate mandibular manipulation (Fig 6-30). The patient's head should be well supported so there is no tension in the neck muscles. The patient should be instructed to relax and to breathe through the nose. All instructions should be provided in a soft, even tone.
2. The patient should be instructed to open widely and to maintain that position for about a minute in an attempt to deprogram the oral musculature. An alternative approach is to have the patient close lightly on cotton rolls for 4 to 5 minutes.
3. If mandibular anterior teeth are present, the dentist's thumb should be positioned on the labial surfaces of these teeth (Fig 6-31). The corresponding index finger should be placed under the patient's chin. The thumb and the index of the opposite hand should be positioned on each side of the maxillary arch opposite the premolars.

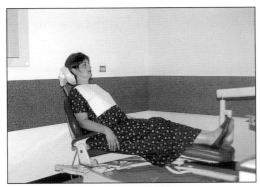

Fig 6-30 When recording the centric relation position, the patient should be comfortably seated. The back of the dental chair should form an angle of 60 degrees with the floor.

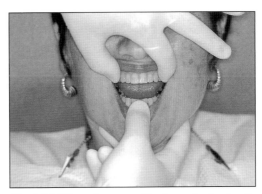

Fig 6-31 When the mandibular anterior teeth are present, the practitioner's thumb should be positioned on the labial surfaces of these teeth.

Fig 6-32 Backward and downward pressure *(single arrow)* is applied as the patient's mandible is guided in a short opening and closing movement. An upward "seating" force *(double arrows)* is placed with the tips of the index and middle fingers.

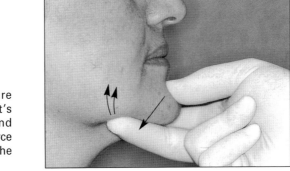

4. Once again, the patient should be reminded to relax and breathe deeply through the nose. It should be emphasized that the dentist will guide movements of the jaw.

5. Slight backward and downward pressure should be applied as the patient's mandible is guided in a short opening and closing movement (Fig 6-32). The teeth should not be allowed to contact because this may activate receptors in the periodontal ligaments and cause the mandible to deviate toward the maximal intercuspal position. Desired retrusion of the mandible is signified by smooth, rotational movement from a distinctly posterior position. Wide opening of the jaws should not be allowed once the mandible is in its most retruded position because it will cause translation of the condyles.

6. When the patient has been rehearsed sufficiently to cooperate and remain relaxed, the centric relation record should be made.

If a freely rotating mandible under control of the operator cannot be achieved, one of the alternative methods of retruding the mandible should be attempted.

### Alternate method one: Alternation of protrusion and retrusion

Frequently, the lateral pterygoid muscles prevent relaxation and free rotation of the mandible. This occurs because one or both lateral pterygoids are in a state of partial contraction. By using alternating protrusion and retrusion of the mandible, the practitioner encourages partially contracted muscle fibers to complete their contraction cycles. When this occurs, the lateral pterygoids are able to relax and return to their resting lengths. In turn, the mandible can move posteriorly toward the centric relation position.

1. Using the same finger position as in the recommended method (see Fig 6-31), the dentist should instruct the patient to "move the chin forward"

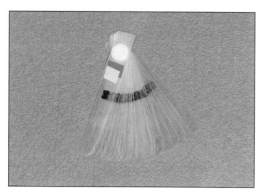

**Fig 6-33** A leaf gauge consists of several small, rectangular sheets of plastic.

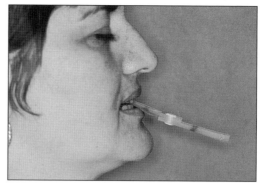

**Fig 6-34** A leaf gauge is positioned between the patient's maxillary and mandibular anterior teeth. The leaf gauge serves as a "deprogramming" device.

and then to "let the chin drop back." This procedure should be repeated until the operator can feel that the patient's mandible freely moves into its most posterior position. At this stage, the mandible should be assisted in rotational closure (see Fig 6-32).

2. This procedure should be practiced until the patient can follow the instructions and the dentist is certain that complete retrusion has been achieved. At this time, a centric relation record should be made.

### Alternate method two: Leaf gauge therapy

The principles employed in leaf gauge therapy may be compared to those described in the previous section. Partially contracted muscle fibers of the lateral pterygoids are encouraged to complete their contraction cycles and return to their resting lengths. When this occurs, the mandible can move posteriorly and superiorly toward centric relation.

A leaf gauge consists of several small, rectangular sheets of plastic (Fig 6-33). The thickness of a leaf gauge may be modified by adding or subtracting these plastic sheets. Clinically, a leaf gauge must be positioned between the patient's maxillary and mandibular anterior teeth (Fig 6-34). The mandible should be gently guided into a retruded position, and the patient should be instructed to close. Plastic sheets should be added or subtracted until the remaining posterior teeth are slightly out of contact. This permits "deprogramming" of the associated musculature and encourages closure that is directed by skeletal components (ie, the

condyles and condylar eminences). The patient should be directed to employ alternating cycles of moderate and heavy masticatory pressure. If the patient notes posterior occlusal contact, additional plastic sheets should be placed between the anterior teeth. The mandible should be posteriorly positioned and the process should be continued. The alternating cycles of moderate and heavy pressure facilitate complete contraction of the lateral pterygoid muscles. Following complete contraction of these muscles, the mandible is free to move toward the centric relation position.

### Alternate method three: Bilateral manipulation of the mandible

Some dentists prefer to use bilateral manipulation of the mandible when recording centric relation. The bilateral manipulation technique is significantly different from those methods previously described.

1. When using bilateral manipulation, four fingers of each hand should be positioned on the lower border of the mandible, and the thumbs should be placed near the prominence of the chin (Fig 6-35). When the mandible is rotating freely, the dentist should exert firm, upward pressure with the fingers. The thumbs should be used to apply pressure in a downward and backward direction. These actions result in a posterior, rotational movement of the mandible.

2. When the dentist is confident that the mandible has been properly positioned, a centric relation record should be made.

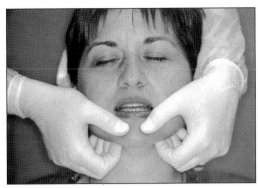

**Fig 6-35** When using bilateral manipulation, four fingers of each hand are positioned on the inferior border of the mandible, while the thumbs are placed near the prominence of the chin.

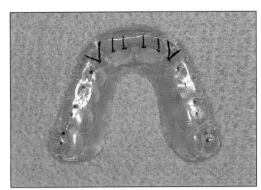

**Fig 6-36** A properly adjusted occlusal device may be used in an attempt to relieve symptoms of temporomandibular joint dysfunction. In turn, the practitioner may obtain a more accurate centric relation record.

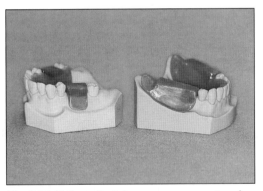

**Fig 6-37** If the edentulous areas are extensive or the teeth are not favorably distributed, record bases and occlusion rims should be used to accurately relate dental casts.

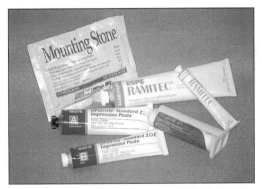

**Fig 6-38** Accurate jaw relation records may be made using accelerated dental stones, zinc oxide–eugenol registration pastes, polyethers, and polyvinylsiloxanes.

### Alternate method four: Use of an occlusal splint

Patients with severe splinting or hypertonicity of the muscles or with acute symptoms of temporomandibular joint dysfunction will usually provide inconsistent and inaccurate results. The construction of an occlusal device to be worn for a time in an attempt to relieve symptoms and to precondition the neuromuscular system is usually indicated for such a patient (Fig 6-36).

### Media for recording centric relation position

A number of media can be used to record centric relation. These include waxes, modeling plastics, acrylic resins, elastomeric impression materials, impression pastes, dental plasters, and dental stones.

The material selected for recording centric relation depends on the number and location of the remaining teeth. If there are a sufficient number of widely spaced occlusal contacts (at least three widely separated areas of contact), record bases are not needed and any recording medium may be used. If the edentulous areas are extensive or the teeth are not favorably distributed, record bases and occlusion rims should be used to accurately relate the dental casts (Fig 6-37). If record bases and occlusion rims are used, the selection of a suitable recording medium becomes critical. A fast-setting, low-viscosity registration material should be used to minimize the danger of record base displacement. Traditionally, accelerated dental stones and zinc oxide–eugenol registration pastes have been used for such records. More recent additions such as polyvinylsiloxane and polyether registration pastes also may be used. These materials are accurate, dimensionally stable, durable, and easy to trim (Fig 6-38).

## Occlusal vertical dimension

In most instances, patients will have two or more teeth that contact at the original occlusal vertical dimension. There are, however, exceptions to this rule. Therefore, a practitioner must be able to use guides such as the physiologic rest position and phonetics in determining an appropriate vertical dimension for restorative treatment. Jaw relation records should then be made at the determined occlusal vertical dimension. A more in-depth discussion of occlusal vertical dimension is included in chapter 13.

Probably the most difficult diagnostic decisions relative to occlusal vertical dimension occur when there is occlusal contact with an apparent overclosure of the mandible (see Fig 5-7). This may be caused by extreme wear or movement of the remaining teeth.

Restoration of a patient's original vertical dimension must be approached with great care. The restorative process must be preceded by a thorough diagnostic workup. A proposed occlusal vertical dimension should be determined, and a diagnostic splint should be constructed. The patient must wear the splint for an extended period to ensure that the proposed change in occlusal vertical dimension can be tolerated. If the patient can tolerate the proposed change in occlusal vertical dimension, definitive treatment may be undertaken.

## Making a centric jaw relation record using wax

Wax is often used as a recording medium when there are sufficient teeth to make an interocclusal registration and relate the casts without the use of a record base. Despite its widespread use, wax also is the most unreliable and unpredictable material used for making centric relation records. Distortion can occur when the record is made, when the records are stored, and when casts are mounted. Consequently, each practitioner must be aware of potential problems and how to avoid them.

Probably the greatest problem associated with wax records is the "memory" exhibited by these materials. Memory may produce warpage of wax records and inaccuracy of the associated mountings. Therefore, the heating, handling, and storage of wax records is critical.

Two distinctly different types of waxes are used for interocclusal records. Hard baseplate wax often is used because it is inexpensive and relatively accurate.

Furthermore, the material is rigid at room temperature. This property minimizes errors that may occur when dental casts are placed into baseplate wax records. The major disadvantages include difficulties in uniformly heating baseplate wax to a passive condition and the large degree of "memory" this material exhibits.

The second type of wax is very soft and contains a metallic filler in the form of finely ground powder (eg, Alu-Wax, Alu-wax Dental Products, Grand Rapids, MI; Coprwax, Heraeus Kulzer, Armonk, NY). The filler permits uniform heating and cooling of the wax. In addition, the metallic powder provides increased heat retention and an extended working time. These properties minimize strains and decrease warpage. Unfortunately, metal-impregnated waxes are relatively soft and may be distorted during mounting procedures.

Considerable care must be exercised when either type of wax is used. Suggested techniques are provided in the following sections.

**Use of hard baseplate wax** The following equipment and supplies are needed to make an interocclusal record with hard baseplate wax:

1. Hard baseplate wax (2 sheets)
2. Water bath at 60°C (140°F)
3. Maxillary and mandibular diagnostic casts
4. Bard-Parker handle with No. 25 blade (Becton, Dickson and Co; Franklin Lakes, NJ)
5. Air syringe
6. Bowl of cool water

The patient should be seated comfortably. Centric jaw relation should be located and the desired occlusal vertical dimension should be identified.

A 100 × 30–mm strip of wax should be placed in a water bath at 60°F (140°C) (Fig 6-39). When the wax is soft, it should be folded lengthwise (Fig 6-40). Using the maxillary diagnostic cast as a guideline, the wax should be formed to the shape of the dental arch (Fig 6-41). Excess wax should be eliminated using a Bard-Parker handle and No. 25 blade.

While it is still warm, the wax should be adapted to the patient's maxillary teeth (Fig 6-42). The mandible should be guided into centric relation and gently closed into the soft wax (Fig 6-43). This maxillo-

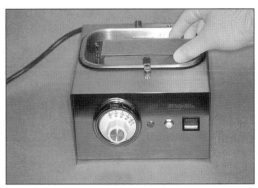

**Fig 6-39** A wax strip of appropriate dimensions is placed in a water bath maintained at 60°C (140° F).

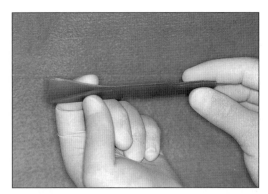

**Fig 6-40** When the wax is pliable, it is folded lengthwise.

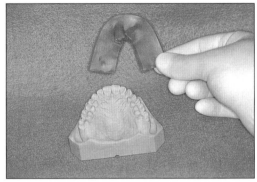

**Fig 6-41** Using the maxillary cast as a guideline, the wax is formed to the approximate shape of the dental arch.

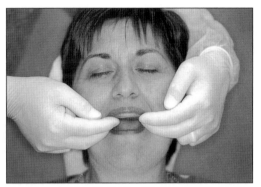

**Fig 6-42** The warm wax is adapted to the occlusal and incisal surfaces of the patient's maxillary teeth.

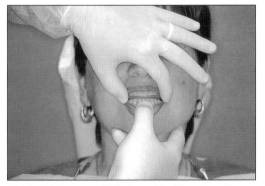

**Fig 6-43** The mandible is guided into centric relation and gently closed into the softened wax.

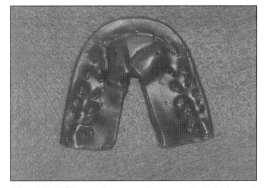

**Fig 6-44** When the wax has cooled, it is removed from the mouth and inspected.

mandibular relationship should be maintained as the wax cools. To speed this process, the practitioner may use a gentle stream of compressed air on the facial surfaces of the wax record.

The record should be removed from the mouth and inspected for thickness (Fig 6-44). The wax record should be approximately 1.0 mm thick. Complete penetration of the wax usually indicates contact of opposing teeth. Tooth contact must be avoided since it may cause the mandible to move away from the desired centric relation position. Hence, the record should be remade if these criteria are not satisfied.

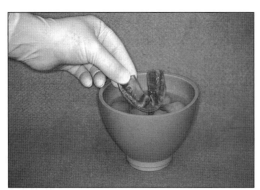

**Fig 6-45** The wax is chilled in a bowl of cool water.

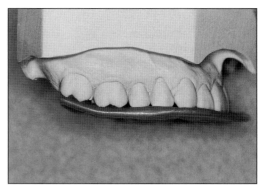

**Fig 6-46** The wax record is gently positioned on the maxillary cast. The cusp tips must fit accurately into the corresponding indentations in the wax record.

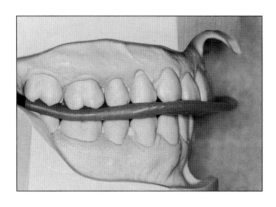

**Fig 6-47** At this stage, the mandibular cast is properly positioned on the record. The mandibular cusp tips also must fit the record accurately.

At this stage, the wax record should be placed into a bowl of cool water (Fig 6-45). Carefully controlled cooling of the wax provides increased rigidity and improved resistance to distortion.

The record should be gently positioned on the maxillary cast (Fig 6-46). The cusp tips of the maxillary cast must fit accurately into depressions created by the patient's teeth. The wax record must not be forced onto the cast and must not rock when light pressure is applied. The cusp tips of the mandibular cast should then be guided into the record. Again, the cusp tips should fit the indentations of the record perfectly (Fig 6-47). If the record fails to fit either cast, the record may be distorted, or the casts may be inaccurate. Accuracy of the record may be tested by placing the wax registration into the patient's mouth and guiding the mandible into a centric relation closure. If the record is accurate, the cusps of the maxillary and mandibular teeth should fit accurately into the record. Records or diagnostic casts that are inaccurate should be remade.

**Use of metal-impregnated wax** The following equipment and supplies are needed to make an interocclusal record with metal-impregnated wax:

1. Metal-impregnated wax (eg, Alu-Wax, Coprwax) (2 sheets)
2. Bunsen burner
3. Maxillary and mandibular diagnostic casts
4. Bard-Parker handle with No. 25 blade
5. No. 7 wax spatula
6. Water bath at 43°C (110°F)
7. Air syringe
8. Bowl of cool water

One sheet of metal-impregnated wax should be passed over a flame until it is slightly softened. The wax should then be folded upon itself to form a double thickness. Using the patient's maxillary cast as a guide, the wax should be trimmed so it extends 2 to 3 mm facial to the surfaces of the remaining teeth (Fig

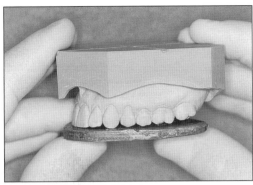

**Fig 6-48** Metal-impregnated wax is heated, folded upon itself, and formed to the approximate size and shape of the maxillary arch. The wax should extend 2 to 3 mm beyond the facial surfaces of the maxillary teeth.

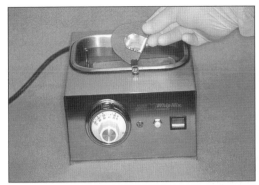

**Fig 6-49** The metal-impregnated wax is softened in a water bath maintained at 43°C (110°F).

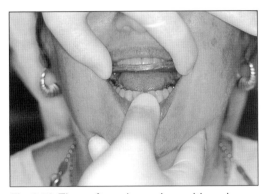

**Fig 6-50** The softened wax is positioned over the occlusal and incisal surfaces of the maxillary teeth.

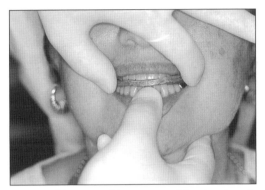

**Fig 6-51** The record is supported by the thumb and index finger of the left hand. The right hand is used to direct the mandible into centric relation and guide mandibular closure.

6-48). The wax should not extend beyond the distal surfaces of the most posterior teeth.

When the wax has been trimmed to the proper dimensions, the edges should be sealed using a heated wax spatula. At this stage, the properly shaped material should be softened in a water bath at 43°C (110°F) (Fig 6-49). The softened record should then be positioned over the occlusal and incisal surfaces of the maxillary teeth (Fig 6-50). For a right-handed operator, the record should be supported by the thumb and index finger of the left hand. The right hand should be used to direct the mandible into centric relation and guide mandibular closure (Fig 6-51). Only light contact of the cusp tips with the softened wax is desired. The teeth must not pass through the wax. While maintaining this maxillomandibular relation-

ship, facial surfaces of the wax record should be cooled using an air syringe.

When the wax record has been sufficiently cooled, it may be removed from the mouth. Upon removal, the wax record should be inspected to ensure it is the proper thickness. The record should then be chilled in a bowl of cool water (Fig 6-52). Upon completion of the cooling process, the record should be removed from the cool water and inspected once again. Areas of soft tissue contact should be eliminated. The record should be returned to the mouth, and the patient should be guided into centric relation closure. This second closure serves to correct slight distortions that may have occurred. In addition, it allows the practitioner to determine whether the patient is closing in a repeatable position.

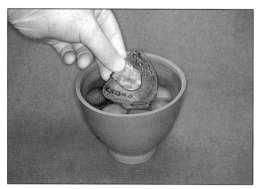

**Fig 6-52** When the wax record has cooled, it is removed from the mouth and chilled in a bowl of cool water.

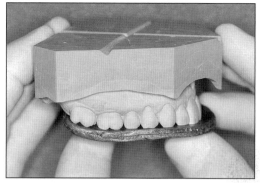

**Fig 6-53** The record is placed on the maxillary cast and carefully inspected to ensure that it accurately fits the cast. This procedure is repeated for the mandibular cast.

Upon completion of record-making procedures, the interocclusal record should be removed from the patient's mouth and placed on the corresponding dental casts (Fig 6-53). The record should be carefully checked to ensure that it fits each of the casts accurately and does not rock. Records or casts that are inaccurate should be remade.

### Use of elastomeric registration materials

During the past 20 years, elastomers such as polyvinylsiloxanes and polyethers have gained increasing popularity as registration materials. These materials generally are supplied as two-paste systems. When mixed, the components form syringeable pastes that may be expressed onto the surfaces of the teeth. The materials then undergo rapid polymerization to form rubbery solids.

Elastomeric registration materials are odorless, tasteless, and easy to use. They are capable of recording fine detail and are dimensionally stable. In addition, they may be trimmed quite easily using surgical blades. Perhaps the greatest disadvantages of these materials are relatively high costs and potential for misuse.

The following equipment and supplies are needed to make an interocclusal record with elastomeric registration materials:

1. Elastomeric registration material in automix cartridge
2. Extrusion device
3. Mixing tips

4. Bard-Parker handle and No. 25 blade
5. Diagnostic casts

The patient should be seated comfortably. Centric relation should be established and the proposed occlusal vertical dimension should be determined. Retrusion and closure should be repeated until the patient is familiar with the process.

The patient should be directed to open the mouth, and the surfaces of the teeth should be dried with gauze. At this point, a ribbon of registration medium should be expressed onto the occlusal and incisal surfaces of the mandibular teeth (Fig 6-54). The mandible should be guided into centric relation closure at the desired occlusal vertical dimension (Fig 6-55). It is essential that the mandible be maintained in this position as polymerization of the registration material occurs.

When the registration material has reached a hardened state, it should be removed from the mouth and inspected. The material should be approximately 1.0 mm thick, with no evidence of complete cuspal penetration, which would indicate tooth contact. If the registration meets these requirements, it should be trimmed using a sharp No. 25 blade attached to a Bard-Parker handle. Due to the fine detail that may be recorded by polyvinylsiloxanes and polyethers, only the cuspal indentations should remain in the record (Fig 6-56).

The record should be seated on maxillary and mandibular diagnostic casts to ensure that it fits passively (Fig 6-57). Records or casts that are inaccurate should be remade.

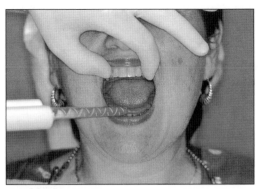

**Fig 6-54** Registration medium is extruded onto the surfaces of the mandibular teeth.

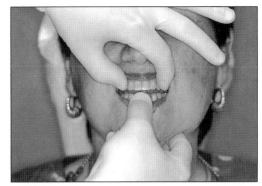

**Fig 6-55** The mandible is guided into centric relation closure at the desired occlusal vertical dimension.

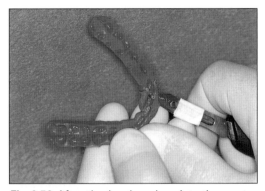

**Fig 6-56** After the hardened registration material has been removed from the mouth and inspected, it is trimmed using a sharp No. 25 surgical blade attached to a Bard-Parker handle. Only the cuspal indentations should remain in the record.

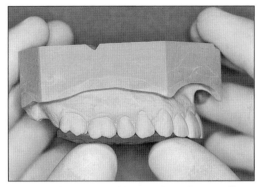

**Fig 6-57** The record is seated on the maxillary cast and inspected to ensure that it accurately fits the cast. This procedure is repeated for the mandibular cast.

### Making centric relation records using record bases with occlusion rims

Record bases with occlusion rims must be used when one or more distal extension areas are present, when tooth-bounded edentulous spaces are large, or when opposing teeth do not meet. Record bases usually are constructed using chemically-activated or light-activated acrylic resins.

Record bases must accurately fit the diagnostic casts and the patient's mouth. In addition, record bases must be comfortable, rigid, and stable when placed in the oral cavity. All surfaces that contact the lips, cheeks, and tongue should be smooth, rounded, and polished. Borders must not interfere with the functional activity of the surrounding tissues. As a result, the borders of a record base should be slightly underextended (Fig 6-58). Overextension of borders

often will produce instability of the record base and inaccuracy of the diagnostic mounting.

Occlusion rims usually are fabricated using baseplate wax. The rims are attached to the surfaces of record bases and are used to support occlusal registration materials (Fig 6-59). This permits a practitioner to record maxillomandibular relations and transfer these positions to a dental articulator.

Without the use of record bases and occlusion rims, it would be extremely difficult (if not impossible) to accurately transfer the horizontal and vertical relationships from a patient to an articulator.

When interocclusal records are obtained using record bases with occlusion rims, it is important to avoid excessive pressure on the underlying soft tissues. If interocclusal records are recorded under pressure, the soft tissues may be compressed. This will produce

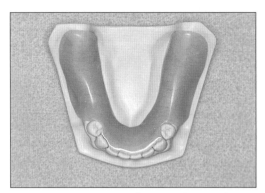

**Fig 6-58** The borders of a record base should be slightly underextended to minimize the likelihood of displacement.

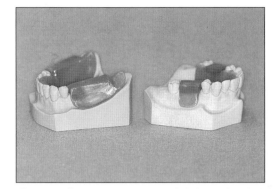

**Fig 6-59** Occlusion rims are fabricated using baseplate wax and serve to support occlusal registration materials.

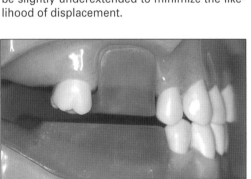

**Fig 6-60** Occlusion rims should be adjusted to provide 1 to 2 mm of clearance between the wax and the opposing teeth or wax rims.

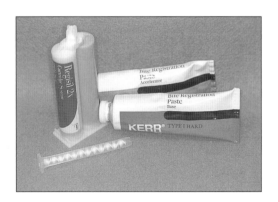

**Fig 6-61** Shallow V-shaped grooves are prepared on the surface of each occlusion rim.

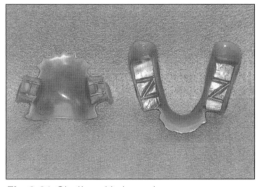

**Fig 6-62** A free-flowing recording medium should be used to make jaw relation records. Zinc oxide–eugenol pastes and polyvinylsiloxane registration media are well suited for this purpose.

movement of the record base and result in an inaccurate registration. Care should be taken to ensure that opposing occlusal surfaces do not contact the occlusion rim. In addition, a soft registration material such as zinc oxide–eugenol or a low-viscosity elastomer should be used.

Clinically, the record base should be placed in the patient's mouth to ensure that it is properly extended, stable, and reasonably comfortable. If a wax

occlusion rim has been added, it should be trimmed to provide 1 to 2 mm clearance between the wax and the opposing teeth or wax rim (Fig 6-60). Subsequently, the record base should be removed from the mouth. Shallow, V-shaped grooves should be prepared on the occlusal surface of each occlusion rim (Fig 6-61). These grooves serve as indices to permit the removal and accurate replacement of registration materials.

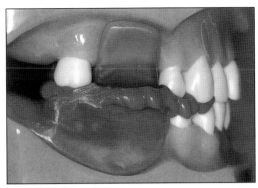

Fig 6-63 Following placement of the registration medium, the patient is guided into centric relation at the desired occlusal vertical dimension.

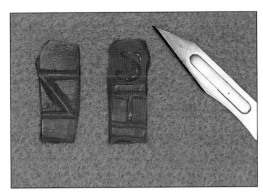

Fig 6-64 The record is removed and properly trimmed.

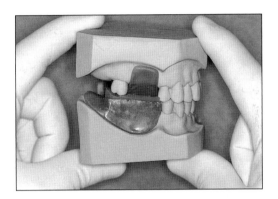

Fig 6-65 Individual record bases are seated on the associated casts. In turn, the record is properly positioned and the casts correctly related.

A free-flowing recording medium such as zinc oxide–eugenol paste or an elastomeric registration material should be prepared and placed on the surface of the occlusion rim (Fig 6-62). The patient should be guided into centric relation closure at the desired occlusal vertical dimension (Fig 6-63). This position should be maintained until the recording material has reached the desired consistency.

Following completion of the setting process, the record should be removed and trimmed until only the imprints of the cusp tips remain (Fig 6-64). The wax occlusion rim should not show through the recording medium indentations. This would indicate contact of the wax with the opposing occlusal or incisal surfaces.

The record base should be completely seated on the appropriate diagnostic cast, and the opposing cast should be properly positioned in the record (Fig 6-65). The cusps should accurately fit the indentations, and the remaining teeth should exhibit the same relationships observed in the mouth. Records or casts that are inaccurate should be remade.

## Preparation of articulator and mounting of mandibular cast

At this stage of the diagnostic mounting procedure, the practitioner should have a properly mounted maxillary cast, an accurate centric relation record, and an unmounted mandibular cast. The practitioner also may have one or more record bases with occlusion rims to facilitate completion of the mounting process. The following procedures should be employed when mounting the mandibular cast.

1. The facebow assembly and cast support should be removed from the articulator if this has not already been accomplished. The mounted maxillary cast should be removed from the articulator.
2. The centric relation record should be placed on the maxillary cast. Care should be taken to ensure that the cusp tips accurately fit the record (Fig 6-66).
3. The base of the mandibular cast should be indexed, and the cusp tips should be guided into the indentations of the centric relation record. The practitioner

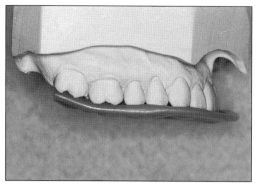

**Fig 6-66** The centric relation record is placed on the maxillary cast. Care is taken to ensure that the cusp tips accurately fit the record.

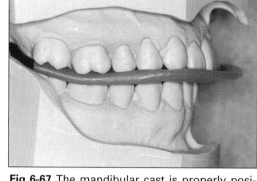

**Fig 6-67** The mandibular cast is properly positioned in the record. Once again, care is taken to ensure that the cusp tips accurately fit the record.

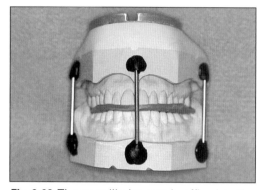

**Fig 6-68** The mandibular cast is affixed to the maxillary cast using wire struts in conjunction with modeling plastic.

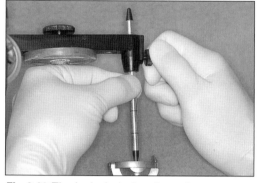

**Fig 6-69** The incisal pin is adjusted to compensate for the thickness of the interocclusal record.

should ensure that the cusp tips accurately fit the record (Fig 6-67). The casts should be maintained in this relationship using light finger pressure.

4. The mandibular cast should be affixed to the maxillary cast using wire struts in conjunction with modeling plastic (Fig 6-68). Metal stabilizing struts can be made by cutting 75-mm lengths of hanger wire. Wooden struts should be avoided since wood may warp in the presence of water. Warpage may produce spatial inaccuracies within the diagnostic mounting.

5. The locking mechanism for the incisal pin should be loosened and the pin opened 2 to 3 mm from its neutral setting (Fig 6-69). This creates increased space between the upper and lower members of the articulator and compensates for the thickness of the interocclusal record.

6. The stabilized casts should be returned to the articulator. The maxillary mounting ring should be at-

tached to the upper member of the articulator, and the mounting screw should be tightened. A clean mounting ring should be attached to the lower member of the articulator. When this has been accomplished, the articulator should be inverted and placed on a firm, horizontal surface.

7. The base of the mandibular cast should be moistened with clear slurry water. Grooves on the base of the cast should then be painted with a gypsum separating medium such as Super-Sep (Fig 6-70).

8. A mix of mounting stone or accelerated dental stone should be prepared. The freshly prepared stone should be applied to the base of the mandibular cast and forced into the openings of the mounting ring (Fig 6-71). The articulator should then be closed. The practitioner should make certain that the incisal pin is in contact with the incisal table. At this stage, the dental stone should be shaped and smoothed (Fig 6-72).

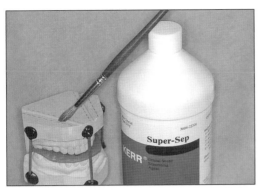

**Fig 6-70** The base of the mandibular cast is moistened with clear slurry water. Subsequently, the grooves are painted with a liquid separating medium.

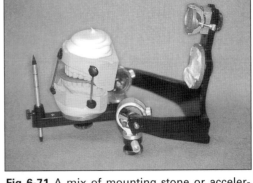

**Fig 6-71** A mix of mounting stone or accelerated dental stone is prepared and used to mount the mandibular cast.

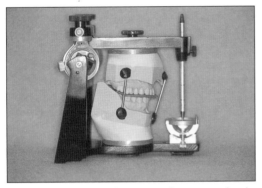

**Fig 6-72** The mounting stone is appropriately shaped and smoothed.

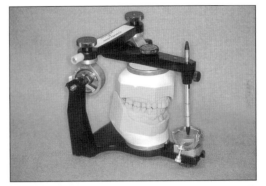

**Fig 6-73** After the dental stone has hardened, the stabilizing struts and interocclusal record are removed. The incisal pin is properly adjusted.

9. After the dental stone has hardened, modeling plastic and metal stabilizing struts should be removed. In turn, the interocclusal record should be removed, and the incisal pin should be properly adjusted (Fig 6-73).

## Verification of mounting

No diagnostic mounting is complete until the centric relation registration has been verified. Occlusal analysis or equilibration should never be attempted on an articulator until the mounting has been proven correct. Therefore, one or more verification records should be made to assess the accuracy of a diagnostic mounting (see procedures for making centric relation records).

Before a verification record is placed between the mounted casts, the incisal guide pin should be removed and the condylar locks should be released. The verification record should be placed very gently onto the maxillary cast. Subsequently, the cusps of the mandibular cast should be guided into the record. Care must be taken to avoid excessive pressure, which could cause distortion of the record.

Following appropriate placement of the verification record, the diagnostic mounting should be carefully inspected. The mounting can be considered correct only if (1) the cusp tips of both casts fit the jaw relation record accurately and (2) the condylar balls remain in contact with their posterior stops on both sides of the articulator (Fig 6-74).

If these conditions are not met, either the original record or the verification record is incorrect. In these instances, additional intraoral records should be made. These records should be used to evaluate the mounting. If the records match the original mounting, the practitioner may proceed with the diagnostic phase of treatment. However, if these records display a consistent pattern of misfit (Fig 6-75), the mandibu-

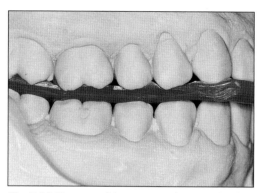

**Fig 6-74** The practitioner must be certain that the maxillary and mandibular cusps are completely seated in the verification record.

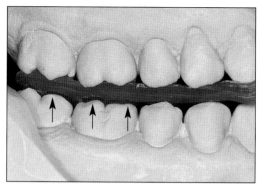

**Fig 6-75** Cusps that are incompletely seated in the verification record *(arrows)* indicate inconsistency or inaccuracy.

lar cast should be remounted using one of the newer records. This procedure must be repeated until the articulator will accept one or more verification records.

When the practitioner is satisfied with the accuracy of the mounting, the verification record should be removed and the articulator closed. As an additional verification, the initial contact of the mounted casts should be compared to the patient's initial occlusal contact at centric relation. These contacts should be identical.

## Improving the appearance of mountings

Following verification of occlusal relationships, both mountings should be removed from the articulator by loosening the screws that secure the mounting rings. The mountings should be soaked in clear slurry water for at least 5 minutes. In turn, a fresh mix of dental stone should be used to smooth the mountings. The mounting stone should not extend onto the lateral surfaces of the cast or onto the outer surfaces of the mounting rings. Stone must not interfere with the complete seating of mounting rings against the associated surfaces of the articulator.

## Setting condylar elements of the articulator

Condylar elements of the articulator may be set using an appropriate protrusive record. Condylar elements also may be set by properly relating wear facets on the remaining teeth. Both techniques are briefly described.

## Use of a protrusive wax record

When using this technique, the patient must be taught to make a straight protrusive movement of 4 to 5 mm. A wax record of several thicknesses of baseplate wax should be fabricated (Fig 6-76). The wax record should then be softened in a water bath and positioned over the occlusal and incisal surfaces of the maxillary teeth. The patient should be instructed to protrude the mandible. When the mandible has moved forward 4 to 5 mm, the patient should be instructed to close into the wax (Fig 6-77). The record should be approximately 1 mm thick at its thinnest point.

When the wax has hardened, the record should be removed and briefly placed in cool water (Fig 6-78). It should be checked for stability on the mounted casts. The record should be repeated if any of the following errors are present:

1. Patient's protrusion is less than 3 mm. (This degree of movement is too small to accurately set the instrument.)
2. Patient's protrusion is greater than 6 mm. (This degree of movement will carry the condyle too far along the articular eminence.)
3. A noticeable lateral component accompanies the protrusive movement.
4. Incisal or occlusal contact of the remaining teeth is evident.
5. The protrusive record is unstable in the mouth or on the casts.

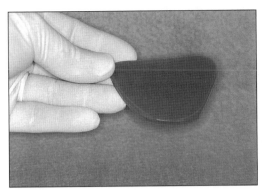

Fig 6-76 The wax form for a protrusive record.

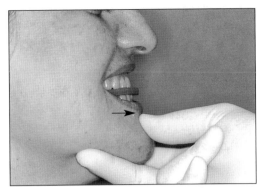

Fig 6-77 When the mandible has moved forward 4 to 5 mm *(arrow)*, the patient is instructed to close into the wax.

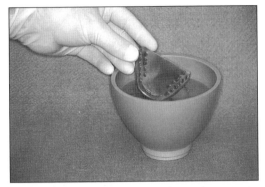

Fig 6-78 Following removal from the mouth, the protrusive record is immersed in cool water.

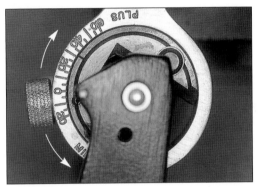

Fig 6-79 Each condylar inclination mechanism is rotated *(arrows)* to determine the appropriate setting.

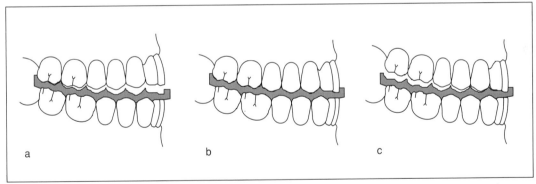

Fig 6-80 *(a)* When the condylar inclination is too shallow, the anterior teeth will not contact the surface of the wax record. *(b)* When the condylar inclination is correct, anterior and posterior teeth will contact the surface of the wax record. *(c)* When the condylar inclination is too steep, the posterior teeth will not contact the surface of the wax record.

When an accurate protrusive wax record has been made and verified, the condylar guidance may be set using the following procedure. The incisal pin should be removed. The centric locks and condylar inclination locking mechanisms should be loosened. The protrusive record should be positioned on the mandibular cast, and an attempt should be made to place the maxillary cast into the appropriate cuspal indentations. The condylar inclination mechanism should be rotated until the maxillary teeth fit accurately into the indentations of the record (Figs 6-79 and 6-80). The condylar inclination locking mechanism should then be tightened (Fig 6-81).

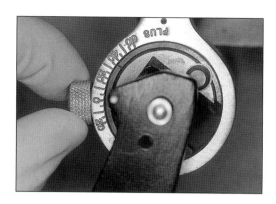

Fig 6-81 When the appropriate condylar inclination has been determined, the associated locking mechanism should be tightened.

This procedure should be repeated, and the results should be compared. The settings for each side should be relatively consistent (ie, within 2 to 5 degrees). The right and left condylar inclination settings should then be compared. These settings should be within 8 degrees of each other.

### Use of wear facets

Wear facets also may be used to determine the condylar settings of an articulator. However, this technique should be used only by experienced operators.

When using this technique, the incisal pin should be removed. In turn, the centric locks and condylar inclination mechanisms should be loosened. The dental casts should be gently guided into eccentric positions. The condylar inclinations should be adjusted to harmonize with the wear patterns displayed on the dental casts.

Upon completion of this process, the practitioner should be able to assess the patient's occlusion.

## ⊡ Definitive Oral Examination

The oral examination must be thorough. The following steps should be included:

1. A thorough examination of the remaining teeth should be performed. Carious lesions and defective restorations should be correlated with radiographs and other diagnostic findings.
2. A complete periodontal examination should be accomplished. Oral structures should be evaluated to determine pocket depths, mobility, soft tissue attachment, furcation involvement, etc.

3. Teeth with suspected pulpal involvement should be tested for vitality.
4. All remaining teeth should be tested for sensitivity to percussion.
5. The oral tissues should be examined for evidence of pathologic changes.
6. The dental arches should be examined for the presence of tori, exostoses, sharp or prominent bony areas, soft or hard tissue undercuts, and/or enlarged tuberosities.
7. A radiographic examination should be performed with special attention focused on proposed abutments and the residual ridge areas.
8. Mounted casts should be examined for the presence of extruded or malposed teeth, reduced interarch space, unfavorable occlusal planes, and any other potential problems.
9. In mandibular applications, a suitable measuring device such as a periodontal probe should be used to determine the distance from the active floor of the mouth to the gingival margins of the mandibular teeth.
10. The diagnostic casts should be analyzed on a dental surveyor and appropriate removable partial denture designs should be generated.

### Evaluation of diagnostic data

All diagnostic data must be collected before an effective evaluation can be made. The practitioner must correlate intraoral findings with those of the radiographic survey, the mounted casts, the survey and analysis of the diagnostic casts, and other relevant information. Results should be used in the development of a sound treatment plan.

## Evaluation of carious lesions and existing restorations

The selection of suitable restorations for partially edentulous patients requires a great deal of thought. A practitioner must examine the remaining teeth for carious lesions. Existing restorations also must be evaluated. The contours of potential abutments should be examined. In addition, the occlusal plane should be evaluated. In some instances, a simple two-surface restoration may be adequate for restoring a carious tooth. In other instances, a cast restoration may be needed to correct discrepancies in the occlusal plane or to provide the tooth with appropriate contours for clasping.

It would be foolish to initiate restorative treatment before completion of a diagnostic mounting and design of the necessary removable partial denture(s). As previously noted, inadequate tooth contours may necessitate the placement of complete-coverage restorations (ie, crowns). If an otherwise satisfactory amalgam restoration is present in an area that is to receive a rest seat, the amalgam restoration must be evaluated to determine whether it is strong enough to withstand the forces it will receive. The outline form of the restoration should be examined to determine whether the entire rest seat will be in amalgam or whether part of the rest seat will contact sound tooth structure. The occlusion should be examined to determine how deep the rest seat must be. Radiographs should be examined to determine the thickness of the amalgam restoration in the area to be prepared. After all these factors have been considered, the most appropriate decision may be to replace the amalgam with a complete-coverage restoration.

Satisfactory amalgam or tooth-colored restorations on the facial surfaces of prospective abutment teeth also must be carefully evaluated. Excessive wear of such restorations may occur if a retentive clasp tip will contact a restoration or cross its margins while moving in and out of the undercut. This wear can result in failure of the restorations or diminished retention of the removable partial denture.

Care must be taken in the placement of margins of cast restorations as well. Frequent movement of a retentive clasp tip may contribute to premature failure of a cast restoration.

Not every tooth that can be saved through restorative procedures should be retained. The more prudent treatment may be removal of the tooth. This is particularly true when retention of a compromised tooth would complicate the design of a prosthesis, or if it would have limited value in the long-term treatment prognosis. Hence, preventive dentistry for a partially edentulous patient does not mean the retention of every retainable tooth.

## Evaluation of pulpal tissues

If warranted, pulp testing should be used to assess the vitality of remaining teeth. It can be inconvenient and expensive for the patient, as well as embarrassing for the dentist, if a pulpal problem is overlooked, and it is discovered that an abutment must be endodontically treated or removed at a later date.

Teeth that have been endodontically treated must be carefully evaluated before selection as abutments. Endodontically treated teeth tend to become more brittle with time, and abutments for removable partial dentures are subjected to considerable stresses. Nevertheless, the selection of endodontically treated teeth as abutments is not contraindicated. If an endodontically treated tooth has a relatively large access opening or an extensive intracoronal restoration, a dowel-and-core restoration and a complete-coverage crown may be indicated to minimize the likelihood of coronal fracture.

## Evaluation of sensitivity to percussion

All remaining teeth should be tested for sensitivity to percussion. Particular attention should be focused on the prospective abutment teeth. The following conditions can contribute to irritation of the periodontal ligament fibers, making a tooth sensitive to percussion:

1. Tooth movement caused by an unstable occlusion or ill-fitting prosthesis
2. A tooth or restoration in traumatic occlusion
3. Periapical or pulpal abscesses
4. Acute pulpitis
5. Gingivitis or periodontitis
6. Cracked tooth syndrome

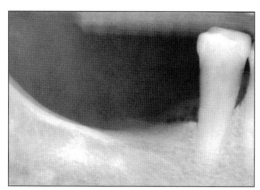

**Fig 6-82** A crown-root ratio greater than 1:1 is unfavorable.

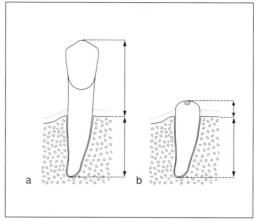

**Fig 6-83** *(a)* This tooth exhibits a crown-root ratio greater than 1:1. *(b)* By performing endodontic therapy and shortening the clinical crown of the tooth, a more favorable crown-root ratio may be achieved.

The exact cause must be determined through the evaluation of other diagnostic data. A removable partial denture should not be constructed until the cause of the discomfort is discovered and the sensitivity is eliminated. The use of a percussion-sensitive tooth as an abutment may result in early failure of the associated prosthesis.

### Evaluation of tooth mobility

Teeth with detectable mobility should be evaluated to determine the causes of such movement. A mobile tooth used as an abutment will have a poor prognosis unless the mobility is markedly decreased. Tooth mobility may be caused by one or more of the following factors:

1. Trauma from occlusion
2. Inflammatory changes in the periodontal ligament
3. Loss of osseous support

In most instances, tooth mobility that results from occlusal trauma usually is reversible. To minimize mobility, the source of occlusal trauma must be identified and corrected. Properly mounted diagnostic casts are useful in the identification of occlusal disharmonies. Correction of occlusal disharmonies may be accomplished by occlusal equilibration or by the placement of one or more restorations.

Tooth mobility caused by inflammatory changes in the periodontal ligament may be reversed if the inflammation is eliminated.

Tooth mobility caused by a loss of osseous support is not reversible in most instances. A tooth with a crown-root ratio greater than 1:1 is not suitable as an abutment for a removable partial denture (Fig 6-82). In these instances, adjacent teeth should be evaluated. If an adjacent tooth is capable of serving as a strong abutment, the practitioner may choose to remove the periodontally weakened tooth. Splinting a weak tooth to a strong tooth must be approached cautiously because splinting frequently weakens the stronger tooth rather than strengthening the weak one.

In some situations, the root of a periodontally weakened tooth may be retained as an overdenture abutment. Overdenture abutments can provide significant support for a removable prosthesis. Clinically, an overdenture abutment should be endodontically treated. In turn, the clinical crown should be reduced and the exposed portion of the root should be gently rounded. The peripheries of the overdenture abutment should be located at the gingival level, while the tallest portion of the "dome" should extend 2 to 3 mm above the gingival margins. This procedure greatly improves the crown-root ratio of a periodontally compromised tooth and often eliminates tooth mobility (Fig 6-83). Hence, this concept of treatment should always be considered when the removal of one

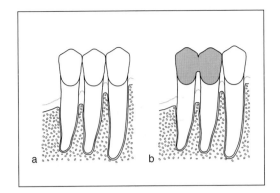

**Fig 6-84** *(a)* In this diagram, the premolars exhibit compromised periodontal support. *(b)* By splinting these teeth with a fixed restoration, it may be possible to provide improved support.

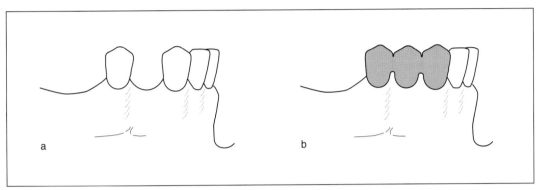

**Fig 6-85** *(a)* In this instance, a first premolar is missing and the second premolar is to serve as a removable partial denture abutment. *(b)* Placement of a fixed partial denture restores the continuity of the arch, thereby creating a more favorable prognosis for the second premolar and the associated removable partial denture.

or more teeth will result in a large edentulous area. A single overdenture abutment is extremely valuable in providing support, particularly in large anterior edentulous areas and distal extension applications.

### Indications for splinting

Splinting may be necessary when the remaining teeth display compromised periodontal support or short, tapered roots. By splinting two or more teeth, it may be possible to provide improved support for a removable prosthesis (Fig 6-84). It is imperative that such restorations be constructed in harmony with the patient's occlusion, temporomandibular joint, and musculature. Furthermore, the removable partial denture must be designed and constructed to place minimal stresses on the splinted teeth.

Splinting with a fixed partial denture is indicated when the first premolar and the molars have been lost and the second premolar is to serve as an abutment. A lone-standing second premolar is likely to be damaged by the forces applied to a distal extension removable partial denture. Placement of a fixed partial denture will restore the continuity of the arch and create a more favorable prognosis for the tooth and the removable partial denture (Fig 6-85).

### *Evaluation of periodontium*

Periodontal disease is one of the primary factors in tooth loss. Therefore, a large percentage of partially edentulous patients show evidence of gingivitis and periodontal disease. A removable partial denture placed in the presence of active periodontal disease may contribute to the rapid progression of the disease and loss of the remaining teeth. If removable partial denture therapy is to be successful, disease processes must be controlled.

The periodontium of partially edentulous patients must be evaluated if any type of prosthodontic treatment is being considered. Evaluation of the periodontium must be based upon thorough clinical and radiographic examinations. The clinical examination must disclose the presence of periodontal pockets, inflammation, infection, furcation involvement(s), and the absence of sufficient attached gingiva.

The health of a patient's periodontium should be evaluated by careful, systematic measurement with a calibrated periodontal probe; by clinical observation of the color, texture, and architecture of the gingival tissues; by observation of any crevicular exudate resulting from probing or the application of digital pressure; and by determination of the width of attached gingiva. A complete radiographic survey should be used to supplement the clinical findings, but should not be considered a substitute for a thorough clinical evaluation.

Examination findings that indicate possible need for periodontal treatment include the following:

1. Pocket depth in excess of 3 mm
2. Furcation involvement
3. Deviations from normal color and contour in gingivae, which indicate gingivitis
4. Marginal exudate upon probing or application of digital pressure
5. Proposed abutment teeth exhibiting less than 2 mm of attached gingiva
6. An inadequate band of attached gingiva associated with the remaining teeth

The selection of abutments in the presence of periodontal disease may present a diagnostic challenge. In many instances, clear-cut choices are not available. A practitioner must consider the periodontal conditions of proposed abutments. The practitioner must recognize that pocket elimination and osseous recontouring will not result in good abutments if the associated teeth are left with inadequate crown-root ratios. Root size, root form, the amount of root in alveolar bone, the number and distribution of remaining teeth, the

patient's age, the type of opposing occlusion, the nature of the residual ridge, and the patient's interest and desire are as important as pocket depth in the selection of suitable abutments. Frequently it is advantageous to sacrifice a periodontally compromised tooth if an adjacent tooth would serve as a better abutment.

From a prosthodontic standpoint, the objective of periodontal treatment of abutment teeth should be restoration of the periodontium to optimum health and creation of contours that will allow the patient to preserve this state of health. Periodontal therapy that falls short of this objective may compromise the prognosis of prosthodontic treatment.

Several types of periodontal treatment are effective in restoring the abutments, as well as the other remaining teeth, to optimum health. Root scaling and root planing in conjunction with good home oral hygiene procedures can dramatically improve the health of the periodontium. Gingivectomy has limited applications. It may provide increased clinical crown length in specific situations. This may permit the use of undercuts that were hidden by the gingival tissues. It can also be used to create longer clinical crowns when tooth preparation is indicated (ie, for surveyed crowns).

Periodontal flap procedures have the widest range of indications in the surgical treatment of periodontal disease. By allowing access to the underlying osseous structures, these procedures permit good visibility and facilitate osseous recontouring.

Free gingival grafts can provide significant advantages when one or more abutments display inadequate zones of gingival attachment. Grafts also may be used to increase vestibular depth, thereby providing room for major connectors, denture bases, and related components.

Ill-fitting prostheses and inadequate oral hygiene measures frequently contribute to the appearance of redundant soft tissues on the proximal surfaces of the remaining teeth. These tissues generally are unhealthy and should be eliminated prior to construction of a new removable partial denture. The introduction of good oral hygiene practices and adequate tissue rest (removal of prostheses for 6 to 8 hours per day) often will allow the affected tissues to return to a state of health. Additional oral hygiene procedures may speed the healing process. Patients may use strips of dampened gauze to clean the proximal surfaces of teeth and

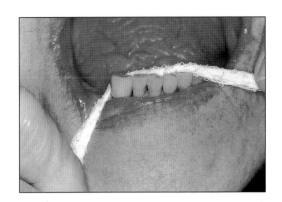

**Fig 6-86** A strip of dampened gauze may be used to clean the proximal surfaces of the teeth and to massage the adjacent soft tissues.

to massage the adjacent soft tissues (Fig 6-86). If there is not sufficient resolution of the redundant tissues in 2 to 3 weeks, surgical intervention may be required.

Patients with long-standing periodontal disease may present difficult diagnostic challenges. These patients often present with extremely long clinical crowns, root caries, oral discomfort, and inadequate oral hygiene. Many patients are discouraged and are seeking complete dentures. A dentist must not be too hasty in complying with such a request. The psychological trauma of becoming completely edentulous can be devastating for some patients. Therefore, the dentist must evaluate all factors that contribute to a patient's ability to successfully wear complete dentures. These factors include the patient's age, psychological condition, neuromuscular capabilities, habits, ridge morphology, and tongue position. The removal of unsalvageable teeth and the construction of a transitional removable partial denture can be useful diagnostic procedures. During this process, many patients change their attitudes about complete edentulism and exhibit improved oral hygiene. As a result, enough teeth can be retained to support conventional removable partial dentures or overdentures.

## Evaluation of oral mucosa

### Pathologic changes

Any ulceration, swelling, or color change that might indicate a malignant or premalignant lesion should be recognized and properly evaluated through biopsy or referral. In spite of the frequency with which the oral cavity is examined by dentists and physicians, approximately 60% of intraoral carcinomas are well advanced

at the time of discovery. In addition, the surgical morbidity of oral cancers is high, and the 5-year survival rate is low (about 30%).

Erythematous (red) lesions seem to be much more indicative of oral cancer than are white lesions. Any persistent red lesion of the floor of the mouth, ventrolateral tongue, or soft palate complex should be considered carcinoma in situ or invasive carcinoma unless these entities are ruled out by biopsy.

Partially edentulous patients usually fall within the cancer-prone age group (40 to 60 years). Therefore, careful examination of the oral soft tissues is essential for these patients. Smokers and drinkers are particularly vulnerable to cancerous and precancerous lesions. As a result, patients who report long-term tobacco or alcohol use should be examined very carefully.

### Tissue reactions related to prosthesis utilization

Tissue reactions related to the use of dental prostheses should be recognized, evaluated, and treated as necessary. The most common tissue reactions related to prosthesis utilization are palatal papillary hyperplasia, denture epulis formation, denture stomatitis, and soft tissue displacement. A brief discussion of these conditions is presented in the following sections.

**Papillary hyperplasia** Papillary hyperplasia is a soft tissue condition that commonly occurs on the anterior hard palate but may affect the remainder of the hard palate and the residual ridges. The condition is caused by an inflammatory response in the submucosa. Clinically, papillary hyperplasia presents as a collection of small, rounded, soft tissue growths (Fig 6-87). Individual growths are separated by distinct crevices. Food

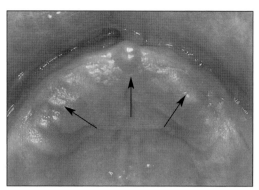

**Fig 6-87** Papillary hyperplasia *(arrows)* presents as a collection of small, rounded, soft tissue growths.

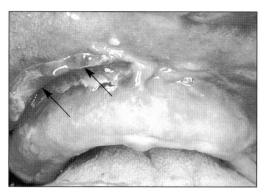

**Fig 6-88** Epulis fissuratum *(arrows)* is a hyperplastic growth caused by an ill-fitting or overextended denture base.

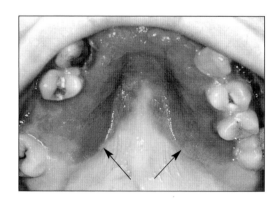

**Fig 6-89** Denture stomatitis *(arrows)* is characterized by erythema. The erythematous tissues are located adjacent to components of a removable prosthesis.

debris, fungi, and bacteria often collect in these crevices and may give rise to secondary infection.

At one time, palatal papillary hyperplasia was considered to be a premalignant lesion. This is no longer thought to be true. Nevertheless, a malignant or premalignant lesion may occupy the same area of the palate.

Palatal papillary hyperplasia usually is associated with poorly fitting prostheses that have been worn for prolonged periods. Inadequate oral hygiene also may contribute to development of this condition.

Tissue conditioning and tissue rest may help resolve some of the edema and inflammation, but only surgical removal will eliminate the hyperplastic papillae. As a result, the affected regions must be evaluated to determine whether they will present oral hygiene problems. If the patient will not be able to properly clean the affected tissues, the hyperplastic tissues should be removed.

**Epulis fissuratum** Epulis fissuratum is a tumorlike hyperplastic growth caused by an ill-fitting or overextended denture base (Fig 6-88). In some instances, it may present as a single fold of tissue adjacent to the border of a denture base. In others, it may appear as a double fold of tissue that projects along the internal and external surfaces of a denture base. The sulcus between the folds may be ulcerated.

In its early stages, an epulis is a soft, flabby growth of tissue that produces moderate discomfort. If left untreated, it assumes a harder, more fibrosed character.

In the past, such lesions were surgically excised. Unfortunately, surgical excision may produce scar tissue in the depth of the vestibule. Scarring may limit border extension and adversely affect denture base adaptation. These factors may adversely affect the stability of a removable prosthesis.

If an epulis has developed at a denture border, its consistency should be determined. A relatively soft

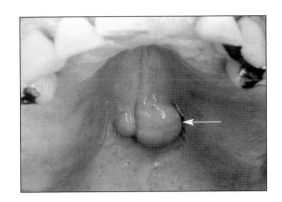

**Fig 6-90** Torus palatinus *(arrow)* is a bony overgrowth arising from the midline of the hard palate.

epulis may resolve if the source of irritation is removed. Hence, the offending border should be adjusted until it no longer contacts the lesion. The more fibrosed the epulis, the longer the time required for healing. Even a badly fibrosed epulis will undergo some degree of healing, thereby decreasing the size of the surgical site if excision becomes necessary.

**Denture stomatitis** Denture stomatitis is characterized by generalized erythema that affects the soft tissues covered by a prosthesis (Fig 6-89). It may occur under metal or acrylic resin denture bases and usually is seen in the maxilla. Frequently the oral mucosa is swollen and smooth. While patients may report burning or itching, they rarely complain of pain.

Research indicates that denture stomatitis is an endogenous infectious disease that affects the tissues and causes the associated lesions. Generally, patients with denture stomatitis display elevated levels of *Candida albicans*. However, treatment with antifungal medications alone will not cause resolution of denture stomatitis.

Trauma from occlusion, poor fit of the prosthesis, poor oral hygiene, and continuous wear of the prosthesis may contribute to this condition. Therefore, tissue rest and tissue conditioning procedures have been effective in treating denture stomatitis.

A treatment prosthesis is usually necessary if tissue conditioning procedures are to be used. Treatment dentures and tissue conditioning materials are discussed in more detail in chapter 18.

**Soft tissue displacement** Displacement of the soft tissues underlying ill-fitting or poorly designed removable partial dentures occurs frequently. Some tissue displacement is usually present in the beaded areas of even a well-fitting prosthesis. Therefore, soft tissues must be allowed to return to normal contours through tissue rest before impressions for master casts are made.

## Evaluation of hard tissue abnormalities

The presence of a torus, exostosis, or bony undercut can severely compromise the treatment of a partially edentulous patient. All areas to be covered by the prosthesis should be palpated to reveal bony protuberances that could interfere with the placement and removal of the prosthesis, as well as with the comfort of the patient. The diagnostic cast should be examined at the selected path of insertion to reveal potential hard tissue problems.

### Torus palatinus

Torus palatinus is a benign, slowly growing protuberance of the palatine processes of the maxilla (Fig 6-90). It occasionally involves the horizontal plates of the palatine bones. Palatal tori occur twice as often in women as in men and can be observed in approximately 20% of the adult population. Such tori serve no useful purpose. Removal of a torus palatinus is not necessary unless it is so large that it interferes with the design and construction of the prosthesis. In many instances, a major connector can be selected and designed to circumvent the torus.

### Torus mandibularis

The torus mandibularis is an exostosis on the lingual surface of the body of the mandible (Fig 6-91). In

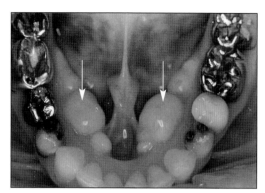

**Fig 6-91** Mandibular tori *(arrows)* are exostoses on the lingual surface of the mandible. In most instances, mandibular tori occur bilaterally.

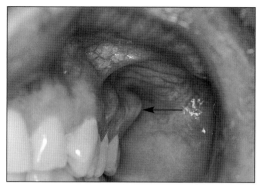

**Fig 6-92** An exostosis *(arrow)* is a bony overgrowth that may occur on any osseous surface. In this instance, the exostosis is located on the lateral aspect of the maxillary tuberosity.

most instances, such tori occur bilaterally. Mandibular tori occur in about 5% to 10% of the adult population and are equally distributed between the sexes. The mucoperiosteum covering such tori is very thin and easily traumatized.

Mandibular tori should be removed if the patient is to wear a removable partial denture with any degree of comfort. Severe compromises have to be made in the design, rigidity, and placement of the major connector if mandibular tori are not removed. Patient satisfaction with a removable partial denture constructed in the presence of a mandibular torus is rare. Most patients discontinue wearing the prosthesis in a short time. Removal of mandibular tori is not difficult and complications are rare if good technique and proper instrumentation are used. Tori can be removed with the patient under local anesthesia and in conjunction with extractions or periodontal surgery.

### Exostoses and undercuts

Exostoses and undercuts that prevent the proper extension of the denture borders should be evaluated and surgically corrected, if necessary (Fig 6-92).

Exostoses are common in the maxillary arch, but occur less frequently in the mandible. The soft tissues covering exostoses are usually thin. Because pressure from the placement and wear of a removable partial denture can cause the patient considerable discomfort, exostoses should be removed.

The maxillary tuberosities, the distolingual areas in the mandibular arch, and recent extraction sites are the most common undercut areas. The effect of some undercut areas may be minimized by a change in the path of insertion of a proposed removable partial denture. Only those undercuts that would seriously compromise the prognosis should be surgically corrected. This decision should be based on whether the denture base can be effectively relieved to accommodate the undercut areas.

Surgical correction of undercuts should be accomplished if relieving the denture base or reducing the length of the denture border would *(1)* significantly reduce support and stability of the prosthesis; *(2)* create a bothersome food impaction area; or *(3)* cause a denture border to be so far away from the underlying tissue that it may affect function, compromise esthetics, or cause discomfort for the patient.

### Evaluation of soft tissue abnormalities

Various soft tissue conditions can present problems in the design and construction of a removable partial denture. Labial and lingual frena, as well as unsupported and hypermobile gingiva should be evaluated to determine whether surgical correction will improve the prognosis.

### Labial frenum

The maxillary labial frenum occasionally presents problems when anterior teeth are replaced with a removable partial denture (Fig 6-93). If the frenum is attached near the crest of the ridge or if it is hyper-

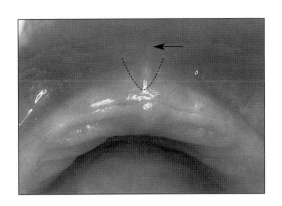

**Fig 6-93** A maxillary labial frenum *(arrow)* that is located near the crest of the ridge may cause difficulties in prosthesis construction and service. The *broken line* depicts denture base contours necessary to accommodate a prominent frenum.

trophic, the notch that must be placed in the denture base to accommodate the frenum may be unsightly. A patient with a short or highly mobile upper lip is most likely to need a frenectomy to correct the condition.

### Unsupported and hypermobile gingiva

Unsupported and hypermobile gingiva occurs more frequently in completely edentulous patients. Nevertheless, atrophy of the residual ridge may occur in partially edentulous patients. In these instances, the gingiva loses its bony support and becomes freely mobile. Adequate support is not provided for the denture base. When this occurs, the area should be evaluated to determine whether removal of the soft tissue would result in an excessively short residual ridge. Vestibular extension or ridge augmentation procedures should be considered.

## Evaluation of quantity and quality of saliva

If the mouth is dry, the patient will probably be uncomfortable wearing a removable partial denture. Denture bases will drag across the tissues during placement and removal of the prosthesis. This may result in irritation or ulceration of the soft tissues and significant discomfort for the patient.

Medications, radiation, advanced age, systemic disturbances, and anxiety can markedly reduce salivary output. Hence, a thorough medical history is essential.

Thick, mucinous saliva and excessive quantities of saliva present problems during impression procedures. These problems and their solutions are discussed in chapter 5.

## Evaluation of space for mandibular major connector

A properly constructed lingual bar major connector must be a minimum of 5 mm in height. The superior margin of the connector should be located 3 mm from the free gingival margins of the mandibular teeth to avoid damage to the gingival tissues. The inferior border of the connector should be positioned at or slightly above the active floor of the mouth to prevent interference with functional movements and to minimize the accumulation of food under the major connector. Therefore, a minimum of 8 mm of vertical space must be available if a lingual bar major connector is planned. A lingual plate major connector should be used if less than 8 mm is available.

It is not possible to accurately determine the position of the active floor of the mouth on a cast because most casts are overextended in this area. The selection of the major connector and the determination of the location of its inferior border can be accomplished most effectively when the distance from the free gingival margins to the active floor of the mouth is measured in the mouth.

Available space can be measured with a calibrated instrument. A periodontal probe with millimeter markings works well. The patient is instructed to raise the tongue toward the palate. This raises the floor of the mouth to its highest level. The tip of the probe is placed to contact the floor of the mouth lightly (Fig 6-94). The millimeter depth is read at the point where the probe contacts the gingival margin. Readings are made and recorded at several positions. The probe is

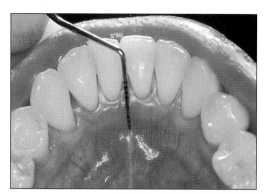

**Fig 6-94** A periodontal probe may be used to measure from the gingival margins to the active floor of the mouth.

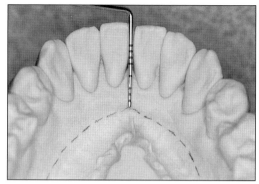

**Fig 6-95** Measurements made in the oral cavity (Fig 6-94) are transferred to the mandibular cast.

then used to transfer the measurements to the diagnostic cast (Fig 6-95). The points are connected by drawing a line that will indicate the position of the active floor of the mouth.

## Evaluation of radiographic survey

An evaluation of the complete radiographic survey is made with special attention focused on prospective abutments and residual ridge areas. All radiolucent and radiopaque areas that vary from normal ranges are carefully examined to determine whether a pathologic condition is present.

The radiographic findings are correlated with the clinical examination to reveal the presence and extent of caries and the relation of the carious lesion to the dental pulp. Existing restorations are evaluated to determine their adequacy.

Root fragments and other foreign bodies are evaluated to determine whether their removal is indicated. Not all retained roots have to be removed. If the roots are deeply embedded and exhibit no evidence of pathologic changes, it is frequently advisable to keep them under observation rather than to remove them. Removing deeply embedded root tips may necessitate the removal of bone and result in a somewhat compromised residual ridge. Root tips not completely enclosed in bone and any retained root or foreign body that shows radiographic evidence of pathologic changes should be removed.

Third molars are evaluated to determine whether they should be retained or removed. Consideration should be given to retaining the third molar as a posterior abutment if its size, shape, and position appear favorable. The greater comfort and stability provided by a tooth-borne removable partial denture (versus a distal extension removable partial denture) make the retention of a possible posterior abutment extremely important. It can be hazardous to retain an unerupted third molar if it is to be covered by a prosthesis. Subsequent eruption can contribute to considerable occlusal and tissue trauma. Therefore, the patient must understand the potential problems and must report the first signs or symptoms of eruption. As an additional measure, frequent clinical and radiographic examinations should be arranged.

Root canal fillings within prospective abutments are evaluated with special emphasis. Root canal fillings should be reaccomplished if the quality or completeness of the fill is questionable. Radiolucent areas on the lateral or apical aspects of the root require careful evaluation. Available radiographs should be examined to determine whether the radiolucency indicates a new pathologic condition or fibrous healing. In most instances, the placement of an extracoronal restoration is indicated on an abutment that has received endodontic treatment, particularly if a large access opening has been made or if the tooth has extensive intracoronal restorations.

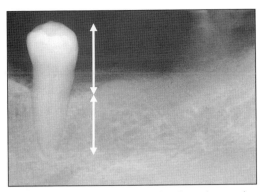

**Fig 6-96** A periodontally involved tooth may be considered for use as an overdenture abutment.

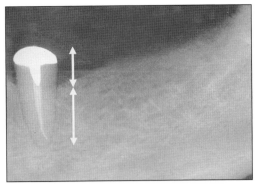

**Fig 6-97** The resultant overdenture abutment displays an improved crown-root ratio (compare with Fig 6-96).

## Radiographic evaluation of prospective abutment teeth

All prospective abutment teeth must be critically evaluated as described in the following discussion.

### Root length, size, and form

Teeth with large or long roots are more favorable abutments because of the greater potential area for periodontal support. However, the relationship between the length of the clinical crown and the amount of root embedded in bone is the most critical factor.

The root form of a prospective abutment has a significant influence on its probable effectiveness. Tapered or conical roots are unfavorable because even a small loss of bone height can greatly diminish the attachment area. Multirooted teeth whose roots are divergent or curved generally are stronger abutment teeth than single-rooted teeth or multirooted teeth whose roots are fused.

The proximity of roots also is important. If the roots of adjacent teeth are in close proximity and display little interproximal bone, even moderate irritation or force may be destructive.

### Crown-root ratio

If the crown-root ratio is greater than 1:1 or if furcation involvement of a multirooted tooth is present, the tooth has a poor prognosis as an abutment. Nevertheless, a tooth with a poor prognosis can still provide support for a prosthesis. Periodontal, endodontic, and restorative treatment can be used to retain one or more roots of a multirooted tooth. Alternatively, endodontic treatment can be used to prepare a tooth with a poor crown-root ratio as an overdenture abutment (Figs 6-96 and 6-97).

### Lamina dura

Partial or total absence of the lamina dura may be found in systemic disorders such as hyperparathyroidism and Paget disease. However, changes in the lamina dura are more frequently caused by function. Resorption or loss of lamina dura occurs where there is pressure, and apposition occurs where there is tension. A tooth that is in the process of tipping because of loss of an adjacent tooth will show evidence of both resorption and apposition. A thickening of the lamina dura may occur if the tooth is mobile, has occlusal trauma, or is under heavy function. Occlusal trauma can also cause partial or total loss of the lamina dura. Evidence of changes in the lamina dura should be correlated with findings of the clinical examination and evaluation of the occlusion. Destructive forces or disease processes causing changes in the lamina dura must be corrected, or the abutment will have a poor prognosis.

### Periodontal ligament space

Changes in the width of the periodontal ligament space must be considered when prospective abutments are evaluated. A widening of the periodontal ligament space with a thickening of the lamina dura

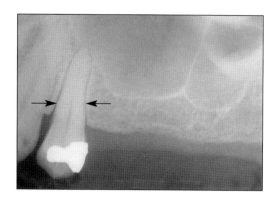

**Fig 6-98** Widening of the periodontal ligament space *(arrows)* usually indicates occlusal trauma and tooth mobility.

usually indicates mobility, occlusal trauma, and heavy function (Fig 6-98). To evaluate these radiographic findings, it is necessary to correlate them with clinical mobility. If the tooth is mobile, these radiographic signs indicate destructive changes. If the tooth is not mobile, these signs may indicate a favorable response to increased occlusal forces. However, the added stress of serving as an abutment may result in severe damage or failure. Therefore, every effort should be made to eliminate heavy occlusal forces on a prospective abutment.

## Evaluation of mounted diagnostic casts

Mounted diagnostic casts can provide important information that may be difficult to obtain by intraoral examination alone. Potential problems such as insufficient interarch space, irregularity or malposition of the occlusal plane, extruded or malposed teeth, and unfavorable maxillomandibular relationships are more apparent when using accurately mounted casts because the lips, cheeks, and skull do not permit good visual access to the teeth in the mouth. Mounted diagnostic casts provide improved visual access from all directions and enable the practitioner to make a detailed analysis of the patient's occlusion.

### Interarch distance

A fairly common finding is lack of sufficient interarch distance for the placement of prosthetic teeth. Frequently the problem is caused by a maxillary tuberosity that is too large (Fig 6-99). A segment of teeth that

has been unopposed for a prolonged period will frequently overerupt, carrying the alveolar process with it. Subsequent removal of the teeth will produce a situation in which it is impossible to establish an acceptable occlusal plane. Surgical reduction of the tuberosity may be necessary if satisfactory replacement of the missing teeth is to be accomplished. The amount and location of tissues to be removed can be indicated on the diagnostic cast. This provides an excellent guide for the practitioner who performs the surgical correction. Radiographs are valuable aids when planning such procedures. The soft tissues overlying each tuberosity are visible on panoramic radiographs and indicate the thickness of coverage in these areas. This helps the practitioner determine whether the surgical procedure can be accomplished by soft tissue correction alone or whether bone removal is also necessary (Fig 6-100). The majority of tuberosity interferences can be corrected by removal of a wedge of soft tissue. Healing is usually complete in 7 to 10 days. The healing period is extended to 2 to 3 weeks when bone removal is necessary.

Maxillary tuberosities also may exhibit unilateral or bilateral mechanical undercuts. These undercuts are carefully evaluated using a dental surveyor. With the cast on the surveying table at the predetermined path of insertion, a determination is made regarding the amount of relief that will be required in the denture if the undercut is not reduced (Fig 6-101). Moderate to severe tuberosity undercuts usually require surgical correction with bone removal.

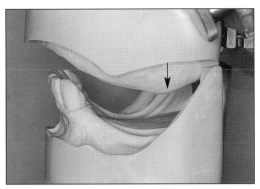

Fig 6-99 Enlargement of the maxillary tuberosities *(arrow)* may yield insufficient room for appropriate prosthetic tooth placement.

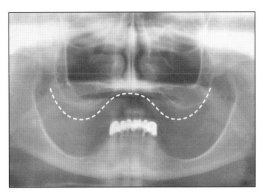

Fig 6-100 A panoramic radiograph is helpful in determining whether tuberosity reduction will require the removal of bone, soft tissue, or a combination of bone and soft tissue. The *broken line* indicates the level of the soft tissue overlying the residual ridge.

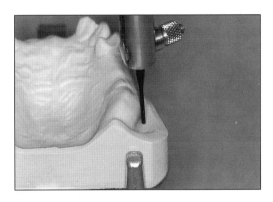

Fig 6-101 Maxillary tuberosities may exhibit lateral undercuts that require relief.

## Occlusal plane

The occlusal plane may be irregular because of extrusion of one or more unopposed teeth. The entire plane may be poorly oriented because of the extrusion of a sizable segment of the dental arch. Both conditions require corrective procedures if an acceptable occlusion is to be developed.

**Irregular occlusal plane** Several courses of treatment are available for correction of an extruded tooth. The treatment will vary depending on the degree of extrusion and the condition of the tooth.

Enameloplasty can be used to reduce a moderately extruded tooth. Approximately 2 mm of enamel can be removed in many situations. At times, such reduction can correct a noticeable discrepancy in the occlusal plane (Fig 6-102).

If the extrusion is greater than 2 mm or if the tooth does not lend itself to enameloplasty, the placement of a crown may be indicated (Fig 6-103). Tooth reduction may be limited by the size of the dental pulp, the length of the clinical crown, or both. If the size of the dental pulp will prevent the required tooth reduction, endodontic therapy should be completed before tooth preparation is undertaken. If clinical crown length is inadequate, crown-lengthening procedures should be completed before tooth preparation is begun (Fig 6-104).

Severely extruded teeth, such as those contacting the opposing ridge, present greater problems. If the alveolar bone has followed the eruption of the offending tooth, it may be necessary to remove the tooth and recontour the surrounding bone. At times endodontic treatment and drastic reduction of the tooth will enable it to be used as an overdenture abutment. This treatment can provide valuable support for a distal extension base.

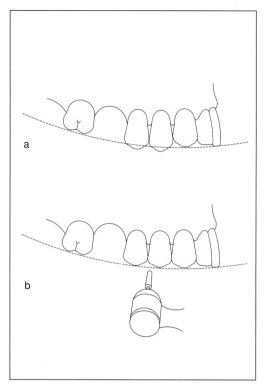

**Fig 6-102** Under certain circumstances, a discrepancy in the occlusal plane *(a)* can be corrected using enameloplasty *(b)*.

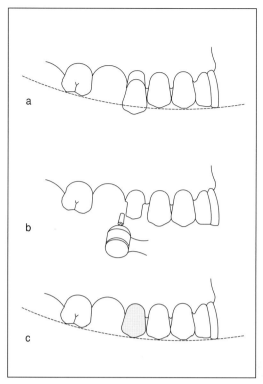

**Fig 6-103** If a tooth has extruded more than 2 mm *(a)*, placement of a crown *(b and c)* may be indicated.

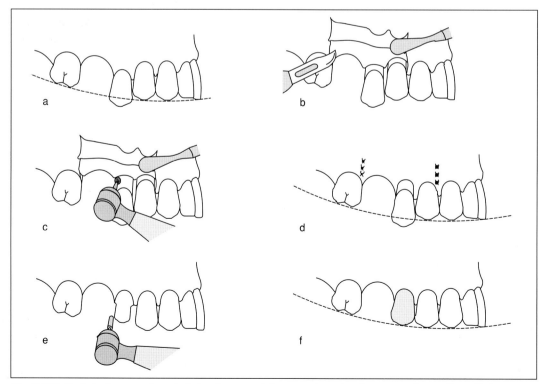

**Fig 6-104** If clinical crown length is inadequate *(a)*, crown-lengthening procedures *(b to f)* should be completed before tooth preparation is begun.

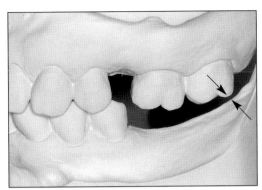

**Fig 6-105** Extruded teeth may approximate or contact the opposing ridge *(arrows)*. This produces distinct difficulties in prosthodontic therapy.

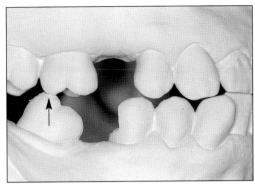

**Fig 6-106** A diagnostic mounting is helpful in identifying occlusal interferences *(arrow)*.

**Malpositioned occlusal plane** In some instances, maxillary premolars and molars may be unopposed on one or both sides of the dental arch. Often this results in extrusion of the unopposed teeth and is accompanied by a downgrowth of the associated alveolar process. The extruded teeth may approximate or contact the opposing residual ridge, causing obvious space problems and malposition of the occlusal plane (Fig 6-105).

One approach to treatment is the removal of the extruded teeth in conjunction with an extensive alveolectomy. However, consideration should be given to corrective (ie, orthognathic) surgical procedures. These procedures are beyond the scope of this text. Therefore, readers are referred to oral and maxillofacial surgery texts for a thorough review of orthognathic surgical procedures and their applications.

## Malrelation of jaws

Severe malrelation of the jaws can preclude the restoration of adequate function and esthetics. Several maxillary and mandibular osteotomy procedures are useful in correcting these problems. The practitioner is referred to oral and maxillofacial surgery texts for a thorough review of these procedures.

## Tipped or malposed teeth

Posterior teeth tend to drift or tip anteriorly when an edentulous space is created immediately mesial to them. Limited orthodontic procedures for minor tooth movement can be used to upright such teeth and permit an improved prosthodontic result.

Remaining teeth also may be buccally or lingually inclined. In many instances, the orientations of these teeth may be corrected via controlled orthodontic movement. In other instances, removal of one or more malposed teeth may simplify the design of the prosthesis.

## Occlusion

Mounted diagnostic casts are commonly used for occlusal assessment. The information obtained during occlusal assessment should be correlated with relevant clinical findings. A common finding is the presence of occlusal interferences (Fig 6-106).

More than 90% of patients display a noticeable discrepancy between centric relation and maximal intercuspal position. Partially edentulous patients have an even greater probability of deflective occlusal contacts because of the drifting and migration of teeth that usually accompany the loss of one or more posterior teeth. Many patients can adapt to imperfections in the occlusion so that deflective contacts do not become traumatic factors. However, there is a limit to physiologic adaptation to the imperfections or disharmony of occlusion. This limit may be surpassed if additional discrepancies are added to the occlusion or if central nervous system tension increases. The result may be increased muscular response leading to bruxism.

Severe bruxism can injure the teeth, the periodontium, and the temporomandibular joint and may initiate muscle spasm and discomfort. The most common causes of bruxism are *(1)* occlusal interferences (ie, deflective contacts) between centric relation and maxi-

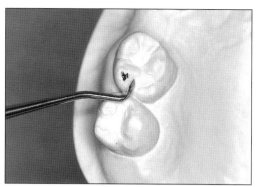

**Fig 6-107** Trial equilibration is performed on mounted diagnostic casts.

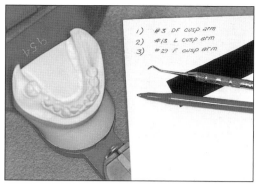

**Fig 6-108** Trial equilibration serves as a blueprint for intraoral adjustment. Therefore, all steps in the trial equilibration process should be recorded.

mal intercuspal position and *(2)* occlusal contacts on the nonworking side of the arch.

The clinical symptoms of traumatic occlusion often present in the following ways:

1. Excessive wear of the teeth, which may include chipping or fracture of their surfaces (see Fig 5-3)
2. A noticeable change in the periodontium, which may result in increased tooth mobility, tooth migration, and discomfort during occlusal contact
3. Involvement of the neuromuscular mechanisms of the temporomandibular joint, which may include muscle spasm, muscle pain, and joint dysfunction

The radiographic signs of traumatic occlusion may include

1. Widening of the periodontal ligament space with increased or decreased thickness of lamina dura
2. Periapical radiolucency
3. Resorption of alveolar bone
4. Root resorption

**Role of occlusal equilibration** Occlusal equilibration is the selective grinding or coronal reshaping of teeth with the intent of producing simultaneous occlusal contacts, minimizing non-axial forces, and/or harmonizing cuspal relations.

Some practitioners believe that all patients should undergo occlusal equilibration to ensure that centric relation and maximal intercuspal position are coinci-

dent. However, occlusal equilibration should not be accomplished for every patient with interferences. Many patients exhibit skeletal and neuromuscular characteristics that minimize dental wear regardless of the occlusal relationships of the teeth. If occlusal equilibration is accomplished on these individuals, an "occlusal awareness" can be developed and may contribute to destructive neuromuscular activity. Faulty occlusal equilibration may induce severe trauma from occlusion.

Extensive occlusal equilibration should never be initiated on a patient with acute temporomandibular joint dysfunction. The symptoms and muscle spasm should be eliminated through the use of an occlusal device before occlusal adjustment is initiated.

Occlusal equilibration should be accomplished only for those individuals who have a definite need for such treatment, such as those with symptoms of traumatic occlusion. Nonworking interferences on natural teeth are particularly destructive and should be eliminated.

If an occlusal equilibration is indicated, the equilibration should be accomplished before restorative procedures are initiated. To determine the feasibility and outcome of this process, an equilibration should first be accomplished on accurately mounted diagnostic casts. This trial equilibration can serve as a blueprint for intraoral adjustment, and, therefore, all steps should be recorded (Figs 6-107 and 6-108). In addition, the diagnostic equilibration may indicate the need for extraction, orthodontic therapy, placement of fixed restorations, or a combination of these procedures.

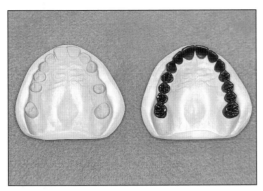

**Fig 6-109** A diagnostic waxup is a valuable diagnostic tool.

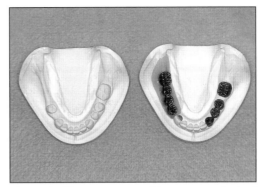

**Fig 6-110** The waxup provides a great deal of information regarding tooth preparation, placement, and occlusion.

### The decision to treat at centric relation or maximal intercuspal position

The decision whether to construct a prosthesis at centric relation or maximal intercuspal position must be made during the diagnostic phase of treatment. The following clinical situations suggest that prostheses should be constructed at centric relation:

1. Coincidence of centric jaw relation and maximal intercuspal position
2. Absence of posterior tooth contacts
3. Situation in which all posterior tooth contacts are to be restored using fixed restorations
4. Few remaining posterior contacts
5. Existing occlusion that can be made acceptable with minor occlusal equilibration
6. Clinical symptoms of occlusal trauma

In the absence of these indications, a removable partial denture should be constructed at maximal intercuspal position. Special care must be taken in the construction and fitting of the prosthesis to make certain that new interferences are not introduced by a removable partial denture.

### Diagnostic waxup

A diagnostic waxup is a valuable diagnostic tool, especially if multiple crowns or fixed partial dentures are planned (Figs 6-109 and 6-110). Problems involving the position and relationship of the remaining teeth become apparent. In addition, the diagnostic waxup provides a guide for tooth preparation and helps indicate problems that may be encountered in establishing the desired occlusal relationships.

## Consultation Requests

Consultation with appropriate medical or dental specialists is often necessary to ensure the safety and suitability of patient treatment. Consultation requests and reports should be clearly written to avoid misunderstandings. Written consultation requests and reports become a permanent part of the patient's record and are available for reference if needed.

The request for medical consultation should include information about the patient's oral condition and should indicate the dental procedures to be used during treatment. Specific questions concerning the need for premedication or supportive medical care may be appropriate.

Consultation requests to dental specialists should indicate whether the patient is being referred for an opinion or for specific treatment. The dentist's evaluation of the present oral condition and the tentative sequence of treatment should also be included. Clear communication and cooperation are essential whenever more than one dentist is responsible for the treatment of the patient.

## ▢ Development of Treatment Plan

The development of an appropriate treatment plan for a partially edentulous patient can be extremely difficult. A great number of factors influence the ultimate success of treatment. An adequate level of oral hygiene is one of the most important factors, and yet it is one of the most elusive.

A patient requiring removable partial denture service but displaying poor oral hygiene presents a dilemma for the dentist. Treatment options may range from maintenance of the existing dentition (no removable partial dentures) to extraction of all remaining teeth and construction of complete dentures. Nevertheless, extremes of treatment are not always appropriate, and some degree of compromise between the ideal and practical considerations becomes necessary. It is in these "gray areas" of decision making that the dentist's clinical judgment is put to its greatest test. Decisions must be based on complete evaluation of all diagnostic data. Properly mounted diagnostic casts are essential in the planning of treatment for a partially edentulous patient. Appropriate removable partial denture designs also are essential. The procedures required to treat the patient should then be placed into a logical treatment sequence.

Treatment of a partially edentulous patient can be divided into five phases. While some phases may overlap, the overall treatment plan should reflect these five phases of treatment. Procedures within each phase should be completed on a priority basis depending upon the patient's needs.

### Phase I

1. Collection and evaluation of the diagnostic data, including a diagnostic mounting and design of diagnostic casts
2. Immediate treatment to control pain or infection
3. Biopsy or referral of patient to an appropriate health professional
4. Development of a treatment plan
5. Education and motivation of patient

### Phase II

1. Removal of deep caries and placement of provisional restorations
2. Extirpation of inflamed or necrotic pulp tissues
3. Removal of periodontally hopeless and nonrestorable teeth
4. Periodontal therapy
5. Construction of interim prostheses for function or esthetics
6. Occlusal equilibration
7. Education and motivation of patient

### Phase III

1. Preprosthetic surgical procedures
2. Definitive endodontic procedures
3. Definitive restoration of teeth, including placement of fixed restorations
4. Fixed partial denture construction
5. Education and motivation of patient

### Phase IV

1. Construction and placement of removable partial denture(s)
2. Oral and written instructions regarding the use and care of removable prostheses

### Phase V

1. Postinsertion care
2. Periodic recall
3. Reinforcement of education and motivation of patient

## ▢ Length of Appointment

The length of this appointment can vary, depending on the complexity of the problems presented by the patient. A dental student should allow 3 to 4 hours to complete these procedures. A more experienced clinician may require 1 to 2 hours to complete the procedures.

## ⊑ Reference

1. Ramfjord SP, Ash MM Jr. Occlusion, ed 2. Philadelphia: Saunders, 1971.

## ⊑ **Bibliography**

Akerly WB. Prosthodontic treatment of traumatic overlap of anterior teeth. J Prosthet Dent 1977;38:26–34.

Alexander JM, Van Sickels JE. Posterior maxillary osteotomies: An aid for a difficult prosthodontic problem. J Prosthet Dent 1979;41:614–617.

Applegate OC. An evaluation of the support for the removable partial denture. J Prosthet Dent 1960;10:112–123.

Bhaskar SN. Synopsis of Oral Pathology, ed 5. St. Louis: Mosby, 1977.

Bollender CL, Swenson RD, Yamane G. Evaluation of treatment of inflammatory papillary hyperplasia of the palate. J Prosthet Dent 1965;15:1013–1022.

Brasher WJ, Rees TD. The medical consultation: Its role in dentistry. J Am Dent Assoc 1977;95:961–964.

Carranza FA Jr. Glickman's Clinical Periodontology, ed 5. Philadelphia: Saunders, 1979.

Christiansen RL. Rationale of the facebow in maxillary cast mounting. J Prosthet Dent 1959;9:388–398.

Epker BN, Bronson J. Surgical-prosthetic correction of dentofacial deformities. J Am Dent Assoc 1978;97:184–192.

Goldman HM, Cohen D. Periodontal Therapy, ed 6. St. Louis: Mosby, 1980.

Langland OE, Sippy FH. Textbook of Dental Radiography. Springfield, IL: Charles C Thomas, 1973.

Mashberg A. Erythroplasia: The earliest sign of asymptomatic oral cancer. J Am Dent Assoc 1978;96:615–620.

Matthews TG. Medication side effects of dental interest. J Prosthet Dent 1990;64:219–226.

McCarthy PL, Shklar G. Diseases of the Oral Mucosa, ed 2. Philadelphia: Lea & Febiger, 1980.

McNeill C, Danzig WM, Farrar WB, et al. Position paper of the American Academy of Craniomandibular Disorders. Craniomandibular (TMJ) disorders—The state of the art. J Prosthet Dent 1980;44:434–437.

Miller EL. Clinical management of denture induced inflammations. J Prosthet Dent 1977;38:362–365.

Miller EL. Sometimes overlooked, preprosthetic surgery. J Prosthet Dent 1976;36:484–490.

Millstein PL, Clark RE, Kronman JH. Determination of the accuracy of wax interocclusal registrations. II. J Prosthet Dent 1973;29:40–45.

Mopsik ER, Buck RP, Connors JO, Watts LN. Surgical intervention to reestablish adequate intermaxillary space before fixed or removable prosthodontics. J Am Dent Assoc 1977;95:957–980.

Palomo F, Kopczyk RA. Rationale and methods of crown lengthening. J Am Dent Assoc 1978;96:257–260.

Pruden WH II. The role of study casts in diagnosis and treatment planning. J Prosthet Dent 1960;10:707–710.

Reynolds JM. Occlusal wear facets. J Prosthet Dent 1970;24:367–372.

Scott AS, Frew AL Jr. Orthognatic surgery: Combined maxillary and mandibular osteotomies with variations of surgical modalities. J Am Dent Assoc 1976;93:98–104.

Sheppard IM, Sheppard SM. Characteristics of temporomandibular joint problems. J Prosthet Dent 1977;38:180–191.

Stafne EC, Gebilisco JA. Oral roentgenographic diagnosis. Philadelphia: Saunders, 1975.

Starshak TJ. Preprosthetic oral surgery. St. Louis: Mosby, 1971.

Turner C, Shaffer FW. Planning the treatment of the complex prosthodontic case. J Am Dent Assoc 1978;97:992–993.

Weinberg LA. An evaluation of basic articulators and their concepts, I and II. J Prosthet Dent 1963;13:622–633.

Weinberg LA. An evaluation of the facebow mounting. J Prosthet Dent 1961;11:32–42.

Wood C Jr, Harrison B, Ackerson D, McCurdy T. Coordination of the goals of orthodontic, surgical, and prosthetic dentistry, anterior maxillary osteotomy. J Am Dent Assoc 1978;97:650–655.

Wood NK. Treatment planning: A pragmatic approach. St. Louis: Mosby, 1978.

Zarb GA, Bergman B, Clayton JA, McKay HF. Prosthodontic Treatment for Partially Edentulous Patients. St. Louis: Mosby, 1978.

# Survey and Design

## ❏ Survey

### Dental surveyor

During the first part of the twentieth century, most removable partial dentures were designed and constructed using arbitrary techniques. Perhaps the most common technique involved viewing dental casts at arm's length and guessing the locations of mechanical undercuts. The associated removable partial denture frameworks would then be designed, constructed, and fitted. As might be expected, the intraoral fitting process was time consuming and often resulted in poorly fitting prostheses.

The turning point in removable partial denture service occurred in 1918. In that year, Dr A. J. Fortunati introduced the dental surveyor at a dental clinic in Boston. Fortunati's surveyor was essentially a parallelometer—an instrument used to determine the parallelism of surfaces. Despite its simplicity, this device changed removable partial denture service from guesswork to an objective, scientifically based procedure.

In 1923 the J. M. Ney Corporation introduced the first commercially available surveyor. In the ensuing years, a number of dental surveyors were introduced. Many of these surveyors were complicated, but all were intended to facilitate the design process and improve treatment outcomes.

Currently, there are a limited number of surveyors on the market. These surveyors vary in design, but most have the following parts (Fig 7-1):

1. A level platform that is parallel to the bench top and on which the cast holder is moved.
2. A vertical column that supports the suprastructure.
3. A horizontal arm that extends at a right angle from the vertical column.
4. A surveying arm that extends vertically from the horizontal arm. The surveying arm is capable of movement in a vertical direction and contains a mandrel at its lower end. This mandrel holds specialized tools that are used in the surveying process.

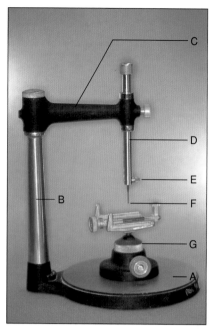

**Fig 7-1** The Ney dental surveyor (Ney Dental, Bloomfield, CT) consists of a surveying platform (A); a vertical column (B); a horizontal arm (C); a surveying arm (D); a mandrel (E), which holds various surveying tools (F); and a surveying table (G).

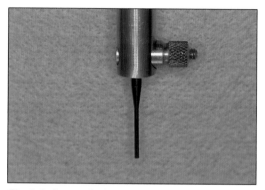

**Fig 7-2** An analyzing rod is positioned in the mandrel of the surveying arm and used to determine relative parallelism of surfaces on a dental cast.

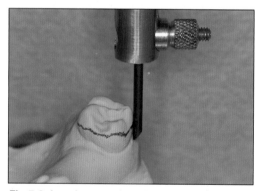

**Fig 7-3** A carbon marker also may be placed in the mandrel. The carbon marker is used to mark the greatest circumference of the teeth. The lines that result are termed *survey lines*.

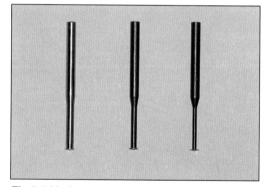

**Fig 7-4** Undercut gauges are used to accurately locate retentive undercuts on proposed abutments. Undercut gauges are commonly supplied in *(left to right)* 0.010-, 0.020-, and 0.030-inch embodiments.

5. Surveying tools that may be placed in the mandrel and used in various surveying applications. These surveying tools include
   - An analyzing rod, which is used to determine relative parallelism of surfaces on a dental cast (Fig 7-2)
   - A carbon marker, which is used to mark the height of contour on one or more surfaces of a dental cast (Fig 7-3)
   - Undercut gauges, which are used to identify the positions of desired undercuts on dental casts (Fig 7-4)

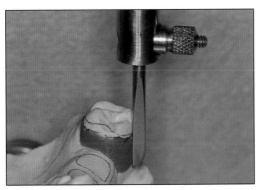

**Fig 7-5** A wax knife is commonly used during blockout procedures and in the construction of surveyed restorations.

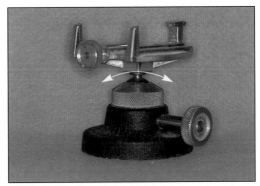

**Fig 7-6** The surveying table includes a ball-and-socket joint, which allows spatial reorientation of the dental cast *(arrows)*.

- A wax knife, which is used during blockout procedures and in the construction of surveyed restorations (Fig 7-5)
6. A surveying table designed to hold a dental cast (Fig 7-6). The surveying table includes a ball-and-socket joint, which permits spatial reorientation of the cast (ie, tipping or tilting).

## Survey process

Partially edentulous arches consist of teeth and edentulous spaces. The dental arches also may present with complicating factors such as soft tissue undercuts and bony prominences (ie, tori or exostoses). When planning a removable partial denture, all of these factors must be considered. The contours of proposed abutments must be analyzed and coordinated with other teeth that will be contacted by the removable partial denture. The contours of the adjacent ridges also must be considered. The best way to evaluate and address these factors is through the use of accurate diagnostic casts and a dental surveyor.

The surveying process is composed of several phases. Each phase is important in successful removable partial denture therapy. As a result, these procedures are described in the following sections.

### Identifying the most favorable tilt

During the initial stages of the surveying process, a cast of the dental arch is affixed to the surveying table (Fig 7-7). The ball-and-socket design of the table permits the practitioner to change the tilt of the cast and to determine the effects of such changes. In this manner, the practitioner may determine the most favorable tilt of the cast.

By convention, the tilt of the cast is described from the viewpoint of a person looking at its posterior surface. Therefore, if the anterior of the cast is lowered, the cast is said to have an anterior tilt. If the posterior is lowered, the cast is said to have a posterior tilt. If the right side is lowered, the cast is said to have a right tilt. And if the left side is lowered, it is said to have a left tilt (Figs 7-8 and 7-9). Any combination of tilts may be used, but extreme tilts should be avoided.

There are four critical factors that must be considered when determining the most favorable tilt of a dental cast. These factors are *(1)* the presence of suitable undercuts; *(2)* the elimination of hard and soft tissue interferences; *(3)* the creation of desirable esthetics; and *(4)* the establishment of appropriate guiding planes. Rarely is it possible to achieve the optimum in all four areas. Therefore, the practitioner must weigh these factors against one another when attempting to determine the best solution.

For purposes of discussion, the foregoing factors have been listed in order of importance. The impact of these factors is more fully described in the following sections.

**Retentive undercuts** The first, unchangeable rule to remember when surveying diagnostic casts for removable partial dentures is that retentive undercuts must

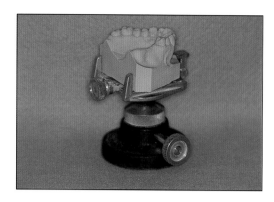

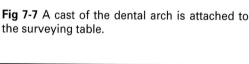

Fig 7-7 A cast of the dental arch is attached to the surveying table.

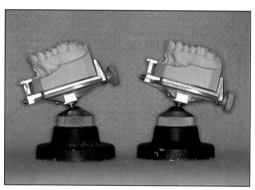

**Fig 7-8** The tilt of a dental cast is described from the viewpoint of a person looking at its posterior surface. Hence, the cast on the left displays an anterior tilt, while the cast on the right displays a posterior tilt.

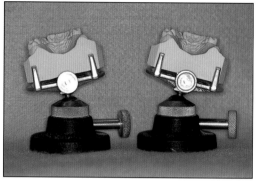

**Fig 7-9** The cast on the left displays a left tilt. The cast on the right displays a right tilt.

be present on the abutment teeth when the cast displays a horizontal tilt. This is essential because dislodging forces are always directed perpendicular to the occlusal plane (Fig 7-10). These forces may include the pull produced by sticky foods or the force of gravity acting on a maxillary denture. Regardless of the cause, resistance to dislodging forces must be present when the dental arch is in a horizontal position. Changing the tilt to produce undercuts is an illusion (Fig 7-11). Unfortunately, in the harsh world of reality, the illusion will vanish and all that will be left is a nonretentive prosthesis of questionable clinical value.

The surveying procedure is always started with the cast firmly attached to the surveying table and the occlusal surfaces parallel to the platform of the surveyor. In turn, each abutment is examined for retentive undercuts. This is accomplished by placing the analyzing rod in the dental surveyor and evaluating the contours of the proposed abutments.

If retentive undercuts are not present, they must be created in the mouth. In most instances, this may be accomplished by carefully recontouring enamel surfaces. In cases requiring more extensive changes, it may be necessary to place fixed restorations (eg, gold crowns or metal-ceramic crowns). If fixed restorations are indicated, these restorations must be carefully planned and completed prior to removable partial denture fabrication. Restorations such as Class V inlays and ceramic veneers may occasionally be used to create retentive undercuts, but they are not as common as complete-coverage restorations. A more thorough description of recontouring is presented in chapter 9.

Ideally, each of the proposed abutments should display a 0.010-inch undercut at the most desirable location. This may be the mesiobuccal line angle, the distobuccal line angle, or the midfacial surface, depending upon the practitioner's clasping philosophy. If a wrought-wire clasp is planned, a retentive under-

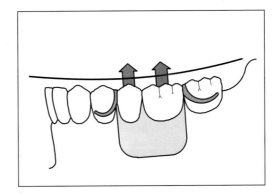

**Fig 7-10** Dislodging forces *(arrows)* are always directed perpendicular to the patient's occlusal plane.

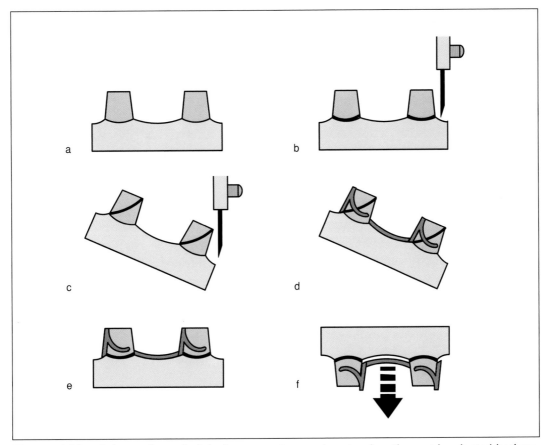

**Fig 7-11** *(a)* Parallel, tapering cylinders that present no undercuts when the cast is oriented horizontally. *(b)* Use of a dental surveyor verifies the absence of mechanical undercuts. *(c)* By tilting the cast, the operator can produce the illusion of usable undercuts. *(d)* A removable partial denture framework may be fabricated based upon the apparent survey lines. *(e)* When the cast is returned to a horizontal orientation, the perceived undercuts disappear. *(f)* This lack of retention becomes evident when the cast is inverted, as would occur in maxillary applications. Such a framework is of questionable clinical value.

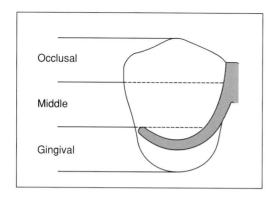

Occlusal

Middle

Gingival

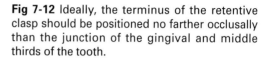

**Fig 7-12** Ideally, the terminus of the retentive clasp should be positioned no farther occlusally than the junction of the gingival and middle thirds of the tooth.

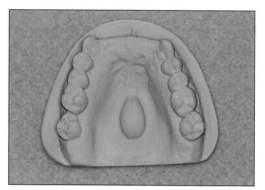

**Fig 7-13** A palatal torus may interfere with the design and construction of a maxillary removable partial denture.

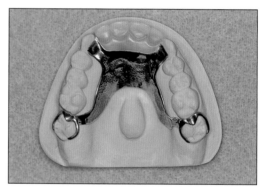

**Fig 7-14** In certain instances, design of the major connector may be altered to accommodate a palatal torus.

cut of 0.015 inches is needed because of the greater flexibility of wrought wire. In all cases, the undercut should be located in the apical third of the clinical crown.

When the existence of retentive undercuts has been verified, the tilt may be changed to optimize the undercut on any tooth. It must be kept in mind that changing the tilt to alter the position of the undercut on one tooth will affect the positions of the undercuts on the remaining teeth. The tilt is normally changed so that a retentive clasp will be positioned no farther occlusally or incisally than the junction of the gingival and middle thirds of the tooth (Fig 7-12). This produces a more esthetic result and may decrease the torquing forces transmitted to the abutment.

**Interferences** Certain structures within the oral cavity may interfere with the insertion of a removable partial denture. These structures may include teeth, bony prominences, soft tissue undercuts, and exostoses. In some instances, difficulties may be avoided by changing the tilt of the cast on the surveying table. In other

instances, surgical intervention may be necessary to correct undesirable contours. It should be a goal of the practitioner to minimize surgical procedures, but never at the expense of compromising restorative outcomes.

As might be expected, maxillary and mandibular interferences present distinctly different challenges to successful removable partial denture therapy. Consequently, these categories are discussed separately.

*Interferences in the maxillary arch.* One of the major sources of interference in the maxillary arch is a palatal torus (Fig 7-13). A prominent palatal torus interferes with placement of the maxillary major connector. As a general rule, changing the tilt of the cast on the surveying table will not solve the problem. In some instances, the design of the major connector may be altered to accommodate the torus (Fig 7-14). If this is not possible, surgical removal of the torus should be accomplished.

Exostoses and undercuts are common on the buccal surfaces of the maxillary arch (Fig 7-15). Buccal ex-

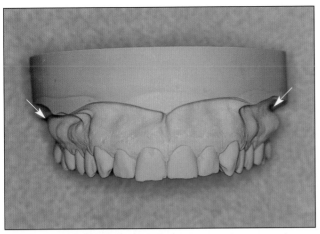

**Fig 7-15** Exostoses and undercuts *(arrows)* commonly appear on maxillary buccal surfaces and may complicate removable partial denture construction.

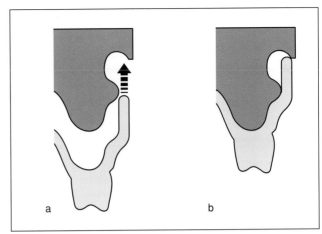

**Fig 7-16** *(a)* Because a removable partial denture displays a linear path of insertion *(arrow)*, the area apical to an exostosis cannot be engaged. *(b)* This results in a void between the soft tissues of the ridge and the internal surface of the prosthesis.

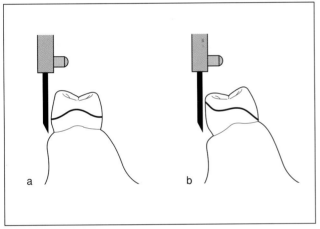

**Fig 7-17** Facial tipping of a maxillary posterior tooth produces noticeable changes in the height of contour. *(a)* The survey line for a representative maxillary premolar is presented. *(b)* As the tooth tips facially, the survey line migrates occlusally on the buccal surface and apically on the lingual surface.

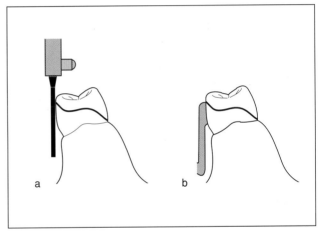

**Fig 7-18** Facial tipping may cause the soft tissues to be in an area of undercut. *(a)* This is evidenced by space between the analyzing rod and the facial aspect of the alveolar ridge. *(b)* The approach arm of an infrabulge clasp also would stand away from the soft tissues of the ridge. An infrabulge clasp should not be used when such a relationship exists.

ostoses and undercuts prevent intimate contact between the removable partial denture and the patient's soft tissues. This may result in an increased accumulation of food beneath the denture base, as well as decreased denture stability (Fig 7-16). Surgical correction of buccal exostoses and undercuts is relatively simple and should be accomplished to provide an improved restorative prognosis.

In addition to the aforementioned factors, facial tipping of posterior teeth may cause significant difficulties. As a maxillary posterior tooth tips facially, the height of contour moves toward the occlusal surface (Fig 7-17). This makes positioning the buccal clasp arm more difficult for esthetic and mechanical reasons. Because the clasp arm must be placed farther from the rotational center of the tooth, the corresponding lever arm is longer, and the resultant forces are likely to be more damaging.

Facial tipping also may cause the associated gingival tissues to be in an undercut (Fig 7-18). This con-

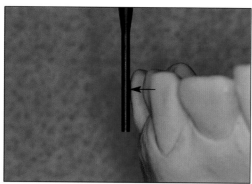

**Fig 7-19** Facial tipping often results in a height of contour *(arrow)* that is located too far occlusally or incisally.

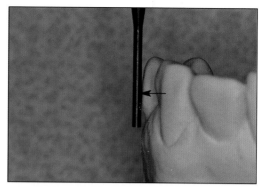

**Fig 7-20** A minor modification in tilt may place the height of contour *(arrow)* at a more desirable level. This may provide a more esthetic result and eliminate the need for mechanical recontouring.

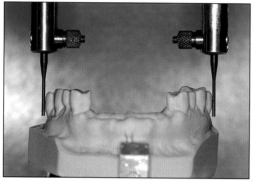

**Fig 7-21** If facially inclined teeth are present on both sides of the arch, changing the tilt of the cast will have no beneficial effect.

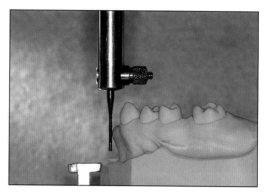

**Fig 7-22** Noticeable undercuts are often encountered in anterior edentulous areas. While these undercuts present certain challenges, surgical intervention is rarely indicated. Maintenance of the hard and soft tissues of the anterior ridge must be given high priority.

traindicates the use of a vertical projection clasp since the approach arm for this clasp must contact the mucosa. If the approach arm for an infrabulge clasp stands away from the gingival tissues, it will act as a food trap and a potential tissue irritant.

If facially inclined teeth are located on just one side of the arch, a minor modification of the tilt may provide an acceptable result (Figs 7-19 and 7-20). If facially inclined teeth are present on both sides of the arch, changing the tilt of the cast will have no beneficial effect (Fig 7-21). If inclination of the maxillary posterior teeth is not severe, the practitioner may be able to move the height of contour to a more appropriate level by recontouring enamel surfaces. As the

severity of the tipping increases, the practitioner may be forced to consider surveyed crowns to satisfy the requirements for clasp placement.

Difficulty also may occur when the maxillary anterior ridge is edentulous and displays a noticeable undercut (Fig 7-22). Most of these undercuts can be controlled by giving the cast a posterior tilt (Fig 7-23). In some instances, anterior undercuts may be avoided by modifying or eliminating the anterior flange of the denture base and butting the replacement teeth directly against the edentulous ridge (Fig 7-24). If hard and soft tissue loss is minimal, this approach can produce excellent esthetic results.

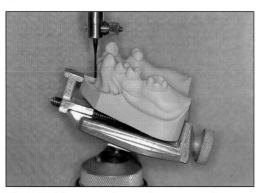

**Fig 7-23** Most anterior undercuts can be controlled by giving the cast a slight posterior tilt.

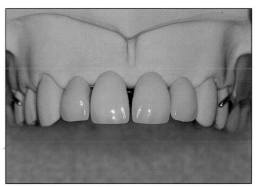

**Fig 7-24** When sufficient ridge height is present, prosthetic teeth may be positioned directly against the edentulous ridge. In carefully selected situations, elimination of the denture base can yield excellent results.

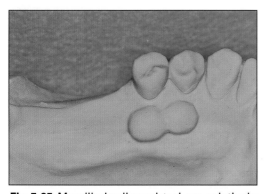

**Fig 7-25** Mandibular lingual tori are relatively common and can produce significant difficulties in removable partial denture therapy.

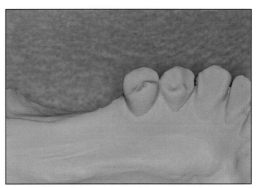

**Fig 7-26** Surgical removal of mandibular lingual tori provides an improved foundation for removable partial denture therapy.

*Interferences in the mandibular arch.* Mandibular tori can produce significant problems in removable partial denture service. Such tori are difficult to avoid because of the anatomy of the mandibular arch. If the delicate tissues overlying mandibular tori must be crossed, space must be created between these tissues and the intaglio surfaces of the major connector. This is accomplished by providing generous relief during framework construction. Unfortunately, this may compromise the thickness of the major connector or interfere with the activities of the tongue and the movable floor of the mouth. Therefore, surgery must be considered for removable partial denture patients exhibiting prominent lingual tori (Figs 7-25 and 7-26).

Unlike maxillary posterior teeth, mandibular posterior teeth frequently display significant lingual tipping. As a result, these teeth may display no undercuts on their facial surfaces and large undercuts on their lingual surfaces (Fig 7-27). Therefore, these teeth may present substantial challenges in removable partial denture design.

The absence of facial undercuts means that lingual retention must be used. Since infrabulge clasps do not lend themselves to such applications, suprabulge clasps are used in the overwhelming majority of these cases. Unfortunately, suprabulge clasps on the lingual surfaces of teeth generally are shorter and more rigid than are clasps located on the corresponding facial

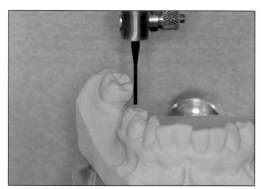

**Fig 7-27** Mandibular posterior teeth frequently display significant lingual tipping. As a result, these teeth may display no undercuts on their facial surfaces and large undercuts on their lingual surfaces.

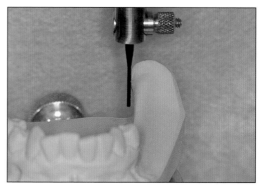

**Fig 7-28** The areas adjacent to the pear-shaped pads may exhibit significant undercuts. If the condition is unilateral, a slight lateral tilt of the surveying table may eliminate the undercut. When the condition is bilateral, tilting the surveying table will have little effect.

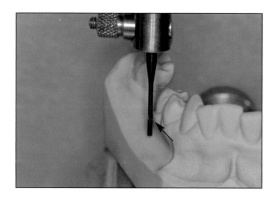

**Fig 7-29** Bony prominences *(arrow)* are often encountered at the facial surfaces of mandibular canines and premolars. These prominences may produce soft tissue undercuts that can interfere with the placement of denture bases and infrabulge clasps. A change in the lateral tilt of the cast may eliminate such interferences.

surfaces. These shorter clasps may exert destructive forces and jeopardize the health of the associated abutments.

Lingual inclination of teeth on both sides of the mandibular arch also may result in a major connector that stands away from the lingual soft tissues and encroaches upon the tongue space. This results in tongue interference and an undesirable space where food and debris may collect.

One solution is to use a labial bar major connector instead of a lingual bar or lingual plate. Unfortunately, experience indicates that the labial bar has poor patient acceptance because of its bulk and location. These factors combine to produce an uncomfortable and unattractive plumping of the lower lip. Therefore, the use of a labial bar major connector should be limited.

The most common solution to this problem involves recontouring the lingual surfaces of the remain-

ing teeth or placing restorations to eliminate the offending undercuts. In some instances, orthodontic movement of the teeth also may be considered.

The areas adjacent to the pear-shaped pads also may produce significant difficulties in removable partial denture design and construction (Fig 7-28). These areas may exhibit significant undercuts on one or both sides of the arch. Tilting the cast is often beneficial in eliminating a unilateral undercut, but has little effect when the arch displays bilateral undercuts. Fortunately, acrylic resin denture bases are located adjacent to these undercuts and may be adjusted to promote patient comfort. Therefore, surgical intervention is rarely indicated to address the existence of such undercuts.

Bony prominences are often encountered at the facial surfaces of mandibular canines and premolars (Fig 7-29). These prominences may produce soft tissue undercuts that can interfere with the placement of den-

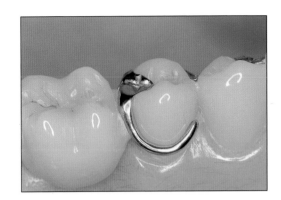

**Fig 7-30** The ideal position for a retentive clasp is in the gingival third of the clinical crown.

ture bases and infrabulge clasps. If these prominences and undercuts are minor, the practitioner may be able to eliminate them by modifying the tilt of the cast. If this does not produce the desired outcome, surgical recontouring should be considered.

**Esthetics** To obtain optimum esthetics in removable partial denture therapy, *(1)* metal components must be concealed as effectively as possible, and *(2)* prosthetic teeth must be selected, appropriately contoured, and properly positioned.

To conceal the metal components of a removable partial denture, the practitioner must pay particular attention to the tilt of the cast. By choosing the appropriate tilt, the practitioner may disguise removable partial denture components while maintaining the health of the associated soft tissues.

The ideal position for a retentive clasp is in the gingival third of the clinical crown (Fig 7-30). This minimizes the likelihood that the clasp will be visible, yet provides enough distance between the clasp and the marginal gingiva to promote and maintain tissue health. A more detailed description of clasp selection is provided later in this chapter.

The second requirement for obtaining optimum esthetics involves the appropriate selection, contouring, and placement of the prosthetic teeth. Appropriate tooth selection requires careful consideration of shade, size, and contour.

Prosthetic teeth also must meet the functional demands of the oral cavity. It is unrealistic to expect that prosthetic teeth supplied by a dental manufacturer will duplicate those lost by the patient. Therefore,

stock teeth should be modified to reflect the esthetic and functional characteristics of the individual.

When teeth are lost and are not replaced immediately, the resulting spaces may become smaller. In most instances, natural teeth will drift mesially to minimize these spaces. Notable exceptions include the mandibular canines and premolars, which tend to move distally if not adequately supported.

Unless something is done to prevent tooth migration, prosthetic teeth will have to display smaller mesiodistal dimensions to fit into the reduced amount of space. This may result in esthetic compromise, particularly in anterior regions.

To address this dilemma, the practitioner should use a dental surveyor. When determining the final tilt of the cast, the space for one or more missing anterior teeth must be given high priority. One or more missing anterior teeth almost always signal that the prosthesis will have a single *path of insertion*. This means that the surveyor must be used to determine whether recontouring of the remaining natural teeth is indicated. Recontouring is necessary not only to produce an acceptable path of insertion, but also to ensure appropriate space for the prosthetic replacement (Fig 7-31). If recontouring the proximal surfaces can produce the desired results, it is the procedure of choice. If contouring the enamel surfaces is not possible, crowns or other suitable restorations should be planned.

Large undercuts on the proximal surfaces of anterior teeth also may create esthetic concerns (Fig 7-32). These undercuts may be caused by the shape of the clinical crown or by tipping of the tooth toward an edentulous space. The undercuts produce triangular

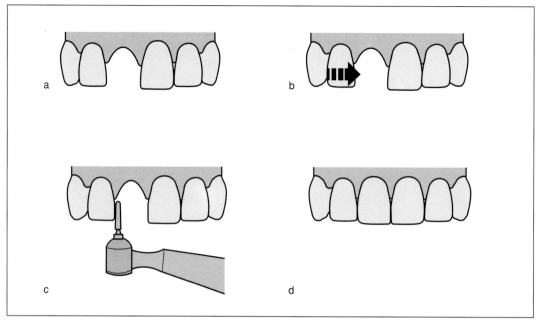

**Fig 7-31** *(a)* The maxillary right central incisor has been lost. *(b)* The adjacent lateral incisor drifts mesially, causing a decrease in the mesiodistal dimension of the edentulous space. *(c)* The mesial surface of the lateral incisor is recontoured to ensure appropriate space for the planned prosthetic replacement. *(d)* An appropriate prosthesis is placed.

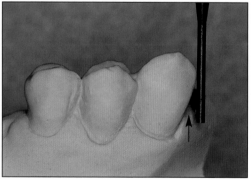

**Fig 7-32** Large undercuts *(arrow)* on the proximal surfaces of anterior teeth may create significant difficulties. These undercuts can produce triangular spaces that detract from the appearance of the prosthesis and act as food traps.

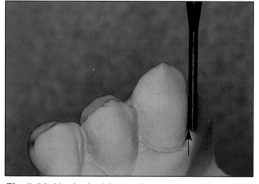

**Fig 7-33** Undesirable undercuts may be minimized or eliminated *(arrow)* by modifying the tilt of the cast.

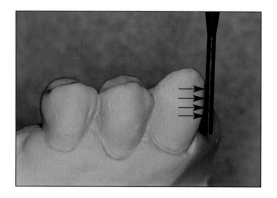

**Fig 7-34** Undercuts also may be minimized or eliminated by reshaping the proximal surfaces of teeth *(arrows)*.

spaces that not only detract from the esthetic value of the removable partial denture, but also act as food traps that can be annoying to the patient. These spaces should by minimized or eliminated by modifying the tilt (Fig 7-33) or recontouring the proximal surfaces of the offending teeth (Fig 7-34). The surveyor is a necessity in determining the amount of recontouring needed to reduce these undesirable undercuts.

**Guiding planes** Guiding planes are parallel surfaces of abutment teeth that direct the insertion and removal of a partial denture. They are formed on the proximal or axial surfaces of the teeth and are contacted by the minor connectors or other rigid elements of the removable partial denture. The surveyor is used to locate surfaces that are parallel to the planned path of insertion or those that can be made parallel to this path by selective grinding. Guiding planes are always parallel to the path of insertion and are rarely greater than 2 to 4 mm in height.

When the partial denture is completely seated in the mouth, the guiding planes are contacted by minor connectors or other rigid components of the partial denture. As a result, guiding planes help stabilize the prosthesis against lateral forces. They also help protect weakened teeth from potentially destructive lateral forces.

Of the four factors considered in determining the most favorable tilt of a cast, the development of guiding planes is the one that can be most easily compromised. Guiding planes can be prepared on most enamel surfaces. If proposed abutments are to receive cast restorations, the removable partial denture should be designed in advance, and preparations for the removable partial denture should be finalized. In turn, the teeth that are to receive cast restorations should be prepared, and wax patterns should be shaped so their guiding surfaces are parallel to the established tilt.

Determination of the most favorable tilt is an important process that requires a thorough understanding of the aforementioned factors. If the tilt of the cast is changed to satisfy any of these factors, the effects of this change on the other factors must be determined. If a change adversely affects any of the remaining factors, a suitable compromise must be reached.

## Path of insertion

The tilt of a cast determines the direction that the partial denture will take during placement and removal. The resultant pathway is termed the *path of insertion*. For practical purposes, the path of insertion and removal will always be parallel to the vertical arm of the surveyor (Fig 7-35).

The path of insertion is often discussed as if it were a single entity. In reality, most removable partial dentures have two or more paths of insertion. The most influential factor in determining whether a prosthesis will have one or more paths of insertion is whether or not edentulous spaces are tooth bounded. In Kennedy Class I arches, the edentulous spaces are bounded by teeth at only one end. Therefore, a prosthesis may enter or exit its intended position at a variety of angles (Fig 7-36).

Like Kennedy Class I arches, unmodified Kennedy Class II arches are bounded at only one end of the edentulous space. Consequently, a prosthesis may enter or exit its fully seated position at a variety of angles. However, if a Kennedy Class II arch exhibits a tooth-bounded modification space on the opposite side of the arch, the modification space will determine the path of insertion. If guiding planes have been prepared on the proximal surfaces of abutments on the tooth-bounded side, the prosthesis will display a single path of insertion (Fig 7-37).

In Kennedy Class III arches, the existing edentulous spaces are entirely tooth bounded. Therefore, if guiding planes have been prepared on the proximal surfaces of the abutments, the associated prosthesis will exhibit a single path of insertion (Fig 7-38).

If a dental arch displays a Kennedy Class IV pattern of edentulism, the associated prosthesis will usually have a single path of insertion. The path of insertion for such a prosthesis will be parallel to the guiding planes on abutment teeth adjacent to the edentulous space (Fig 7-39).

The components of a removable partial denture that govern the path of insertion are the minor connectors, which join the clasps to the major connector. These minor connectors are normally the only components that contact the guiding planes of the teeth. It is essential that the minor connectors remain in contact with the guiding planes throughout the insertion and removal processes.

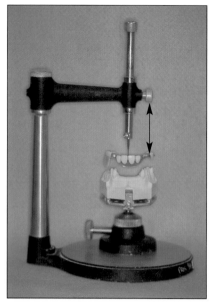

**Fig 7-35** The path of insertion *(arrow)* is the route that the removable partial denture takes during placement and removal. This path is determined during survey and design procedures and is parallel to the vertical arm of the surveyor.

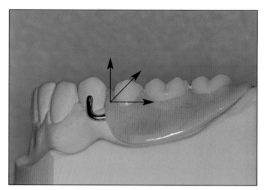

**Fig 7-36** A Kennedy Class I prosthesis may enter or exit its intended position at a variety of angles *(arrows)*.

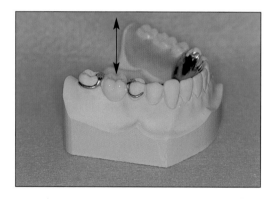

**Fig 7-37** The path of insertion for a Kennedy Class II prosthesis with a modification space is determined by the modification space. If guiding planes have been prepared on the proximal surfaces of abutments on the tooth-bounded side, the prosthesis will display a single path of insertion *(arrow)*.

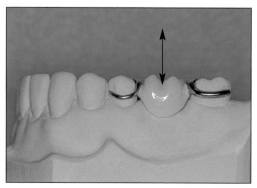

**Fig 7-38** In Kennedy Class III arches, the existing edentulous spaces are entirely tooth bounded. Guiding planes on the proximal surfaces of abutment teeth define a single path of insertion *(arrow)*.

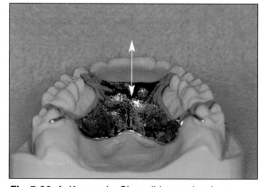

**Fig 7-39** A Kennedy Class IV prosthesis generally exhibits a single path of insertion *(arrow)*. This path is defined by guiding planes on the proximal surfaces of abutments lying adjacent to the edentulous space.

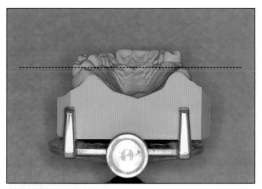

Fig 7-40 When the proposed path of insertion has been finalized, the tilt of the cast must be recorded. This is accomplished by clearly marking three points in the same horizontal plane *(broken line)*. When these points are re-aligned in the horizontal plane, the cast will display the prescribed orientation.

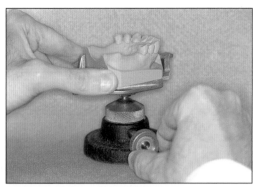

Fig 7-41 After ensuring that the proper tilt has been selected, the surveying table is locked in position.

Fig 7-42 For purposes of tripodization, the 0.030-inch undercut gauge is positioned in the mandrel.

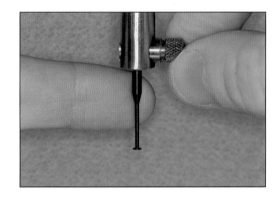

The body and shoulders of a clasp assembly may exert some influence on the path of insertion. However, the effect is limited because these segments are positioned above the height of contour and lie on sloping surfaces. In the event that guiding planes have been prepared on the lingual surfaces of the remaining teeth, reciprocal elements in the form of clasp arms or plating may exert a definite influence on the path of insertion.

### Tripoding the cast

After the most favorable tilt of the cast has been selected, it must be recorded for future reference. This procedure is referred to as *tripoding* or *tripodization*. The simplest method consists of placing crossmarks at three widely spaced points on the dental cast while the

vertical arm of the surveyor is held at a fixed vertical position. This will establish three points on the same horizontal plane and permit the cast to be accurately repositioned (Fig 7-40).

There are a number of acceptable methods for tripodization of dental casts. One technique involves the use of an undercut gauge to mark the surface of the cast. This is the technique preferred by the authors and described in the following paragraph.

After ensuring that the proper tilt has been selected, the surveying table is locked in position (Fig 7-41). A suitable undercut gauge is placed in the vertical arm of the surveyor, and the mandrel is tightened (Fig 7-42). The vertical arm of the surveyor is adjusted to contact the cast at three easily identifiable locations on the lingual surface of the cast (Fig 7-43). The practitioner

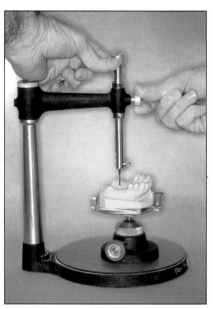

**Fig 7-44** The vertical arm of the surveyor is locked into position. This ensures that the tip of the undercut gauge defines a single horizontal plane.

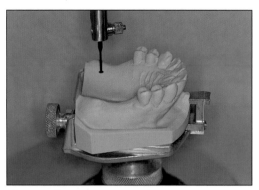

**Fig 7-43** The vertical arm of the surveyor is adjusted to permit contact between the head of the undercut gauge and the cast. The practitioner should ensure that the undercut gauge contacts the cast at three easily identifiable locations on the lingual surface of the cast.

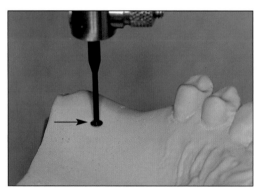

**Fig 7-45** The surveying table is moved to bring the cast into contact with the undercut gauge at three widely separated points. At each location, contact between the undercut gauge and the cast should produce a shallow groove *(arrow)*.

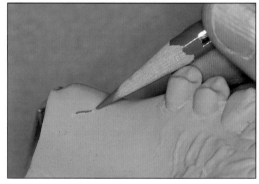

**Fig 7-46** A red pencil is used to indicate the position of each horizontal groove. Each red line should be approximately 4 mm long and relatively narrow.

should ensure that these locations are widely spaced and that they are on anatomic areas that are not likely to change from cast to cast. At this stage, the vertical arm of the surveyor is locked in position (Fig 7-44). The surveying table is then moved to bring the cast in contact with the undercut gauge at the desired positions. Contact between the cast and the undercut gauge

should produce three shallow grooves in the surface of the cast (Fig 7-45). To enhance visibility, a red pencil is used to record the positions of these grooves. Resultant lines should be about 4 mm long and relatively narrow (Fig 7-46). Tripod marks are completed by creating a crosshair configuration at each position (Figs 7-47 and 7-48).

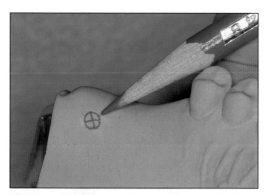

**Fig 7-47** Each horizontal line is crossed and then circled, resulting in a crosshair configuration.

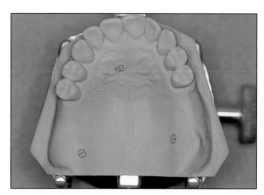

**Fig 7-48** When tripodization is complete, tripod marks should be positioned at three widely spaced anatomic areas of the cast and should be readily identifiable.

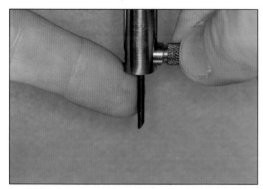

**Fig 7-49** To place survey lines, a carbon marker is positioned in the surveyor's mandrel, and the mandrel is tightened.

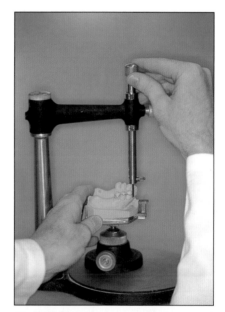

**Fig 7-50** The surveying table is moved along the surface of the platform until the cast comes into light contact with the carbon marker. This is accomplished by controlling the surveyor's vertical arm with one hand while guiding movement of the surveying table with the opposite hand.

## Placing survey lines

The surveyor is also used to scribe survey lines on the teeth and soft tissues. Proper placement of survey lines is essential to the design process and must be accomplished with great care.

To place survey lines, a carbon marker is positioned in the surveyor's mandrel, and the mandrel is tightened (Fig 7-49). The vertical arm of the surveyor is unlocked to ensure free movement in a supero-inferior direction. The surveying table is then moved along the surface of the platform until the cast comes into light contact with the carbon marker. The practitioner may accomplish this by controlling the surveyor's vertical arm with one hand while guiding movement of the surveying table with the opposite hand (Fig 7-50).

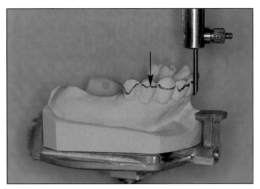

**Fig 7-51** Survey lines *(arrow)* are transferred to the teeth as a result of contact between the dental cast and the side of the carbon marker. These lines represent the most prominent contours of individual teeth at a chosen orientation. Areas located occlusal or incisal to survey lines do not display undercuts. Areas located apical to survey lines are undercut relative to the chosen path of insertion.

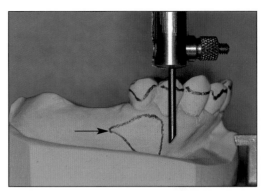

**Fig 7-52** Survey lines *(arrow)* are transferred to soft tissue areas that may be contacted by components of a removable partial denture. These commonly include soft tissue areas that may be contacted by infrabulge (bar-type) clasps.

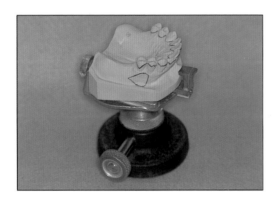

**Fig 7-53** The clinician must ensure that survey lines have been transferred to all facial and lingual surfaces.

Survey lines are transferred to the teeth by moving the surveying table across the platform while maintaining light contact between the carbon marker and the cast (Fig 7-51). Survey lines are transferred to soft tissue areas in a similar manner (Fig 7-52). This process is continued until the required survey lines have been clearly marked on facial and lingual surfaces of the cast (Fig 7-53).

### Locating and marking measured undercuts

Mechanical undercuts must be accurately located and appropriately marked to permit correct placement of retentive clasps. Therefore, procedures for locating and marking retentive undercuts warrant particular attention. The depth and position of the desired undercut will vary with the material and clasping system to be used. As a result, the practitioner must be familiar with the requirements for each system. This will allow the practitioner to choose the appropriate undercut gauge and identify the position of the required undercut.

Upon selection of the appropriate undercut gauge, the gauge is inserted into the mandrel and locked into place (Fig 7-54). The surveying table is then positioned so that the selected abutment tooth contacts the shank of the undercut gauge (Fig 7-55). The vertical arm of the surveyor is raised until the head of the undercut gauge lightly contacts the infrabulge area of the tooth (Fig 7-56). The point of contact should appear as a very light "scrape" on the surface of the cast. The apical border of this contact should be clearly marked

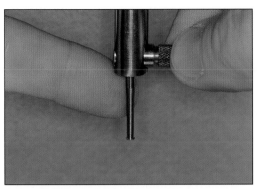

**Fig 7-54** The appropriate undercut gauge is placed into the mandrel. For most clasp assemblies, a 0.010-inch undercut gauge is indicated.

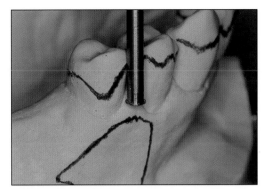

**Fig 7-55** The dental cast is brought into light contact with the shank of the undercut gauge. At this stage of the procedure, the head of the undercut gauge does not contact the surface of the cast.

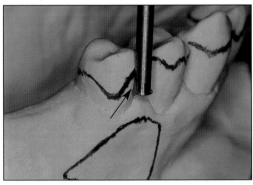

**Fig 7-56** The vertical arm of the surveyor is raised until the head of the undercut gauge contacts the infrabulge area of the tooth. The point of contact should appear as a very light "scrape" *(arrow)* on the surface of the cast.

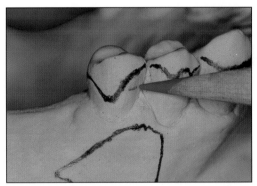

**Fig 7-57** The apical border of this contact is clearly marked using a red pencil. The pencil mark should appear as a thin, horizontal line approximately 2 mm in length.

using a red pencil and should appear as a thin, horizontal line approximately 2 mm in length (Fig 7-57).

## ▢ Design

During the survey process, the practitioner determines the most favorable tilt for a dental cast, completes the tripodization process, places survey lines, and accurately marks the desired mechanical undercuts. At this stage, the practitioner is ready to begin the design process.

The completed design will serve as a blueprint for removable partial denture construction. Therefore, the design process must be completed with great care.

The mechanical characteristics of the removable partial denture must be considered. Components must be neatly drawn and accurately positioned. Most importantly, the completed design must convey essential information to the laboratory personnel responsible for prosthesis construction.

### Principles of design

Authorities in the field of removable partial prosthodontics may differ in their approaches to the design of individual prostheses. There is, however, complete agreement that the correct design must be based upon accepted mechanical and biological principles. Proper application of these principles permits the supporting teeth and soft tissues to withstand those forces placed on a removable partial denture during function.

It would be gratifying to be able to say that partial denture design is based upon the results of scientific research accomplished under rigid and repeatable conditions. Regretfully, this is not so, although there have been a number of important investigations that have contributed to the knowledge of removable partial denture design.

Ongoing clinical and laboratory research continues to add to the body of knowledge in removable partial prosthodontics. This is a positive step, and one that should contribute to improved removable partial denture service in the future.

In considering removable partial denture design, the dentist should bear in mind the following basic principles expounded by Dr A. H. Schmidt in 1953.[1] These principles remain as true and accurate today as the day they were proposed.

1. The dentist must have a thorough knowledge of both the mechanical and biological factors involved in removable partial denture design. In addition, the dentist must have a background in the basic and applied sciences and a working knowledge of the laws of physics and engineering, particularly as they relate to levers.
2. The treatment plan must be based on a complete examination and diagnosis of the individual patient.
3. The dentist must correlate the pertinent factors and determine a proper plan of treatment. This is an area in which the profession has functioned poorly in the past. The tendency, all too often, has been to submit casts to a laboratory and allow the technician to produce a removable partial denture. The dentist alone can modify the conditions in the mouth to enhance the success of the treatment.
4. A removable partial denture should restore form and function without injury to the remaining oral structures. In restoring occlusion, the prosthesis should also restore a normal or desirable facial contour and not impede the normal movement of the tongue and other tissues. The prosthesis must be planned so the remaining oral structures are not stressed beyond their physiologic capabilities.
5. A removable partial denture is a form of treatment and not a cure. The responsibility of the dentist

does not end with the final placement of the prosthesis in the patient's mouth. Oral tissues never remain static, but are constantly undergoing change, reflecting the general health and age of the patient. The patient should be recalled periodically to prevent any deleterious changes from taking place. The prosthesis should be planned with the knowledge that future corrections may be required. The design should be such that modifications may be made to compensate for changes that can be expected in oral tissues.

These principles are indeed basic, but if they are properly applied, the probability of successful removable partial denture therapy will be greatly increased.

## Philosophy of design

Of the various philosophies relating to removable partial denture design, none is backed by overwhelming scientific evidence. They are the ideas of experienced dentists who have formulated rules for the design of removable partial dentures. There is little evidence to indicate that one of the existing philosophies has a real advantage over any other except in the mind of the follower. In fact, all philosophies can lead to excellent clinical results if properly applied. It is not so much the theoretical side of partial denture design that is critical, but appropriate execution of clinical and laboratory procedures. Nearly any removable partial denture design can be made to work successfully if respect for the physiologic limits of the supporting structures is observed.

In partial denture design, the main concern is for prostheses that are partially supported by teeth and partially supported by soft tissues. Prostheses that are entirely supported by teeth (ie, those used in the treatment of Kennedy Class III arches) are generally very straightforward. Because these partial dentures derive all of their support from the remaining teeth, a single impression may be used to record the teeth and soft tissues. Since the edentulous ridge does not offer support, it may be recorded in its anatomic form. Because noticeable rotational forces do not occur, indirect retention or flexible direct retention is not required. Retentive clasping is based on convenience; in other words, the simplest possible clasping systems are used. The chal-

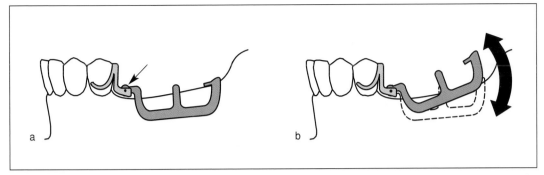

**Fig 7-58** *(a)* A stress director may take the form of a hinge *(arrow)*. *(b)* The hinge is activated by a lifting force that allows the denture base to rotate away from the ridge *(arrow)*. This minimizes the application of torquing forces to the abutments.

lenge in design, then, lies primarily in Class I and Class II arches and to some extent in Class IV arches.

There is ongoing controversy about the design requirements for free end or extension base removable partial dentures (ie, Class I, Class II, and long-span Class IV applications). The debate centers upon the amount of support that should be derived from the edentulous ridge and that which should be derived from the remaining teeth. As might be expected, differences in opinion have given rise to a variety of design philosophies. These philosophies are based upon three approaches to force distribution. These approaches may be described as follows:

1. Stress equalization
2. Physiologic basing
3. Broad stress distribution

There are obviously some design concepts that may attempt to take advantage of more than one of these basic goals, but nearly all can be grouped into one of the aforementioned categories.

The three basic design philosophies are discussed in the following sections. The reader should note that the advantages presented for the different concepts are those cited by the advocates of that particular school of thought.

## Stress equalization

Advocates of the stress equalization approach to partial denture design emphasize that the vertical displaceability of a natural tooth is not as great as that of the soft tissues covering the edentulous ridge. Advocates of this school believe that forces applied to a removable partial denture are transmitted to the abutments. As a result, proponents believe that rigid connections between denture bases and direct retainers are damaging, and that stress directors are essential to protect the abutments (Fig 7-58).

Stress directors may take several forms. The most commonly used stress directors are simple hinges interposed between the denture bases and the adjacent clasping assemblies. These hinges are designed to permit vertical movement of the denture bases without causing undue loading of the abutments. In addition, many of these devices can be adjusted to control the amount of vertical travel that is permitted.

**Advantages** Stress director designs usually call for minimal direct retention because the denture bases operate more independently than do those used in conventional removable partial denture applications.

Stress directors are sometimes used in conjunction with intracoronal attachments. This is particularly true in Kennedy Class I and Class II applications because of the unyielding nature of intracoronal retentive elements. Theoretically, stress directors minimize the tipping forces on abutment teeth, thereby limiting bone resorption.

**Disadvantages** Stress directors are comparatively fragile and their incorporation into removable partial denture frameworks can be costly. In addition, these devices require constant maintenance and may be difficult or impossible to repair.

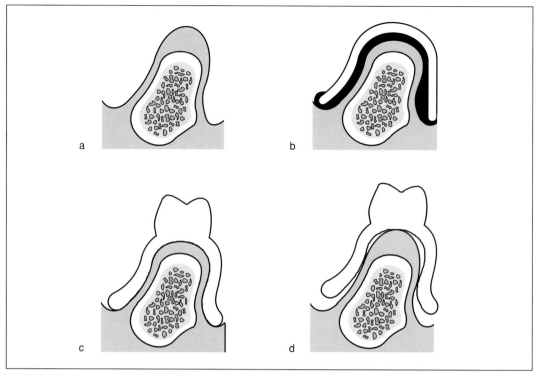

**Fig 7-59** *(a)* Cross-sectional view of the mandibular ridge in its anatomic form. *(b)* Functional form of the mandibular ridge during impression procedure (physiologic basing philosophy). *(c)* Adaptation of denture base during function. *(d)* Adaptation of denture base at rest. When at rest, the denture base is displaced occlusally.

Of the three schools of thought of partial denture design, the stress equalization school has the fewest advocates.

### Physiologic basing

Proponents of physiologic basing also believe that there is a significant disparity between the apical displaceability of teeth and the compressibility of the soft tissues. However, these practitioners do not believe that stress directors are necessary to account for this difference. These practitioners believe that equalization can best be accomplished by recording the anatomy of the edentulous ridge in its functional form and ensuring that the associated denture base accurately reflects this anatomy. This may be accomplished by depressing the mucosa during impression-making procedures or by relining the denture base after it has been constructed.

Advocates of this theory believe that denture bases formed over compressed tissues will show an increased ability to withstand vertical forces. These prac-

titioners also recognize that the prosthetic teeth and occlusal rests will be positioned above the existing occlusal plane when the prosthesis is not in function (Fig 7-59). To permit vertical movement of the partial denture from its rest position to its functioning position, the number of direct retainers must be limited. Furthermore, these direct retainers must be designed to provide minimal retention.

**Advantages** Proponents of this theory believe that denture base movement occurring as a result of soft tissue compression and recovery exerts a physiologically stimulating effect on the tissues of the residual ridges. They also believe that this action promotes tissue health and reduces the necessity for frequent relining or rebasing procedures.

The minimal retention requirements associated with physiologic basing result in lightweight prostheses requiring minimal maintenance and repair. The forgiving nature of retentive clasps (eg, combination clasps with wrought-wire retentive arms) produces a

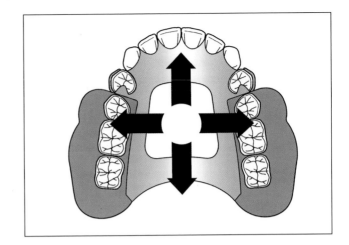

**Fig 7-60** Proponents of broad stress distribution believe in extensive coverage of the teeth and soft tissues. The purpose is to distribute applied forces over as large an area as possible *(arrows)*.

significant reduction in the forces transmitted to the abutment teeth. As a result, advocates of this theory believe that abutments are retained for longer periods.

**Disadvantages** Because the artificial teeth are slightly above the occlusal plane when the denture is not in function, there will always be premature contacts between the opposing teeth and the prosthesis during closure. This may be somewhat annoying to the patient and may result in some discomfort.

It is difficult to produce effective indirect retention because of the vertical movement of the denture and the minimal retention provided by the direct retainers. By the time the indirect retainers engage the associated rest seats, the direct retainers may have lost contact with their respective abutments. In such instances, indirect retention is of little consequence.

In addition to the foregoing factors, prostheses constructed in accordance with physiologic basing principles are not well stabilized against lateral forces. This is related to the minimal number of direct retainers used in conjunction with these designs.

### Broad stress distribution

Advocates of broad stress distribution believe that trauma to the remaining teeth and residual ridges can be prevented by distributing forces over as many teeth and as much of the soft tissue area as possible. This is accomplished by using additional rests and clasp assemblies and by ensuring that the associated denture bases provide broad coverage (Fig 7-60).

**Advantages** Proponents of this philosophy believe that forces transmitted to the supporting teeth and residual ridges may be minimized by distributing these forces over a greater number of teeth and a larger soft tissue area. For example, occlusal forces distributed among five or six teeth may physiologically stimulate them to a state of health, whereas the same load applied to two teeth may exceed the physiologic limits of these teeth and result in resorption of the associated alveolar bone.

Advocates of this philosophy also believe that increased contact with the remaining teeth and soft tissues minimizes the lateral forces on the remaining structures. The use of multiple clasp assemblies is not intended to increase retention. Instead, these components are intended to provide additional resistance to horizontal movement. This is particularly important when some or all of the remaining teeth have lost some periodontal support. This approach constitutes a form of removable splinting and may allow the remaining teeth to be retained for longer periods.

In addition to the advantages already listed, proponents of this philosophy believe that the resultant prostheses are easier and less expensive to construct. There are no moving parts, so there is less danger of fracture and distortion. In addition, the rigid components minimize rotational movements and provide excellent horizontal stabilization. Because of this decreased movement and increased stability, the residual ridges do not bear as much of the occlusal load, and these partial dentures do not require frequent relining or rebasing.

**Disadvantages** The increased coverage provided by such prostheses may not be accepted by some patients. This coverage also may complicate oral hygiene. As a result, preventive dental programs must be instituted and oral hygiene must be carefully monitored.

## Summary

It must be remembered that any of the aforementioned philosophies can be successful if applied under the appropriate circumstances. Likewise, any or all of these philosophies may fail if applied under inappropriate circumstances. Therefore, the practitioner must display a thorough understanding of those factors that will impact the design process. To achieve success in removable partial denture therapy, nothing can replace good judgment coupled with the knowledge of the fundamental principles of partial denture design. Essential considerations are summarized in Box 7-1. This summary is intended to help the student remember which components must be used in designing removable partial dentures for Kennedy Class I, Class II, Class III, and Class IV arches. The outline most closely follows the principles for broad stress distribution, but is also valid for the remaining philosophies.

---

**Box 7-1  Essentials of design**

I. Kennedy Class I and Class II partially edentulous arches
  A. Direct retention
    1. Retention should not be considered a primary objective of removable partial denture design. The main objectives should be the restoration of function and appearance, the maintenance of comfort, and the preservation of remaining oral structures.
    2. Although clasp assemblies are largely responsible for direct retention, they are supplemented by close adaptation of the framework to properly prepared guiding planes on the remaining teeth. Proper extension and adaptation of one or more denture bases also contribute to retention of a removable partial denture.
  B. Clasps
    1. The practitioner should use the simplest clasps that will satisfy the design objectives.
    2. All clasps should have good stabilizing qualities, remain passive until activated by functional stresses, and accommodate a minor amount of movement without transmitting torque to the associated abutment teeth.
    3. Clasps should be strategically positioned in the arch to achieve the greatest possible control of applied forces.
      a) A Class I prosthesis usually requires only two clasp assemblies. One clasp assembly should be located on the most posterior tooth on the right side of the arch. The remaining clasp assembly should be located on the most posterior tooth on the left side of the arch (Fig 7-61).
        (1) If a distobuccal undercut is present, an infrabulge clasp (T or ½T) is preferred (Figs 7-62 and 7-63).
        (2) If a mesiobuccal undercut is present, a wrought-wire clasp is indicated (Figs 7-64 and 7-65). A cast circumferential clasp should not be used.
        (3) The reciprocal elements must be rigid. These components may be in the form of bracing arms or lingual plating (Figs 7-66 and 7-67).

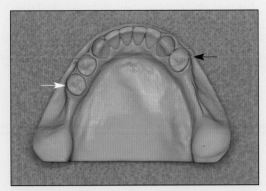

**Fig 7-61** A Kennedy Class I removable partial denture usually requires only two clasp assemblies. One clasp assembly is located on the most posterior tooth on the right side of the arch *(black arrow)*. The remaining clasp assembly is located on the most posterior tooth on the left side of the arch *(white arrow)*.

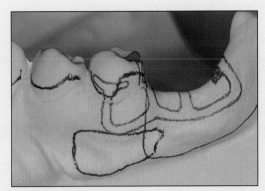

**Fig 7-62** A representative T-clasp engaging a distobuccal undercut.

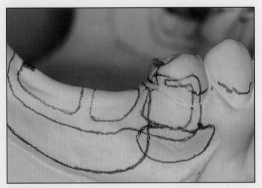

**Fig 7-63** A representative ½T-clasp engaging a distobuccal undercut.

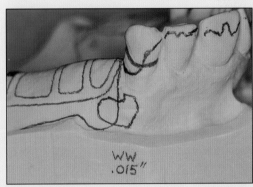

**Fig 7-64** A wrought-wire clasp arm engaging a mesiobuccal undercut. (Note that unlike other retentive clasps, a wrought wire is drawn as a solid brown line.)

**Fig 7-65** A wrought-wire clasp should be attached to the framework as far from the proximal plate as is practical to minimize the adverse effects of heating and preserve the desirable qualities of the wrought structure. Here, wrought wire *(arrows)* is extended onto the transverse struts lingual to the crest of the ridge. This allows the wire to be attached to the transverse struts using common soldering procedures.

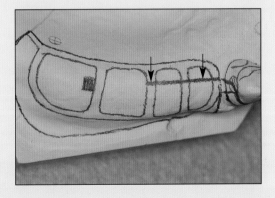

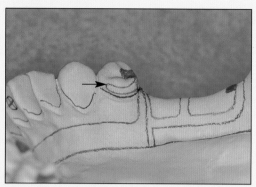

**Fig 7-66** A representative reciprocal arm or bracing arm *(arrow)*.

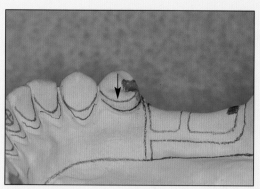

**Fig 7-67** Reciprocation in the form of lingual plating *(arrow)*.

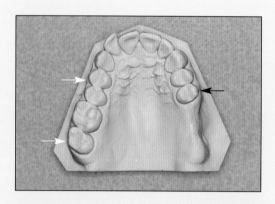

**Fig 7-68** A Kennedy Class II removable partial denture should have three clasp assemblies. One of these should be located adjacent to the distal extension area *(black arrow)*. The remaining clasp assemblies should be located on the opposite side of the arch and should be positioned with regard to structural and esthetic considerations *(white arrows)*.

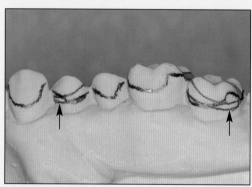

**Fig 7-69** For a Kennedy Class II application with no modifications, clasp assemblies should be positioned as far posterior as is practical and as far anterior as esthetics will permit. In this instance, direct retainers have been placed on the second molar and first premolar *(arrows)*.

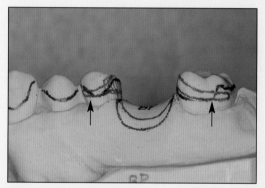

**Fig 7-70** For a Kennedy Class II application with a modification space on the opposite side of the dental arch, clasp assemblies are often placed adjacent to the edentulous space. In this instance, direct retainers have been placed on the second molar and second premolar *(arrows)*.

*b)* A Class II prosthesis should usually have three retentive clasp assemblies (Fig 7-68).

    (1) The distal extension side should be designed with the same considerations as described for a Kennedy Class I arch.

    (2) The opposite side of the arch should have two retentive clasp arms: one as far posterior and one as far anterior as tooth contours and esthetics permit (Fig 7-69). If a modification space is present, it is most convenient to clasp the teeth adjacent to the edentulous space (Fig 7-70).

**Fig 7-71** In a Kennedy Class II application, the primary axis of rotation passes through the most posterior abutment on each side of the dental arch (ie, the right second molar and left second premolar). To minimize movement of the distal extension base away from the supporting tissues, an indirect retainer should be placed opposite the distal extension base and as far from the rotational axis as practical. In this instance, the indirect retainer would be positioned on the mesio-occlusal surface of the first premolar or the lingual surface of the canine.

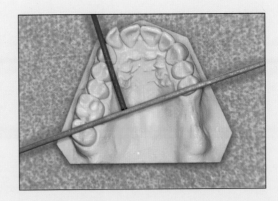

(a) The type of clasp and position of the retentive undercut can be selected for convenience. In most instances, circumferential clasps should be used.

(b) Rigidity is required for all reciprocal elements. Reciprocation may be provided via bracing arms or lingual plating.

C. Rests

1. Abutments should be selected to provide maximum support for a prosthesis.

2. Rest seats should be prepared so that forces will be directed within the long axes of the abutments.

3. In most instances, rests should be placed adjacent to the edentulous space(s).

D. Indirect retention

1. Indirect retention should be employed to neutralize unseating forces.

a) Each indirect retainer should be located as far from the fulcrum line as is practical. Indirect retainers should not be placed more anterior than the canines.

b) Two indirect retainers should generally be used in a Class I design, whereas one indirect retainer is generally adequate in a Class II design. The indirect retainer in a Class II design should be located on the side opposite the distal extension base (Fig 7-71).

c) Indirect retainers should direct forces within the long axes of the associated teeth.

2. Lingual plating may be used to augment indirect retention. It is important to remember that lingual plating must be supported by appropriate rest–rest seat combinations.

E. Major connectors

1. The practitioner should select the simplest connector that will accomplish treatment objectives.

a) The major connector must be rigid.

b) The major connector must not impinge on gingival tissues.

2. In the maxillary arch, a broad major connector may be used to derive additional support from the hard palate. The greater the palatal coverage, the greater the support that may be derived.

3. Extension of the major connector onto the lingual surfaces of the teeth may be used to increase rigidity, distribute lateral stresses, improve indirect retention, and/or eliminate potential food impaction areas. Lingual plating should always be accompanied by appropriately positioned rests and rests seats.

F. Minor connectors

1. Minor connectors must be rigid.

2. Minor connectors should be positioned to enhance comfort, cleanliness, and the placement of artificial teeth.

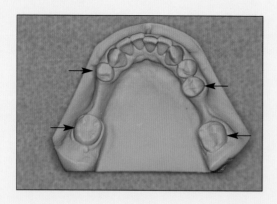

**Fig 7-72** In a Kennedy Class III application, four clasp assemblies *(arrows)* are considered ideal.

G. Occlusion

1. If possible, maximum intercuspation should coincide with centric relation.

2. A harmonious occlusion should be established. All eccentric movements should be dictated by, or occur in harmony with, the remaining natural teeth.

3. Prosthetic teeth should be selected and positioned to minimize stresses on the prosthesis.

*a)* The practitioner may choose to place fewer teeth and/or teeth that are narrower buccolingually.

*b)* Prosthetic teeth should be placed over the crest of the residual ridge when possible.

*c)* Prosthetic teeth should display sharp cutting edges and ample escapeways.

H. Denture bases

1. Denture bases should be designed to provide broad coverage. This permits the distribution of forces over a greater area and minimizes the probability of stress concentration.

*a)* Border extensions must not interfere with functional movements of the surrounding tissues.

*b)* Selective pressure impressions are recommended for extension base areas of Kennedy Class I and Class II arches.

2. The external (ie, cameo) surfaces of a denture base should enable the patient to exercise maximum neuromuscular control.

II. Kennedy Class III partially edentulous arches

A. Direct retention

1. Because these prostheses are entirely tooth borne, the transmission of harmful forces to the abutment teeth and residual ridges can be minimized.

2. Positions of the retentive undercuts on individual abutment teeth are not critical.

B. Clasps

1. Quadrilateral positioning of direct retainers is considered ideal (Fig 7-72).

2. Tooth contours, soft tissue contours, and esthetics should be considered, and the simplest possible clasps should be selected. In most instances, simple circlet clasps are chosen.

3. Reciprocal elements must be rigid.

C. Rests

1. When possible, rests and/or rest seats should be positioned adjacent to the edentulous space(s).

2. Rests should be used to support major connectors and lingual plating.

D. Indirect retention

1. Indirect retention is usually not required in Kennedy Class III applications.

2. In many instances, Kennedy Class III arches display bilateral tooth loss (ie, Kennedy Class III, Modification 1). If one or both of the posterior abutments are used solely for vertical support and not for retention, the entire design must satisfy the requirements described for Kennedy Class I or Class II arches.

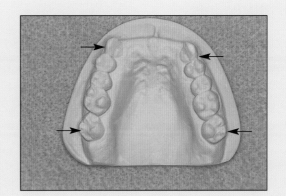

**Fig 7-73** Four clasp assemblies *(arrows)* should be used in Kennedy Class IV applications. Two clasp assemblies should be placed as far anterior as possible. The remaining clasp assemblies should be placed as far posterior as possible.

E. Major and minor connectors

   1. Major and minor connectors must be rigid and must meet the same requirements described for Kennedy Class I and Class II arches.

F. Occlusion

   1. The requirements for occlusion are the same as for Kennedy Class I and Class II arches.

G. Denture bases

   1. Functional impressions are not required. Because these prostheses are entirely tooth borne, anatomic impressions are indicated.

   2. Coverage of the residual ridge areas should be determined by appearance, comfort, and the avoidance of food impaction.

III. Kennedy Class IV partially edentulous arches

  A. The movements of removable partial dentures fabricated for Kennedy Class IV arches and the stresses transmitted to the associated abutment teeth are unlike those seen in Kennedy Class I, Class II, and Class III applications.

  B. The arrangement of prosthetic teeth to satisfy esthetic and phonetic requirements may place these teeth anterior to the ridge crest. This may result in "tipping" of the prosthesis and application of rotational forces to the associated abutments. Every effort should be made to minimize these stresses. To accomplish this, the following guidelines should be observed.

   1. Every effort should be made to preserve the hard and soft tissue components of the anterior edentulous ridge.

   2. If possible, a central incisor or other tooth should be retained to serve as an intermediate abutment or as an overdenture abutment. Rotation of the prosthesis can be minimized by retaining serviceable teeth. This may serve to minimize harmful forces.

   3. A quadrilateral configuration of direct retainers is considered ideal (Fig 7-73). For mechanical purposes, the anterior clasp assemblies should be placed as far anterior as possible, and the posterior clasp assemblies should be placed as far posterior as possible.

  C. The major connector should be rigid, and broad palatal coverage should be used in the maxillary arch.

  D. Indirect retention should be located as far posterior to the fulcrum line as possible.

   1. An ideal quadrilateral configuration of clasping may preclude the need for additional indirect retainers.

  E. A functional impression may be indicated if the edentulous area is extensive.

## Design procedures

Design procedures for removable partial denture service are the responsibility of the dentist. Failure to accomplish these procedures represents a breach of professional ethics and exposes the dentist to potential litigation.

In the past, reluctance to design removable partial dentures may have been caused by a lack of knowledge. It is the goal of this text to present the basic principles of removable partial denture design. Simplicity is of prime concern in the following discussion, but simplicity should never be placed above the biological and mechanical standards that are necessary for maintenance of patient health.

Criticism may come from proponents of other design philosophies. This criticism is to be expected, and it is welcome if other methods provide viable and defensible methods of patient care. On the other hand, criticism for the sake of controversy may represent the primary reason that dentists have avoided design procedures.

It is the responsibility of the dentist to know the various components used in removable partial denture design, to understand the functions of those components, and to select the components that will provide the best possible service for the patient. Seldom, if ever, is there a single best way to design any partial denture. More often than not, several completely acceptable designs may be generated for a given partially edentulous arch.

It must be stressed once again that a thorough knowledge of components is essential in the removable partial denture design process. Each component is capable of performing well under certain conditions, but may not perform well under other conditions. Each component has definite indications and contraindications. These must be known or the design process will become a guessing game rather than a controlled procedure.

A few words also should be said about the quality of dental casts and the overall neatness of partial denture designs. Before casts are forwarded to a laboratory, they should be checked for accuracy and neatness. Removable partial denture designs should be clearly and accurately drawn. The more presentable the work submitted to the dental laboratory, the greater the probability that quality prostheses will be fabricated.

### Armamentarium

The armamentarium needed to accomplish survey and design procedures is shown in Fig 7-74. This equipment should be readily available to prevent wasted time and effort.

The practitioner should ensure that the dental surveyor is maintained in a usable condition. The surface of the platform tends to oxidize over time. Oxidation prevents the surveying table from gliding smoothly over the surface of the platform and makes the surveying process much more difficult. This can be corrected by wiping the surface of the platform with an alcohol- or acetone-soaked gauze pad. The base of the surveying table should be cleaned in a similar manner. A small amount of acrylic resin powder may then be spread on the surface of the platform to facilitate movement of the surveying platform (Fig 7-75).

The vertical arm of the surveyor tends to collect debris over time and become difficult to move. It should be cleaned with alcohol or acetone to improve its action. Lubricants generally are not needed. If necessary, an extremely thin film of light machine oil may be applied to the vertical arm of the surveyor.

Other essential items include the analyzing rod, carbon markers, and undercut gauges (Fig 7-76). The 0.010-inch undercut gauge is used to position retentive clasps constructed from chrome alloys and titanium alloys. The 0.020-inch undercut gauge may be used to position retentive clasps made from wrought wire. Nevertheless, the majority of wrought-wire clasps should be placed in 0.015-inch undercuts. The 0.030-inch undercut gauge is rarely used for the placement of retentive clasps. This undercut gauge is more likely to be used to scribe the surface of the cast during tripodization procedures.

A plasterless articulator also may be included in the armamentarium (Fig 7-77). Opposing casts are related by means of a jaw relation record and held in place by adjustable clamps. When the casts have been properly aligned, the remaining controls may be locked into position. The occlusion may be studied at maximum intercuspation or centric relation depending upon the clinical requirements of treatment.

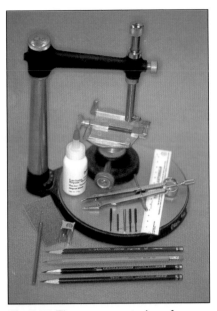

**Fig 7-74** The armamentarium for survey and design procedures includes a surveyor, surveying table, surveying tools, polymethyl methacrylate powder, colored pencils, pencil sharpener, sandpaper, a carving instrument, millimeter rule, and calipers.

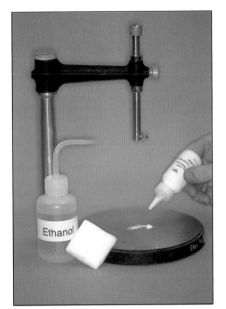

**Fig 7-75** The platform of the surveyor and the base of the surveying table should be cleaned using an acetone- or alcohol-soaked gauze pad. A small amount of polymethyl methacrylate powder may be placed on the platform to minimize friction. The spherical particles of the polymethyl methacrylate serve as tiny ball bearings and thereby facilitate movement of the surveying table across the platform.

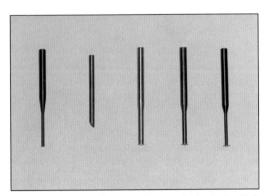

**Fig 7-76** Required surveying tools include *(left to right)* an analyzing rod; carbon marker; and 0.010-, 0.020-, and 0.030-inch undercut gauges.

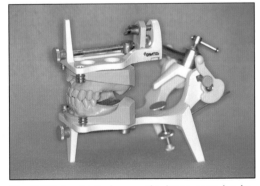

**Fig 7-77** A plasterless articulator may be included in the armamentarium. Such an articulator allows rapid mounting of casts for initial assessment.

The practitioner must be aware of potential difficulties presented by the patient's occlusion. Interarch space may dictate the placement of various components, particularly occlusal rests, retentive elements, and reciprocal elements. In many cases, components that create interferences cannot be adjusted without mutilating the associated metal frameworks. This may present additional restorative problems and may necessitate construction of additional frameworks. The practitioner can avoid countless hours of clinical effort and frustration by spending a few minutes on the planning process.

## Color coding

A consistent color coding system should be used in the removable partial denture design process. Color coding permits improved communication between the dentist and the dental laboratory technician and generally results in improved laboratory service. Currently, there is not a single, universally accepted color coding system. As a result, any system agreed to by a dentist and a dental laboratory is considered acceptable.

The authors prefer the color coding system presented in this chapter. This system requires the use of red, black, blue, and brown pencils (Fig 7-78). Each color represents a specific action or material.

Red is used to denote a required action and for the placement of tripod marks. It is also used to identify those areas of the teeth and soft tissues that must be prepared, recontoured, or relieved (Fig 7-79). For design purposes, rest seats are drawn in solid red. Surfaces that must be recontoured are outlined in red and filled with evenly spaced diagonal lines. Soft tissue areas that require relief are outlined in red and accompanied by the word *relief*.

Black lines are used to denote survey lines on the teeth and soft tissues (Fig 7-80). Black also may be used to enter information on the base of the cast. Such entries may include the type of tooth replacement, the type of clasp, or the depth of undercut to be used.

Blue denotes those portions of the removable partial denture that will be made of acrylic resin (Fig 7-81). This is most often used to identify denture bases, but also may be used to identify individual tooth replacements such as reinforced acrylic pontics.

Brown is used to outline the metallic portions of the partial denture (Fig 7-82). This includes all components of the framework (eg, major connectors, minor connectors, rests, and clasp assemblies).

This color system will be used for all designs presented in this text.

## Step-by-step procedure

The following list provides a step-by-step technique for removable partial denture design. The accompanying photographs illustrate the design process for maxillary and mandibular arches (Fig 7-83).

1. Examine the occluded diagnostic casts (Figs 7-84 to 7-86):

- Indicate proposed rest areas by using short, black lines on the bases of the dental casts (Figs 7-87 and 7-88). The authors' philosophy requires placement of a rest seat adjacent to each edentulous space. Additional rest seats are placed for indirect retention, additional support, etc.
- Using a red pencil, outline those areas that must be reshaped to provide adequate space for rests (Fig 7-89). Such recontouring should be used sparingly and should never be performed where it will produce tooth movement or instability of opposing tooth surfaces.
- Examine the occluded casts from the lingual aspect. Using a black pencil, record the vertical overlap of the anterior teeth. This should be accomplished using the incisal edges of the mandibular anterior teeth as a guide and scribing a thin, continuous line on the lingual surfaces of the maxillary anterior teeth (Fig 7-90). The resultant line indicates the incisal limit of proposed metal extensions such as lingual plating (Fig 7-91).

2. Using a black pencil, indicate the proposed tooth replacements on the base of the cast. The following designations should be used:
- Denture tooth/teeth on a denture base—no symbol indicated
- Reinforced acrylic pontic—RAP (Fig 7-92)
- Braided post—BP (Fig 7-93)
- Tube tooth—T
- Metal pontic—M

One symbol should be used for each tooth replacement.

3. Place the selected cast on the surveying table and lock the cast into place. Orient the cast so the occlusal plane is horizontally positioned. Examine proposed abutments for favorable retentive undercuts. Examine edentulous areas for esthetic considerations. Examine proximal and lingual tooth surfaces for existing or prospective guiding planes. Be aware of soft tissue undercuts that may interfere with placement of the partial denture. After considering these factors, select the most favorable tilt and tighten the surveying table's locking mechanism (Figs 7-94 to 7-101).

4. Tripod the cast (Figs 7-102 and 7-103).

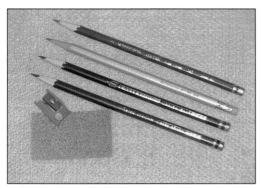

**Fig 7-78** Red, black, blue, and brown pencils are used for survey and design procedures. A pencil sharpener and sandpaper should be available to ensure that lines are crisp and well defined.

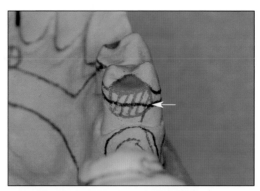

**Fig 7-79** Red is used to denote action. Proposed rest seats are indicated by solid red. Areas that require recontouring are outlined in red and filled with evenly spaced diagonal lines *(arrow)*.

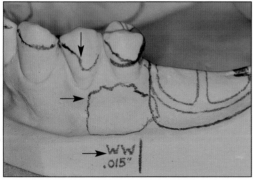

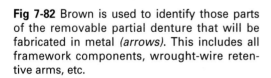

**Fig 7-80** Black is used to place survey lines and to provide written instructions on the base of the cast *(arrows)*. Written instructions may include the type of tooth replacement, the type of clasp, or the depth of undercut to be used.

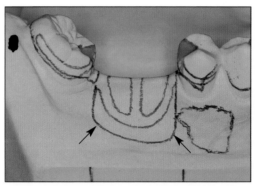

**Fig 7-81** Blue is used to identify portions of the removable partial denture that will be made of acrylic resin *(arrows)*.

**Fig 7-82** Brown is used to identify those parts of the removable partial denture that will be fabricated in metal *(arrows)*. This includes all framework components, wrought-wire retentive arms, etc.

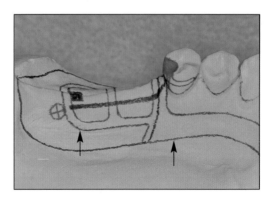

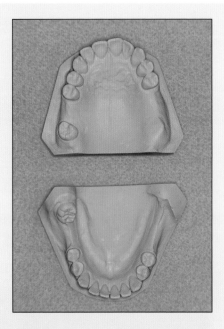

**Fig 7-83** Maxillary and mandibular diagnostic casts.

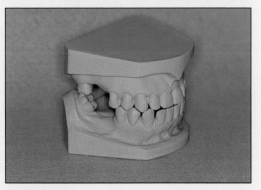

**Fig 7-84** Properly related diagnostic casts (right lateral view).

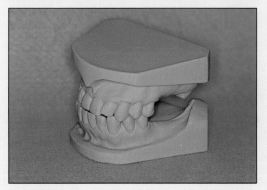

**Fig 7-85** Properly related diagnostic casts (left lateral view).

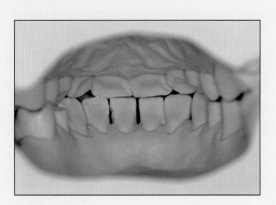

**Fig 7-86** Properly related diagnostic casts (lingual view).

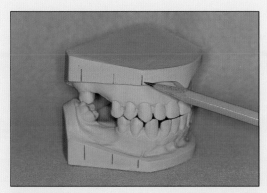

**Fig 7-87** Proposed rest seats are identified by placing vertical black lines on the bases of the maxillary and mandibular casts. On the maxillary right, rest seats are planned for the mesio-occlusal surface of the third molar and the disto-occlusal surface of the second premolar. An additional rest seat is planned for the canine and will serve as an indirect retainer. On the mandibular right, rest seats are planned for the mesio-occlusal surface of the third molar and the disto-occlusal surface of the second premolar. An additional rest seat is planned for the mesio-occlusal surface of the first premolar and will be used for indirect retention.

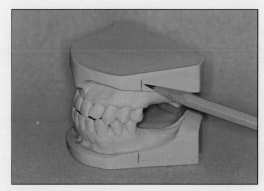

**Fig 7-88** On the maxillary left, a rest seat is planned for the distal fossa of the second premolar. On the mandibular left, a rest seat is planned for the disto-occlusal fossa of the second premolar.

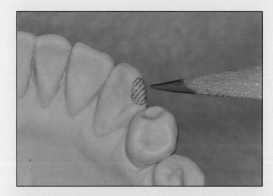

**Fig 7-89** In some situations, it is necessary for the practitioner to reshape teeth to permit adequate space for rests. For ease of identification, these areas should be outlined in red and filled with evenly spaced diagonal lines.

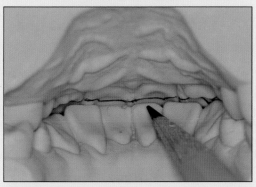

**Fig 7-90** Vertical overlap of the anterior teeth must be recorded to facilitate design procedures. This is accomplished by properly relating the dental casts and using a black pencil to scribe a continuous line on the lingual aspects of the maxillary teeth. The position of this line is dictated by the incisal edges of the mandibular anterior teeth.

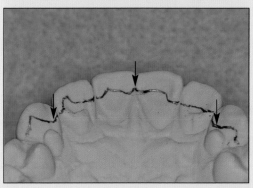

**Fig 7-91** The line scribed in Fig 7-90 *(arrows)* clearly indicates the vertical overlap of anterior teeth and defines the incisal limit for extension of the removable partial denture framework.

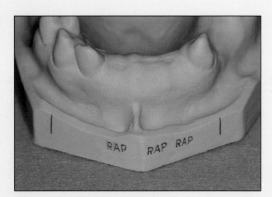

**Fig 7-92** A black pencil is used to indicate proposed tooth replacements on the base of the cast. In this instance, three reinforced acrylic pontics (RAPs) have been indicated. Reinforced acrylic pontics are commonly used for the reinforcement of anterior tooth replacements.

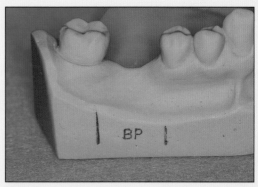

**Fig 7-93** In this instance, a braided post has been selected for reinforcement of a prosthetic tooth in the mandibular right first molar position. Braided posts are commonly used in posterior applications.

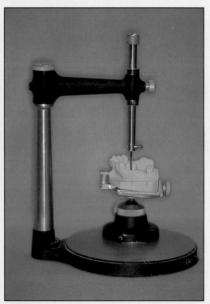

**Fig 7-94** The maxillary cast is placed on a surveying table. During initial evaluation, the occlusal plane is oriented parallel to the bench top.

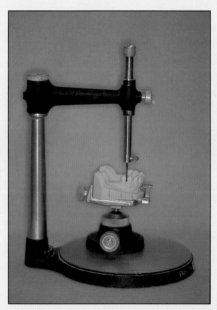

**Fig 7-95** The mandibular cast is placed on a surveying table and locked in position. The practitioner should ensure that the occlusal plane is oriented parallel to the bench top.

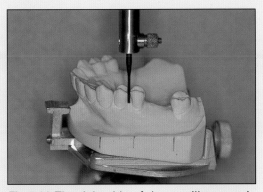

**Fig 7-96** The right side of the maxillary cast is evaluated. The analyzing rod permits rapid visual assessment of cast contours. In this instance, undercuts are available at the distofacial line angle of the third molar and the mesiofacial line angle of the second premolar.

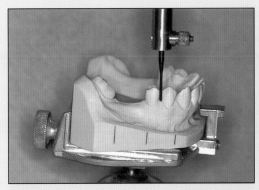

**Fig 7-97** The right side of the mandibular cast is evaluated using an analyzing rod in the vertical arm of the surveyor. Undercuts are available at the distolingual line angle of the third molar and the mesiofacial line angle of the second premolar.

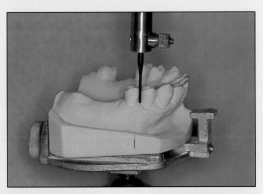

**Fig 7-98** The left side of the maxillary cast is evaluated. Undercuts are available at the mesiofacial and distofacial line angles of the second premolar. Soft tissue contours adjacent to this tooth will permit placement of an infrabulge clasp.

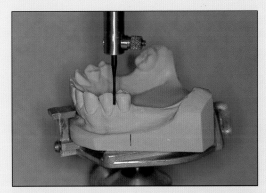

**Fig 7-99** The left side of the mandibular cast is evaluated. An undercut is available at the mesiofacial and distofacial line angles of the second premolar. Soft tissue contours adjacent to this tooth do not favor placement of an infrabulge clasp. Hence, the practitioner must consider a combination clasp (wrought-wire retentive element in conjunction with a cast reciprocal component).

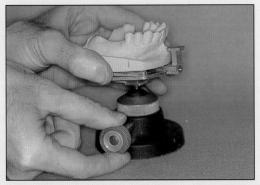

**Fig 7-100** Following determination of the most favorable tilt, the surveying table is locked in position. This maintains the spatial orientation of the maxillary cast.

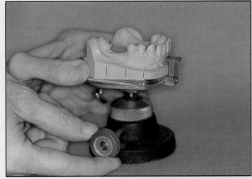

**Fig 7-101** When the most favorable tilt for the mandibular cast has been finalized and verified, the surveying table is locked in position. This maintains the spatial orientation of the mandibular cast.

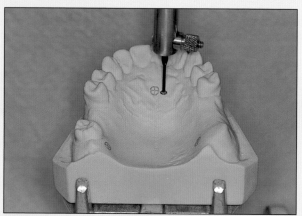

**Fig 7-102** Tripod marks are placed to record the orientation of the maxillary cast. Tripod marks must be within a single horizontal plane. In addition, the tripod marks must be widely spaced and they must be on easily identifiable anatomic areas of the cast. These marks should never be placed on areas that will be inconsistent from cast to cast. Hence, the base and land areas should be avoided.

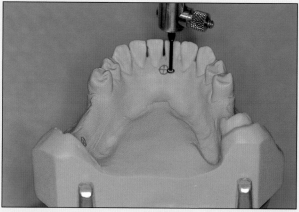

**Fig 7-103** Tripod marks are placed on the mandibular cast. These marks are essential in recording the proposed path of insertion for the prosthesis. They also allow accurate spatial reorientation of the cast following removal from the surveying table.

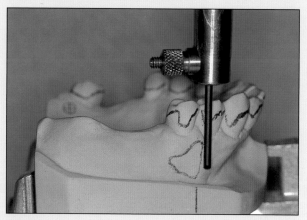

**Fig 7-104** Survey lines are transferred to the surfaces of the maxillary teeth. Survey lines are also required on soft tissue areas adjacent to proposed abutments. Soft tissue contours are often primary determinants in the ability or inability to use infrabulge clasps.

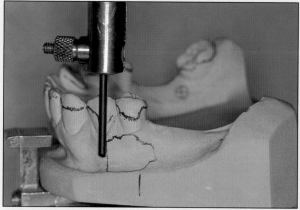

**Fig 7-105** Survey lines are transferred to the exposed surfaces of all mandibular teeth. In addition, survey lines are transferred to soft tissue areas adjacent to proposed abutments. The position of the soft tissue survey line adjacent to the second premolar would prevent the use of an infrabulge clasp arm. When an infrabulge clasp is being considered, it is desirable to have at least 3 mm of attached tissue between the gingival margin and the soft tissue survey line.

5. Place a carbon marker in the vertical arm of the surveyor and scribe survey lines on the teeth and soft tissues that will be contacted by the partial denture (Figs 7-104 and 7-105).

6. Replace the carbon marker with the appropriate undercut gauge. Carefully identify the desired undercuts on the proposed abutment teeth and mark the positions of these undercuts using a red pencil. The resultant marks should appear as thin, horizontal lines approximately 2 mm in length (Figs 7-106 and 7-107).

7. With a red pencil, identify those areas where rest seats will be prepared. Rest seats should be solid red (Figs 7-108 and 7-109).

8. Using a red pencil, outline tooth surfaces that will require recontouring to produce the desired results. Place evenly spaced diagonal lines to ensure that these areas are highly visible (Figs 7-110 and 7-111).

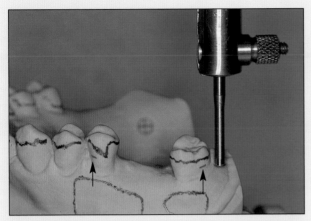

Fig 7-106 The desired undercuts are identified using appropriate undercut gauges. Undercuts are clearly marked using a red pencil *(arrows)*. Undercut marks should be approximately 2 mm long and relatively thin.

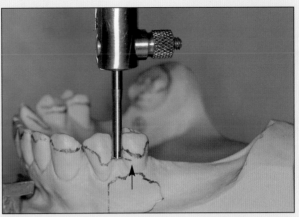

Fig 7-107 Desired undercuts are identified in the mandibular arch. Undercuts are identified using a sharply defined, red line approximately 2 mm in length *(arrow)*.

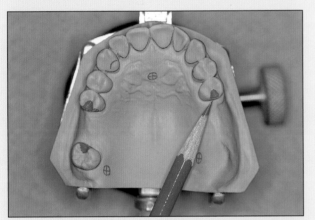

Fig 7-108 Rest seats are drawn using a red pencil. The locations of the rest seats should correspond to the black lines drawn on the base of each cast (see Figs 7-87 and 7-88). Rest seats should be solid red and should display the appropriate size and shape. In this instance, occlusal rest seats are located on the right second molar, right third premolar, and left second premolar. A cingulum rest seat is indicated on the lingual surface of the right canine.

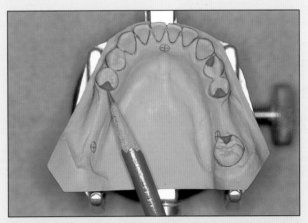

Fig 7-109 Mandibular rest seats are clearly indicated using a red pencil. For this arch, occlusal rest seats are located on the left second premolar, the right first premolar, the right second premolar, and the right third molar.

Areas of soft tissue relief should be outlined in red and accompanied by the word relief.

9. Using a blue pencil, outline the exact position of each acrylic resin denture base (Figs 7-112 and 7-113).

10. With a brown pencil, draw the outline of the major connector, minor connectors, and indirect retainers when present. Ensure that all components are in harmony with each other and display smoothly flowing contours (Figs 7-114 to 7-121).

11. Using a brown pencil, draw the retentive and reciprocal elements to the desired sizes, shapes, and locations (Figs 7-122 to 7-127). If wrought-wire clasps are to be used, ensure that they are appropriately drawn and properly identified. This may be accomplished by placing the symbol WW on the land area adjacent to each wrought-wire clasp.

12. The design should now be complete (Figs 7-128 to 7-133). The practitioner should examine all aspects of the design for accuracy and clarity.

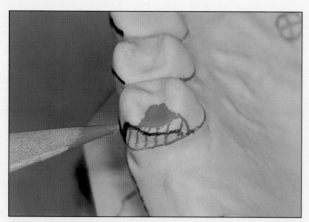

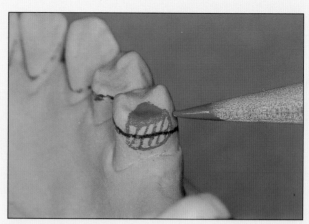

**Fig 7-110** Maxillary tooth surfaces that require recontouring are identified. This is accomplished by outlining these areas in red and filling the designated areas with evenly spaced diagonal lines.

**Fig 7-111** Mandibular tooth surfaces that require recontouring also are identified using a red pencil.

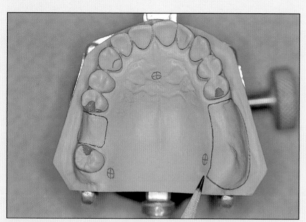

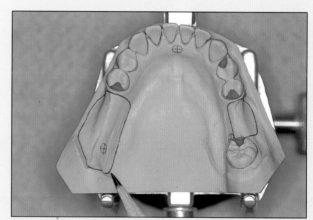

**Fig 7-112** The outline of each maxillary denture base is drawn using a blue pencil. Denture bases should be properly extended in all directions. Buccal extensions should reach the depth of the vestibule. Lingual extensions should be consistent with the lingual surfaces of the remaining teeth (as viewed from an occlusal perspective). Distal extension bases should always extend to the depth of the hamular notch posteriorly.

**Fig 7-113** Using a blue pencil, the outline of each mandibular base is drawn. Buccal extensions should reach the depth of the vestibule. Lingual extensions for tooth-bounded areas should follow the arc established by the lingual surfaces of the remaining teeth. In distal extension areas, denture bases should be extended to the depth of the lingual sulcus. Posteriorly, distal extension bases should cover the pear-shaped pads.

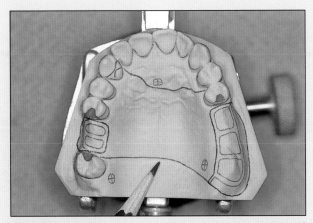

**Fig 7-114** A brown pencil is used to draw the outline of the maxillary major connector, minor connectors, and auxiliary components. In this instance, a wide palatal strap was selected. Under different clinical circumstances, a complete palate or anteroposterior palatal strap may have been chosen. The selection of a major connector may be driven by a number of factors, including patient desires, periodontal conditions, phonetics, etc.

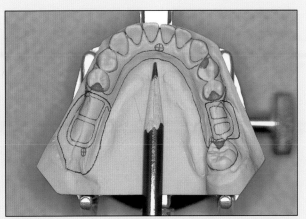

**Fig 7-115** The mandibular major connector, minor connectors, and auxiliary components are outlined using a brown pencil. A lingual bar major connector was selected in this situation. This selection was based upon adequate depth of the lingual sulcus (a minimum distance of 8 mm between the gingival margins and the active floor of the mouth) and the presence of obvious diastemata between the remaining anterior teeth. Nevertheless, a modified lingual plate may have been selected under different clinical conditions.

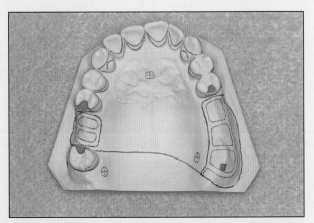

**Fig 7-116** Occlusal view of an alternative maxillary major connector design. This major connector is classified as a complete palate. Note the additional cingulum rest seat placed on the left canine.

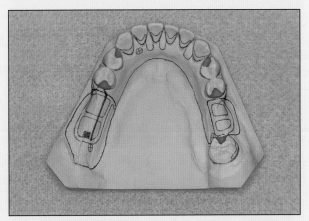

**Fig 7-117** Occlusal view of an alternative mandibular major connector design. This major connector is classified as a modified lingual plate because of the "drop aways" or step backs in the anterior region. Notice the additional occlusal rest seat located in the mesial fossa of the left first premolar.

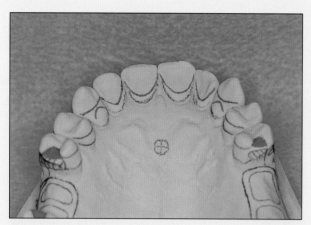

**Fig 7-118** Closer view of Fig 7-116 showing the scalloped appearance that should be displayed by lingual plating. Plating should extend from the cingula to the proximal contacts in a series of connected arcs.

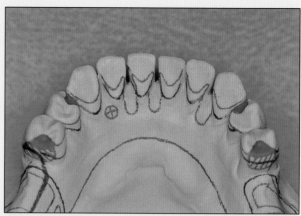

**Fig 7-119** Closer view of Fig 7-117 showing the modifications of lingual plating that are often necessary to avoid the display of metal interproximally. In this instance, lingual plating includes a series of drop aways. It is important to recognize that a minimum vertical height (5 mm) of the major connector must be maintained or rigidity will be compromised.

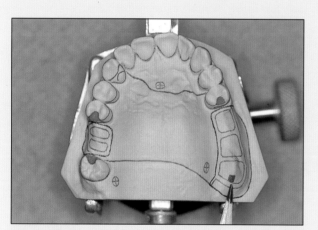

**Fig 7-120** Cast stops are represented as projections originating from distal extension areas of a maxillary framework. Cast stops should be solid brown and should be located on relatively horizontal areas of the cast. These auxiliary components are necessary to prevent distortion of framework components during resin-packing procedures.

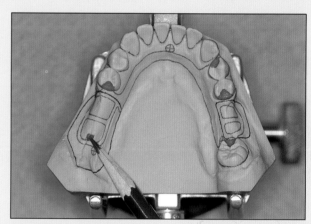

**Fig 7-121** Cast stops also are included for distal extension areas of mandibular frameworks. As previously noted, cast stops should be solid brown and should be located on relatively horizontal areas of the cast.

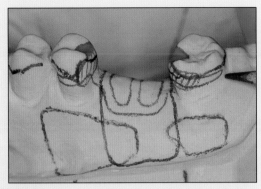

**Fig 7-122** At this stage, maxillary retentive elements are drawn using a brown pencil. For circumferential clasp assemblies, only the terminal third of each retentive arm should enter the undercut. It is important to note the position of each clasp relative to the red line that identifies the measured undercut. Only the apical border of the clasp terminus should contact the red mark.

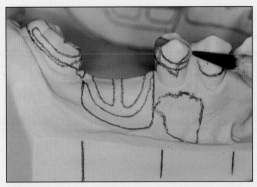

**Fig 7-123** The mandibular retentive elements should be drawn using the guidelines described in Fig 7-122. Note that a retentive arm is located on the facial surface of the second premolar, while a reciprocal arm is located on the facial surface of the third molar. The retentive element for the third molar clasp assembly is located on the lingual surface of the abutment (see Fig 7-125).

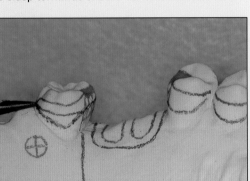

**Fig 7-124** Maxillary reciprocal elements also are drawn using a brown pencil. A reciprocal clasp arm has been used on the third molar, while lingual plating has been employed on the second premolar. Notice that the entire reciprocal arm is located occlusal to the survey line. Lingual plating is an extension of the major connector and also extends occlusal to the survey line.

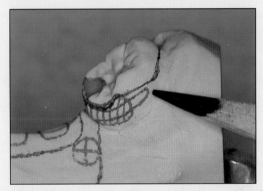

**Fig 7-125** A retentive element has been placed on the lingual surface of the mandibular right third molar. Such retentive elements are commonly used for mandibular molars.

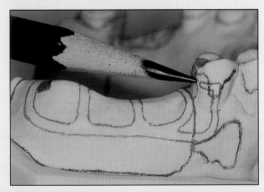

**Fig 7-126** A distal ½T retentive arm is placed on the maxillary left second premolar. The approach arm originates from the resin-retaining component, travels anteriorly, and then turns occlusally. After passing occlusal to the survey line, the clasp arm turns distally to engage a 0.010-inch undercut at the distofacial line angle.

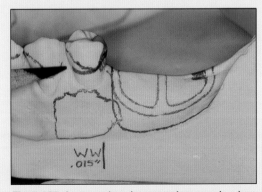

**Fig 7-127** A wrought-wire retentive arm is placed on the mandibular left second premolar. Unlike other clasp arms, a wrought-wire retentive arm is drawn as a solid brown component. When using a wrought wire, the symbol *WW* must be placed on the base of the cast and must be accompanied by the prescribed undercut.

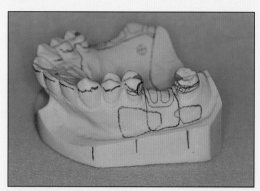

**Fig 7-128** Right lateral view of the completed maxillary design.

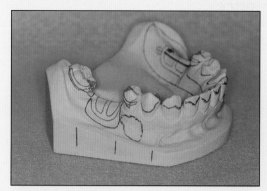

**Fig 7-129** Right lateral view of the completed mandibular design.

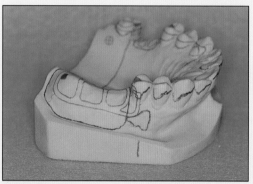

**Fig 7-130** Left lateral view of the completed maxillary design.

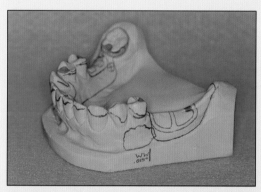

**Fig 7-131** Left lateral view of the completed mandibular design.

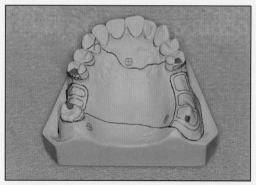

**Fig 7-132** Occlusal view of the completed maxillary design.

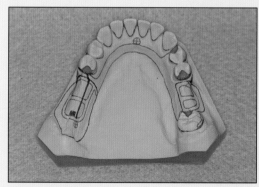

**Fig 7-133** Occlusal view of the completed mandibular design.

## ⌑ Reference

1. Schmidt AH. Planning and designing removable partial dentures. J Prosthet Dent 1953;3:783–806.

## ⌑ Bibliography

Applegate OC. Use of paralleling surveyor in modern partial denture construction. J Am Dent Assoc 1940;27:1317–1407.

Atkinson HF. Partial denture problems: Designing about a path of withdrawal. Aust J Dent 1953;37:187–190.

Atkinson HF. Partial denture problems: Surveyors and surveying. Aust J Dent 1955;59:28–31.

Atkinson RA, Elliot RW. Removable partial denture designed for laboratory fabrication by recent dental school graduates. J Prosthet Dent 1969;22:528–543.

Beaumont AJ, Bianco HJ. Microcomputer-aided removable partial denture design. J Prosthet Dent 1989;62:417–421.

Black GV. A Work on Operative Dentistry, ed 4. Chicago: Medico-Dental, 1920.

Blatterfein L. A new approach to partial denture design for unilaterally remaining lower teeth. J Prosthet Dent 1972;23:145–163.

Boero E, Forbes WG. Considerations in design of removable prosthetic abutments. J Prosthet Dent 1972;23:253–263.

Boitel RH. The parallelometer, a precision instrument for the prosthetic laboratory. J Prosthet Dent 1962;12:732–736.

Bolouve A. Removable partial denture design for a few remaining natural teeth. J Prosthet Dent 1978;39:346–348.

Burns DR, Ward JE, Nance GL. Removable partial denture design and fabrication survey of the prosthodontic specialist. J Prosthet Dent 1989;62:303–307.

Chistner SB. A methodical approach to the analysis of study casts. J Prosthet Dent 1954;4:622–624.

Christidou L, Osborne J, Chamberlain JB. The effects of partial denture design on the mobility of abutment teeth. Br Dent J 1973;135:9–18.

Coy RE, Arnold PD. Survey and design of diagnostic casts for removable partial dentures. J Prosthet Dent 1974;32:103–106.

Craddock FW. Clasp surveying and mysticism. Aust J Dent 1955;59:205–208.

DeBoer J. The effects on function of distal-extension removable partial dentures as determined by occlusal rest position. J Prosthet Dent 1988;60:693–696.

Dental Laboratory Technician's Manual, Department of the Air Force. Washington, DC: US Government Printing Office, 1959.

Dunn BW. Treatment planning for removable partial dentures. J Prosthet Dent 1961;11:247–255.

Elliot FC. A method that simplified the design of partial dentures. J Am Dent Assoc 1940;27:1263–1268.

Fish, EW. A new principle in partial denture design. Br Dent J 1952;92:135–144.

Frantz WR. Variations in a removable maxillary partial denture design by dentists. J Prosthet Dent 1975;34:625–633.

Frechette AR. The influence of partial denture design on distribution of force to abutment teeth. J Prosthet Dent 1956;6:195–212.

Girardot RI. History and development of partial denture design. J Am Dent Assoc 1941;28:1399–1408.

Goodkind RJ. The effects of removable partial dentures on abutment tooth mobility: A clinical study. J Prosthet Dent 1973;30:139–145.

Hanson JG. Surveying. J Am Dent Assoc 1975;91:826–828.

Hardy I. Partial lower denture design. Dent Dig 1938;44:57–71.

Jordan LG. Designing removable partial dentures with external attachments. J Prosthet Dent 1952;2:716–722.

Kaires AK. A study of partial denture design and masticatory pressure in a mandibular distal extension case. J Prosthet Dent 1967;17:472–478.

Katulski EM, Appleyard WN. Biological concepts of the use of the mechanical cast surveyor. J Prosthet Dent 1959;9:629–634.

Kelley EK. The physiologic approach to partial denture design. J Prosthet Dent 1953;3:699–710.

Kratochvil FJ. Influence of occlusal rest position and clasp design on movement of abutment teeth. J Prosthet Dent 1963;13:114–124.

LaVere AM. A simplified procedure for survey and design of diagnostic casts. J Prosthet Dent 1977;37:680–683.

Lazarus AH. Partial denture design. J Prosthet Dent 1951;1:438–442.

McCracken WL. Contemporary partial denture designs. J Prosthet Dent 1958;8:71–84.

McCracken WL. Survey of partial denture designs by commercial dental laboratories. J Prosthet Dent 1962;12:1089–1110.

McKinstry RE, Minsley GE, Wood MT. The effect of clinical experience on dental students' ability to design removable partial denture frameworks. J Prosthet Dent 1989;62:563–566.

Maxfield JB, Nicholls JI, Smith DE. The measurement of forces transmitted to abutment teeth of removable partial dentures. J Prosthet Dent 1979;41:134–142.

Moore DS. Some fundamentals of partial denture design to conserve the supporting structures. J Ont Dent Assoc 1955;32:238–240.

Neurohr FG. Health conservation of the periodontal tissues by a method of functional partial denture design. J Am Dent Assoc 1974;31:58–70.

Osborne J, Lammie GA. The bilateral free-end saddle lower denture. J Prosthet Dent 1954;4:640–653.

Perry C. A philosophy of partial denture design. J Prosthet Dent 1956;6:775–784.

Potter RB, Appleby RC, Adams CD. Removable partial denture designs: A review and a challenge. J Prosthet Dent 1967;17:63–68.

Rudd KD, Dunn BW. Accurate removable partial dentures. J Prosthet Dent 1967;18:559–570.

Ryan J. Technique of design in partial denture construction. J Dent Assoc S Afr 1954;9:123–133.

Ryback SA Jr. Simplicity in a distal extension partial denture. J Prosthet Dent 1953;3:783–806.

Scott DD. Suggested designs for metal partial dentures. Dent Tech 1954;2:21.

Solle W. An improved dental surveyor. J Am Dent Assoc 1960;60:727–731.

Steffel VL. Current concepts in removable partial denture service. J Prosthet Dent 1968;20:387–395.

Steffel VL. Fundamental principles involved in partial denture design. J Am Dent Assoc 1951;42:534.

Sykora O, Calikkocaoglu S. Maxillary removable partial denture designs by commercial dental laboratories. J Prosthet Dent 1970;23:633–640.

Tench RW. Fundamentals of partial denture design. J Am Dent Assoc 1936;23:1087–1092.

Thompson WD, Kratochvil FJ, Caputo AA. Evaluation of photoelastic stress patterns produced by various designs of bilateral distal-extension removable partial dentures. J Prosthet Dent 1977;38:261–273.

Trainor JE, Elliott RW Jr, Bartlett SO. Removable partial dentures designed by dentists before and after graduate level instruction: A comparative study. J Prosthet Dent 1972;27:509–514.

Trapozzano VR, Winter GR. Periodontal aspects of partial denture design. J Prosthet Dent 1952;2:101–107.

Wagner AG, Forgue EG. A study of four methods of recording the path of insertion of removable partial dentures. J Prosthet Dent 1976;35:267–272.

Wills NG. Practical engineering applied to removable partial denture designing. Prosthet Dent Centenary 1940:319–331.

Yilmaz G. Optical surveying of casts for removable partial dentures. J Prosthet Dent 1975;34:292–296.

# I-bar Removable Partial Dentures

**Michael A. Mansueto**, DDS, MS, FACP

Distal extension removable partial dentures are supported by the remaining teeth and soft tissues. The teeth are less displaceable and less compressible than is the alveolar mucosa. Consequently, the practitioner must design distal extension prostheses that distribute forces evenly without overloading the teeth or soft tissues. This presents a dilemma for the practitioner, who must restore function without endangering the remaining oral structures. As a result, numerous philosophies for the treatment of Kennedy Class I and Class II arches have been introduced. Indisputable scientific evidence establishing the superiority of one philosophy over others does not exist, even though proponents of individual philosophies cite years of clinical experience and empirical evidence of success.

As might be expected, the effects of clasping have received a great deal of attention. Historically, teeth serving as distal extension abutments were at increased risk for early tooth loss. The two most commonly cited causes for abutment loss were overloading and periodontal disease. Overloading was of particular significance because it could be directly related to removable partial denture design, and more specifically to clasp design. This led to the introduction of numerous clasp-

ing philosophies for use in distal extension applications. For years, the majority of philosophies were based upon common suprabulge clasping systems. Then, in 1963, Kratochvil introduced the I-bar design philosophy.[1] This philosophy was based upon use of an I-bar retentive element, a mesial rest, and a distal proximal plate. Proponents of the I-bar philosophy claimed that the resultant clasp design minimized torquing forces and directed occlusal loads parallel to the long axes of abutments. Years of in vivo and in vitro experimentation followed, with researchers attempting to establish the ideal clasp assembly—one that would proportionately load the teeth and soft tissues. Test results were often unclear, conflicting, or dismissed because of flaws in experimental design. Still, the I-bar rationale, especially the use of a mesial rest, emerged as a popular by-product of Kratochvil's design principles.

Although the I-bar system can be applied to tooth-supported partial dentures, the following text addresses Kennedy Class I and Class II patterns of edentulism in order to demonstrate basic design principles. An explanation of design changes to Kratochvil's concepts that have been advocated by some is also offered.

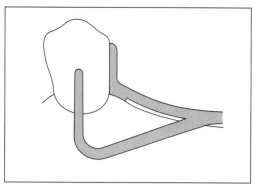

**Fig 8-1** I-bar clasp assembly, buccal view. Note the long distal guiding plane.

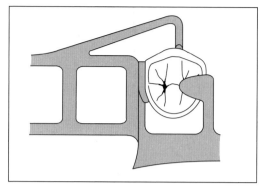

**Fig 8-2** I-bar clasp assembly, occlusal view. The I-bar is positioned at or mesial to the mesiodistal height of contour.

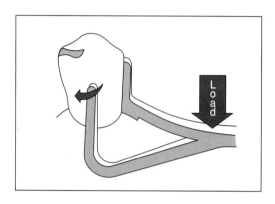

**Fig 8-3** Occlusal force on the distal extension base causes rotation about the mesial rest. The retentive terminus disengages into the mesial undercut, minimizing torque at the abutment.

## ☐ Components of the I-bar System

Kratochvil's I-bar system includes a mesial rest, I-bar retainer, and a long distal guiding plane that extends to the tooth-tissue junction. Each component must function properly to ensure success of the I-bar system. Unfortunately, the importance of the I-bar retentive clasp has been overemphasized. The practitioner must understand that the I-bar retentive clasp is only one element in the design equation (Figs 8-1 to 8-3). For this clasping system to function effectively, all components must be properly designed, constructed, and fitted.

## ☐ Design Concepts

Successful removable partial denture therapy requires careful evaluation of the patient, astute treatment planning, and an organized design sequence. As might be expected, the principles involved in examina-

tion and diagnosis (see chapters 5 and 6) also apply to I-bar designs. The practitioner must assess radiographic information, determine pertinent periodontal conditions, and examine occlusal relationships using properly mounted diagnostic casts. With this information, ideal partial denture design may be considered (Fig 8-4). In turn, diagnostic casts may be surveyed to determine whether this tentative design can be used without modification (Fig 8-5). Required tooth preparation or design modifications are then planned.

The I-bar partial denture components will be discussed in the order of the design sequence advocated by Kratochvil and Vig[2]: rests, proximal plates, major connectors, minor connectors, denture base connectors, and retainers.

### Rests

Rests provide vertical support against occlusal forces and control the vertical relationship between the pros-

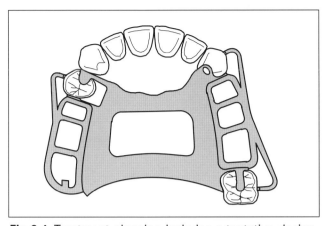

**Fig 8-4** Treatment planning includes a tentative design. Rests are placed on the mesio-occlusal surfaces of abutments adjacent to the distal extension bases. Rests are placed adjacent to modification spaces. Reciprocation for distal extension applications is provided by long guiding planes and properly positioned minor connectors. Reciprocation for tooth-bounded applications may be provided by lingual plating, as depicted on the canine and molar.

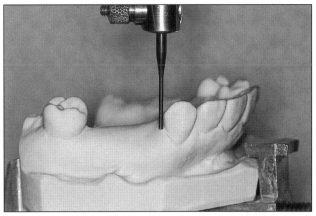

**Fig 8-5** Diagnostic casts are surveyed to determine the amount of tooth modification necessary to provide retention and establish appropriate guiding planes. Tipping of abutments or the presence of soft tissue undercuts may mandate modification of the "ideal" design.

thesis and the supporting structures. To perform these functions, rests must display excellent adaptation to the corresponding abutments and must possess sufficient bulk to withstand applied loads.

In addition to the strength and positive-seating requirements shared by all rests, anterior rests must satisfy esthetic requirements. Cingulum rests are ideal for anterior applications (Fig 8-6). A cingulum rest places forces closer to the rotational center of the associated tooth and provides maximum stabilization.

Cingulum rest seats can be prepared directly in the enamel of bulky canines and maxillary central incisors (Fig 8-7), or they may be included in cast restorations (Fig 8-8). Mandibular anterior teeth generally lack sufficient enamel for appropriate preparation of cingulum rest seats. Therefore, incisal rest seats should be used on mandibular anterior teeth when esthetics permit (Fig 8-9).

Posterior rests are designed to direct forces within the long axes of the associated abutments. In I-bar applications, premolar rest seats are prepared in

marginal and triangular ridges, and molar rest seats extend into the central fossae. Each rest should display a gently rounded bearing surface that allows ball-and-socket movement around the axis of rotation (Fig 8-10).

In distal extension applications, the most posterior rests are placed on the mesial surfaces of the abutment teeth for the following reasons:

1. During the application of occlusal loads, rests serve as rotational centers. As the distance from the rotational center to the denture base is increased, the associated radius becomes larger, and the accompanying arc becomes more linear. Consequently, anterior placement of rests helps direct the forces vertically onto the bearing tissues beneath the extension bases (Fig 8-11).
2. Mesial rests direct tipping forces toward the mesial surfaces. This places the abutments in firm contact with adjacent teeth, providing a "buttressing" effect (Fig 8-12).

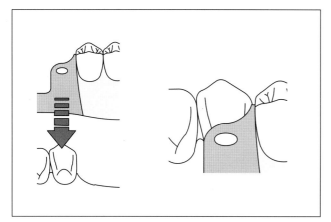

**Fig 8-6** The cingulum rest is advocated for maxillary canines. An opening in the framework allows the practitioner to evaluate seating and adaptation of the framework.

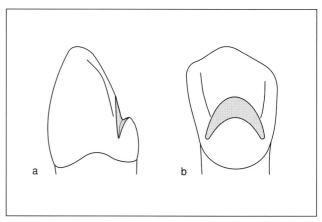

**Fig 8-7** A cingulum rest seat can be prepared in enamel if the abutment is large enough. The preparation provides a positive seat *(a)* and is rounded mesiodistally *(b)* to permit rotation of the framework.

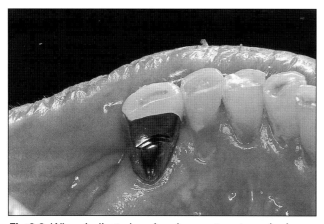

**Fig 8-8** When indicated, a cingulum rest seat can be incorporated into a surveyed crown. This is particularly helpful when the abutment lacks appropriate contours or sufficient enamel.

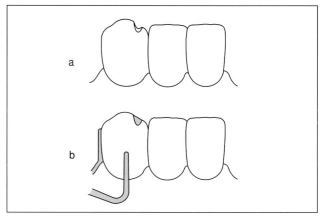

**Fig 8-9** Incisal rests may be used on mandibular anterior teeth when esthetics permit. Incisal rests also may be used to splint periodontally weakened teeth. *(a)* Abutment preparation must permit a bulk of metal for strength, yet it must not lead to overcontouring. *(b)* The rest engages a short facial bevel to prevent facial displacement of the tooth.

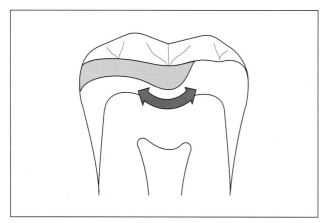

**Fig 8-10** Posterior rests direct vertical forces along the long axes of teeth. Rests must be strong, yet must not interfere with the patient's existing occlusion. Rests and rest seats must display rounded contours that permit ball-and-socket rotation.

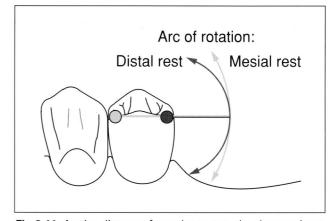

**Fig 8-11** As the distance from the rest to the denture base is increased, the associated radius becomes larger, and the arc of rotation becomes more linear. Hence, anterior placement of the rest helps direct the forces more vertically onto the tissues of the residual ridge.

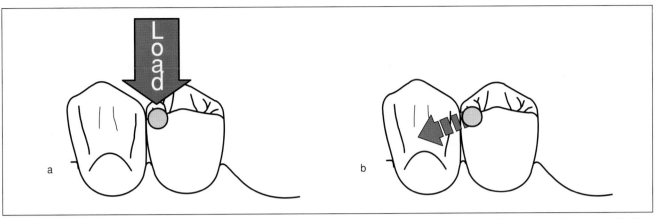

**Fig 8-12** *(a)* Functional loading of the mesial rest directs tipping forces toward the mesial surface of the abutment. *(b)* The resultant force vector places the abutment in firm contact with the adjacent tooth and results in a more favorable distribution of forces.

## Proximal plates

While retentive elements have been overemphasized in the execution of Kratochvil's design, the significance of the guiding planes and proximal plates has been underemphasized. Guiding planes are prepared on proximal tooth surfaces adjacent to edentulous spaces. Proximal plates cover these guiding planes from marginal ridge to tooth-tissue junction and extend onto the attached gingiva for 2 mm. This configuration

1. Permits improved stabilization of the prosthesis
2. Reunites and stabilizes remaining teeth within the dental arch
3. Improves retentive characteristics by limiting/defining the path of insertion and removal
4. Protects the tooth-tissue junction by reducing food impaction between the tooth and the proximal plate
5. Provides reciprocation during insertion and removal of the prosthesis
6. Distributes occlusal forces throughout the arch

Despite the advantages offered by long guiding planes, many practitioners are hesitant to make the required tooth reductions. It is important to note that in the Kratochvil technique, underprepared guiding planes compromise the stability and function of the prosthesis.

The path of insertion is chosen in consideration of smaller anterior teeth that may otherwise be over-reduced. Cast restorations are placed on tipped teeth that require severe axial reduction.

## Major connectors

Major connectors are designed for maximum rigidity and optimum gingival health. An anteroposterior strap is preferred in the maxillary arch, while a lingual bar is preferred for mandibular applications (Figs 8-13 and 8-14). A maxillary major connector should be positioned 6 mm away from tooth-tissue junctions. A mandibular major connector should be placed on unattached mucosa or at least 3 mm away from the gingival margins.

Design modifications are made to address anatomic variations, such as a shallow anterior lingual sulcus that does not provide an adequate dimension to allow both a rigid lingual bar and 3 mm of space for gingival health. A lingual plate major connector is advocated when space is inadequate for a lingual bar or when tooth or soft tissue contours promote food impaction. Relief is not provided at the intaglio surface of a major connector because close adaptation is needed to prevent soft tissue hypertrophy and food impaction. Tissue impingement is minimized by providing adequate vertical support for the major connector.

## Minor connectors

Minor connectors join rests, proximal plates, and retainers to the major connector. Minor connectors also

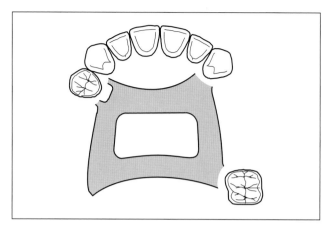

**Fig 8-13** Maxillary major connector. An anteroposterior strap is advocated for maxillary removable partial dentures. Lateral borders of the major connector should be positioned at least 6 mm from tooth-tissue junctions, allowing adequate stimulation of the gingivae and preventing gingival hypertrophy.

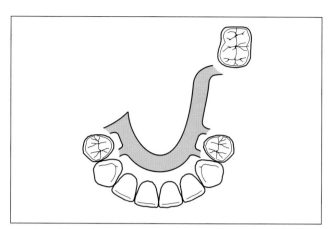

**Fig 8-14** Mandibular major connector. A lingual bar is recommended for mandibular removable partial dentures. Borders of the major connector should be positioned at least 3 mm from tooth-tissue junctions. If lingual tori are present or if the lingual sulcus is shallow, a lingual plate design may be substituted.

help provide horizontal stability. Because minor connectors are usually located in lingual embrasures, they have considerable potential for disrupting the food-deflecting morphology of the natural dentition. With this in mind, the connectors are designed to cross tooth-tissue junctions at right angles, minimizing food impaction. The intended areas of placement for minor connectors are surveyed, and tooth contours are altered, eliminating gross undercuts and allowing increased thickness of metal for improved strength.

### Denture base connectors

Denture base connectors are designed to provide strength, adequately retain acrylic resin denture bases, and avoid interference with placement of prosthetic teeth. One millimeter of relief is provided between denture base connectors and the dental cast. This permits acrylic resin to encompass the connectors, thereby providing strong mechanical attachment.

Since the acrylic resin is subject to deterioration under stress at the tooth-tissue junction, this area is covered with metal. The acrylic resin then forms a butt joint with metal 2 mm from the abutment teeth.

Altered cast impressions are made for all extension bases. The interface between the impression material and the metal that covers the tooth-tissue junction serves as an indicator of proper framework orientation during impression procedures.

### Direct retainers

Following Kratochvil's guidance, direct retention is provided by clasp assemblies featuring I-bar retentive elements. The I-bars engage mechanical undercuts on the surfaces of abutments (Fig 8-15). Retention is augmented by the parallelism of long guiding planes that define a relatively precise path of insertion and removal.

Each I-bar is designed to minimize the coverage of teeth and soft tissues, thereby promoting tissue health. The approach arm is long and tapering and displays a half-round cross-sectional geometry. The clasp terminus engages an undercut at the height of mesiodistal contour or slightly mesial to it. This position of the I-bar in relation to the height of contour allows the clasp terminus to move passively toward the mesial embrasure space when a load is applied to the denture base.

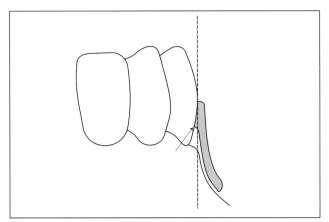

**Fig 8-15** The I-bar engages a 0.010-inch undercut *(arrow)* and terminates at or slightly above the height of contour, reducing tooth abrasion and preventing the clasp from snapping into place. *Broken line* indicates the path of insertion.

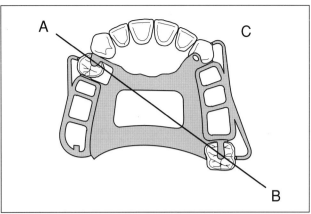

**Fig 8-16** I-bar retainers should be positioned at or mesial to the mesiodistal height of contour (A and B). I-bars distant to the axis of rotation (C) are not placed in retentive undercuts and provide frictional retention and horizontal stabilization.

The following important advantages are gained with the I-bar configuration:

1. Food accumulation is minimized because tooth contours are not significantly altered.
2. The clasp terminus disengages from the tooth when an occlusal load is applied to the adjacent distal extension base.
3. Because the approach arm does not contact the abutment, lateral forces are minimized.

Disadvantages of the I-bar stem from its minimal tooth contact and small clasp terminus. The following are of consequence only if the design concept is not properly executed:

1. Less horizontal stability than other types of clasp assemblies
2. Less retention

When used in tooth-supported situations, I-bar retainers can be placed for convenience. In distal extension applications, retentive I-bars should be positioned with regard to the axis of rotation (Fig 8-16).

## *Indirect retainers*

Indirect retention is provided by rests placed on secondary abutments located as far as is practical from the axis of rotation and the extension base. Although some studies have cast doubt on the effectiveness of indirect retention to improve the retentive function of the clasp assembly, indirect retainers have been shown to be very effective in redistributing occlusal forces throughout the entire dentoalveolar structure.

One of the more convenient indirect retention sites is the mesial fossa of a mandibular first premolar because the tooth form accommodates the rest and because there is usually no opposing occlusion. Similarly, in the maxillary arch, the cingulum rest seat on a canine is a popular indirect retainer site.

## ◻ Physiologic Adjustment of Extension Base Removable Partial Dentures

To allow movement of the partial denture around the axis of rotation and to better distribute an occlusal

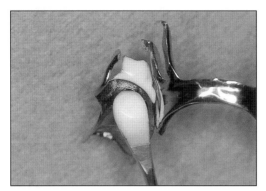

**Fig 8-17** Disclosing wax is applied to the framework prior to seating in the oral cavity to indicate areas that bind as a result of functional loading.

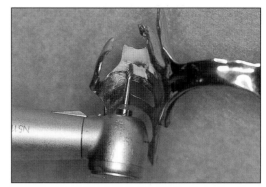

**Fig 8-18** After the framework is seated in the oral cavity and moderate pressure is applied to the distal extension base, the framework is removed and carefully inspected. Metal show-through indicates an area that requires adjustment.

load to the edentulous ridge, it is necessary to reduce binding between the framework and the abutments. This is accomplished by precise adjustment of the removable partial denture framework under physiologic loading conditions.

Physiologic adjustment is a chairside procedure and is accomplished only after the fit of the framework has been verified. A disclosing medium such as disclosing wax or gold rouge is placed on all parts of the framework that contact tooth surfaces (Fig 8-17). The framework is seated in the mouth, and moderately heavy finger pressure is placed on the latticework of extension bases. The framework is then removed and inspected for evidence of binding (Fig 8-18). Areas of binding are relieved, and the process is repeated until the framework moves freely under moderately heavy pressure. Initially, the guiding planes and proximal plates may provide so much frictional retention that rotational movement is not possible. Careful adjustment increases the rotational freedom of the framework. Throughout the adjustment process, care must be taken to ensure that the rotation is occurring through the action of the rests in the rest seats. If a non-rest contact is identified, the interference is eliminated by adjusting the intaglio of the framework. The surface of the framework is adjusted until the rests serve as the fulcrum points for rotation. The rests of a properly adjusted framework should rotate in their rest seats without lifting.

Altered cast impressions are made of all extension areas to provide maximum support from the residual ridges. In the passive state, the rests make full contact with the rest preparations, and extension bases are closely adapted to the soft tissues. In function, movement is dependent upon the resiliency of the supporting soft tissues.

## ◻ Design Variations

### Physical considerations and alternate components

In spite of the versatility of the I-bar system, there are situations that defy successful application of the basic design. In these situations, the practitioner must make design modifications without violating the basic principles of removable partial denture therapy. Commonly encountered difficulties include tipped abutments, unfavorable soft tissue contours, and poorly positioned frenum attachments.

Tipping of abutments may complicate retention and clasping in several ways. Buccolingual tipping frequently creates excessive undercuts or eliminates undercuts entirely. When tipping creates an excessive undercut, the solutions include *(1)* enameloplasty to reduce the undercut or *(2)* the placement of a cast restoration to provide improved abutment contours.

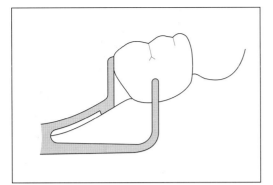

Fig 8-19 Tipped teeth may require endodontic therapy and cast restorations to provide appropriate guiding planes. If this is not possible, the practitioner should ensure that guiding planes are restricted to the enamel. Proximal plating should be kept away from the marginal tissues to reduce food impaction.

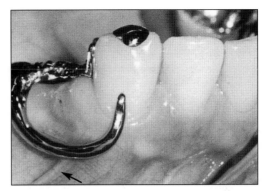

Fig 8-20 Frena (arrow) do not preclude the use of infrabulge retainers as long as the tissue to be crossed by the clasp arm is loosely attached and mobile.

When tipping results in an inadequate undercut, the solutions are (1) preparation of an undercut via enameloplasty or (2) use of an existing undercut on the opposite surface (ie, lingual vs buccal). Mesiodistal tipping affects the resistance and retention provided by opposing guiding planes.

Severe tipping is most effectively controlled with cast restorations. Endodontic therapy should be considered if adequate preparation of the guiding plane risks pulpal exposure. If the tooth in question is not critical to the function of the removable partial denture, it may be better to design the framework to avoid the tipped tooth, especially if adequate retention can be obtained from other retentive elements. If the tipped tooth is used as an abutment, the long guiding surface of the clasp assembly can be sacrificed as long as the retentive demands on the tooth are minimal. When this alternative is chosen, the framework should be kept well away from the tooth-tissue junction to prevent food impaction (Fig 8-19).

Frena, high muscle attachments, lack of attached gingiva, and tissue undercuts all interfere with placement of infrabulge retentive elements. However, the presence of frena does not categorically preclude the placement of I-bars. If attachments are loose enough to allow the vertical portion of the I-bar to be at least 5 mm long for flexure and hygiene, I-bar placement is possible (Fig 8-20). When a frenum attachment also contributes to gingival recession, the patient's inter-

ests may be best served with a frenectomy or graft procedure.

The attachment of the buccinator muscle adjacent to mandibular molars will occasionally obliterate the vestibule. The lack of attached gingiva further complicates I-bar placement. An alternative to placement of a buccal I-bar is the use of a lingual I-bar for retention and a buccal rest extension for reciprocation.

## Rest, proximal plate, and I-bar (RPI)

Krol, who was in agreement with Kratochvil's basic design but philosophically opposed to its extensive tooth preparation, developed a design modification requiring less tooth alteration. Krol's stated emphasis is stress control with minimal hard and soft tissue coverage. Krol cites inflammation in the presence of stress as the key to vertical bone loss around abutment teeth. His concept is intended to minimize plaque accumulations that may endanger the health of the teeth and their vesting structures.[3-5]

Krol's clasp assembly includes the three elements of Kratochvil's system: mesial rest, proximal plate, and I-bar (Fig 8-21). Each element, however, has undergone significant change to meet "minimal coverage" criteria. Rest preparations are less extensive in the RPI system. Rests extend only into the triangular fossa, even in molar preparations, and canine rest

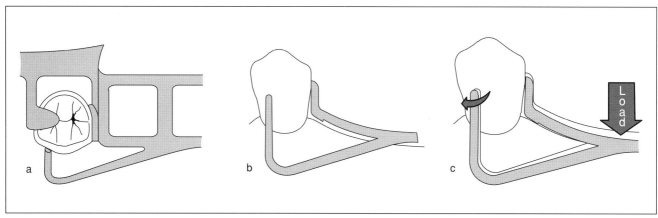

**Fig 8-21** The RPI system, with modification of each component, includes the basic I-bar elements proposed by Kratochvil. *(a)* The rest is positioned on the mesial aspect of a distal extension abutment, but is slightly smaller than that described by Kratochvil. *(b)* The retentive tip is positioned mesial to the mesiodistal height of contour. The proximal plate is diminished in all directions and does not terminate on the soft tissues. *(c)* When a functional load is applied to the extension base, the proximal plate disengages from the guiding plane, and the I-bar moves toward the mesial embrasure.

seats are often circular, concave depressions prepared in mesial marginal ridges.

The proximal plate makes the greatest departure from Kratochvil's design. The prepared guiding plane is 2 to 3 mm high occlusogingivally, and the proximal plate contacts only the apical 1 mm of the guiding plane. Relief is provided at the tooth-tissue junction to allow the proximal plate to disengage when loaded. The stated purpose for reducing the proximal plate is to improve gingival health by opening embrasure spaces as much as possible. An anticipated problem is impaction of food into the space above the proximal plate.

Modifications in I-bar configuration and placement are needed to compensate for reduced tooth contact by the proximal plate. The I-bar terminus is pod shaped to allow additional tooth contact, and the vertical portion of the clasp arm assumes a more mesial position to achieve efficient reciprocation from the smaller proximal plate. As with Kratochvil's design, occlusal force on the extension base disengages the retentive tip toward the mesial embrasure.

## ⌑ Conclusion

Despite the controversies that have surrounded clasp design and rest placement for extension base applications, it appears that the most valid indicators of distal extension removable partial denture success are *(1)* abutment teeth that are periodontally healthy and well maintained; *(2)* a partial denture framework that fits the teeth well; and *(3)* a denture base that fits the supporting soft tissues well, ideally derived from an altered cast technique.

The I-bar design meets all of the requirements of a partial denture clasp system: vertical support, horizontal stabilization, retention, reciprocation, and passivity. Successful use of the I-bar system requires careful analysis and planning of each component, skillful abutment preparation, and precise fitting of the framework.

# References

1. Kratochvil FJ. Influence of occlusal rest position and clasp design on movement of abutment teeth. J Prosthet Dent 1963;13:114–124.
2. Kratochvil FJ, Vig RG. Principles of Removable Partial Dentures. Los Angeles: UCLA School of Dentistry, 1979.
3. Krol AJ. Clasp design for extension-base removable partial dentures. J Prosthet Dent 1973;29:408–415.
4. Krol AJ. Removable Partial Denture Design: An Outline Syllabus, ed 2. San Francisco: University of the Pacific, 1976.
5. Krol AJ. RPI (rest, proximal plate, I-bar) clasp retainer and its modification. Dent Clin North Am 1973;17:631–649.

# Bibliography

Bates JF. Retention of partial dentures. Br Dent J 1980; 149(6):171–174.

Becker CM, Kaiser DA, Goldfogel MH. Evolution of removable partial denture design. J Prosthodont 1994;3(3):158–166.

Benson D, Spolsky VW. A clinical evaluation of removable partial dentures with I-bar retainers, Part I. J Prosthet Dent 1979; 41:246–254.

Berg E. Periodontal problems associated with use of distal extension removable partial dentures—A matter of construction? J Oral Rehabil 1985;12:369–379.

Berg T. I-bar: Myth and countermyth. Dent Clin North Am 1979;23:65–75.

Berg, T, Caputo AA. Anterior rests for maxillary partial dentures. J Prosthet Dent 1978;39:139–146.

Cecconi BT, Asgar K, Dootz E. Clasp assembly modifications and their effect on abutment tooth mobility. J Prosthet Dent 1972;27:160–167.

Clayton JA, Jaslow C. A measurement of clasp forces on teeth. J Prosthet Dent 1971;25:21–43.

Frank RP, Nicholls JI. An investigation of the effectiveness of indirect retainers. J Prosthet Dent 1977;38:494–506.

Gomes BC, Renner RP, Bauer PN. Periodontal considerations in removable partial dentures. J Am Dent Assoc 1980;101: 496–498.

Holmes JB. Influence of impression procedures and occlusal loading on partial denture movement. J Prosthet Dent 1965; 15:474–481.

Igarashi Y, Ogata A, Kuroiwa A, Wang CH. Stress distribution and abutment tooth mobility of distal-extension removable partial dentures with different retainers: An in vivo study. J Oral Rehabil 1999;26:111–116.

Kapur KK, Deupree R, Dent RJ, Hasse AL. A randomized clinical trial of two basic removable partial denture designs. Part I: Comparisons of five-year success rates and periodontal health. J Prosthet Dent 1994;72:268–282.

Kratochvil FJ, Caputo AA. Photoelastic analysis of pressure on teeth and bone supporting removable partial dentures. J Prosthet Dent 1974;32:52–62.

Leupold RJ. A comparative study of impression procedures for distal extension removable partial dentures. J Prosthet Dent 1966;16:708–720.

McDowell GC. Force transmission by indirect retainers during unilateral loading. J Prosthet Dent 1978;39:616–621.

Ogata K. Longitudinal study on torque around the sagittal axis in lower distal-extension removable partial dentures. J Oral Rehabil 1993;20:203–211.

Pezzoli M, Rossetto M. Evaluation of load transmission by removable partial dentures. Panminerva Med 1984;26(2):83–86.

Potter RB, Appleby RC, Adams CD. Removable partial denture design: A review and a challenge. J Prosthet Dent 1967;17: 63–68.

Tebrock OC, Rohen RM, Fenster RK, Pelleu GB Jr. The effect of various clasping systems on the mobility of abutment teeth for distal-extension removable partial dentures. J Prosthet Dent 1979;41:511–516.

Thompson WD, Kratochvil FJ. Evaluation of photoelastic stress patterns produced by various designs of bilateral distal-extension removable partial dentures. J Prosthet Dent 1977; 38:261–273.

# Mouth Preparation and Master Cast

The treatment plan for a patient who is to receive removable partial dentures can only be finalized after a thorough diagnostic assessment. To accomplish this, diagnostic casts must be accurately mounted using an appropriate articulator. Diagnostic casts must then be surveyed and proposed removable partial dentures must be designed. Upon completion of these processes, the practitioner should have a thorough understanding of required mouth preparation procedures. These procedures may include relief of pain and infection, preprosthetic surgeries, supporting restorative therapies, and a variety of adjunctive processes.

Mouth preparation appointments must be planned with the goal of conserving as much time as possible. The following discussion is arranged in the order that mouth preparation procedures are normally performed.

## ▢ Relief of Pain and Infection

Dental conditions that are causing discomfort should be addressed as soon as possible. Necessary endodontic and surgical procedures should be completed.

Carious lesions should be treated to decrease the likelihood that an acute episode of pain will occur during the course of treatment. Gingival tissues should be treated to minimize the probability that periodontal abscesses and other inflammatory responses will occur. Scaling, root planing, and prophylaxis should be performed, and a rigorous oral hygiene program should be established and carefully monitored.

Once the potential emergency-causing conditions have been addressed, the definitive treatment plan may be formulated.

## ▢ Completion of Required Surgical Procedures

As a general rule, conditions requiring surgical intervention are addressed early in the treatment process. Such conditions include teeth that have been deemed unrestorable, teeth that have insufficient periodontal support, and those that are unerupted or impacted. Surgery also may be required to eliminate tori or prominent exostoses that would complicate removable partial denture construction.

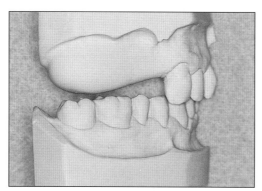

**Fig 9-1** Maxillary tuberosities often display downward migration. As a result, interarch space may be limited.

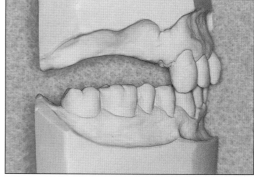

**Fig 9-2** Surgical reduction of the tuberosities may be needed to provide adequate space for a removable partial denture.

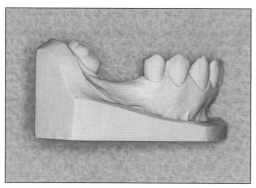

**Fig 9-3** The mandibular right second molar exhibits noticeable mesial tipping.

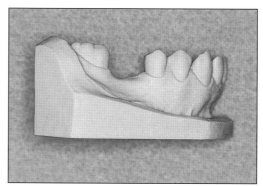

**Fig 9-4** The mandibular right second molar following orthodontic correction.

Preprosthetic procedures such as implant placement, ridge augmentation, and vestibular extension should be performed early in the treatment process to allow for adequate healing and to ensure that the desired results have been achieved. These procedures are valuable adjuncts in removable partial denture therapy. Consequently, these procedures must be meticulously planned and executed. The clinical and laboratory procedures for the aforementioned therapies are described in a number of excellent texts and will not be addressed here.

## ❑ Correction of Occlusal Plane Discrepancies

The occlusal plane in most partially edentulous mouths will be uneven. The severity of this unevenness will determine the treatment needed to correct the condition. Teeth that have been unopposed for a prolonged period tend to supraerupt. Unopposed maxillary teeth tend to move inferiorly, while unopposed mandibular teeth may move superiorly. If supraeruption is relatively minor, the occlusal plane may be corrected by carefully recontouring the surfaces of the teeth. If moderate supraeruption has occurred, correction of the occlusal plane may require the placement of cast restorations such as onlays or crowns. If supraeruption is extreme, extraction of the offending teeth may be the only logical solution.

In maxillary posterior regions, supraeruption also may be accompanied by a downward migration of the tuberosities (Fig 9-1). As a result, the interarch space may be extremely limited and may preclude the placement of an acceptable prosthesis. Surgical reduction of the tuberosities may be required to provide adequate restorative space (Fig 9-2).

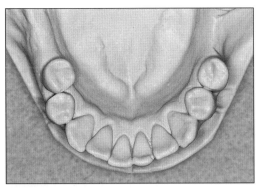

**Fig 9-5** The mandibular right second premolar is lingually positioned.

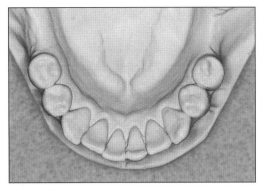

**Fig 9-6** The mandibular right second premolar following orthodontic therapy.

Tipped molars may present significant problems in removable partial denture therapy. The loss of premolars often allows adjacent molars to drift mesially. This mesial migration may be accompanied by tipping (Fig 9-3). The ideal solution is to upright such teeth orthodontically (Figs 9-4). Unfortunately, orthodontic correction is not always possible, nor is it always desired by the patient. In these situations, the occlusal plane may be reestablished in a number of ways. If migration and tipping are minor, the occlusal plane may be corrected via enameloplasty. If migration and tipping are more severe, onlays or crowns may be indicated for correction of the occlusal plane.

Severe discrepancies in the occlusal plane may require surgical intervention. A variety of maxillary and mandibular surgical procedures may be used in the correction of such discrepancies. As might be expected, these procedures are quite invasive and should be reserved for situations that cannot be addressed with more conservative therapies. Nevertheless, the practitioner should be aware of what can be accomplished for patients with severe occlusal plane discrepancies.

## ☐ Correction of Malalignment

Teeth that are out of alignment may create significant difficulties in removable partial denture service. Malaligned teeth compromise the contours and posi-tions of removable partial denture components. Because these teeth are often tipped facially or lingually, they also complicate clasping procedures.

While it is possible to alter the design of a removable partial denture to accommodate minor malalignments, it is recommended that malalignments be corrected. Orthodontic movement of malpositioned teeth should be the first option (Figs 9-5 and 9-6). Unfortunately, orthodontic therapy may not be possible for patients with few remaining teeth. In some instances, the number, distribution, and periodontal conditions of the remaining teeth may not provide sufficient anchorage for orthodontic treatment. Other patients may be unable or unwilling to undergo orthodontic therapy.

When orthodontic therapy is not an option, the practitioner must consider other forms of treatment. Minor malalignments may be corrected by recontouring the axial surfaces of the malposed teeth (Fig 9-7). Moderate malalignments may be treated by placing crowns (Fig 9-8). When this option is chosen, the practitioner must ensure that tooth preparation permits correction of the malalignment. Failure to provide adequate tooth reduction will result in insufficient room for restorative materials. This will result in improper crown contours or require revision of the preparation.

In some instances, a proposed crown preparation may encroach upon the pulpal tissues (Fig 9-9). When this occurs, the practitioner should opt for endodontic therapy prior to tooth preparation. A dowel and core

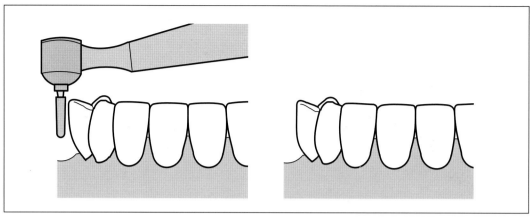

**Fig 9-7** Some dental malalignments may be corrected using enameloplasty procedures.

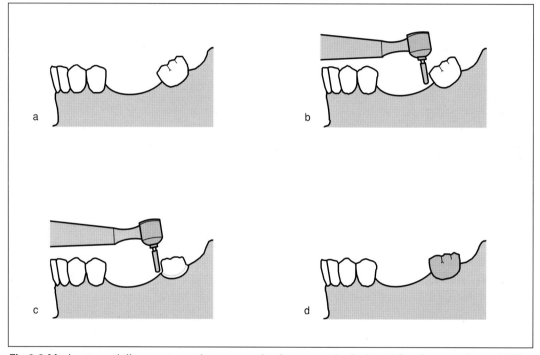

**Fig 9-8** Moderate malalignment may be corrected using properly designed fixed restorations. *(a)* The mandibular left second molar displays noticeable tipping. *(b)* Tooth preparation is intended to correct malalignment. (Notice the angulation of the bur.) *(c)* The finished preparation permits placement of a suitable crown. *(d)* The resultant crown displays the desired angulation and contours.

may be used to place the preparation in a more suitable position. Subsequently, a crown with desirable contours may be fabricated. When restoring a tooth in this manner, the practitioner should remember that the long axes of the crown and remaining root must not be significantly different, or undesirable forces will be placed on the root and associated periodontium.

Therefore, such restorations should not be used to treat severe malalignment.

When malalignment is so severe that it renders a tooth unusable, the practitioner should consider extraction of the malposed tooth. Nevertheless, all reasonable possibilities should be exhausted before extraction is chosen.

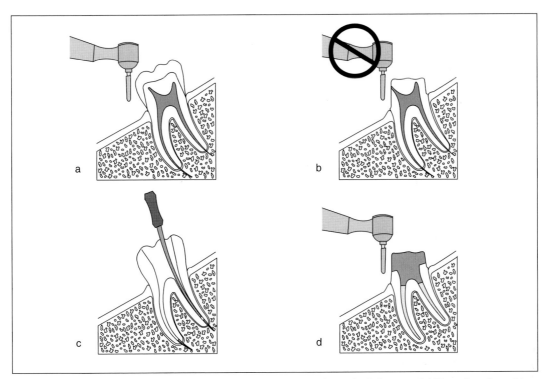

**Fig 9-9** In some instances, tooth preparation may threaten the pulpal tissues. *(a)* Tipped molar with a prominent mesial pulp horn. *(b)* The likelihood of mechanical exposure contraindicates tooth preparation. *(c)* The tooth is endodontically treated before preparation. *(d)* A core is placed and the preparation is completed. In turn, a properly contoured crown will be placed.

## ⬚ Provision of Support for Periodontally Weakened Teeth

In many partially edentulous mouths, some or all the remaining teeth may display decreased periodontal support. These teeth may require some form of splinting to provide adequate support and stabilization for a removable partial denture. Splinting may be accomplished using fixed restorations or designing the removable partial denture to join teeth as a functional unit.

Fixed splinting is accomplished by joining teeth with complete- or partial-coverage restorations. These restorations may be cast as a single unit or they may be cast individually and joined via soldering procedures. The objective is to gain improved resistance to applied forces.

It is important to recognize that fixed splinting of posterior teeth will provide additional resistance to anteroposterior forces, but not mediolateral forces

(Fig 9-10). To obtain improved resistance to mediolateral forces, fixed splinting must be extended to include one or more anterior teeth (Fig 9-11). Inclusion of the canine is particularly important since this tooth occupies a position at the "corner" of the arch. Teeth located distal to the canine are oriented anteroposteriorly, while the canine and the remaining anterior teeth assume a mediolateral orientation. Due to its position, the canine provides a buttressing effect that yields significant lateral resistance.

A major drawback of fixed splinting centers upon inability of the patient to adequately clean the splinted teeth. The inability of a patient to pass floss through interproximal spaces may lead to inadequate oral hygiene (Fig 9-12). This is particularly disconcerting when one considers that splinting is performed where periodontal compromise already exists. Cost and projected longevity of such restorations also must be considered when deciding whether to employ fixed splinting.

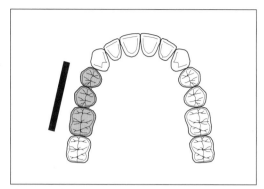

**Fig 9-10** Splinting of posterior teeth provides additional resistance to anteroposterior forces, but not mediolateral forces. This is due to the linear arrangement of posterior teeth *(bar)*.

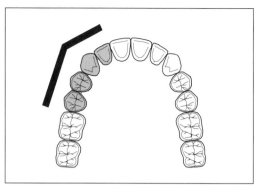

**Fig 9-11** To obtain improved resistance to mediolateral forces, splinting must include one or more anterior teeth. This places the restoration in an additional plane and provides an L-beam effect *(bar)*.

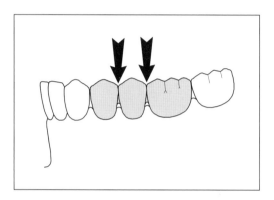

**Fig 9-12** Fixed splinting results in closure of the interproximal contacts *(arrows)*. Hence, oral hygiene may be complicated.

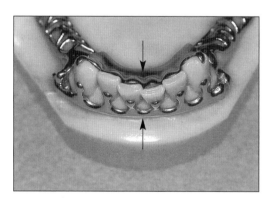

**Fig 9-13** Splinting *(arrows)* may be provided by removable partial dentures. The Swing-Lock removable partial denture is particularly useful in such applications.

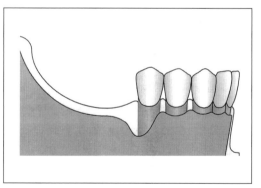

**Fig 9-14** A tooth that has lost more than 50% of its bony support is a poor candidate for fixed splinting. In such a situation, fixed splinting weakens the stronger tooth rather than strengthening the weaker tooth.

As previously noted, splinting also may be accomplished using properly designed removable partial dentures. This may be performed in a number of ways, but usually involves the use of lingual plating in conjunction with multiple facially positioned clasp arms. The encompassment provided by these components joins the teeth as a functional unit. This permits the even distribution of applied forces over an increased number of

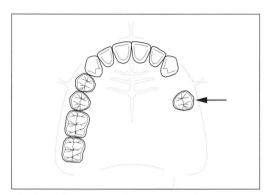

**Fig 9-15** A lone-standing tooth adjacent to an extension base area is termed a *pier abutment (arrow)*. Experience indicates that placing a clasp on such a tooth leads to periodontal destruction and abutment loss. Consequently, pier abutments may receive rests, but generally are not clasped.

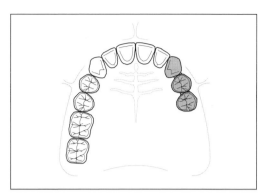

**Fig 9-16** When a lone-standing abutment is present (see Fig 9-15), the practitioner should determine whether the patient would benefit from the placement of a fixed partial denture.

teeth and may improve the longevity of the remaining teeth. Specialized prostheses such as Swing-Lock removable partial dentures (Fig 9-13) are commonly used in such applications. A description of Swing-Lock removable partial dentures is included in chapter 19.

When considering fixed or removable splinting, the practitioner must carefully assess the existing oral conditions. For purposes of discussion, consider a tooth that has lost more than 50% of its bony support and occupies the most posterior position in a Kennedy Class I or Class II arch (Fig 9-14). Such a tooth is a poor candidate for fixed splinting because of its position and its questionable periodontal support. Even if the adjacent tooth displays adequate support, fixed splinting is contraindicated. Fixed splinting in such a situation generally weakens the stronger tooth rather than strengthening the weaker tooth. Addition of a removable partial denture complicates the scenario and often leads to the accelerated loss of both teeth. Such an outcome is unacceptable and should be avoided.

A second option involves retaining both teeth and fabricating a removable partial denture with a direct retainer on the periodontally compromised tooth. This generally leads to accelerated failure of the periodontally compromised tooth and renders the removable partial denture unusable.

A third option involves extraction of the periodontally compromised tooth. The adjacent tooth may then be used as a removable partial denture abutment. Experience indicates that this option usually is the most suitable. Nevertheless, each case must be evaluated on its own merits and no sweeping generalizations regarding ideal treatment should be made.

## Reestablishment of Arch Continuity

There are times when a tooth stands alone at the distal aspect of a Kennedy Class I or Class II partially edentulous arch (Fig 9-15). This presents an interesting challenge in removable partial denture therapy. Clinical experience indicates that placing a direct retainer on such a tooth (often termed a *pier abutment*) may lead to the rapid destruction of the supporting periodontium and loss of the tooth. For this reason, lone-standing abutments may receive rests, but generally are not clasped.

When a lone-standing abutment is present, the practitioner should carefully examine the remainder of the arch to determine whether the patient would benefit from placement of a fixed partial denture (Fig 9-16). An appropriately constructed fixed partial denture may be used to reestablish continuity of the den-

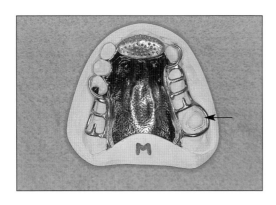

**Fig 9-17** Despite moderate bone loss, strategically positioned teeth may serve as overdenture abutments *(arrow)*. This is particularly helpful in extension base applications.

tal arch and greatly improve the prognosis for removable partial denture therapy.

## ◻ Additional Considerations

Teeth that have lost a moderate amount of supporting bone but display minimal mobility and are strategically positioned in the arch may be retained to provide support for removable partial dentures (Fig 9-17). These teeth are intended to resist movement of removable partial dentures toward tissues during function. If teeth that are located at the posterior end of a distal extension base, the prosthesis will function as a Class III removable partial denture rather than a Class I or Class II prosthesis. This change improves the function and patient acceptance of the removable partial denture.

## ◻ Reshaping Teeth

Tooth surfaces often need to be recontoured to accomplish specific purposes. The recontouring process may be accomplished in the enamel, on the surface of an existing restoration, or by placing a new restoration.

### Enameloplasty

Conservatism must be the rule when recontouring enamel surfaces. The practitioner must ensure that recontouring accomplishes the desired objectives, but never at the expense of overcutting the tooth. If the danger of overcutting is apparent, recontouring

should first be accomplished on a diagnostic cast. In most instances, this procedure will reveal whether reshaping of enamel surfaces is possible. If it appears that recontouring will result in substantial tooth reduction, the practitioner should consider the placement of properly contoured crowns.

If the desired recontouring can be accomplished in enamel, this procedure should be completed intraorally. In turn, the prepared enamel surfaces should be highly polished. To accomplish this, a carborundum-impregnated rubber wheel or point should be placed in a low-speed handpiece. Light, intermittent pressure and moderate speed should be used during polishing procedures. Dangerously high heat can be generated if care is not exercised.

### Developing guiding planes

Guiding planes are surfaces on proximal or lingual surfaces of teeth that are parallel to each other and, more importantly, to the path of insertion and removal of a removable partial denture. The characteristics of guiding planes are described in chapter 4. A description of intraoral preparation procedures is included in the following sections.

It is essential that the diagnostic cast with the proposed removable partial denture design be available during mouth preparation procedures. The diagnostic cast should be properly positioned on the surveying table and should be oriented at the tilt used during survey and design procedures. During the mouth preparation process, the surveying table and cast should be readily accessible to the practitioner. This permits the practitioner to visualize the desired relationship between a given dental bur and the tooth to

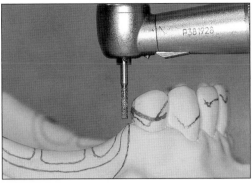

**Fig 9-18** The design cast should be properly oriented on the surveying table during mouth preparation procedures. This permits the practitioner to visualize the desired relationship between a dental bur and the teeth to be recontoured.

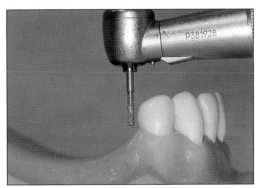

**Fig 9-19** The relationship between the bur and the dental cast (see Fig 9-18) may then be duplicated in the patient's mouth.

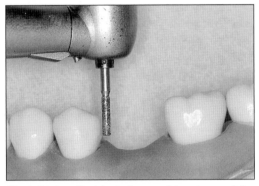

**Fig 9-20** A cylindrical diamond bur is used for the preparation of guiding planes.

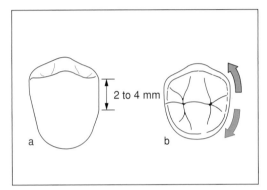

**Fig 9-21** *(a)* A guiding plane adjacent to a tooth-supported segment should be 2 to 4 mm in height. *(b)* The prepared surface should not resemble a straight "slice," but should follow the natural curvature of the tooth surface *(arrows)* when viewed from an occlusal/incisal perspective.

be recontoured (Fig 9-18). The same relationship can then be duplicated in the patient's mouth (Fig 9-19). This process allows the practitioner to create guiding planes and other contours that are in harmony with the planned path of insertion.

**Abutment teeth adjacent to tooth-supported segments** A cylindrical diamond or carbide bur is generally used for the preparation of guiding planes (Fig 9-20). The chosen bur is placed in a high-speed handpiece. A light, sweeping stroke from the facial line

angle to the lingual line angle is then used to create a gently curving plane. This surface should be 2 to 4 mm in occlusogingival height, but should not resemble a straight slice when viewed from the occlusal or incisal surface. Instead, it should follow the natural curvature of the tooth surface (Fig 9-21).

At this stage, prepared surfaces are polished with a carborundum-impregnated rubber point or wheel in a low-speed handpiece (Fig 9-22). Light, intermittent pressure is recommended to avoid undue generation of heat.

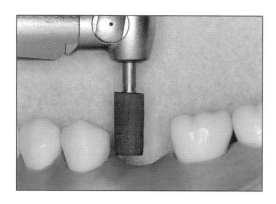

**Fig 9-22** Prepared surfaces are polished with a carborundum-impregnated rubber point or wheel in a low-speed handpiece.

**Abutment teeth adjacent to distal extension edentulous spaces** The preparation of guiding planes adjacent to distal extension spaces is accomplished using the same armamentarium described in the previous section. A cylindrical diamond or carbide bur is used in conjunction with a high-speed handpiece to prepare surfaces that are parallel to the proposed path of insertion.

A guiding plane prepared adjacent to a distal extension space should be slightly shorter than a guiding plane prepared adjacent to a tooth-supported segment. Typically, a guiding plane adjacent to a distal extension space is 1.5 to 2.0 mm in height (Fig 9-23). The reduced height results in decreased contact with the associated minor connector (ie, proximal plate) and permits greater freedom of movement for the associated removable partial denture (Fig 9-24). As a result, potentially destructive torquing forces are minimized.

**Lingual surfaces of abutment teeth** There are a number of reasons for placing guiding planes on the lingual surfaces of abutments. One of the most important reasons is to enhance reciprocation (Fig 9-25). As a clasp assembly travels to or from its fully seated position, the retentive arm must pass over the height of contour. This places lateral forces on the abutment. Unless effective reciprocation is provided, these forces will lead to destruction of the supporting periodontal tissues. To prevent this destruction, the practitioner must ensure that the reciprocal element is in contact with the tooth as lateral forces are generated. This may be accomplished by using a vertical reciprocal element such as a lingual plate or by using a lingual guid-

ing plane in conjunction with a reciprocal clasp arm. When a clasp arm is the reciprocal element of choice, a lingual guiding plane should be prepared to achieve effective reciprocation.

A second reason for preparing lingual guiding planes is to minimize the number of pathways by which the prosthesis may enter and exit its fully seated position. Therefore, the practitioner may enhance retention by preparing guiding planes on the lingual surfaces of the remaining teeth.

A third reason for preparing guiding planes on the lingual surfaces of the remaining teeth is to provide maximum resistance to lateral forces. The more teeth that are used to stabilize the removable partial denture, the less stress will be transmitted to any individual tooth.

As might be expected, tooth preparation is accomplished in the same manner described for guiding planes adjacent to tooth-supported edentulous areas. A cylindrical diamond or carbide bur may be used for this purpose.

A lingual guiding plane should be 2 to 4 mm in occlusogingival height and should be located in the middle third of the clinical crown as viewed from the mesial or distal surfaces (Fig 9-26). The practitioner should take special care to avoid changing the contour of the gingival third of the tooth because a significant alteration of contour may produce improper shunting of food and result in damage to the marginal gingivae.

**Anterior abutment teeth** Guiding planes may be prepared on anterior teeth to enhance stabilization of the prosthesis, to decrease undesirable space between the

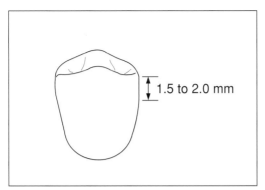

**Fig 9-23** A guiding plane adjacent to an extension base segment should be 1.5 to 2.0 mm in height.

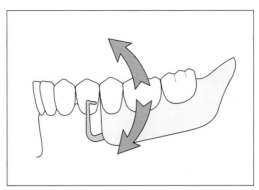

**Fig 9-24** Reduced height results in decreased contact with the minor connector and permits greater freedom of movement *(arrows)* for the removable partial denture. Hence, potentially damaging forces are minimized.

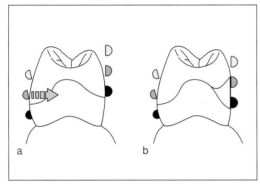

**Fig 9-25** The timing and effectiveness of reciprocation is very important in removable partial denture service. A reciprocating element must brace the abutment as the retentive element passes to and from its fully seated position. *(a)* If reciprocation is ineffective, potentially destructive lateral forces *(arrow)* will be transferred to the abutment. *(b)* A properly prepared guiding plane permits sustained contact between the reciprocal element and the abutment and prevents the application of unopposed lateral forces.

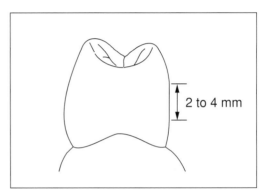

**Fig 9-26** A properly prepared lingual guiding plane should be 2 to 4 mm in occlusogingival height and should be located in the middle third of the clinical crown.

prosthesis and an abutment tooth, and to increase retention through frictional resistance.

Another important purpose of such guiding planes is to reestablish the normal width of an edentulous space. If one or more anterior teeth are lost, adjacent teeth tend to drift or tip into these spaces. Both actions result in reduced space and make esthetic replacement of the missing teeth much more difficult. Tipping is relatively common and often results in a large undercut apical to the height of contour (Fig 9-27). If the tooth is not recontoured, this undercut will appear as an unsightly space between the tipped tooth and the removable partial denture. Such a space detracts from the esthetic value of the removable partial denture and acts as a food trap. Recontouring should be performed to minimize the effects of tipping and to improve the esthetic and functional results of the removable partial denture service (Fig 9-28) This recontouring should be performed with the proposed path of insertion in mind, and the resultant guiding planes should be parallel to the planned path of insertion.

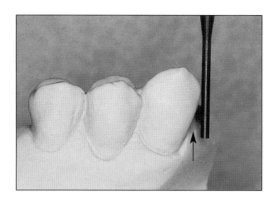

**Fig 9-27** Tipping of a maxillary canine results in a large undercut *(arrow)* apical to the height of contour.

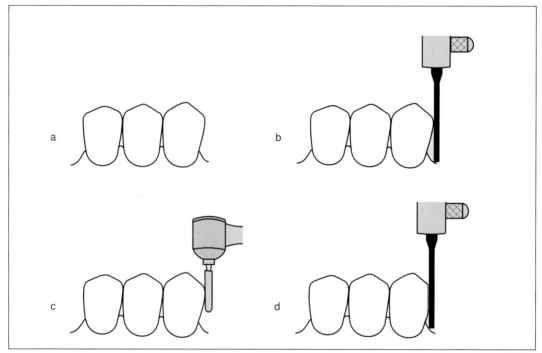

**Fig 9-28** *(a)* Maxillary canine that displays mesial tipping. *(b)* When surveyed at the proposed path of insertion and removal, a large mesial undercut is evident. *(c)* The tooth is recontoured to minimize the mesial undercut. *(d)* The resultant contours are favorable for removable partial denture construction.

A cylindrical diamond or carbide bur may be used to create the desired guiding planes. If the required changes cannot be made without penetrating into the dentin, an appropriate restoration should be planned.

### Changing height of contour

The height of contour is often changed to provide more favorable positions for clasp arms or lingual plating. Ideally a retentive clasp arm should be located no

farther occlusally (or incisally) than the junction of the gingival and middle thirds of the crown. This not only improves the esthetic qualities of the clasp, but also places the clasp nearer the tooth's center of rotation. As a result, both the appearance and mechanical characteristics of the prosthesis are improved.

Enameloplasty is necessary when teeth have drifted or tipped. Maxillary posterior teeth often tip in a facial direction, while mandibular teeth generally tip in a lin-

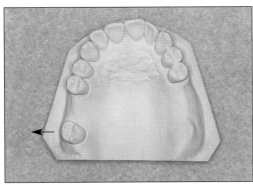

**Fig 9-29** Maxillary teeth often tip in a facial direction *(arrow)*.

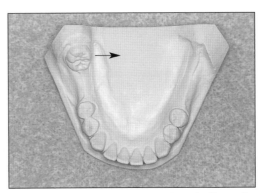

**Fig 9-30** Mandibular teeth tend to tip lingually *(arrow)*.

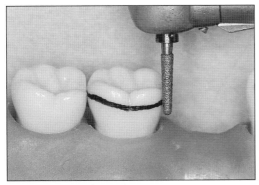

**Fig 9-31** The height of contour before alteration using a tapered diamond bur in a high-speed handpiece.

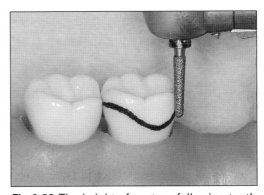

**Fig 9-32** The height of contour following tooth modification. (Note the change in survey line.)

**Fig 9-33** Prepared surfaces are smoothed using a carborundum-impregnated rubber point or wheel.

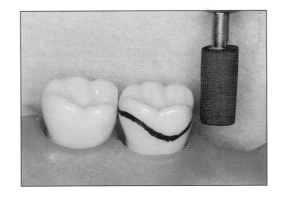

gual direction (Figs 9-29 and 9-30). These movements produce distinct changes in the heights of contour. In these situations, enameloplasty is performed to place partial denture components in more desirable positions.

The amount of correction that can be accomplished by enameloplasty is limited by the thickness of the enamel. Care must be taken not to penetrate the enamel and expose the underlying dentin. In the event that dentin is exposed, a restoration must be placed to protect the tooth.

The height of contour is best lowered by using a tapered diamond bur in a high-speed handpiece (Figs 9-31 and 9-32). Tooth surfaces should be smoothed using a carborundum-impregnated point or wheel in a low-speed handpiece (Fig 9-33).

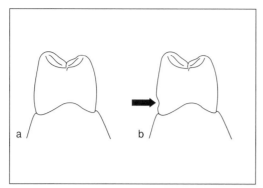

**Fig 9-34** *(a)* The facial and lingual surfaces of the tooth are relatively vertical. *(b)* As a result, a gentle depression *(arrow)* may be created. In this instance, the depression has been created on the facial surface.

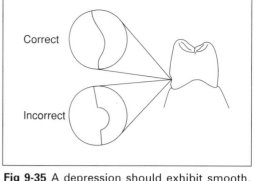

**Fig 9-35** A depression should exhibit smooth, flowing contours. Sharply defined dimples and pits should be avoided since retentive clasps cannot flex into and out of these indentations.

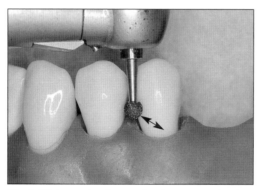

**Fig 9-36** A gentle depression is prepared using a round diamond bur in a high-speed handpiece. The bur is moved in an anteroposterior direction *(arrow)*.

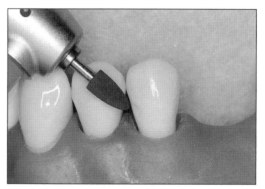

**Fig 9-37** The preparation is smoothed using a carborundum-impregnated rubber point in a low-speed handpiece. Care must be taken not to obliterate the depression.

## Enhancing retentive undercuts

Occasionally, a proposed abutment tooth has an insufficient retentive undercut. Under certain conditions, tooth contours may be modified to enhance an existing undercut or create a conservative undercut. While this technique may be used in some instances, it does not have universal applications. Under no circumstances should this technique take the place of well-executed survey and design procedures.

For this technique to be successful, the facial and lingual surfaces of the tooth must be nearly vertical. Under these circumstances, a gentle depression may be created on one of these surfaces (Fig 9-34). This depression should exhibit smooth, flowing contours. Gentle variations in contour permit retentive clasps to enter and exit a depression with relative ease. Sharply defined dimples and pits should be avoided since re-

tentive clasps cannot flex into and out of these indentations (Fig 9-35).

A suitable depression may be prepared using a round or football-shaped diamond bur in a high-speed handpiece. The bur should be moved in an anteroposterior direction near the line angle of the tooth (Fig 9-36). The resultant depression should be parallel to the gingival margin and as close to the margin as is practical. The depression should be approximately 4 mm in mesiodistal length and 3 mm in occlusogingival height. More importantly, it should establish an undercut of 0.010 inches relative to the proposed path of insertion.

The preparation should be polished with a carborundum-impregnated rubber point (Fig 9-37). Extreme care must be exercised during the polishing procedure since poor polishing technique may obliterate the depression.

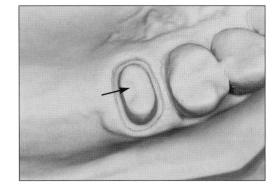

**Fig 9-38** Preparations must follow established guidelines for taper and reduction. Notice that a rest seat has been included in the preparation *(arrow)*.

## Complete- and partial-coverage restorations

Restorations may be required for teeth displaying caries lesions, defective restorations, fracture, or endodontic therapy. If the remaining teeth do not possess usable contours and the enamel surfaces cannot be modified to produce these contours, complete- or partial-coverage restorations also may be required. These restorations must be carefully planned and constructed and must include the appropriate undercuts, guiding planes, and rest seats. To accomplish these objectives, accurate diagnostic casts must be made and carefully analyzed. In turn, a definitive removable partial denture design must be drawn. At this stage, mouth preparations must be carefully planned and executed.

From a clinical perspective, it is essential that recontouring procedures be completed before crown and onlay preparations are begun. Recontouring must include the preparation of guiding planes and rest seats. Guiding planes define the path of insertion and removal for a removable partial denture. By establishing guiding planes on teeth that will not receive fixed restorations, the practitioner clearly defines the path of insertion and removal for the proposed removable partial denture. At this stage, the practitioner may prepare teeth that are to receive complete- or partial-coverage restorations. The master cast should accurately represent those contours established during the various preparation procedures. Subsequently, the wax patterns for fixed restorations should be appropriately contoured. Guiding surfaces should be created on the wax patterns and should be parallel to the guiding planes on the remaining teeth. Restorations may then be completed, adjusted, and inserted. This technique results in improved parallelism between the guiding planes and provides an improved restorative result. Therefore, the placement of guiding planes should always precede the preparation of teeth that are to receive fixed restorations.

All preparations should follow established guidelines for taper and reduction (Fig 9-38). The practitioner must pay particular attention when preparing malpositioned teeth for fixed restorations. A tooth with a noticeable lingual inclination must be prepared so that a greater amount of tooth structure is removed from the lingual surface than from the facial surface. This will permit the development of suitable contours in the wax pattern and the associated restoration. Similar precautions must be taken for teeth that are tipped facially, mesially, or distally. The ultimate aim in preparing and restoring a malpositioned tooth is to produce a restoration with the best possible alignment.

### Shaping the wax pattern

To create a wax pattern with the desired contours, an accurate cast is essential. This cast must include a properly prepared die that is correctly related to the remainder of the dental arch (Fig 9-39). The cast must be firmly attached to a surveying table and positioned at the prescribed tilt (see chapter 7). When this has been accomplished, the cast may be analyzed using a dental surveyor.

To accurately assess the contours of the wax pattern, the pattern is dusted with a thin layer of powdered wax or zinc stearate (Fig 9-40). The height of contour is then marked using the analyzing rod in the vertical arm

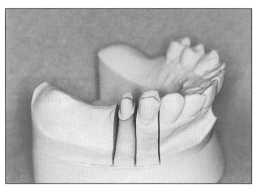

Fig 9-39 An accurate, properly trimmed cast is essential.

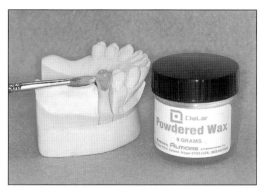

Fig 9-40 The wax pattern is dusted with a thin layer of powdered wax.

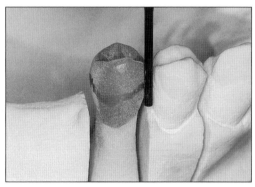

Fig 9-41 The cast is properly oriented on a surveying table. The height of contour is marked using an analyzing rod in the vertical arm of a dental surveyor.

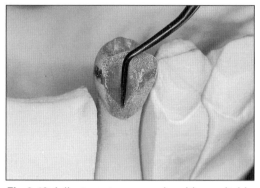

Fig 9-42 Adjustments are made with a suitable carving instrument.

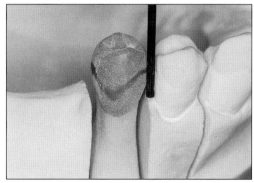

Fig 9-43 Powdered wax or zinc stearate is reapplied and contours are reassessed until they are ideal.

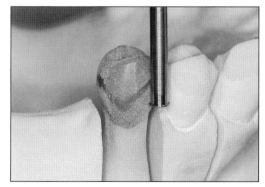

Fig 9-44 The position of the undercut is verified. Required changes are made.

of the surveyor (Fig 9-41). Following evaluation of contours, the pattern is reshaped using wax carving instruments (Fig 9-42). Contours created during this process should be as ideal as possible (Fig 9-43).

The desired undercut is developed and its depth is verified using the appropriate undercut gauge. A 0.010-inch undercut is recommended for the majority of removable partial denture alloys. The undercut should be

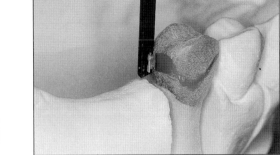

**Fig 9-45** Guiding planes are created and refined using a wax knife in the vertical arm of a dental surveyor.

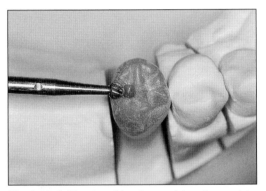

**Fig 9-46** A No. 4 or No. 6 round bur is used to begin preparation of the rest seat. For convenience and control, the bur is rotated in the operator's fingers.

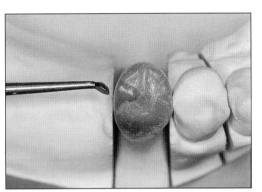

**Fig 9-47** A discoid instrument is used to finalize rest seat contours.

located at the mesial line angle or the distal line angle in most instances (Fig 9-44). When using an I-bar clasping system, the undercut may be positioned at the midfacial (or, rarely, at the midlingual) line angle.

At this stage, the required guiding planes are prepared on the wax pattern. These surfaces generally are created and refined using a wax knife in the vertical arm of the surveyor (Fig 9-45). Extreme care must be taken to ensure that these surfaces are parallel to the guiding surfaces previously prepared on the remaining natural teeth.

When the practitioner is satisfied with the axial contours of the wax pattern, required rest seats are placed. This is most easily accomplished using a small, round bur in conjunction with a discoid carver (Figs 9-46 and 9-47). Each rest seat should display the appropriate geometry, depth, and contour.

As a final measure, the wax pattern is reexamined. The occlusion is evaluated to ensure its suitability. Rest seats are carefully inspected for proper form and depth.

Axial contours are assessed and refined as necessary. At this stage, the wax pattern is gently cleaned with damp cotton. All contours are inspected once again, and the pattern is prepared for the casting process.

### Refining the cast restoration

Restorations are cast using standard techniques. After the casting has been made, it is carefully recovered and finished. Contours that were established in the wax pattern should be preserved.

To ensure that the proper anatomy has not been lost, the casting is fitted to the master die and properly positioned on the accompanying cast. The cast is returned to the surveying table and positioned at the prescribed tilt. The height of contour and guiding planes are examined using the analyzing rod in the vertical arm of the surveyor (Fig 9-48). The position and depth of the undercut are verified using an appropriate undercut gauge (Fig 9-49). If changes in contour are noted, these changes must be corrected using

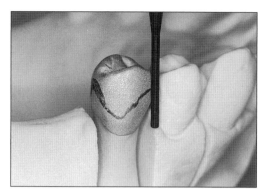

**Fig 9-48** Crown contours are examined using an analyzing rod in the vertical arm of a dental surveyor.

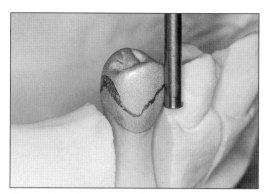

**Fig 9-49** The location of the undercut is verified using an appropriate undercut gauge.

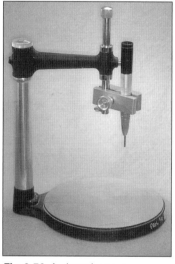

**Fig 9-50** A dental surveyor may be used as a milling device. A handpiece holder is attached to the vertical arm of the surveyor. A straight handpiece is then secured parallel to the vertical arm of the surveyor in the handpiece holder.

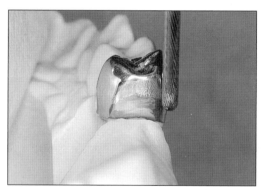

**Fig 9-51** A cylindrical bur or stone is placed in the handpiece for machining purposes. At this stage, guiding planes are refined.

carefully controlled finishing and polishing techniques. If changes are so great that the appropriate contours cannot be reestablished, the waxing and casting procedures must be reaccomplished.

If the restoration displays the appropriate contours, it may be finished and polished. Techniques for finishing and polishing cast restorations are available in a variety of fixed prosthodontics textbooks and will not be presented here.

Upon completion of polishing procedures, guiding planes are refined once again. This may be accomplished using a variety of milling devices, which may be relatively simple or quite complex. The most common embodiment is a simple modification of the dental surveyor. In this configuration, a handpiece holder is attached to the vertical arm of the surveyor. A straight handpiece is then secured in the handpiece holder (Fig 9-50). The handpiece holder positions the handpiece parallel to the vertical arm of the surveyor. A cylindrical bur or stone is then placed in the handpiece for machining purposes (Fig 9-51). The surveying table is moved to bring the guiding plane of the restoration in contact with the rotating bur or stone. The milling process should provide a smooth, even surface that is

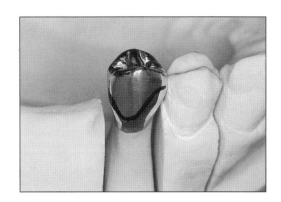

**Fig 9-52** The completed restoration is shown. The survey line has been added to permit improved visualization.

parallel to the established path of insertion (Fig 9-52). No additional finishing and polishing is indicated at this point. Additional finishing and polishing often disrupts established guiding planes.

## Metal-ceramic and all-ceramic crowns

Metal-ceramic and all-ceramic restorations have gained widespread acceptance in dentistry. These restorations are commonly used to provide improved esthetic results in anterior and posterior regions of the oral cavity. Nevertheless, metal-ceramic and all-ceramic restorations exhibit certain physical properties that may contraindicate their use in removable partial denture applications.

As a rule, ceramic materials are relatively strong in compression, but weak in tension (Fig 9-53). Forces that cause "wedging" or "elongation" of a ceramic surface often lead to fracture. In dental applications, such fracture may render a restoration unusable. If the fractured restoration serves as an abutment for a removable partial denture, the removable partial denture also may be unusable. Hence, the practitioner must carefully consider all characteristics of fixed restorations to be used in conjunction with removable partial dentures.

Oftentimes, fixed restorations provide supporting surfaces for removable partial dentures. As might be expected, these supporting surfaces will always exhibit one or more rest seats. Rest seats on ceramic surfaces warrant particular attention since they may be subjected to undesirable tensile forces. Consider the interaction between a ceramic rest seat and the associated metal rest. When viewed in cross section, the rest seat appears as a shallow cup with gently sloping walls. If

the associated rest does not fit well, it may bind against the walls of the rest seat. This will result in a wedging effect and create tensile forces that are likely to produce failure of the restoration (Fig 9-54). As a result, the authors do not believe that all-ceramic restorations should be used to support removable partial dentures.

Unlike all-ceramic restorations, metal-ceramic restorations allow the practitioner to place potentially damaging tensile forces on metal surfaces. These surfaces can withstand tensile stresses easily and enhance the survivability of such restorations. Therefore, it is recommended that rest seats for metal-ceramic restorations be constructed entirely in metal. The metal borders should extend at least 1 mm beyond the borders of the proposed rest (in all directions) (Fig 9-55). Surfaces that are to exhibit guiding planes also should be fabricated in metal. These features should be established during waxing procedures and may be refined after the casting process.

After the metal has been adequately shaped, the ceramic is added. This requires precise placement and contouring of the surface. Therefore, the designed diagnostic cast must be available to guide the laboratory technician.

Following addition of the ceramic, crown contours are analyzed using the dental surveyor (Fig 9-56). The ceramic surface is adjusted to provide the desired height of contour, as well as the prescribed position and depth of the retentive undercut. At this stage, the restoration is thoroughly cleaned and then glazed. Crown contours are evaluated and modified as necessary. When all modifications have been completed, metal surfaces are finished and polished (Fig 9-57).

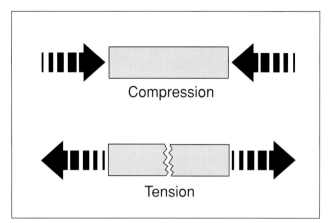

**Fig 9-53** Dental ceramics are strong in compression, but weak in tension.

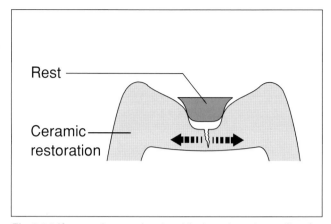

**Fig 9-54** If a rest is permitted to bind against the walls of a rest seat, wedging forces will result. The accompanying tensile forces may result in failure of a ceramic restoration.

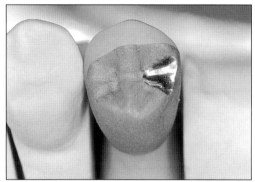

**Fig 9-55** If possible, a rest seat should be constructed entirely in metal. To minimize the likelihood of fracture, metal borders should extend at least 1 mm beyond the borders of a proposed rest. For photographic purposes, the rest seat has been finished using a carbide bur. The remainder of the occlusal surfaces have been abraded to provide a textured finish.

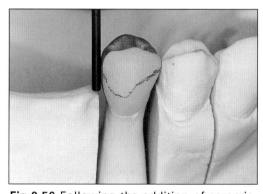

**Fig 9-56** Following the addition of ceramic, crown contours are evaluated using a dental surveyor. A wax pencil is used to mark the height of contour. Graphite is difficult to remove from the ceramic surface and should not be used.

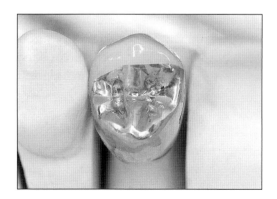

**Fig 9-57** The occlusal surface of the completed restoration is shown. Note the gently rolling contours of the rest seat.

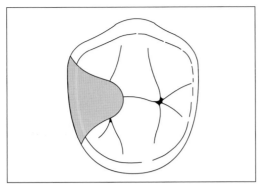

**Fig 9-58** An occlusal rest seat is basically triangular, with the base of the triangle located at the marginal ridge and the apex pointing toward the center of the tooth. All features of the rest seat are gently rounded.

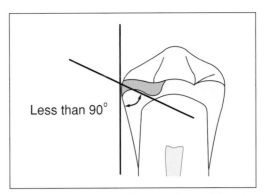

Less than 90°

**Fig 9-59** The enclosed angle formed by the floor of the rest seat and the proximal surface of the tooth must be less than 90 degrees.

## Rest Seat Preparations for Posterior Teeth

The purposes and functions of rests are described in chapter 3. Basically, the function of a rest is to direct the forces of mastication parallel to the long axis of the associated abutment. A rest also prevents the gingival displacement of a removable partial denture and maintains the intended relationship between a clasp assembly and the associated tooth. In certain applications, a rest may be used as an indirect retainer. In addition, a rest may be used to close a small space between teeth, thereby restoring continuity of the arch and preventing food impaction. Finally, a rest may be used to establish a more acceptable occlusal plane and to help prevent the extrusion of one or more teeth.

To fulfill the requirements described in the preceding paragraph, each rest must be positioned in a properly prepared rest seat. These rest seats must be prepared before final impressions and master casts are made. If rest seats are not adequately prepared, the forces transmitted from the prosthesis to the abutments may not be directed within the long axes of these teeth. This may result in irreparable damage to the abutments.

The remainder of this discussion is centered upon the preparation of rest seats in removable partial denture therapy.

### Occlusal rest seats in enamel

The outline form of an occlusal rest seat is basically triangular, with the base of the triangle at the marginal ridge and the apex pointing toward the center of the tooth. The apex of the triangle should be rounded, as should all external margins of the preparation (Fig 9-58).

The floor of the occlusal rest seat must be inclined toward the center of the tooth and should display gently rounded contours. The enclosed angle formed by the floor of the rest seat and the proximal surface of the tooth must be less than 90 degrees (Fig 9-59).

An occlusal rest should be at least 1 mm thick at its thinnest point. Therefore, the practitioner must ensure that sufficient tooth structure is removed during rest seat preparation. Failure to achieve sufficient reduction may make a rest more susceptible to fracture.

An occlusal rest seat may be prepared using a variety of rotary instruments. Many practitioners use round diamond burs, while others prefer diamond burs with rounded ends and tapering sides (Fig 9-60). While round diamond burs may be used successfully, care must be taken to ensure that mechanical undercuts are not created at the peripheries of the preparation (Fig 9-61). Burs with rounded ends and tapering sides are less likely to produce such undercuts and therefore provide distinct advantages (Fig 9-62).

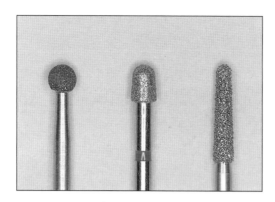

Fig 9-60 A variety of burs may be used in the preparation of rest seats. These include round burs *(left)* and tapered cylinders *(middle and right)*.

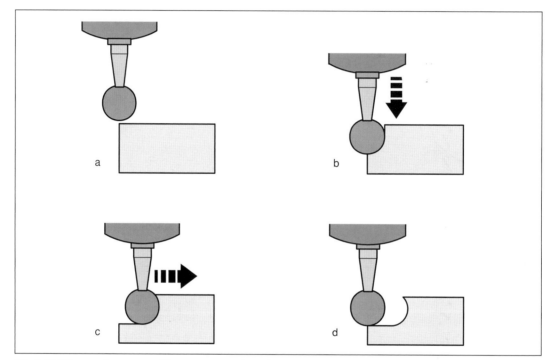

Fig 9-61 When using a round bur, care must be taken to ensure that mechanical undercuts are not created. *(a)* Round bur positioned above enamel surface. *(b)* Round bur moved vertically into enamel. *(c)* Bur moved laterally. *(d)* Upon removal of the bur, a distinct overhang is present.

In a clinical setting, the chosen bur is placed in a high-speed handpiece and used to establish the outline of the rest seat preparation. The same bur is then used to create the appropriate depth of the preparation (Fig 9-63). The borders of the preparation are carefully inspected to ensure that no undercuts exist.

At this stage, the preparation is examined to ensure that the floor of the rest seat is properly inclined and that the preparation displays adequate depth.

An effective method for evaluating the anatomy and depth of the preparation involves the use of red boxing wax (Figs 9-64 to 9-67). A small piece of boxing wax is formed into a disk and firmly pressed against the occlusal surface of the prepared tooth. Subsequently, the patient is instructed to close firmly and to maintain closure for 5 seconds. At this stage of the procedure, the patient is directed to open and the wax is gently removed. The surface of the wax is in-

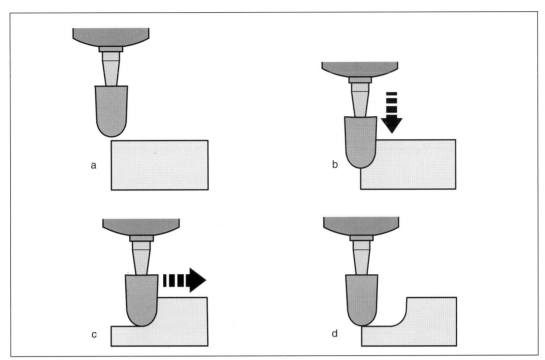

**Fig 9-62** A tapered cylinder may help eliminate mechanical undercuts. *(a)* Tapered bur positioned above enamel surface. *(b)* Tapered bur moved vertically into the enamel. *(c)* Bur moved laterally. *(d)* Upon removal of bur, no overhang is present.

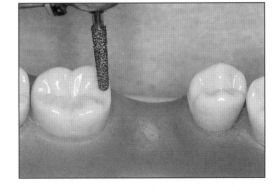

**Fig 9-63** The outline form for an occlusal rest seat is established using a rounded-end, tapering bur in a high-speed handpiece. The same bur is used to establish the correct depth of the preparation.

spected to determine the anatomy of the rest seat preparation. The depth of the rest seat is determined by carefully measuring the thickness of the wax. If necessary, changes in the anatomy and depth of the preparation are accomplished. The form and depth of the rest seat preparation are evaluated once again using boxing wax. When the practitioner is satisfied with the preparation, finishing and polishing procedures are instituted.

Finishing procedures are performed using a green stone in a low-speed handpiece (Fig 9-68). The green stone is intended to gently round sharp angles and eliminate scratches produced by the diamond bur.

Polishing is performed using a small, carborundum-impregnated rubber point in a low-speed handpiece (Fig 9-69). Polishing procedures are intended to provide smooth surfaces that will not retain plaque and debris (Fig 9-70).

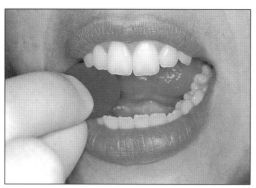

**Fig 9-64** The form and depth of an occlusal rest seat is evaluated using red boxing wax. To accomplish this, boxing wax should be formed into a disk approximately 4 mm in thickness and 15 mm in diameter.

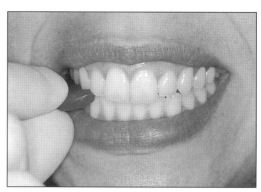

**Fig 9-65** The disk is pressed against the prepared surface or surfaces, and the patient is asked to close firmly.

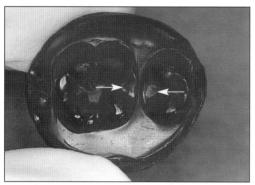

**Fig 9-66** After the patient is directed to open and the wax disk is carefully removed, the form of each rest seat *(arrows)* is carefully inspected.

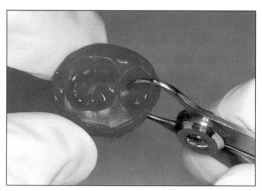

**Fig 9-67** Available space is evaluated by measuring rest seat areas with a wax thickness gauge. The boxing wax should be at least 1 mm thick in rest seat areas.

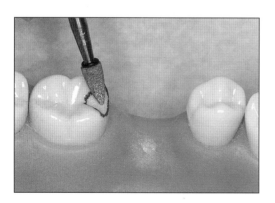

**Fig 9-68** Finishing procedures are performed using a green stone in a low-speed handpiece. The green stone is intended to round sharp angles (represented by the solid line at periphery of preparation) and to eliminate scratches produced by the diamond bur.

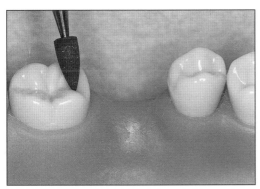

**Fig 9-69** Polishing is performed using a carborundum-impregnated rubber point in a low-speed handpiece.

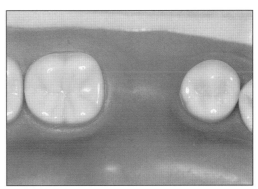

**Fig 9-70** The completed rest seat should exhibit smooth, gently rounded surfaces.

## Occlusal rest seats as part of a new cast-metal restoration

When one or more fixed restorations will be placed in conjunction with removable partial denture therapy, these restorations must be carefully planned and fabricated. Accordingly, occlusal rest seats for cast gold restorations should always be placed during the wax pattern stage.

Required rest seats are carved into the wax pattern following placement of guiding planes. A round carbide bur (No. 4 or 6) is used to perform the initial shaping procedure for each rest seat. The bur is rotated between the finger and thumb or placed in a handpiece and rotated at a slow speed (see Fig 9-46). Minimal pressure is used to prevent fracture of the wax pattern. The rest seat is then refined with a rounded carver (see Fig 9-47). At this stage, the wax pattern may be sprued, invested, and cast in an appropriate alloy.

Upon completion of the casting process, the restoration is recovered, finished, and polished. Special care is taken to ensure that the rest seat is not altered during the process.

## Occlusal rest seats on the surface of an existing cast-metal restoration

Sometimes a removable partial denture is indicated for a patient with one or more cast restorations on proposed partial denture abutments. Although it would be ideal to replace these restorations, such treatment may not be feasible. If the existing restorations demonstrate marginal integrity and occlusal harmony, the practitioner should try to contour these restorations to satisfy the requirements of the proposed removable partial denture.

It is usually not too difficult to prepare acceptable guiding planes on the axial surfaces of existing restorations. The necessary thickness of gold is normally present in these positions. The greatest problem arises in developing adequate rest seats. Often there is insufficient gold to permit adequate preparation. This may result in perforation of the casting and exposure of the underlying tooth structure. Patients must be informed of this possibility and also must be told that perforated restorations must be replaced.

When preparing rest seats in existing cast restorations, the establishment of sufficient space should be the practitioner's highest priority. Inadequate tooth preparation often results in insufficient framework thickness and failure of the removable partial denture. Therefore, adequate tooth preparation is essential.

The instrumentation and procedures for preparing rest seats on existing fixed restorations are identical to those for preparing rest seats on enamel surfaces.

## Occlusal rest seats on an amalgam restoration

A rest seat preparation on a multiple-surface amalgam restoration is less desirable than a rest seat preparation on sound enamel or a cast restoration. Amalgam

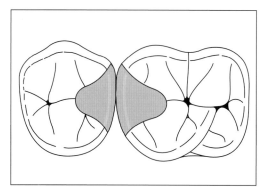

**Fig 9-71** An embrasure rest seat consists of adjacent occlusal rest seats.

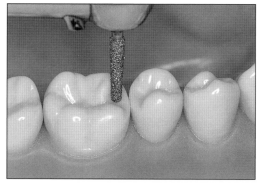

**Fig 9-72** The outline form for an embrasure rest seat is established using a rounded-end, tapering bur in a high-speed handpiece. The practitioner must ensure appropriate reduction at the facial and lingual extensions.

alloys tend to deform when a sustained load is applied. Clinically, this may result in fracture of the material and failure of the restoration.

It is the practitioner's responsibility to decide whether a rest seat should be placed on an amalgam restoration. When making this decision, the practitioner must consider the amount and distribution of remaining tooth structure, the depth and breadth of the amalgam restoration, the physical properties of the alloy used in the restoration, and the size and position of the proposed rest seat. If the practitioner is not familiar with all of these factors, the existing amalgam restoration should be removed, the preparation should be optimized, and a new amalgam restoration should be placed.

Conservative amalgam restorations are quite capable of providing support for removable partial dentures. Therefore, rest seats may be prepared on conservative single- and multiple-surface amalgams. Larger amalgam restorations present greater difficulties for the practitioner because of their flow characteristics and increased susceptibility to fracture. Experience indicates that rest seats should not be placed entirely on amalgam. If a substantial portion of the rest seat cannot be placed on sound tooth structure, then a complete- or partial-coverage casting should be considered.

The instrumentation and procedures for preparing rest seats on amalgam restorations are the same as those for preparing rest seats on enamel surfaces.

## Embrasure rest seats

This preparation crosses the occlusal embrasure of two approximating posterior teeth, from the mesial fossa of one tooth to the distal fossa of the adjacent tooth (Fig 9-71). There is probably more difficulty encountered in making this preparation than any other. In most instances, the practitioner fails to remove sufficient tooth structure at the facial and lingual surfaces of the abutments. As a result, these areas of the removable partial denture framework are extremely thin and susceptible to fracture. Hence, the practitioner must ensure that sufficient tooth structure is removed at the facial and lingual extensions of these preparations.

A diamond bur with a rounded end and tapering sides is ideal for preparing embrasure rest seats. The bur is placed in a high-speed handpiece and the outline form of the rest seat is established. The diamond bur is then used to create the appropriate depth of the preparation (Fig 9-72). Contact between the teeth should not be broken since this may result in tooth migration or food impaction.

The same bur is used to prepare the facial and lingual extensions of the embrasure rest seat. As a rule, obtaining sufficient reduction at the facial surface is much more difficult than obtaining sufficient reduction at the lingual surface. Therefore, the practitioner must pay particular attention to the form and depth of the facial extension. Clearance may be evaluated by placing two pieces of 18-gauge wire across the prepa-

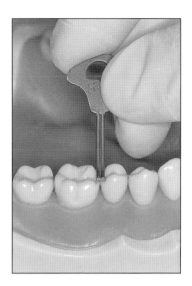

Fig 9-73 Occlusal clearance is evaluated by placing two pieces of 18-gauge wire across the preparation. The patient should be able to close without contacting these wires.

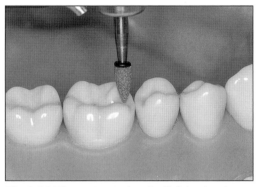

Fig 9-74 The preparation is finished using a green stone in a low-speed handpiece. A carborundum-impregnated rubber point is used to polish the preparation.

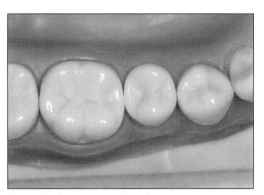

Fig 9-75 A completed embrasure rest seat is shown.

ration (Fig 9-73). The patient should be able to close without contacting these wires.

The form and depth of the rest seat is evaluated using red boxing wax and a wax-thickness gauge. At the facial and lingual embrasures, the embrasure rest seat should be 3.0 to 3.5 mm wide and 1.5 to 2.0 mm deep. All contours should be gently rounded and no undercuts should be present.

When the practitioner is satisfied with the form and depth of the rest seat, the prepared surfaces are finished using a green stone in a low-speed handpiece (Fig 9-74). A carborundum-impregnated rubber point is then used to polish the preparation. The completed preparation is shown in Fig 9-75.

## ☐ Rest Seat Preparations for Anterior Teeth

In most instances, an occlusal rest seat on a posterior tooth is preferred over a cingulum or incisal rest seat on an anterior tooth. Because of its size and position, an occlusal rest seat permits forces to be directed along the long axis of the tooth. Cingulum and incisal rest seats often present inclined surfaces that may result in off-axis loading. Posterior teeth also present large, divergent roots that can withstand more loading than the small, conical roots of anterior teeth. Despite these considerations, cingulum and incisal rest seats are essential elements of removable partial denture

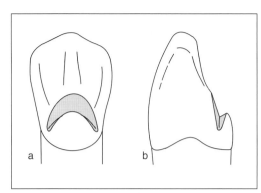

**Fig 9-76** A cingulum rest seat as viewed from the lingual surface *(a)* and the proximal surface *(b)*.

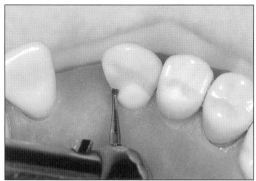

**Fig 9-77** An inverted cone bur is used to establish the outline form of a cingulum rest seat. The preparation begins on one marginal ridge, passes over the cingulum, and terminates on the opposite marginal ridge.

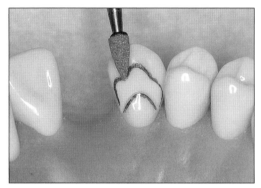

**Fig 9-78** The preparation is finished using a green stone in a low-speed handpiece. Care must be taken to round sharp angles (denoted by solid line). The preparation is then polished using a carborundum-containing rubber point in a low-speed handpiece.

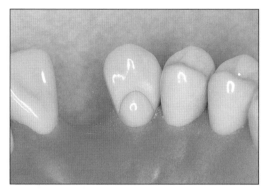

**Fig 9-79** A completed cingulum rest seat is shown.

therapy. In some clinical situations, posterior teeth are missing or are poorly positioned. In other cases, the placement of rest seats on posterior teeth would adversely affect functional or esthetic results. When these conditions exist, cingulum and incisal rests provide useful treatment alternatives.

When a rest seat must be placed on an anterior tooth, a canine is preferred to a lateral or central incisor. This preference is related to the greater length and root surface area for a representative canine. When a canine is not present, the practitioner must consider the placement of rest seats on two or more incisors. The locations for these rest seats are commonly dictated by occlusal and esthetic considerations.

In clinical applications, a cingulum rest seat is preferred to an incisal rest seat. The cingulum rest seat can be prepared nearer the rotational center of the tooth, thereby minimizing the tipping action produced by the rest. A cingulum rest is also more esthetic and less subject to breakage and distortion.

### Cingulum rest seats in enamel

A cingulum rest seat may be prepared in the enamel surface of an anterior tooth if tooth contours are favorable, sufficient enamel is present, and the patient exhibits good oral hygiene.

The outline form of a cingulum rest seat should be crescent shaped when viewed from the lingual aspect

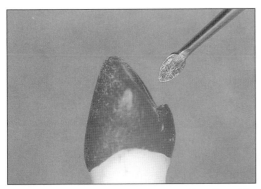

**Fig 9-80** A cingulum rest seat may be placed in a wax pattern. This is easily accomplished using a cleoid-discoid carver.

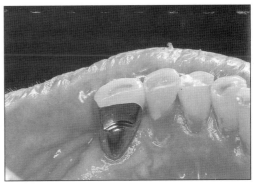

**Fig 9-81** A mandibular metal-ceramic restoration with a cingulum rest seat.

(Fig 9-76). The rest seat should form a smooth curve from one marginal ridge to the other. When viewed in profile, the rest seat should be V-shaped. Sharp angles should be avoided because they serve as stress concentrators and also may interfere with the fit of the partial denture framework.

Preparation of a cingulum rest seat is accomplished using a No. 38 carbide bur in a high-speed handpiece. The No. 38 bur is an inverted cone with side- and end-cutting surfaces. Consequently, it may be used to prepare both walls of the rest seat in an efficient manner. During the preparation process, the bur is oriented at a slight angle to the lingual surface of the tooth. The bur is then used to create a crescent-shaped rest seat that begins on one marginal ridge, passes over the cingulum, and terminates on the opposite marginal ridge (Fig 9-77). The practitioner must be certain that the walls of the rest seat are relatively smooth and that they do not present any mechanical undercuts. The practitioner must also ensure that the cingulum rest seat is placed apical to the contact level of the opposing teeth. If this is not accomplished, there will not be adequate room for the partial denture framework.

The preparation is finished using a green stone in a low-speed handpiece (Fig 9-78). Polishing is accomplished using a carborundum-impregnated rubber wheel or point in a low-speed handpiece. The finished preparation should be smooth and gently rounded (Fig 9-79).

## Cingulum rest seats in a new cast-metal or metal-ceramic restoration

If a fixed restoration is to be placed on an anterior abutment, a cingulum rest seat should be incorporated into the wax pattern. This rest seat should exhibit ideal contours and should direct forces along the long axis of the abutment.

Waxing procedures are identical to those used for other fixed restorations. The practitioner must be careful to develop the appropriate contours and occlusion. Guiding planes are established in the wax pattern. The rest seat is then developed using a cleoid-discoid carver or similar instrument (Fig 9-80). The wax pattern is then sprued and invested, and a casting is made.

Following completion of the casting process, the restoration is finished and polished using established techniques. Care is taken to ensure that desirable contours are retained in the completed restoration. Restoration contours are reevaluated using a dental surveyor. In turn, the restoration is adjusted and cemented (Fig 9-81).

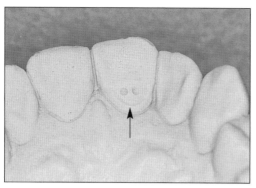

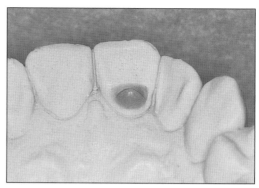

**Fig 9-82** The preparation for a bonded cingulum rest seat includes a shallow indentation *(arrow)* and two or three circular indentations. The depression helps disguise the thickness of the metal, while the circular indentations guide placement of the completed restoration.

**Fig 9-83** The wax pattern must exhibit a properly contoured cingulum rest seat and excellent adaptation at its margins.

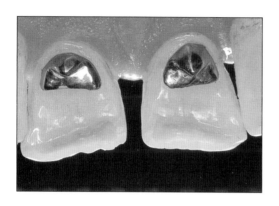

**Fig 9-84** Bonded cingulum rest seats are shown. (Courtesy of Dr Scott Schmitt.)

### Placement of cingulum rest seats using dental bonding techniques

Maxillary canines usually exhibit characteristics that will permit the placement of cingulum rests. Unfortunately, most mandibular canines do not exhibit properties that will permit the placement of properly formed cingulum rest seats. In most instances, mandibular canines do not display prominent cingula, nor do they have appreciable thicknesses of enamel on their lingual surfaces. Attempts to prepare cingulum rest seats on mandibular canines often result in exposure of the underlying dentin and greatly increase the risk of caries. As a result, practitioners have devised other methods

for the placement of cingulum rest seats. Among these are the placement of cingulum rest seats using conservative castings and composite resin materials.

When abutment contours will not permit the preparation of a conventional cingulum rest seat, the practitioner may bond a small metal casting to the lingual surface of the tooth. This may be accomplished rather easily using minimal tooth preparation, a relatively small cast, and a suitable bonding agent.

The initial stages of tooth preparation are accomplished using a small, tapering diamond bur in a high-speed handpiece. A limited area on the lingual surface of the proposed abutment is prepared to a depth of 0.5 to 0.7 mm. This minimizes tooth reduction and

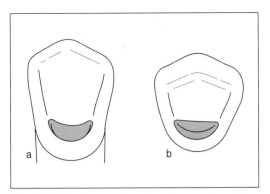

Fig 9-85 An alternative cingulum rest seat as viewed from the lingual surface *(a)* and the incisal surface *(b)*.

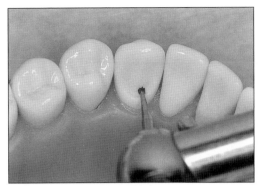

Fig 9-86 An inverted cone bur is used to prepare an alternative cingulum rest seat.

permits the surface of the casting to be positioned at the level of the adjacent tooth structure. Two or three circular indentations are then prepared within the borders of the previous tooth reduction (Fig 9-82). These indentations are prepared using a No. 2 carbide bur and should be no deeper than one third to one half the bur's diameter. The indentations assist in placement of the restoration and also provide vertical support for the cast. At this stage, an impression is made and a cast is generated.

A wax pattern is generated in the dental laboratory. This pattern is contoured to include an appropriate cingulum rest seat and excellent adaptation at its margins (Fig 9-83). In turn, the pattern is sprued and invested, and a casting is made. Upon recovery, the casting is finished and polished using accepted laboratory procedures.

Following clinical adjustment, the casting is cleaned and prepared for cementation. The surface of the tooth is treated and the casting is cemented using an appropriate luting agent (Fig 9-84).

Cingulum rest seats also may be constructed using composite resin materials. This is accomplished by bonding composite resin to the lingual surface of the tooth, then shaping the resin in the manner described for rest seats prepared in enamel. Evidence indicates that composite resin rest seats are susceptible to wear and may lose their effectiveness over a relatively short period. Consequently, composite resin rest seats are not recommended.

## An alternative cingulum rest seat

As previously noted, mandibular canines usually do not display sufficient enamel to allow preparation of conventional cingulum rest seats. This led to the introduction of an alternative cingulum rest seat. The alternative cingulum rest seat may be described as a crescent-shaped depression located in the middle and apical thirds of the clinical crown (Fig 9-85). In many ways, this rest seat resembles an inverted cingulum rest seat.

The alternative cingulum rest seat is prepared using a No. 38 carbide bur or a small diamond disk in a high-speed handpiece. The preparation begins within the enamel of one marginal ridge, progresses apically to the level of the cingulum, and then sweeps incisally within the enamel of the remaining marginal ridge (Fig 9-86). Finishing and polishing are accomplished using a green stone and carborundum-impregnated rubber point, respectively (Fig 9-87). The finished preparation appears as a smooth, gently arcing depression within the lingual enamel (Fig 9-88).

While the alternative cingulum rest seat may be used in certain applications, these applications are limited. For the rest seat to be effective, it must be relatively well defined. Attempts to create adequate depth often result in exposure of the underlying dentin and complicate restorative therapy. Therefore, the alternative cingulum rest seat should be used very sparingly.

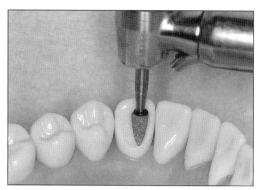

**Fig 9-87** Finishing procedures are performed using a green stone, while polishing is accomplished using a carborundum-impregnated rubber point.

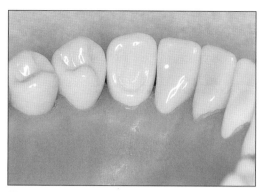

**Fig 9-88** A completed alternative cingulum rest seat on the mandibular left canine.

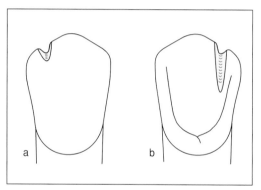

**Fig 9-89** An incisal rest seat as viewed from the facial surface *(a)* and lingual surface *(b)*.

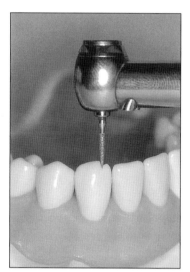

**Fig 9-90** The outline form for an incisal rest seat is established using a flame-shaped diamond bur.

## Incisal rest seats in enamel

Incisal rest seats are the least desirable rest seats for anterior teeth. The accompanying rests are unesthetic and may interfere with occlusion. More importantly, incisal rests are located far from the rotational centers of the abutments. Hence, these teeth may be damaged by tipping or torquing forces (see chapter 2).

Despite their shortcomings, incisal rest seats may be used successfully if they are properly positioned and adequately prepared. Incisal rest seats are commonly used on mandibular canines, but may be used on other anterior teeth as well. The placement of in-

cisal rest seats on incisors should be considered a last resort because of the esthetic and mechanical compromises that must be made.

Incisal rest seats should be used only on enamel surfaces. If a cast restoration is planned for an anterior abutment, a cingulum rest seat should be included in the restoration. This places the accompanying rest in a more desirable esthetic and mechanical position.

An incisal rest seat is usually placed near a proximal surface (Fig 9-89). In most instances, the disto-incisal surface is selected for esthetic purposes, but the mesio-incisal surface also may be used.

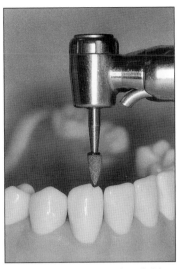

**Fig 9-91** Finishing and polishing are accomplished using a green stone and carborundum-impregnated rubber point, respectively.

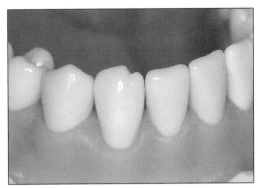

**Fig 9-92** A completed incisal rest seat.

The incisal rest seat preparation is begun with a flame-shaped diamond bur in a high-speed handpiece. The bur is oriented parallel to the proposed path of insertion, and a notch is created (Fig 9-90). This notch should be located 2 to 3 mm from the proximal angle of the tooth and should be 1.5 to 2.0 mm in depth. The notch is extended slightly onto the facial surface of the tooth. This provides a method to prevent facial movement of the abutment. On the lingual surface of the tooth, a small channel is created. This channel helps disguise the thickness of the associated minor connector.

The preparation is finished using a green stone in a low-speed handpiece. A carborundum-impregnated rubber point or wheel is used to finish the prepared surfaces (Fig 9-91). The completed preparation should be smooth and comfortable to the patient (Fig 9-92).

## Making the Impression for the Master Cast

Dental professionals often discuss the difference between "making an impression" and "taking an impression." While the difference in terms may seem minimal, there is a substantial difference in meaning. The expression "making an impression" implies that the practitioner is an active participant in the impression process. In contrast, the expression "taking an impression" implies that the impression material accomplishes the task, and the practitioner's only responsibility is removal of the impression from the mouth.

In reality, the practitioner is responsible for numerous factors, including patient position, moisture control, tray selection, material selection, and impression technique. Therefore, when speaking about impression procedures, the expression "making an impression" should be used.

There are a number of impression materials and techniques that may be used to make final impressions for removable partial denture construction. Impression materials include alginates, polysulfides, polyvinlysiloxanes, and polyethers. Each of these materials has inherent advantages and disadvantages related to accuracy, surface detail, cost, etc. Impression techniques also may affect the accuracy of the impression and the resultant cast. Therefore, it is the responsibility of the dentist to choose the material and technique that will provide the best result under a variety of clinical conditions.

## Impression materials

The properties and handling characteristics of irreversible hydrocolloid (alginate) are covered in chapter 5. A few important points are repeated here for the convenience of the reader.

Alginate impression material is the most widely used and possibly the most versatile of the dental impression materials. The material is readily available, relatively inexpensive, easy to use, and dimensionally accurate. The primary drawback of alginate impression material is the inability to store the material for an appreciable length of time. Although manufacturers and some investigators may advocate storing a completed impression in a humid environment, alginate impressions should be poured within 12 minutes of removal from the mouth.

Another advantage of alginate impression material is that a custom tray is not required for most impressions. A custom tray is only used when a stock tray will not fit the dental arch. This may occur when the arch is extremely large or extremely small, or when tooth alignment precludes the use of a stock tray. The presence of tori or exostoses also may necessitate the construction of a custom tray.

### Using a stock tray

When a stock tray is to be used for a final impression for a removable partial denture, the tray must be modified to ensure a consistent thickness of alginate. If the impression material is not supported during the gelation process, it may slump. Slumping produces inaccuracies in the impression that are reflected in the master cast. This is a common problem in the palatal region of the maxillary arch and may account for the poor adaptation of many major connectors. Therefore, stock trays should be properly modified before final impressions are made.

The simplest and most accurate method of modifying a stock impression tray is by using modeling plastic. The modeling plastic is softened in a water bath at 60°C (140°F) and molded over the area of the tray that requires modification. While the modeling plastic is still soft, the surface is heated with an alcohol torch, tempered in the water bath, and seated in the mouth. This should result in a relatively accurate impression of the corresponding oral tissues.

Following removal from the mouth, the tray is immersed in an ice-water bath. The modeling plastic is then trimmed to provide adequate space for the alginate impression material. The internal aspects of the modified impression tray are then coated with an appropriate adhesive and allowed to dry for 5 minutes. Subsequently, the impression is made.

## Impression procedure

The impression procedure for a master impression is the same as that described for a diagnostic impression, with the exception that special care must be shown in recording the rest seat preparations that have been made in the abutment teeth. A complete description of the impression procedure is presented in chapter 5. A brief review of the procedure is provided in the following text.

1. Ensure that the patient is properly positioned for the impression procedure to be performed.
2. Select and modify the required impression tray or trays.
3. Rehearse the operator position and tray placement several times so that the patient is aware of his or her responsibilities.
4. Have the patient rinse and then place gauze pads.
5. Measure and mix the impression material according to the manufacturer's directions. Load the tray in small increments to avoid trapping air.
6. Remove gauze pads from the oral cavity and paint or inject impression material into critical areas (eg, peripheries, hard palate). Forcibly wipe the impression material onto all tooth surfaces.
7. Seat the tray as rehearsed. Manipulate the lips and cheeks to ensure that the peripheries are properly extended and that air is not trapped in the vestibules. For the mandibular impression, ensure that the patient's tongue is raised and then gently protruded.
8. Support the tray until the impression material has set. Never leave a patient unattended with an impression in the mouth.
9. Following gelation, remove the impression with a rapid, sustained tug in the direction of the long axes of the teeth.
10. Clean the impression by placing it under a gentle stream of cool water. If necessary, saliva and

other contaminants may be removed by sprinkling dental stone onto the surface of the impression and lightly brushing with a soft camel-hair brush.

11. Examine the impression to determine whether all details are accurately recorded. If there is any doubt regarding accuracy, reject the impression.

12. Spray the impression using an appropriate chemical disinfectant. Allow the disinfectant to remain in contact with the impression for the period prescribed by the manufacturer.

### Reasons for rejecting an impression

The following are specific reasons for rejecting and repeating an impression:

1. Bubbles or voids in and around rest seat preparations

2. Contact of cusps with the tray, especially when the teeth are involved in the framework design

3. Show-through between teeth and modeling plastic or modeling plastic and hard palate if the tray has been modified for an alginate impression

4. Voids or bubbles in the palatal vault when palatal major connectors are to be constructed

5. Peripheral underextension when a denture base has been designed and a corrected cast impression is not planned

6. Interproximal tearing of the impression material when coverage of those teeth has been designed

7. Lack of detail on the impression surface

8. Any doubt as to the accuracy of the impression

## ⌨ Pouring the Master Cast

The technique for pouring the master cast is the same as that for the diagnostic cast (chapter 5), except that a minimal expansion, improved artificial stone should be used.

1. After the impression has been cleaned of saliva, examined for defects, and sprayed with disinfectant, pour the cast immediately. Under no circumstances should a final alginate impression go unpoured for more than 12 minutes.

2. Never allow the impression to rest on a bench top or in a rubber bowl. Suspend it by the tray handle.

3. Do not make the second, or opposing, impression before pouring the first.

4. Have pre-weighed stone available before the start of the appointment.

5. Make the stone mix, preferably under vacuum, according to directions and complete the first pour.

6. Be certain all peripheries are covered by at least 6 mm of stone. Leave the stone surface rough.

7. After the initial set (10 to 12 minutes), wet the base of the first pour with slurry water and add the second pour. Invert the impression with the first pour on a pad of stone and shape the base.

8. Between 45 and 60 minutes after the first pour, separate the impression from the cast if hydrocolloid material has been used.

9. Wet the cast thoroughly in slurry water by partially submerging it. Do not completely immerse the cast because this would prevent air from escaping from the stone and the cast will never be thoroughly wet.

10. Trim the cast. The base of the cast should be trimmed so that the occlusal surfaces of the teeth will be as parallel to the base as possible. The thickness of the cast should be determined at this time also. The cast should be 10 mm thick at its thinnest point—usually the center of the hard palate for the maxillary cast and the depth of the lingual sulcus for the mandibular cast.

The posterior border of the cast is trimmed next. It must form an angle of 90 degrees with the base and should be perpendicular to a line passing between the central incisors.

The sides of the cast are trimmed so that they are parallel to the buccal surfaces of the posterior teeth or to the crest of the edentulous ridge. Do not trim so close as to obliterate the vestibule or the buccal shelf. A land area or periphery at least 3 mm wide should be maintained around the entire cast.

The sides and the posterior borders are joined by trimming just posterior to the hamular notch or retromolar pad. Be careful not to overtrim and thereby remove the hamular notch or the retromolar pad. These are essential landmarks and must be preserved.

The anterior borders of the maxillary cast are formed by trimming from the canine area on each side to a point anterior to the interproximal area of the central incisors, being careful again to maintain the vestibule and the land area.

The anterior border of the mandibular cast is formed by creating a curving wall from the canine on one side to the canine on the other. The curve should be kept constant (ie, harmonious).

The tongue space of the mandibular cast must be trimmed flat, but the integrity of the lingual frenum, sublingual fold space, and the lingual sulcus must be maintained.

11. Identify the casts with the patient's name. Do not put any foreign material on the master cast.

12. Casts must not be subjected to running water, brushing, or soaking in any solution other than clear slurry water. If they are allowed to dry, they must be resoaked in clear slurry water before being shaped on the model trimmer.

## 📖 Bibliography

Anusavice KJ (ed). Philllips' Science of Dental Materials, ed 10. Philadelphia: Saunders, 1996.

Breeding LC, Dixon D, Caughman WF. An articulator and surveyor remount technique for surveyed abutment crowns. J Prosthet Dent 1987;58:708–710.

Craig RG (ed). Restorative Dental Materials, ed 10. St Louis: Mosby, 1997.

Ivanhoe JR. Alternative cingulum rest seat. J Prosthet Dent 1985;54:395–396.

Kahn AE. Partial versus full coverage. J Prosthet Dent 1960;10:167–178.

Krokos AA. Artificial undercuts for teeth which have unfavorable shapes for clasping. J Prosthet Dent 1969;22:301–306.

Leupold RJ. A comparative study of impression procedures for distal extension removable partial dentures. J Prosthet Dent 1966;16:708–720.

Mann AW. A critical appraisal of the hydrocolloid technique: Its advantages and disadvantages. J Prosthet Dent 1951;1:733–749.

McCracken WL. Mouth preparations for partial dentures. J Prosthet Dent 1956;6:39–52.

Mills M. Mouth preparation for removable partial dentures. J Am Dent Assoc 1960;60:154–159.

Mitchell JV, Dameles JJ. Influence of tray design upon elastic impression materials. J Prosthet Dent 1970;23:51–57.

Paffenbarger GC. Hydrocolloid impression materials: Physical properties and a specification. J Am Dent Assoc 1940;27:373–388.

Perry CF, Applegate SG. Occlusal rest: An important part of a partial denture. J Mich Dent Soc 1947;29:24–25.

Philips RW. Factors affecting the surface of stone dies poured in hydrocolloid impressions. J Prosthet Dent 1952;2:390–400.

Samson BP, Flinton RJ, Parks VJ, Pallen GB, Kingman A. Rest seat designs for inclined posterior abutments: A photoelastic comparison. J Prosthet Dent 1987;58:57–62.

Schorr L, Clayton LH. Reshaping abutment teeth for reception of partial denture clasps. J Prosthet Dent 1954;4:625–633.

Seiden A. Occlusal rests and rest seats. J Prosthet Dent 1958;8:431–440.

Skinner EW, Hoblit NE. A study of the accuracy of hydrocolloid impressions. J Prosthet Dent 1956;6:80–86.

Solle W. The Parallelo-facere: A parallel drilling machine for use in the oral cavity. J Am Dent Assoc 1961;63:344–352.

Stern WJ. Guiding planes in clasp reciprocation and retention. J Prosthet Dent 1975;34:408–414.

# Laboratory Procedures for Framework Construction

**Raymond G. Koeppen,** DDS, MS, FACP
**Michael A. Mansueto,** DDS, MS, FACP

## ☐ Dentist-Laboratory Relations

The fabrication of a removable partial denture framework in contemporary dental practice is routinely delegated to a commercial dental laboratory. Dental schools rarely provide practical experience in framework construction techniques. Therefore, most dentists possess only a superficial understanding of the exacting procedures required to produce a quality casting. Unfortunately, this combination of factors often leads to a situation in which the dentist delgates framework design as well as construction to the dental laboratory.

To fully understand the relationship between a dentist and a dental laboratory, one must understand that a dental laboratory is a business. For a prearranged cost, a dental laboratory technician constructs a prosthesis or appliance according to the dentist's instructions. In most instances, the dental laboratories that construct removable partial denture frameworks are large, serve many dentists, and produce as many as 50 frameworks per day. Were it not for a large volume, the cost of the equipment used in the fabrication of removable partial denture frameworks would be prohibitive. Framework-fabricating laboratories usually are not collocated with dental offices. In fact, they are usually not located in the same city, which puts a strain on communication between dentist and technician. Therefore, a properly completed work authorization is a critical component in the overall success of removable partial denture service.

The dentist's expectation that the technician perform tasks requiring clinical judgment is unfair and may be illegal if the technician is asked to design the partial denture framework as well as construct it. In any case, it does not reflect well on the profession when removable partial denture design responsibility is inappropriately delegated. Even with years of experience in the construction of partial dentures, the technician has no experience in assessing the clinical results of prosthodontic treatment and has no firsthand clinical data from which to personalize therapy. When placed in a position where a clinical judgment must be made, the technician is likely to think only of construction issues and not the long-term effects of removable partial denture service.

The dentist must provide the clinical and professional components of patient treatment, allowing the technician to perform those technical duties for which training has been received. Manipulation of dental materials, casting and finishing techniques, and repair of existing partial dentures are but a few examples of where the technician's knowledge may exceed that of the dentist. By franchising the materials and techniques for the construction of the partial denture frameworks, dental manufacturers provide laboratories with technical information that may not be common knowledge for dentists. A good working relationship between the dentist and the dental laboratory technician permits the construction of quality prostheses and the delivery of quality care.

## Training of Laboratory Technicians

Traditionally, the road to becoming an accomplished technician was long and often discouraging because technicians had to learn the trade through on-the-job training. This began to change when the great demand for dental care that resulted from the military buildup of the 1940s provided the impetus for an expanded dental laboratory service. For the first time, the military services provided training for laboratory technicians on a large scale. Formal dental laboratory technology education, in response to the training needs of advanced dental technologies such as ceramics and implants, continued to increase rapidly during the 1960s and reached its height in the 1980s.

In addition to military training programs, formal dental laboratory training is offered at more than 25 accredited institutions in the United States. Following formal training and on-the-job experience, technicians desiring certification by the National Board for Certification in Dental Laboratory Technology may be examined voluntarily in one or more of five areas of expertise in the laboratory field: complete dentures, removable partial dentures, fixed partial dentures, ceramics, and orthodontics. Although certification is not required by any state, it does serve as an indicator of technical proficiency. Certification also may play a part in workforce dynamics, where a certified technician may command a higher salary.

## Registration of Laboratories

Periodic attempts have been made to require certification of dental laboratories. The purpose of the certification would be to control the quality of technical work performed. These attempts have never been successful, and the need for such control has never been demonstrated. Competition forces laboratories to maintain quality standards. Where quality is inadequate, the laboratory suffers the same consequences as any business that does not satisfy its customers—ultimate failure. However, most states do require the registration of dental laboratories and individual dental laboratory technicians.

## Work Authorizations

All states require that requests for dental laboratory services be accompanied by written instructions (Fig 10-1). The minimum information required by most states includes (1) the signature and license number of the dentist, (2) the date the authorization was signed, (3) the name and address of the patient (because of privacy laws, some states require only a patient identification number), and (4) a description of the service or material ordered.

A written request for dental laboratory services is termed a *work authorization* and is equivalent to a prescription. If the work authorization is used correctly, it represents an excellent line of communication between dentist and laboratory. The dentist should supply dental laboratory personnel with the information needed to produce the requested prosthesis. In turn, laboratory personnel should not hesitate to contact the practitioner if the instructions are vague or if additional information is needed. Once this avenue of communication is established, the quality of dental products submitted by the dentist and returned by the laboratory can be significantly improved.

In addition to providing instructions to the laboratory, the written work authorization serves as a legal document in the event of a lawsuit. For this reason, most states require both the dentist and the dental laboratory to maintain a copy of each work authorization for a period of 2 years. The written authorization

## WORK AUTHORIZATION NUMBER 12345

DATE SUBMITTED _December 2, 2002_     DATE REQUESTED _December 16, 2002_

**PATIENT'S NAME AND CHART NUMBER**

①   John Doe
    Chart number 12256

**DENTIST'S NAME AND OFFICE ADDRESS**

Dr. Hale MacKown
57 Laboratory Way
San Antonio, TX 78284

**TYPE OF PROSTHESIS / ADA CODE**

☐ Maxillary Complete Denture / 05110    ☒ Maxillary RPD / 05213    ☐ Other
☐ Mandibular Complete Denture / 05120    ☐ Mandibular RPD / 05214    _____

**FRAMEWORK MATERIAL**

☐ Co-Cr alloy    ☒ Ni-Cr alloy    ☐ Ti alloy    ☐ Other _____

②

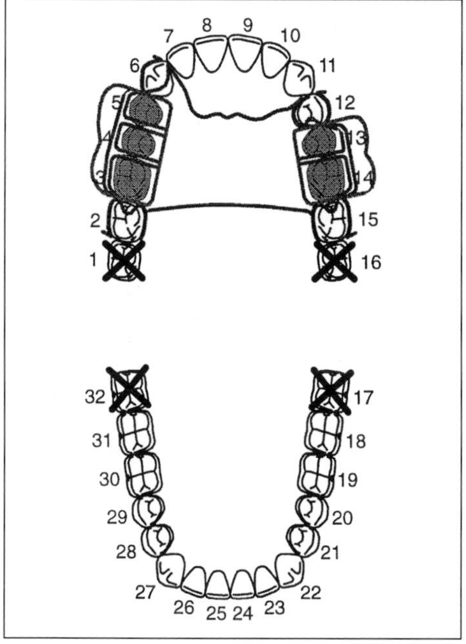

**CLASPING**

③

| Tooth | Clasp type | Undercut |
|-------|------------|----------|
| 2 | Simple circlet | 0.010 in. |
| 6 | Simple circlet | 0.010 in. |
| 12 | Simple circlet | 0.010 in. |
| 15 | Simple circlet | 0.010 in. |
| | | |
| | | |
| | | |
| | | |

**PROSTHETIC TOOTH SELECTION**

Material: ☐ Plastic    ☐ Porcelain

④

| Location | Shade | Mold |
|----------|-------|------|
| Maxillary anterior | | |
| Mandibular anterior | | |
| Maxillary posterior | | |
| Mandibular posterior | | |

**DENTURE BASE MATERIAL**

Type: ☐ Standard     Shade: ☐ Light    ☐ Bluish pink
      ☐ High impact         ☐ Light reddish pink    ☐ Other _____
                             ☐ Reddish pink

**REMARKS AND SPECIAL INSTRUCTIONS**

⑤

Please fabricate maxillary RPD framework as indicated.
If you have questions, concerns, etc., please contact me at (210) 555-7222.

                              Thank you for your assistance.
                                    HM

Dentist's signature: _Hale MacKown_       License number _57057_

**Fig 10-1** A representative work authorization order.

also clearly establishes the separate lines of responsibility for the dentist and the laboratory technician.

## Design of written work authorizations

Teaching institutions, the military services, large commercial dental laboratories, and many practicing dentists have developed standardized forms that suit their communication requirements. Forms are designed to be uncomplicated and to minimize the necessity for additional writing. Most forms are generated using pressure-sensitive papers so that copies of work authorizations are immediately available for the dentist and dental laboratory personnel.

To be useful, a work authorization order must be legible, concise, and easily understood. Information that is of little value to the technician should be avoided. Unfortunately, a common problem with work authorizations is the lack of essential information. In many instances, the only instructions are such statements as "Make partial denture" or "Don't use too many clasps." Insufficient information, coupled with the dentist's potentially unrealistic expectations, often leads to clinical disappointment and inadequate prosthetic service.

During the course of patient treatment, it is often necessary to submit the same prosthesis to the laboratory more than once. Casts for removable partial dentures may be submitted for framework construction, resubmitted for arrangement of prosthetic teeth, and submitted yet again for processing and finishing the denture bases. Attempting to use the same work authorization form for all steps is a potential problem since the technician may have difficulty in determining the appropriate instructions. Therefore, it is wise to use a new work authorization order each time the cast is submitted to the dental laboratory.

To help the laboratory identify the cast as it passes through the laboratory, the form should have the doctor's and patient's names prominently displayed. In addition, the work authorization number assigned by the laboratory and the type of prosthesis should be clearly indicated (see section 1 in Fig 10-1).

The work authorization order should accurately communicate the positions of all removable partial denture components. To accomplish this, the removable partial denture design should be drawn on the appropriate portion of the work authorization order (see section 2 in Fig 10-1). Though done with care, the drawing is not a substitute for properly designed diagnostic casts, which should always accompany the master casts to the laboratory. The drawing should identify all missing teeth. Teeth to be replaced by the removable partial denture should be darkened using a pen. Teeth that are not to be replaced should be identified by placing a large X through the crown form. The major connector should be drawn to the desired size and shape, and the configuration of the clasps should be included. The placement of denture bases should be accurately indicated. Among the purposes of the diagrammed design are (1) to remind the technician of the prescribed design and (2) to provide a form of identification in the event that the dental casts and the case pan become separated while in the dental laboratory.

The work authorization order should clearly identify the major connector to be used. In addition, the practitioner should list the teeth to be clasped, the type of clasp to be used (eg, cast circumferential clasp, combination clasp, I-bar, or T-bar), and the amount of undercut that each clasp assembly must engage (see section 3 in Fig 10-1).

The selection of prosthetic teeth must be handled very carefully (see section 4 in Fig 10-1). The dentist should indicate the size and number of artificial teeth to be used as pontics. The type of artificial tooth and the material from which it is made, such as porcelain or resin, must be indicated. The desired tooth shade and the manufacturer of the shade guide should be listed.

Perhaps the most important portion of the written work authorization is the "Remarks and Special Instructions" section (see section 5 in Fig 10-1). In this section, the dentist must delineate the prosthodontic requirements needed to satisfy the patient's unique biologic conditions. Any portion of the design that deviates from the norm should be listed in this section. Communications should be complete yet succinct.

The dentist should use a polite and respectful tone when submitting a work authorization order to the dental laboratory. This fosters a spirit of cooperation and is essential if the dentist and dental laboratory personnel are to work as a team.

Whether or not the dentist assumes the proper degree of responsibility in designing and supervising the laboratory phases of partial denture construction, the legal weight of patient treatment rests entirely on the dentist, not on the technician.

## ❑ Infection Control for the Dental Laboratory

Dental laboratories must establish and maintain appropriate infection control programs. The following sections provide guidelines regarding infection control for dental laboratories.

### Receiving area

A strict barrier system is the most effective and practical method for protection from contamination and cross-contamination within the dental laboratory. This system provides a series of cleaning and disinfection procedures designed to rid a prosthesis (device, appliance, impression, etc) of organic debris and microorganisms before it enters or leaves the main portion of the laboratory. The result is a product that can be safely handled by laboratory personnel with a minimum of personal protective equipment.

The laboratory's receiving area should be established in a location separate from the main work area. The receiving area should be disinfected daily by spraying the countertops and other working areas with an approved disinfectant. Personnel in the receiving area should wear disposable gloves and masks when unpacking incoming cases. All materials should be placed into clean, clearly identified case pans. To prevent cross-contamination, case pans should be disinfected after each use.

Items that have been in the oral cavity (impressions, dentures, occlusion rims, trial dentures, cast frameworks, etc) should be disinfected with a 0.55% sodium hypochlorite solution spray. The disinfecting spray should be left in contact with the item for 2 minutes. At the end of this period, the item should be thoroughly rinsed with water.

### Production area

Work surfaces and equipment should be kept free of debris. Provided the barrier system is in effect, no dis-

infection of instruments, equipment, or materials is required. To ensure cleanliness, pumice solutions should be discarded at the end of each workday.

## ❑ Laboratory Procedures

Framework fabrication is almost always delegated to a technician located outside the dental office. Therefore, effective communication between the clinician and the technician is essential if a quality product is to be provided. To facilitate this process, the practitioner must understand the laboratory phases of removable partial denture construction.

For successful construction of a removable partial denture, the dentist must provide dental laboratory personnel with the following: *(1)* a written work authorization describing the desired prosthesis (see Fig 10-1), *(2)* a properly surveyed diagnostic cast with an appropriate removable partial denture design, and *(3)* a properly articulated master cast that provides an accurate reproduction of existing hard and soft tissue contours. Anything less will compromise quality and adversely impact patient care.

Before framework construction can begin, the dental laboratory technician must transfer the prescribed design from the diagnostic cast to the master cast. The preferred method for design transfer is described in the following sections.

### Retripoding the master cast

During the survey and design process, the clinician determines a specific path of insertion and removal for the partial denture. This path is recorded by placing tripod marks on the diagnostic cast. In turn, the clinician prepares both hard and soft tissues of the mouth in harmony with this path. The technician must ensure that all framework fabrication steps are based upon this path of insertion and removal.

As noted in chapter 7, tripodization is accomplished by placing three easily identifiable marks on the same horizontal plane. These marks must be widely separated and must be positioned on anatomic portions of the diagnostic cast. Because these marks define a single horizontal plane, they allow rapid orientation and reorientation of the diagnostic cast.

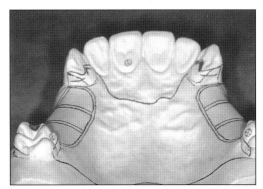

**Fig 10-2** Tripod marks allow precise orientation and reorientation of diagnostic and master casts.

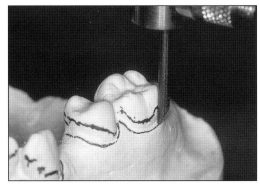

**Fig 10-3** The height of contour is scribed using a surveyor and carbon marker.

Transfer of these marks also permits orientation of the master cast. This allows the technician to position the diagnostic and master casts in the same spatial orientation, thereby reproducing the prescribed path of insertion and removal (Fig 10-2).

## Heights of contour

With the master cast properly oriented on the survey table, the technician uses a dental surveyor and carbon marker to indicate the heights of contour for the teeth and soft tissues (Fig 10-3). To accomplish this, the survey table is gently guided along the horizontal platform of the dental surveyor. The technician must ensure that the carbon marker remains in contact with the master cast throughout the process. This results in the transfer of distinct black survey lines to the master cast. These lines represent the heights of contour at the selected orientation.

## Design transfer

Without removing the master cast from the survey table or changing the tilt, the technician transfers the design from the diagnostic cast to the master cast (Figs 10-4 and 10-5). Each laboratory has its own methods for identifying finish lines, resin-retention areas, clasp positions, etc. Areas of special consideration, such as undercut depths for retentive clasp arms,

gauges of wrought-wire clasps, cast clasps' pattern sizes, and other critical items should be transferred to the master cast with extreme care and clearly marked to avoid confusion.

## Blockout and relief

Blocking out is the act of placing wax and other materials into undesirable undercuts on the master cast. Since the framework is waxed and cast on a duplicate of the master cast, undercuts that would prohibit the framework from going into place must be eliminated. Specifics of the blockout process are described in the following sections.

### Cast preparation

Before the addition of the blockout wax, a maxillary cast is beaded (Fig 10-6). *Beading* is the act of scraping the outline of the major connector into the master cast. The bead line is approximately 0.5 mm deep and becomes less distinct as it approaches the gingival margins. The bead line produces a raised edge at the border of the major connector and ensures positive contact of the major connector with the palatal tissues. This feature reduces packing of food beneath the major connector. Bead lines are not used in conjunction with mandibular major connectors because these connectors rest on thin gingival tissues that cannot tolerate the associated pressures.

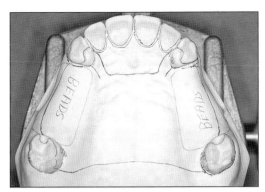

**Fig 10-4** The master cast is shown immediately following design transfer.

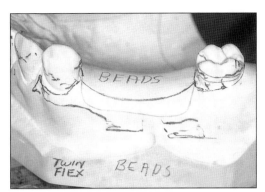

**Fig 10-5** Upon completion of the design transfer, notes are made on the base of the master cast. In this instance, notes indicate the use of a twin-flex clasp and bead retention on the metal base.

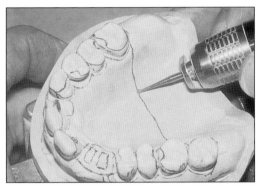

**Fig 10-6** Bead lines are carefully prepared on a maxillary dental cast.

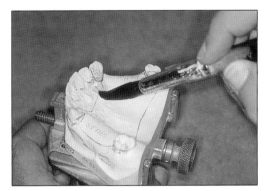

**Fig 10-7** The master cast is sealed using an acetone-based liquid.

Before further progress is made, the master cast must be treated with a surface sealer. The sealer is a mixture of acetone, diethyl phthalate, and cellulose acetate. The material provides an almost imperceptible film that protects the design throughout the blockout and duplication processes.

Surface sealer may be applied using a brush (Fig 10-7) or an aerosol spray. In either case, application should be performed in a fume hood or in front of a suction vent. Careful application is required to prevent a buildup of material, which could create false contours and affect the accuracy of the associated prosthesis. Following application of sealer, the cast must be allowed to dry for a minimum of 5 minutes. Blockout wax then may be applied to the cast.

## Blockout technique

Blockout wax can be purchased as a commercially prepared product or it can be mixed to the technician's personal preference by using a combination of common dental waxes. Most formulas employ a mixture of hard baseplate wax, gutta percha, sticky wax, and a colorant for visual contrast against the dental cast.

Blockout wax is normally kept fluid in an electrically heated pot. The molten wax can be applied to the dental cast using a spatula. Wax is placed apical to the height of contour and is not applied in areas where intimate metal contact is desired. Wax that is inadvertently positioned occlusal or incisal to the height of contour must be removed, or it will add to the dimension of the refractory cast and result in a poorly fitting framework.

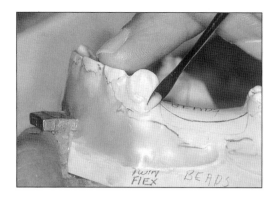

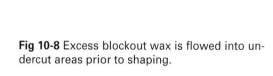

**Fig 10-8** Excess blockout wax is flowed into undercut areas prior to shaping.

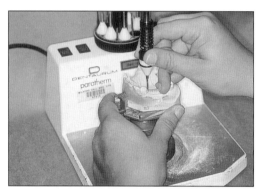

**Fig 10-9** A dental surveyor is used to shape the blockout wax.

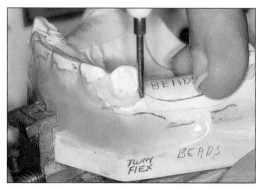

**Fig 10-10** Excess wax is removed with a parallel-sided instrument.

During this stage of the procedure, a slight excess of blockout wax is placed into all undercut areas (Fig 10-8). In turn, definitive shaping of the blockout wax can begin.

**Tapered versus parallel blockout** Blockout wax is contoured in a predetermined relation to the prescribed path of insertion. Excess wax is removed with a metallic blockout instrument mounted in the dental surveyor (Figs 10-9 and 10-10). Normally the surface of the blockout instrument is held perpendicular to the surveyor base. This results in a 0-degree blockout (ie, a blockout that is parallel to the path of insertion). Other blades are available and offer blockouts that range from 2 to 6 degrees from the path of insertion.

The decision to block out the undercuts exactly parallel to the path of placement or to allow some degree of taper is a clinical one and should be determined by the dentist. All tooth-supported removable partial dentures should be blocked out parallel to the path of in-

sertion. Tooth-tissue–supported removable partial dentures may be blocked out in a similar manner, or they may be given a tapered blockout to allow increased freedom of movement in function. Personal design philosophy generally determines the degree of blockout.

**Contouring the blockout wax** With the blockout instrument properly positioned, excess wax is carefully removed until the entire undercut area has been shaped (Fig 10-11). Blockout tools may be electrically heated or warmed over a flame. The use of a warm instrument makes the contouring process easier and more efficient.

Areas associated with retentive clasp tips are critical to the success of the prosthesis and warrant special consideration. Blockout wax can be shaped with hand instruments to provide a slight ledge just apical to the clasp terminus (Fig 10-12). This ledge guides the placement of the wax or plastic pattern and ensures that the clasp tip is accurately positioned in the desired undercut.

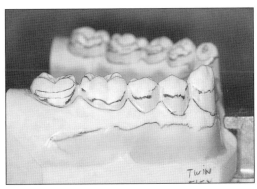

**Fig 10-11** The blockout process creates a smooth vertical surface apical to the height of contour.

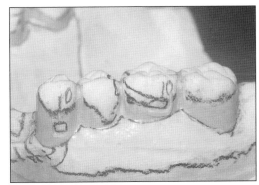

**Fig 10-12** A soft tissue undercut is blocked out under the approach arm of an infrabulge clasp for the maxillary right first premolar. A ledge is present at the distofacial aspect of the first molar. This ledge aids in placement of the circumferential clasp's retentive terminus.

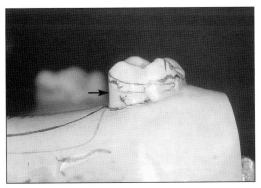

**Fig 10-13** An undesirable undercut *(arrow)* at the origin of the retentive clasp on the maxillary right second molar is blocked out.

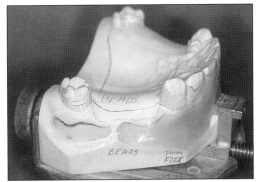

**Fig 10-14** Undercut areas that are not involved with framework are blocked out to minimize distortion during duplication.

In some instances, mechanical undercuts may be present where the body and shoulder of the clasp arm are to be placed. Since only the terminal third of the retentive clasp arm should be placed into an undercut, the body and shoulder areas commonly require blockout. An example is seen at the mesiobuccal surface of the maxillary right second molar in Fig 10-13. Appropriate blockout permits placement of the clasp. Failure to accomplish this represents a compromise in removable partial denture design and construction. The clinician is responsible for evaluating tooth contours prior to master cast submission and should ensure the adequacy of mouth preparation procedures.

**Arbitrary blockout** Areas of undercut that are not directly involved with framework fabrication also must be addressed. These areas should be recontoured to minimize distortions that may occur during cast duplication (Fig 10-14). Duplicating materials such as reversible hydrocolloids can rebound from relatively small undercuts (< 3 mm), but distort or tear when larger undercuts are present. To prevent distortion and tearing, areas of gross undercut should be eliminated. Because these areas do not directly affect framework construction, blockout can be somewhat arbitrary. Soft wax, clay, and mortite are commonly used in such applications (Fig 10-15). These materials are pressed

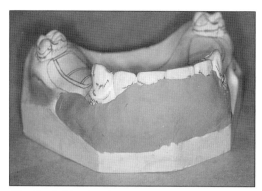

**Fig 10-15** Clay is often used to block out areas of gross soft tissue undercut.

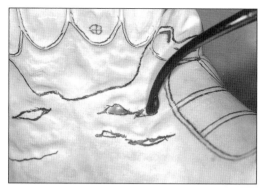

**Fig 10-16** Palatal clefts and other irregularities in areas to be covered by the maxillary major connector are filled with wax.

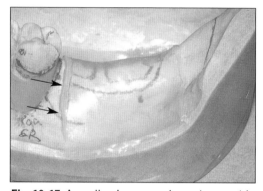

**Fig 10-17** An adhesive wax sheet *(arrows)* is sealed at the finish line, approximately 1.5 mm distal to the premolar abutment.

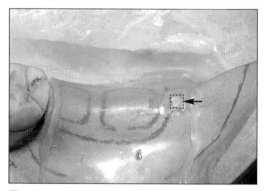

**Fig 10-18** A 2-mm square of wax *(box, arrow)* is removed from the relief pad to allow placement of a cast stop.

into position and manually shaped, thereby eliminating the need for blockout instruments.

On a maxillary cast, deep palatal clefts and irregularities are filled with wax to eliminate potentially sharp areas on the intaglio of the major connector (Fig 10-16). The same approach is used for a mandibular cast. Since intimate soft tissue contact is not desirable in the anterior mandible, a thin film of wax is applied to the major connector area. The wax is then smoothed by flaming or by polishing it with gauze or cotton batten. As an alternative, relief wax of known (usually 28-gauge) thickness can be placed over this critical area.

## Relief

Removable partial denture frameworks usually display intimate contact with the teeth and soft tissues. However, there are certain areas where contact is not desir-

able. In these areas, frameworks are shaped to stand away from the underlying tissues. This is accomplished by adding one or more wax spacers of known dimension to the master cast. Any addition of wax intended to make the framework stand away from the master cast is termed *relief*. In removable partial denture applications, relief is most commonly used in conjunction with denture bases. The retentive latticework must be raised above the edentulous area to allow resin to completely surround the longitudinal and transverse struts. For practical purposes, 1 mm of space should be created between these struts and the surface of the master cast. This allows resin to encompass the latticework, thereby forming an effective mechanical attachment.

In addition to serving as a spacer, one margin of the relief wax forms the internal finish line of the framework. It is essential that this finish line be sharply

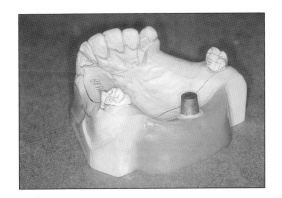

**Fig 10-19** A tapered metal cylinder is positioned on the master cast, thereby establishing the location for the main sprue on the refractory cast.

defined. A properly formed internal finish line permits formation of a butt joint between the framework and the acrylic resin denture base. This allows a smooth transition from metal to resin and minimizes the likelihood of trauma to the adjacent soft tissues. As a rule, the finish line should be placed 1.5 mm from the neighboring abutment or abutments. This distance ensures that the porous resin will not contact the marginal gingivae.

One thickness of baseplate wax makes an ideal relief pad for latticework and mesh components. The baseplate wax is softened over a flame and placed on the corresponding area of the cast. The wax is then luted in position with a hot spatula. This prevents lifting or displacement of relief wax during cast duplication. Special wax sheets with an adhesive on one side also are available to facilitate the adherence of the relief pad (Fig 10-17).

After the relief wax is firmly attached to the cast, it is trimmed with a sharp instrument. This instrument must be held at 90 degrees to the surface of the cast so that the internal finish line of the cast will be sharp and the resin will join the metal at a right angle. If indicated, a 2 × 2–mm section is removed at the prescribed location of the cast stop (Fig 10-18). Again, the blade is held at 90 degrees to the cast.

Trimming any other part of the mesh relief wax is unnecessary. The sheet only needs to cover the design and can end anywhere peripheral to the denture base area.

Relief for small or inoperable tori may be provided using a thin, uniform wax covering. Both the work au-

thorization and the diagnostic cast design should indicate the location and amount of relief needed. When providing relief for tori, the wax borders should be blended with contours of the cast. No sharp demarcation should be visible.

## Sprue guide placement

Some removable partial denture alloys are sprued with an overjet sprue former and reservoir. This technique requires the placement of a small tapered cylinder on the master cast. This cylinder may be made from wax, plastic, or metal and must be placed in the exact position that the main sprue will occupy on the refractory cast (Fig 10-19). Placement of the overjet sprue former is a laboratory procedure and is governed by recommendations from the company that markets the alloy.

## Duplication

Blockout philosophies and techniques are similar regardless of the chosen alloy. In contrast, duplication materials and techniques are alloy specific. As a result, each step is critical and must be followed exactly because refractory cast expansion determines the ultimate fit of the framework. For example, low-heat alloys are used with gypsum-bound refractory materials. In these situations, reversible hydrocolloid with a water base is used for the impression to create the refractory cast. On the other hand, high-heat alloys use phosphate-bound investments and glycerin-based colloids for duplication.

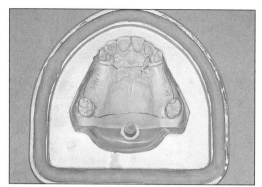

**Fig 10-20** The blocked out master cast is positioned on the base of the duplicating flask.

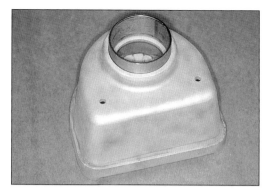

**Fig 10-21** The flask is assembled in preparation for the duplication process.

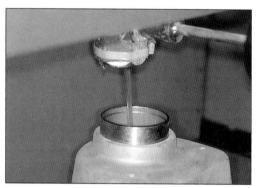

**Fig 10-22** The duplicating flask is slowly filled with reversible hydrocolloid.

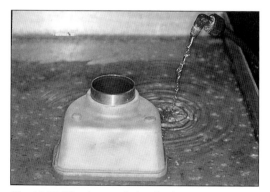

**Fig 10-23** The base of the flask rests in a container of cool, running water.

## Impression

Many similarities exist between duplication techniques, and the following instructions are appropriate regardless of the alloy used. To make the impression, a blocked-out master cast is placed on the base of a duplicating flask (Fig 10-20). The flask is assembled (Fig 10-21), and a steady stream of reversible hydrocolloid is poured into the flask (Fig 10-22). Once filled, the flask is placed in a regulated cooling tank (Fig 10-23). Up to an hour may be required to fully set the colloid. The flask is then disassembled. The master cast is carefully removed with the aid of two knife blades engaging the sides of the cast. Alternatively, the master cast may be removed by directing compressed air at the cast-colloid junction. In either instance, removal of the master cast must be followed by careful examination of the colloid impression (Fig 10-24).

Duplicating colloids can be reused repeatedly. Most laboratories have special equipment to remelt and store the colloid (Fig 10-25). Colloids also can be prepared with less sophisticated equipment. To employ such techniques, clean colloid is cut into small pieces and heated in a double boiler until the material reaches a fluid consistency. The resulting sol is then allowed to cool to working temperature, ensuring suitable flow of the material without melting the blockout wax. A breakdown temperature of 100°C (212°F) and a working temperature of 63°C (145°F) are suitable for most duplicating materials.

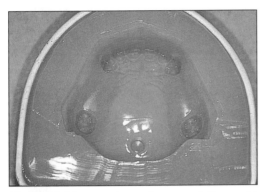

**Fig 10-24** After master cast removal, the mold is carefully inspected for flaws in the hydrocolloid.

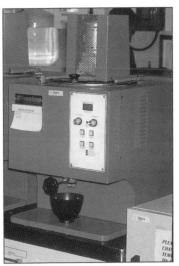

**Fig 10-25** An automated duplicating machine is used in the preparation and storage of reversible hydrocolloid impression material.

### Equipment

During the duplication process, the master cast is centered on the base of a metal duplicating flask and held in place with a claylike material (ie, plasticene). The remainder of the duplicating flask is then positioned on the base, and the flask is filled with warm colloid material. At this stage, the duplicating flask is placed in a cooling bath. The cooling bath is designed so that only the base of the duplicating flask is submerged in cold water. As a result, heat is drawn from the base, causing the colloid to shrink toward the master cast and resulting in an accurate impression.

The water in the cooling bath must be shallow so that only the base of the duplicating flask is cooled. Some manufacturers avoid potential difficulties by creating flasks with sidewalls that are nonconductors, thereby ensuring that setting shrinkage occurs toward the metal base. Other manufacturers market flasks that are completely metal, but since the sides are insulated from the metal base by clay, the setting pattern of the material is the same.

The ideal water bath, used by large commercial laboratories, has a cooling system that circulates water at a regulated temperature. Cold tap water flowing through a sink drain will accomplish the same end, but if the water is too warm, it will take longer to produce complete gelation of the duplicating material.

### Refractory cast

Refractory materials (also termed *investments*) must be measured and mixed according to the manufacturer's instructions if mold expansion is to match the shrinkage of the associated alloy.

Gypsum-bonded refractory materials, commonly called *low-heat investments*, are used for casting Type IV partial denture gold and Ticonium (CMP Industries, Albany, NY). These refractory materials can be heated to 704°C (1,300°F) without causing breakdown of the investment.

Refractory materials used for Vitallium (Austenal, Chicago, IL), Nobillium (CMP Industries), Jelenko's LG (Heraeus Kulzer, Armonk, NY), other chrome-cobalt alloys, titanium, and titanium alloys are termed *high-heat investments* and may be heated to temperatures approximating 1,037°C (1,900°F). These high-heat investments are phosphate bonded and usually

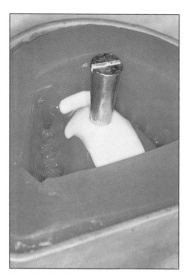

**Fig 10-26** Refractory material is carefully flowed into the mold.

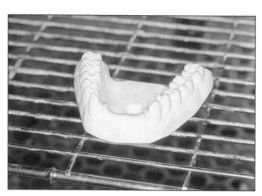

**Fig 10-27** The refractory cast is dried in an oven at 93°C (200°F) for 1 hour.

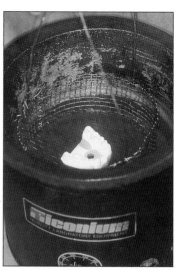

**Fig 10-28** The refractory cast is dipped in hot beeswax.

require a special, silica-containing liquid to mix with the refractory powder.

In removable partial denture fabrication, a cast made from refractory material serves as the foundation for waxing and casting procedures. After the master cast has been removed from the colloid mold, refractory material is carefully introduced into the resultant impression (Fig 10-26). The mold is then placed in a humidor to prevent water loss, which would result in distortion of the colloid.

The time required for complete set of the refractory material is provided by the manufacturer. At the end of this period, the refractory cast is retrieved. This is accomplished by cutting the colloid away from the refractory cast rather than pulling the delicate cast out of the uncut mold. Following removal, the refractory cast is placed in a drying oven at 93°C (200°F) for 30 to 60 minutes (Fig 10-27). When dry, the cast is trimmed to within 6 mm of the proposed design. This is an essential step in ensuring the escape of gases during the casting process. Trimming is usually done on a dry cast trimmer to eliminate the possibility of a slurry mixture accumulating on the cast, changing its contours and dimensions.

## Beeswax dip

The refractory cast is dipped in hot beeswax to ensure a smooth, dense surface and to eliminate the need for soaking the cast prior to the investment process (Fig 10-28). To achieve these objectives, the dry refractory cast is dipped into beeswax at 138°C to 149°C (280°F to 300°F) for 15 seconds. Once dipped, the cast is positioned on its end to allow excess wax to run off. The framework may be waxed when the cast reaches room temperature.

## Waxing the framework

### Design transfer

Before waxing can begin, the design must be transferred from the master cast to the refractory cast. Every effort is made to precisely transfer the outline of the framework to the refractory cast (Fig 10-29). Care is taken to draw with a minimum of pressure so the surface of the refractory cast is not damaged.

The position of individual clasp tips is the most critical part of the transfer. If appropriate ledges were created during blockout procedures, the placement of

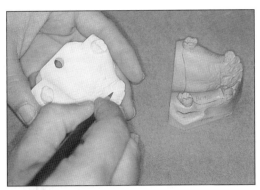

**Fig 10-29** The design is carefully transferred from the master cast to the refractory cast.

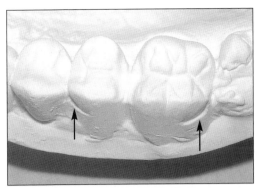

**Fig 10-30** The ledges created in blockout wax *(arrows)* delineate the positions of the retentive clasp tips.

retentive clasp tips is much easier and more precise (Fig 10-30). Other areas of the design outline are not as critical and can be accurately transferred with reasonable care.

## Materials

The availability of prefabricated plastic patterns has dramatically reduced the amount of freehand waxing that must be performed during framework construction. Manufacturers provide a variety of patterns that are alloy specific. The most helpful of these patterns are the clasp arms. As might be expected, pattern choices are greatly influenced by clasp length. A retentive clasp that is longer than 10 mm can be thicker than a shorter clasp, while maintaining the same degree of flexibility. When the clasp is shorter, it must be thinner to ensure adequate flexibility.

Manufacturers also market prefabricated patterns for the construction of major connectors. Some experience is required to evaluate the rigidity of these patterns. In general, those having the recommendation of the manufacturer will have sufficient rigidity for the average situation. The clinician has the responsibility of evaluating the connector and informing the laboratory if design changes are required to improve rigidity.

## Waxing technique

The plastic patterns are "glued" to the refractory cast with a mixture of acetone and plastic pattern scraps

mixed to a watery consistency. This solution, called *tacky liquid*, is painted onto the design outline with a fine brush and allowed to dry for just a few seconds (Fig 10-31). The pattern can then be adapted to the desired position on the refractory cast. Should the pattern separate from the refractory cast, the accuracy of the casting will be lost. Consequently, there is a tendency for the inexperienced technician to apply a thicker coat of the tacky liquid. Although this increases the likelihood that the pattern will stick to the cast, too much tacky liquid will result in a flash of metal around the casting. This excess metal increases the amount of finishing required and may render the casting unusable.

The manufacturer provides plastic patterns arranged on easy-release cards (Fig 10-32). Some care is required to remove these prefabricated patterns without distorting them. If the cards are kept cold (eg, in a standard refrigerator) the patterns can be removed with a quick snap. It is particularly important that retentive clasp patterns are not distorted because the shape of the clasp greatly affects flexibility. Therefore, each clasp pattern should be cut to the desired length using a surgical blade. In turn, the pattern should be separated from the underlying card with a quick lateral motion.

After the plastic patterns have been placed on the refractory cast, they must be adapted without distortion. A pattern adapter purchased through a dental

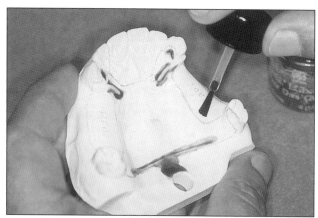

**Fig 10-31** Tacky liquid is painted onto the areas of the cast that will be covered by plastic patterns.

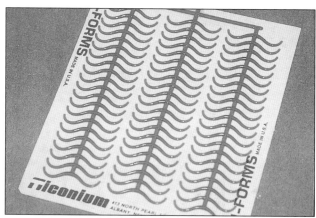

**Fig 10-32** Many manufacturers supply prefabricated plastic patterns that may be applied to the refractory cast.

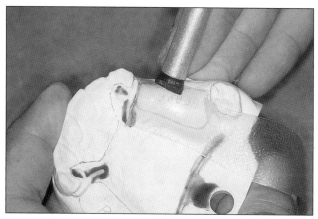

**Fig 10-33** A pattern adapter is used to place plastic patterns onto the cast.

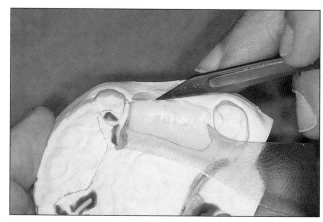

**Fig 10-34** Plastic patterns may be trimmed using a surgical blade.

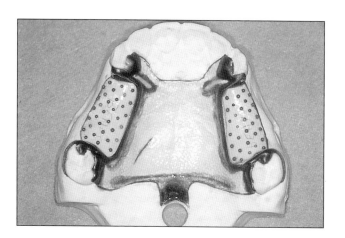

**Fig 10-35** The waxup is completed by joining prefabricated patterns using inlay wax.

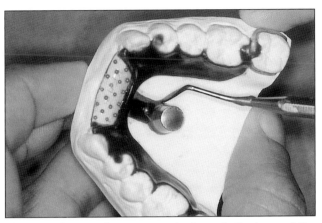

**Fig 10-36** A sprue former extends through the base of the cast and is connected to the waxup.

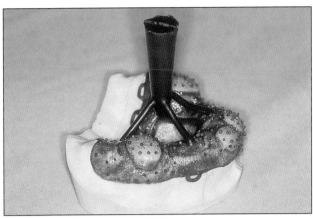

**Fig 10-37** An example of overhead spruing with multiple secondary sprue formers.

manufacturer or a soft rubber pencil eraser shaped into a wedge is most useful in this adaptation (Fig 10-33). Each pattern is placed on the refractory cast at its tip and lightly pressed against the previously applied tacky liquid. The pattern is then carefully positioned along the design outline with the placement tool. At every step of this operation, the technician must exercise extreme care not to stretch the pattern. A blade is used to trim pattern material that extends beyond the outline drawn on the cast (Fig 10-34). While major connector patterns are not normally distorted during this process, retentive clasp patterns often are.

Once the plastic patterns are in place on the refractory cast, these patterns must be joined using wax (Fig 10-35). A wax with a formulation similar to blue inlay wax is indicated because it sets hard and polishes easily. This wax is also used to seal the margins of the major connector and to create the minor connectors and rests. Areas where the resin-retentive elements join the major connector are usually reinforced.

For final contouring, each technician develops his or her own set of instruments. Carvers with small, rounded blades are often used. A standard Hanau torch (Waterpik, Fort Collins, CO) may be too bulky and hot for removable partial denture wax finishing. A smaller, more controlled torch can be made from a hypodermic needle and a piece of rubber hose attached to a natural gas outlet. The flame provided can be used to smooth even the finest details of the wax pattern.

## Spruing the framework

### Technique

The location and geometry of the sprue former is based upon recommendations of the alloy manufacturer. Ticonium is cast using a single sprue former that approaches through the refractory cast (Fig 10-36). Type IV gold and a number of high-heat, chrome-cobalt alloys are cast using a sprue that approaches from above and gives rise to a number of smaller, accessory sprues (Fig 10-37). Regardless of the technique used, special care must be taken to round all sprue connections. Sharp edges in the refractory material can be broken off as molten alloy enters the mold. These displaced fragments can be carried deep within the mold and may ruin the casting.

### Size of sprue former

The dimensions used for sprue formers are critical, and the manufacturer's directions must be followed exactly. Sprue formers must not contain constrictions that would cause the molten metal to flow from a thick to a thin area and then back to a thick area. The turbulence set up by this type of sprue former often results in internal mold deformation and castings that contain unwanted inclusions.

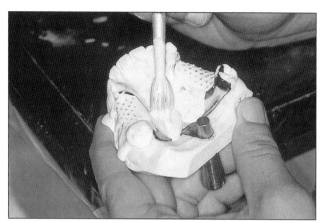

**Fig 10-38** The first layer of investment is painted onto the wax pattern.

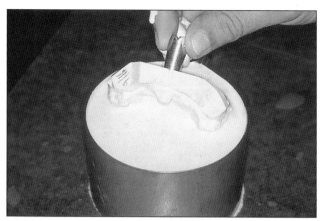

**Fig 10-39** The refractory cast is carefully placed into freshly mixed investment in the mold former.

### Auxiliary sprue formers

Any area that is separated from the bulk of the framework by a long span of latticework or meshwork requires a secondary sprue former. The secondary sprue former is a large-diameter wax cylinder that emerges from the main sprue former to ensure that molten alloy reaches remote areas of the mold cavity (see Fig 10-37). Secondary sprue formers are also required to support heavy metal pontics where the molten metal might be required to flow from thinner areas into the thicker metal pontics. These secondary sprue formers should be one third to one fourth the diameter of the main sprue former and should be gently curved.

## *Investing the refractory cast*

### Two-part mold

Some systems require a two-part investment process, the first part being a 3- to 4-mm "paint-on" layer (Fig 10-38). This layer is carefully brushed onto the waxed refractory cast to ensure that no voids are present.

As soon as the first layer reaches its initial set, the second part of the investment procedure begins. An investment ring large enough to accommodate the refractory cast and its first layer is selected. An appropriate amount of refractory material is measured, mixed, and placed into the investment ring. Subsequently, the refractory cast is moistened, held by the sprue base, and worked into the freshly mixed refractory material (Fig 10-39). Some skill is required to place the cast in

the proper relation to the bottom of the ring, allowing an adequate thickness of investment for the escape of gas during casting without sacrificing mold strength. The position of the sprue former is marked on the outside of the mold to ensure proper orientation in the casting machine.

### Mold storage

Some alloy manufacturers recommend removal of the investment ring before the mold is placed in the furnace for wax elimination. Other manufacturers recommend leaving the ring in place. In either situation, the sprue former is removed and the entrance of the mold is carefully inspected. Any debris or sharp edges that might break off are carefully eliminated. While waiting for wax elimination, the mold is stored in a sealed plastic bag to prevent unnecessary drying of the refractory material.

## *Wax elimination or burnout*

### Time and temperature

The time and temperature required to eliminate wax from the mold cavity is specific to the refractory-alloy system that is being used. Each system is developed to provide mold expansion that closely matches the anticipated shrinkage of the alloy as it solidifies. Since the ultimate fit of the restoration is dependent upon this relationship, the manufacturer's directions must be carefully followed.

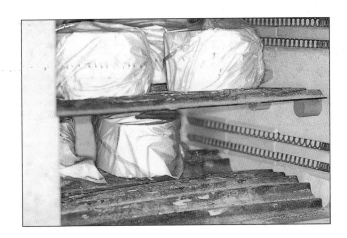

**Fig 10-40** Plastic bags containing molds are placed in a burnout furnace.

## Furnaces

Burnout furnaces can be either electric or gas and must be vented to allow the escape of noxious fumes resulting from this process. Furnaces vary greatly in capacity. Large, industrial-type gas furnaces are capable of holding 25 molds, while small electric furnaces may hold only one or two molds.

Most modern furnaces permit electronic control of both time and temperature. The ovens are often programmable, allowing for a delayed start to the burnout. Using this feature, the wax elimination process can be started at night, preparing the molds for a morning casting cycle. Molds placed into the furnace at the end of the workday should be placed inside sealed plastic bags to prevent dehydration (Fig 10-40). When the furnace starts the burnout cycle hours later, the plastic bags will be consumed by heat.

Although insufficient burnout can result in technical problems such as incomplete casts and insufficient mold expansion, there is little that the clinician can do to influence laboratory management of these areas. Fortunately, most laboratories follow the manufacturer's recommendations.

Heating the mold beyond the intended range inevitably results in a breakdown of the binder and destruction of the mold. Again, modern furnaces protect against this potential problem.

## Casting

Induction casting of removable partial denture frameworks has become the method of choice for contemporary dentistry. Since removable partial denture alloys are cast in the 1,371°C (2,500°F) range, they are particularly technique sensitive. However, expensive induction casting machines allow technicians with minimum experience to cast these alloys successfully (Fig 10-41).

Induction casting is based on the electric currents in a metal core induced from a magnetic field. A heating coil of copper tubing is shaped to fit closely around the casting crucible and is attached to an alternating current source. The alternating current in the coil sets up eddy currents of electrons in the crucible and the alloy. The movement of these currents melts the alloy. The heating coil, also at risk for melting during the heating cycle, is internally cooled by water.

An electronic sensor directly above the crucible measures the temperature of the alloy throughout the heating process (Fig 10-42). This optical sensor activates the casting mechanism at the temperature selected by the operator. Some of these sensing devices, classified as optical pyrometers, are driven by the infrared wavelengths emitted by the molten metal.

The casting arm's spin rate and the temperature required to initiate casting are programmable features on most casting machines. Casting machines have the capability to revolve at up to 600 rpm.

The placement of the alloy ingot into an uncontaminated crucible begins the casting sequence (Fig 10-43). Activation of the alternating current source starts the heating process. While the alloy is heating, the mold is removed from the furnace and placed in the casting arm's holding mechanism (Fig 10-44). This device varies from machine to machine, but in every

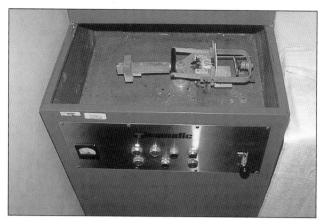

**Fig 10-41** An example of an induction casting machine.

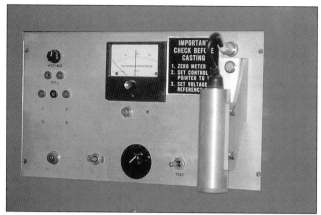

**Fig 10-42** An electronic sensor measures the temperature of the molten metal. When the chosen alloy reaches the appropriate temperature, this sensor activates the casting process.

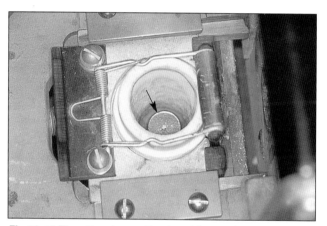

**Fig 10-43** The alloy *(arrow)* is placed into a clean crucible.

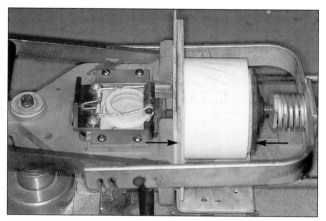

**Fig 10-44** The mold is positioned in the holding mechanism *(arrows).*

case the mold must be balanced by placing a counterweight on the casting arm.

Modern induction casting machines are normally programmed to cast when the alloy has reached the desired temperature. Some alloys require a heat-soak period of up to 3 seconds, during which time the alloy is kept at the casting temperature by a rapid cycling of the alternating current. In addition, some machines allow the operator to determine the exact moment to cast. Technicians who cast using this method require both experience and a means to view the molten metal. Looking directly into the crucible is never recommended unless approved eye protection is used.

## Casting recovery

When the casting process is complete, the mold is removed from the casting machine and allowed to cool according to the manufacturer's instructions. At the appropriate time, the outer layer of refractory material is removed by tapping it with a mallet (Fig 10-45). The remaining investment is then removed by airborne particle abrasion in a self-contained machine manufactured for this purpose (Fig 10-46). Subsequently, the casting is examined for defects. If the casting is deemed satisfactory, finishing and fitting procedures are begun.

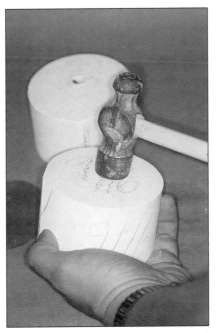

**Fig 10-45** The framework is recovered by lightly tapping the investment with a hammer.

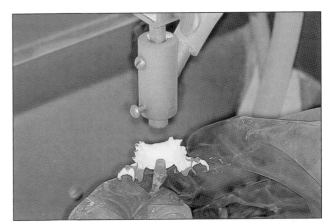

**Fig 10-46** Residual investment is removed using an airborne particle abrasion device.

## Finishing the framework

### Sprue removal

Using high-speed lathes and large abrasive disks, the sprue leads are cut from the casting (Fig 10-47).

### Rough finishing and shaping

Before fitting the framework to the master cast, the major connector is shaped to its ultimate form. In turn, rubber wheels and points are used to give the framework a "satin" finish. Nodules are removed from the surfaces that will contact the teeth. This step must be performed carefully to avoid destroying the frictional fit of the casting.

The casting is then adjusted and finished in an orderly sequence. An experienced technician uses coarser disks and stones and then proceeds to finer grinding agents (Fig 10-48). The intaglio surfaces of critical framework components such as rests, retentive clasp tips, and proximal plates must receive an absolute minimum of finishing (Fig 10-49). The clinician should carefully inspect these areas when the framework is returned from the laboratory and has every right to be concerned if evidence of overfinishing exists.

Electropolishing, a form of electrolytic stripping, is usually the first step in polishing the framework. In this process, atoms of metal from rough projections on the framework go into solution before those in smooth areas do. This results in a very consistent, satin-like surface. The unit pictured in Fig 10-50 is the Ti-Lectro Polisher (CMP Industries). The polishing occurs in a bath of 85% orthophosphoric acid, which is heated to 49°C (120°F) to 60°C (140°F). The anode is attached to the cast and the cast is immersed in the solution (Fig 10-51). Each square inch of metal surface area requires 2 amperes of current for 6 minutes. The average setting is 6 amperes for 6 minutes.

## Fitting the framework

At this stage of the procedure, the technician carefully seats the metal framework on a duplicate master cast. The technician tries to identify areas that prevent seating of the framework. Because the retentive clasp

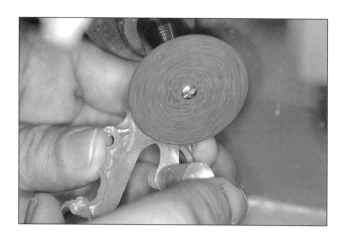

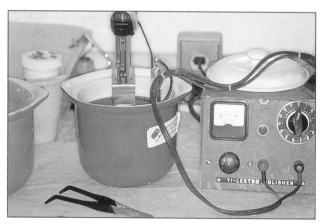
Fig 10-47 The sprue lead is removed using an abrasive disk.

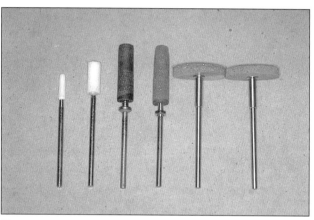
Fig 10-48 White stones, rubber wheels, and rubber disks are included in the finishing armamentarium.

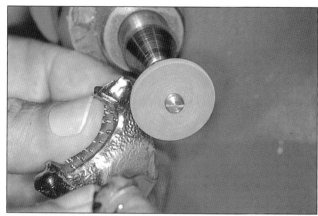
Fig 10-49 Finishing procedures are accomplished on a high-speed lathe.

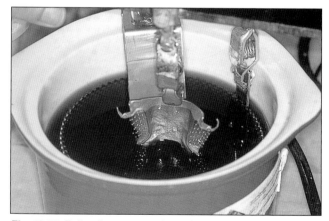
Fig 10-50 The Ti-Lectro Polisher produces a satin-like surface.

Fig 10-51 Following connection of the electrical leads, the framework is lowered into the deplating solution.

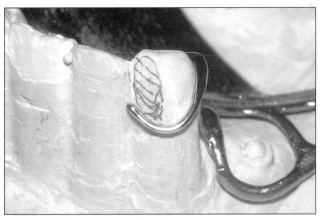

**Fig 10-52** The fitting cast is relieved in the areas that correspond to the retentive clasp tips. This allows the framework to seat without undue binding.

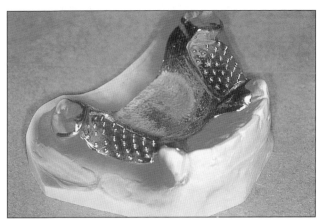

**Fig 10-53** Occlude spray (Pascal, Bellevue, WA) is an excellent disclosing medium used to detect interferences when seating the framework.

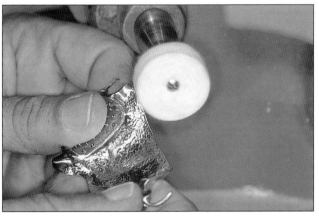

**Fig 10-54** The framework is polished using felt wheels and fine-grit polishing agents.

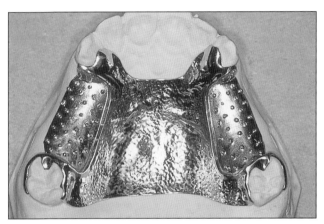

**Fig 10-55** The completed maxillary framework is shown on the duplicate master cast.

tips engage undercut areas, they will be among the first areas to bind. Therefore, the technician carefully relieves the cast in these areas (Fig 10-52). This allows the clasps to pass over the height of contour without binding and simplifies the fitting process.

Following modification of the cast, the fitting process is continued. Special powdered sprays and liquid disclosing media are commercially available to aid in this process (Fig 10-53). An appropriate disclosing medium is selected and applied to the cast. The framework is then seated and subsequently removed. Areas that interfere with seating are identified and relieved using spot-grinding techniques. This process of seating and spot grinding is repeated until the rests are completely seated on the cast.

### Rubber wheeling and final polish

When the casting is completely seated on the master cast and shows no evidence of rocking or distortion, the technician may proceed with rubber wheeling and polishing operations. Alloy manufacturers sell a variety of polishing compounds especially suited to their respective alloys. Rag and felt wheels are used on high-speed lathes to apply polishing agents (Fig 10-54).

Ultrasonic cleaning of the framework is commonly used to remove residual polishing materials. The framework is inspected and, if acceptable, returned to the clinician on the master cast or duplicate master cast (Fig 10-55).

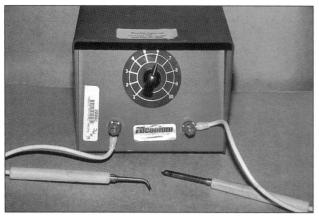

**Fig 10-56** An electrosoldering unit is commonly used to attach wrought wires and metallic loops to a cast framework.

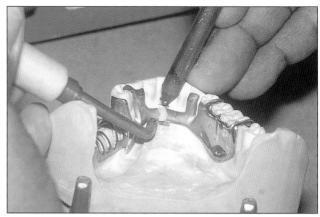

**Fig 10-57** Foil is placed between the cast and the components to be soldered. Electrosoldering tips are placed on each side of the joint to heat the solder.

## Sectioning and soldering the framework

It is strongly suggested that each framework be fitted to the oral cavity before denture bases and prosthetic teeth are added. If the framework cannot be seated, the clinician must (1) decide to have a new framework made or (2) attempt to correct the fit of the existing framework via sectioning and soldering procedures. Although the latter approach is commonly used in the fabrication of fixed partial dentures, it is much more difficult to accomplish with removable partial dentures. This is largely due to the size and complexity of removable partial denture castings.

Minor connectors and some major connectors can be sectioned and soldered with either precious or nonprecious brazing alloys. This type of soldering is normally done with an electrosoldering device (Fig 10-56), a common piece of equipment in many removable partial denture laboratories.

Sectioned segments must be satisfactorily related in the mouth and then transferred with either a plaster index or a resin matrix to the laboratory. At this stage, the technician carefully pours a soldering cast against the properly related segments. Foil is placed over the area of the proposed solder joint (Fig 10-57), and the soldering operation is completed.

## Adjusting occlusion

Preliminary adjustments to the occlusion of a removable partial denture framework should be accomplished in the laboratory. To increase adjustment accuracy and to maximize technician efforts, the clinician should provide an opposing cast and suitable interocclusal records.

Occlusal and incisal rests are sometimes made excessively thick to ensure complete casting. In many instances, the rests are waxed into hyperocclusion to develop needed bulk. Once cast, these areas are adjusted to return to the proper occlusal vertical dimension. This procedure requires properly articulated maxillary and mandibular casts.

Although the clinician has the responsibility of creating sufficient space for the framework, there are occasions when the technician will be called upon to make adjustments for inadequate occlusal clearance. Once the framework has been adjusted to the minimum required dimensions, the interfering part of the opposing cast should be relieved and clearly marked with a red pencil. In this way, a potential problem area is called to the attention of the clinician. This approach allows the clinician the option of performing the final framework adjustment personally, reducing the opposing tooth, or both.

## Wrought-wire retentive clasp arms

Retentive clasp arms can be constructed of wrought wire as well as cast alloy. Many clinicians prefer wire clasps, believing they are more adjustable and adaptable than are cast clasps. Since wrought wire is normally round, it has the potential to flex equally in all directions. This uniform flexibility is thought to apply less force than a half-round clasp, which flexes in only one plane.

Wires available for removable partial dentures normally range from 17 through 20 gauge. These wires may be made of precious (gold, palladium, platinum, silver) or nonprecious (stainless steel, nickel-chromium, nickel-chromium-cobalt) alloys. Because of the high cost of precious metals, 18- and 19-gauge nickel-chromium-cobalt wires are currently the most popular. While nonprecious wires are not as resilient as precious wires, they have proven to be clinically dependable.

Wrought-wire clasps are commonly used on a variety of interim and transitional prostheses and as repair additions for fractured or distorted cast clasps (Fig 10-58). The clinician should develop and maintain skill in the manipulation of the wrought-wire clasp.

Wire-bending skills vary greatly, with few concrete rules to guide the student. In general, the best results occur when the wire is held with pliers and bent with the fingers (Fig 10-59). Rather than attempting to start at the clasp tip to form the entire clasp from that point, the beginning student may find it easier to estimate and bend the wire in a basic curve that corresponds to the surface of the tooth to be clasped. The wire curve can then be moved along the tooth until it coincides with the desired clasp position (Fig 10-60). Any part of the wire extending beyond the intended clasp tip can be identified and subsequently removed (Fig 10-61). This technique is most applicable to nonprecious wires because of their low cost. The same approach is indicated for clasp forms other than circumferential.

Wire clasps can be attached to the removable partial denture in four ways. The first of these is to embed the wire into the resin of the denture base. This method is most commonly used in repair situations. Another method calls for the wire clasp to be incorporated into the wax pattern. Metal is then cast to the wire, a procedure that can adversely affect clasp longevity.

The most dependable results are achievable by soldering the wire clasp to the framework after the framework is completed. If the clasp is soldered at the rest–minor connector junction, the heat of the soldering operation will adversely affect the physical characteristics of the wire. As a result, the best method of attaching a wrought-wire clasp to the framework is by soldering it on the latticework, well away from the area where it will be required to flex (Fig 10-62). In this manner, the destructive potential of the soldering operation will be limited to an area covered by denture base resin. The soldering itself is best done with an electrosoldering device and nickel-based industrial alloys (solders). Precious metal solders can be used, but they give no particular advantage unless the joint area will not be covered with resin. Should the joint be exposed to the oral fluids, the ability of the precious metal solders to withstand corrosion and tarnish makes them the materials of choice. The electrosoldering technique is far easier to master than is torch soldering and permits the use of very high-fusing solders. Fluxes containing fluoride must be used in this procedure. The electrosoldering machine is basically a step-up transformer with two terminals, one copper and one carbon. When the carbon tip is placed on the solder and the copper tip on the framework a short distance from the soldering area, the electric circuit is completed through the framework and the electric energy, dissipated as heat (resistance), melts the solder.

Laser welding represents a fourth method for joining a wire to the framework. The laser welder shown in Fig 10-63 is a pulsed, solid-state neodymium:yttrium-aluminum-garnet (Nd:YAG) unit. Objects to be welded are placed into the unit through the sleeve arms located on the sides. The operator holds the appliance and focuses crosshair sights through a 12-power stereomicroscope onto the area that will be exposed to the laser. The unit is foot controlled. When the aiming beam is properly aligned, the operator activates the foot control, sending a laser pulse to the metal (Fig 10-64). An automatic shield in the unit protects the operator's eyes from accidental exposure. The operator controls the length and energy intensity with adjustment dials on the front of the unit. Argon gas within the unit improves the quality of the weld by reducing the effects of oxygen in the immediate atmosphere. The laser pulse is 0.5 mm in diameter and the

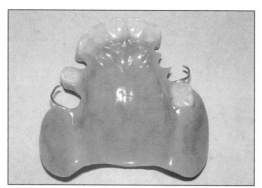

**Fig 10-58** Wrought-wire clasps are frequently used in interim prostheses.

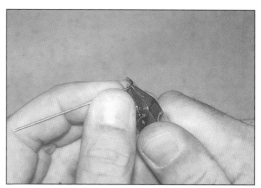

**Fig 10-59** For best results, a wire should be held with pliers and bent with the fingers.

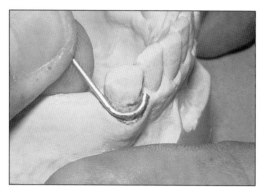

**Fig 10-60** The contoured wire is positioned on the cast to coincide with the desired clasp position.

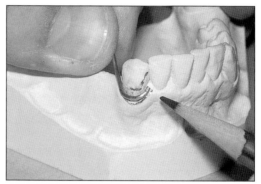

**Fig 10-61** The wire is marked with a pencil to indicate the tip of the clasp. Excess wire then will be removed using wire cutters.

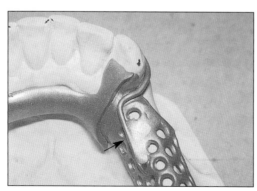

**Fig 10-62** The ideal soldering location for a wrought-wire clasp is on the retentive latticework or meshwork *(arrow)*, far away from the area of clasp flexure.

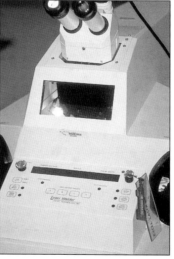

**Fig 10-63** A laser welder can be used to join components of a removable partial denture.

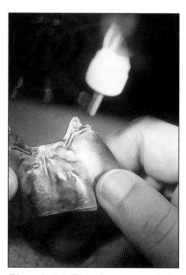

**Fig 10-64** The framework is placed within the chamber of the laser welder. Welding occurs in an argon-rich environment, which improves the quality of the weld.

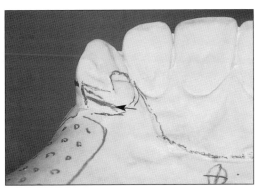

**Fig 10-65** The partial denture design shows the prescribed position of the twin-flex clasp *(arrow)*.

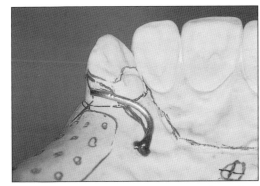

**Fig 10-66** A wrought-wire clasp is adapted to the master cast.

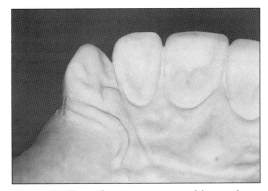

**Fig 10-67** The refractory cast provides a channel to facilitate placement of the wrought-wire clasp.

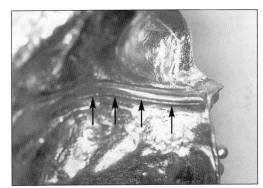

**Fig 10-68** The twin-flex clasp *(arrows)* is soldered into the channel.

energy generated can produce temperatures of 10,000°C (18,000°F). Normally, no finishing is needed on the soldered or laser-joined clasp if the joint is to be enclosed within denture base resin.

## Twin-flex clasp

The twin-flex clasp is a unique application of wrought wire. This clasp can provide a flexible clasp that is less noticeable to the patient. In the twin-flex technique, a Ticonium 19-gauge wrought wire is adapted into a measured undercut area on the proximal surface of an abutment on the master cast (Figs 10-65 and 10-66). A small amount of wax is added around the clasp, ultimately creating a channel in the tissue surface of the major connector following standard duplication and refractory cast procedures (Fig 10-67). After framework

casting and finishing, the original wrought wire is removed from the master cast and soldered into the channel (Fig 10-68). The outcome is a flexible, hidden clasp that engages an interproximal undercut.

## ▢ Conclusions

Although the clinician's direct involvement with construction phases of the removable partial denture framework is impractical, each dentist should be aware of the techniques and processes used in prosthesis fabrication. The dentist who has the confidence to guide framework construction and maintain a rational dialogue with laboratory personnel is certain to benefit. The information in this chapter, broad as it is, can serve as the basis for improved dentist-laboratory relations.

## ▢ Bibliography

Belles DM. The Twin-Flex clasp: An esthetic alternative. J Prosthet Dent 1997;77:450–452.

Henderson CW, Schwartz RS, Herbold ET, Mayhew RB. Evaluation of the barrier system, an infection control system for the dental laboratory. J Prosthet Dent 1987;58:517–521.

Hickey JD. Responsibility of the dentist in removable partial dentures. J Ky Dent Assoc 1965;17:70–87.

Mansueto MA, Phoenix RD. The Twin-Flex removable partial denture: Design, fabrication, and clinical usage. J Prosthodont 1998;7:268–272.

Olin PS, Clay DJ, Look JO. Current prosthodontic practice: A dental laboratory survey. J Prosthet Dent 1989;61:742–745.

Rudd KD, Morrow RM, Rhoads JE. Dental Laboratory Procedures. Vol 3: Removable partial dentures, ed 2. St Louis: Mosby, 1986.

St Arnault FD, Allen DL. Dental laboratory work authorization forms: A survey. J Prosthet Dent 1990;64:497–501.

United States Air Force Medical Service. Dental Laboratory Technology. Vol 2: Removable prosthodontics [Air Force Pamphlet 162-6]. Washington, DC: Department of the Air Force Medical Service, 1991.

# Fitting the Framework

There are three phases in removable partial denture service. The first phase begins with examination of the patient and concludes with design of the proposed prosthesis. The second phase involves mouth preparation and construction of the removable partial denture. The third phase involves fitting the prosthesis to the patient. This chapter deals with the initial stages of the fitting process. More specifically, it addresses the process for fitting the metal framework to the mouth.

No matter how much care is taken during the clinical and laboratory phases of removable partial denture service, some discrepancies in the fit of the framework will occur. Improvements in materials and techniques have reduced the number and size of these discrepancies, but have not eliminated them. As might be expected, controlling these errors can be a monumental task. It is hoped that discrepancies can be held to a minimum, but these discrepancies must be corrected if the practitioner is to provide the health service that the patient deserves.

It has been estimated that as many as 75% of removable partial dentures do not fit the mouth on the day of insertion. Improper fit may contribute to move-ment of the associated teeth and may result in discomfort. Improper fit also may be the primary reason that many removable partial dentures are not worn.

The practitioner must ensure that each framework fits extremely well. This requires patience, careful examination, and precise adjustment. Each completed removable partial denture must be completely passive in the mouth. When the prosthesis is fully seated, it should not exert forces on the teeth or the soft tissues. Uncontrolled forces can produce movement of the remaining teeth and cause damage to the soft tissues and supporting bone.

The practitioner must remember that the tip of each retentive clasp is designed to lie passively in a measured undercut. If the tip of a retentive clasp cannot reach this undercut, it will not be passive. Instead, it will exert potentially damaging forces on the associated abutment (Fig 11-1). The usual result is that the tooth becomes sore. Radiographs also may indicate crestal bone loss and widening of the periodontal ligament space. To prevent periodontal complications, the practitioner must ensure that all components of the removable partial denture are properly fitted to the teeth and soft tissues.

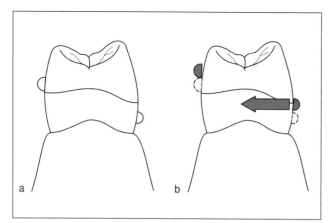

**Fig 11-1** *(a)* When completely seated, a properly fabricated clasp assembly will not apply lateral forces to the associated abutment. *(b)* If the clasp assembly is incompletely seated, the retentive arm will apply potentially damaging lateral forces *(arrow)* to the abutment.

The metal framework should be fitted to the mouth shortly after it is returned from the dental laboratory. This will decrease the likelihood of tooth movement and simplify the fitting process. Movement of the teeth is not likely to occur unless there is a long delay between making the master impression and fitting the metal framework. Periodontal therapy and extractions adjacent to the abutment teeth may increase the likelihood of migration and should be considered when planning treatment and scheduling appointments.

## ▢ Examination of Framework

The metal framework should be carefully examined upon its return from the dental laboratory. The practitioner should ensure that all directions have been followed and that the metal framework accurately fits the master cast. The importance of this examination sequence cannot be overemphasized.

Although most schools no longer require students to perform the laboratory procedures necessary to construct removable partial dentures, it is imperative that the practitioner be able to recognize deficiencies in a completed framework. To expedite the examination of the completed laboratory work, the following questions should be addressed.

## *Was the proposed design closely followed?*

1. Has the major connector been positioned as requested?
2. Are the finish lines for acrylic resin denture bases properly positioned?
3. Have the required rests been included?
4. Are the designated clasp assemblies present and complete?
5. Do the retentive clasp arms display the appropriate sizes, shapes, and positions?
6. Have soft tissue undercuts been handled as directed?

Dental laboratory personnel should never alter a design without consulting the dentist who submitted the work authorization order. If any discrepancy exists between the prescribed design and the framework returned by the laboratory, the reason for the difference should be determined.

## *Does the framework fit the master cast accurately?*

A properly constructed framework should fit tightly against the cast (Fig 11-2). In fact, it may be difficult to remove the framework from the underlying cast because of the roughness of the dental stone. If the framework accurately fits the stone cast, the practitioner may adjust the stone teeth to facilitate framework placement and removal.

1. *Are the rests fully seated in their preparations?* The rests should be closely adapted to the contours of the associated rest seats (Fig 11-3). If the margins of the rests are not flush with contours of the rest seats, the reason(s) should be determined. If a framework does not fit the master cast, it is highly unlikely that it will fit the mouth.
2. *Are reciprocal clasp arms and/or lingual plating in intimate contact with tooth surfaces?* If the blockout, waxing, and metal finishing were correctly done, there should be no space between the metal framework and the surfaces of the associated teeth (Fig 11-4). Spaces that exist in these locations are potentially damaging because debris can collect between the framework and the teeth. This may result in decalci-

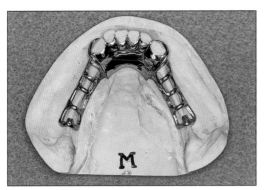

**Fig 11-2** The completed framework must be examined to ensure that it fits the cast accurately.

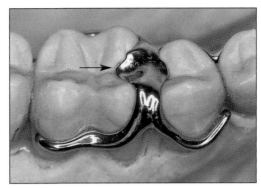

**Fig 11-3** Rests must be completely seated in the corresponding rest seats *(arrow)*.

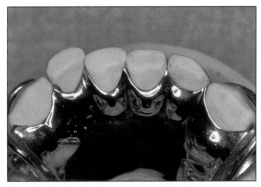

**Fig 11-4** Lingual plating should be closely adapted to the surface of the cast.

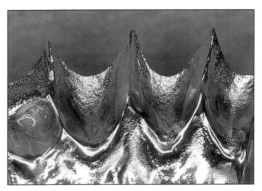

**Fig 11-5** The tissue surface of the framework should exhibit a fine matte texture. This surface should not be highly polished.

**Fig 11-6** The external surface of the framework should be extremely smooth and should be polished to a high shine.

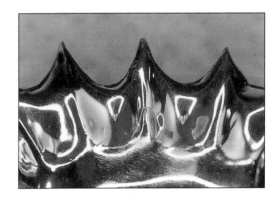

fication of the teeth or inflammation of the soft tissues.

3. *Have finishing and polishing procedures been carried out correctly?* The tissue surface of the framework should be finished to a fine matte texture (Fig 11-5). Polishing of the tissue surface is not indicated because removal of additional metal adversely affects the fit of the framework.

The external surface of the framework should be finished and subsequently polished to a high shine (Fig 11-6). The highly polished external surface provides increased comfort and is less likely to retain plaque and debris.

Both the internal and the external surfaces of the framework should be examined for nodules and other artifacts that may prevent complete seating or

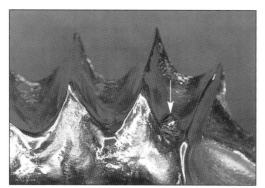

**Fig 11-7** All surfaces should be checked for nodules *(arrow)*, which may produce discomfort and prevent complete seating of the framework.

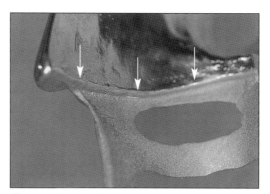

**Fig 11-8** Internal finish lines *(arrows)* should be sharply defined.

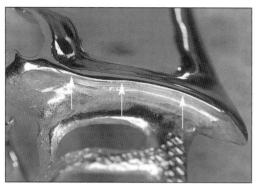

**Fig 11-9** External finish lines *(arrows)* should be sharply defined and slightly undercut to permit improved retention of acrylic resin denture bases.

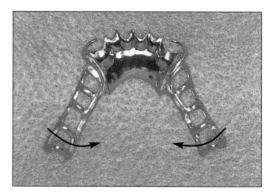

**Fig 11-10** Finger pressure should be applied to both sides of the framework simultaneously *(arrows)*. The framework should be rigid enough to resist flexure.

produce patient discomfort (Fig 11-7). These surfaces should also be checked for pits and scratches that may retain oral debris. These irregularities should be eliminated before the framework is transferred to the patient's mouth.

Internal and external finish lines should be sharply defined and slightly undercut to provide firm mechanical locks for acrylic resin denture bases (Figs 11-8 and 11-9). These areas also should be checked to ensure that the metal framework is thick enough to resist fracture. Excessive thinning sometimes occurs because of the proximity of internal and external finish lines. If the metal is unduly thinned, fracture of the metal framework may occur.

Clasps also should be examined to ensure that they are free from nicks and notches, which could predispose them to fracture. Retentive clasps should display smoothly tapering contours, while reciprocal clasps should display consistent thicknesses.

4. *Is the major connector sufficiently rigid?* The rigidity of the major connector should be tested using light-to-moderate finger pressure (Fig 11-10). If the framework displays significant flexure during this process, it should not be used. Rigidity is the first and most important requirement of a major connector. Lack of rigidity can result in the localization of destructive forces and may cause traumatic injury to the teeth, soft tissues, and underlying bone.

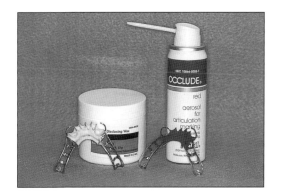

**Fig 11-11** A variety of disclosing media are available. These are commonly supplied as waxes and sprays.

## ◻ Clinical Procedures

This appointment has two separate objectives. The first is to fit the framework to the teeth and soft tissues of the supporting arch. The second is to adjust the framework to the opposing occlusion. The framework always must be fitted to the supporting arch before occlusal adjustments are made.

### Fitting the framework to supporting teeth and soft tissues

In most instances, a metal framework will fit the supporting arch reasonably well with little or no adjustment. Nevertheless, the fit of a framework must never be taken for granted. It is almost always possible to improve the fit of a framework by judicious grinding of the metal.

Frameworks that are close to being accurately fitted can be as damaging to the oral structures as poorly fitting frameworks. A partial denture that is not quite seated can produce discomfort and destruction beyond what might be expected. Therefore, the practitioner must always remember that "near fit" is not sufficient. An accurate fit is essential for prosthodontic success. The few minutes required to improve the adaptation of a framework will be more than offset by the increased level of patient satisfaction and the decreased need for subsequent adjustments.

#### Disclosing media
To properly adjust a removable partial denture framework, the practitioner must identify areas of interference and binding. This may be accomplished using a number of commercially available disclosing media (Fig 11-11). Spray-type disclosing media are often used during fitting procedures. While sprays are convenient, they are often messy and difficult to control in the presence of moisture. Consequently, spray-type disclosing media should not be used for intraoral fitting procedures.

Disclosing wax is easy to use and will provide excellent results if it is properly read. The practitioner must learn to differentiate between areas of excessive pressure and those caused by the intimate adaptation of guiding surfaces. The practitioner also must learn to recognize the displacement of wax on retentive clasps, as well as the "tearing" that occurs as the result of adherence to the teeth. The ability to differentiate between these phenomena must be developed via careful thought and observation.

The greatest advantage of disclosing wax over other disclosing agents is its three-dimensional nature. Because the wax is translucent, it provides clear visual evidence regarding framework adaptation. In thin films, disclosing wax takes on the grayish appearance of the removable partial denture framework. In thicker films, the wax appears white. Therefore, disclosing wax will indicate not only whether a framework is well adapted to the associated teeth, but also areas of binding and areas that display substantial misfit. While a cursory clinical examination may indicate that the framework fits adequately, disclosing wax may demonstrate a 1- to 2-mm space between the internal surface of a rest and the corresponding rest seat. Such errors must be addressed if removable partial denture therapy is to be successful.

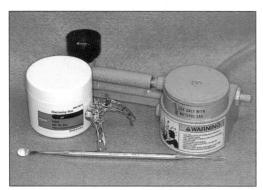

**Fig 11-12** The armamentarium for wax application includes the wax itself, a heat source, and a waxing instrument.

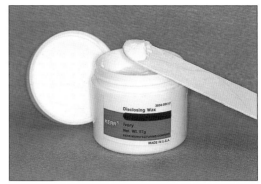

**Fig 11-13** To prevent contamination of the remaining material, disclosing wax is removed from its container using a clean tongue depressor.

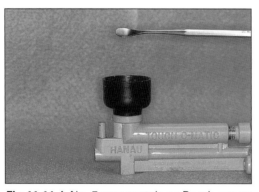

**Fig 11-14** A No. 7 wax spatula or Roach carver is heated over a laboratory burner.

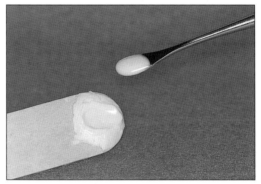

**Fig 11-15** The heated instrument is used to gather disclosing wax.

**Application and use of disclosing wax** The armamentarium for wax application includes the disclosing wax itself, a heat source, and a suitable waxing instrument (Fig 11-12). Disclosing wax generally is supplied in a glass or plastic container. To prevent contamination of the remaining material, a small amount of disclosing wax is removed from the container using a clean tongue depressor (Fig 11-13). A No. 7 wax spatula or a Roach carver is then heated and used to gather disclosing wax (Figs 11-14 and 11-15). In turn, the melted disclosing wax is applied to framework surfaces that will contact the teeth (Fig 11-16). A thin, even coat of wax is desired.

Following application of the disclosing wax, the framework is aligned over the teeth. Finger pressure is applied in the planned path of insertion (Figs 11-17 and 11-18). If significant resistance is met, the framework should be removed and examined for signs of distortion. A framework should never be forced into position if significant resistance is encountered.

During insertion, the practitioner should pay particular attention to the clasp assemblies. It is very easy to trap the buccal mucosa between a clasp and the corresponding tooth. This can result in severe discomfort and can shake the patient's confidence in the dentist.

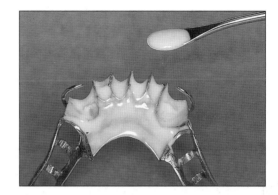

**Fig 11-16** Disclosing wax is applied to the intaglio of the framework.

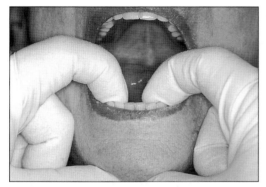

**Fig 11-17** The framework is properly aligned and gentle finger pressure is applied.

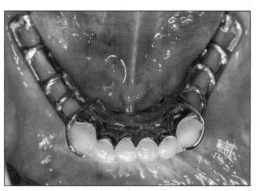

**Fig 11-18** A well-fitting framework should go into place with relative ease.

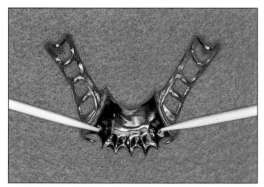

**Fig 11-19** In this instance, cingulum rests were employed. Therefore, pressure was applied over the lingual surfaces of the canines *(indicators)*.

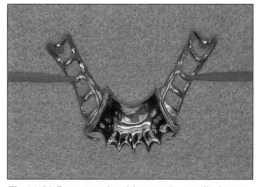

**Fig 11-20** Pressure should never be applied to extension base areas of a framework *(indicators)*.

When the framework is in place, firm vertical pressure is applied to rests (Fig 11-19). A mirror handle may be used to apply this seating force, but care must be taken to ensure that the instrument does not slip and cause injury to the patient.

In the case of a distal extension framework, no pressure should be applied over the distal extension area (Fig 11-20). This would cause the framework to rock and would produce misleading results in the disclosing wax.

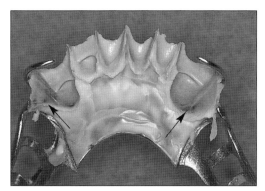

**Fig 11-21** Upon removal of the framework, the disclosing wax is carefully examined. Areas of show-through *(arrows)* are identified.

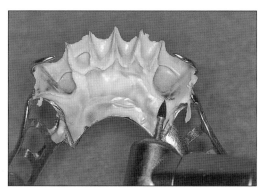

**Fig 11-22** Areas that have been identified as true interferences are carefully modified using a multifluted finishing bur in a high-speed handpiece.

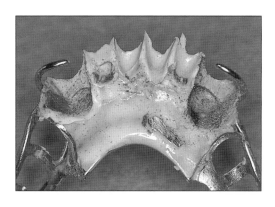

**Fig 11-23** Metal shavings often become embedded in the disclosing wax as a result of grinding procedures. If the contaminated wax is not removed, these particles will interfere with seating of the framework.

## Correcting discrepancies

The framework is carefully removed from the mouth to avoid damaging the surface of the disclosing wax. The surface of the wax is examined for areas of metal show-through (Fig 11-21). Areas of show-through represent interferences that prevent complete seating of the framework. The most common areas of interference occur at the shoulders of circumferential clasps and at the interproximal extensions of lingual plating. As a result, the practitioner should pay particular attention to these areas.

During the fitting process, the practitioner must differentiate between true areas of interference and those areas that represent guiding surfaces. Guiding surfaces produce thinning of the wax due to pro-

longed contact between prominent tooth surfaces and the internal aspects of the corresponding framework. Although the disclosing wax appears thin, the framework should not be relieved in these areas. These surfaces define the path of insertion and removal and, in many cases, provide reciprocation for clasp assemblies.

Areas that have been defined as true interferences must be carefully machined. This is accomplished using a multifluted carbide bur in a high-speed handpiece (Fig 11-22). Machining produces metal shavings that become embedded in the remaining wax (Fig 11-23). As a result, all remaining wax is removed and fresh wax is applied. The most efficient way to remove the wax is by gently heating the framework and then

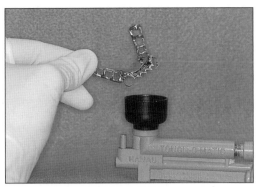

**Fig 11-24** The framework is heated over a laboratory burner to facilitate removal of contaminated disclosing wax.

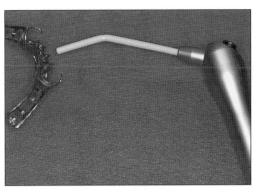

**Fig 11-25** Melted wax is eliminated from the framework using an air syringe.

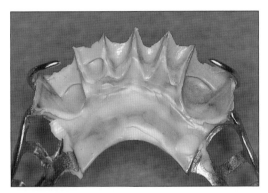

**Fig 11-26** When the framework has been properly adjusted, the disclosing wax displays a grayish hue.

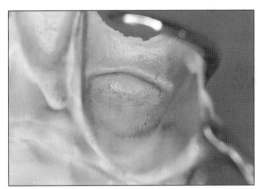

**Fig 11-27** Inspection of a properly adjusted framework reveals a thin, even layer of disclosing wax on the intaglio surface.

using an air syringe to blow the melted wax from the framework (Figs 11-24 and 11-25). The entire sequence is repeated until all interferences have been removed and the framework is fully seated.

The framework fits properly when the disclosing wax is evenly displaced. If cobalt-chromium, nickel-chromium, or titanium alloys are used, the wax will have a characteristic grayish hue (Figs 11-26 and 11-27).

In addition to changes in the appearance of the disclosing wax, adjustment also produces noticeable changes in the feel of partial denture placement. Instead of a "grating" sensation, which is often present at the beginning of the appointment, proper adjustment yields a distinct "gliding" sensation.

The time required to properly adjust the framework to the supporting teeth will vary depending on the amount of grinding that must be done. An experienced practitioner should be able to complete this portion of the adjustment process in 15 to 20 minutes. If adjustment requires unusual time and effort, the practitioner must determine whether correction is possible. If the practitioner determines that adjustment of the framework will not yield a suitable result, a new impression should be made and a new master cast should be generated. The previous master cast should be discarded since it represents an inaccurate reproduction of the dental arch. In addition, it may have been marred by placement of the ill-fitting framework.

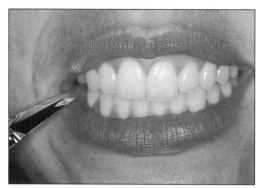

**Fig 11-28** Shim stock is used to identify the patient's existing occlusal contacts. This pattern of occlusal contacts also must be present following insertion and adjustment of removable partial denture framework.

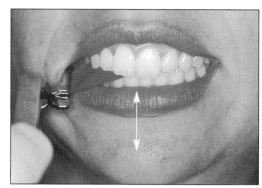

**Fig 11-29** Thin articulating paper is used to evaluate centric contacts as the patient taps the teeth together in a vertical motion *(arrow)*.

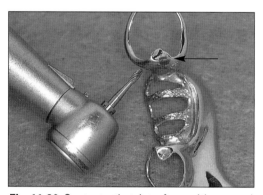

**Fig 11-30** Contacts that interfere with normal closure *(arrow)* are eliminated using a multifluted carbide bur in a high-speed handpiece.

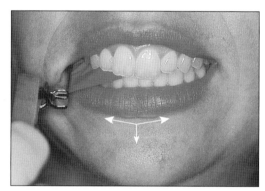

**Fig 11-31** Articulating paper is used to evaluate eccentric contacts. This is accomplished by having the patient make right lateral, left lateral, and protrusive movements *(arrows)* with the articulating paper between the teeth.

## Fitting the framework to the opposing occlusion

After the framework has been fitted to the teeth, it must be adjusted to the opposing occlusion. The framework must not keep the natural teeth from making normal occlusal contacts in centric or eccentric closures.

The simplest and most reliable method for correcting occlusal errors is to have the patient close into the desired position with nothing in the mouth. In this position, the relationships of the maxillary and mandibular teeth can be noted. Most patients have one or more occlusal contacts at this position (Fig 11-28). The practitioner must ensure that the same pattern of contact exists when each framework is placed individually. This pattern also must exist when maxillary and mandibular frameworks are placed in the mouth simultaneously.

In a clinical setting, one framework is positioned in the mouth and the patient is guided into the appropriate closure. The amount of occlusal interference is determined by observing the amount of space between the remaining natural teeth. Thin articulating paper is then placed over the teeth on one side of the arch, and the patient is directed to tap the teeth together with a light vertical force (Fig 11-29). This procedure is then repeated for the opposite side of the arch. Contact produces a transfer of ink from the articulating paper to those areas that are touching during closure.

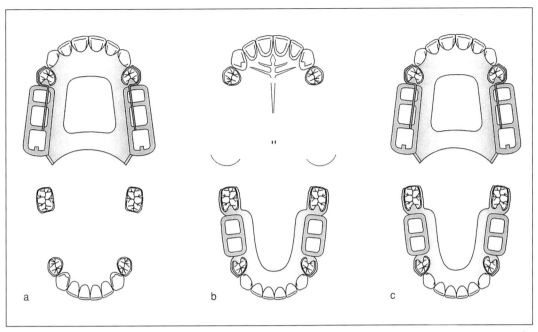

**Fig 11-32** *(a)* The maxillary framework is fitted and the occlusion is adjusted. *(b)* The mandibular framework is fitted and the occlusion is adjusted. *(c)* Frameworks are placed simultaneously and the occlusion is adjusted.

Contact that occurs on the framework interferes with normal closure. Undesirable contact is eliminated by grinding the offending area or areas of the metal framework. To promote patient comfort, all adjustments should be accomplished with the framework out of the mouth. Reduction of the framework is best accomplished using a multifluted carbide bur in a high-speed handpiece (Fig 11-30). The framework is then returned to the mouth and the procedure is repeated until the patient's original contacts have been reestablished.

When the patient's original contacts have been reestablished, the practitioner should evaluate all eccentric movements. This is accomplished by having the patient make lateral and protrusive movements with articulating paper between the teeth (Fig 11-31). Eccentric interferences are corrected using the same armamentarium and techniques described in the preceding paragraphs.

If maxillary and mandibular frameworks have been constructed, the frameworks should be fitted individually. After each framework has been corrected individ-

ually, maxillary and mandibular frameworks should be placed simultaneously (Fig 11-32). Any interference will occur between the metal of the opposing frameworks. Therefore, a final correction is made using articulating paper to locate the points of interference. Adjustments are performed using a multifluted carbide bur in a high-speed handpiece.

## Important considerations

Corrective grinding procedures should always be performed with great care. The practitioner must avoid overcutting the metal surfaces, since this process may weaken important elements of the removable partial denture framework. If an occlusal rest is removed as a result of overcutting, support will be compromised. This necessitates repair or refabrication of the framework. Undue thinning of a clasp also may result in mechanical failure and require repair or refabrication.

To avoid undue thinning of a framework, the practitioner should use a metal thickness gauge (Fig 11-33). A metal thickness gauge allows the practitioner to rapidly and accurately evaluate the dimen-

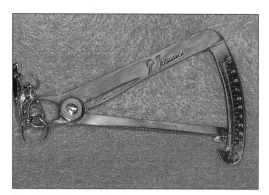

**Fig 11-33** A metal thickness gauge is used to ensure that the framework is not thinned excessively.

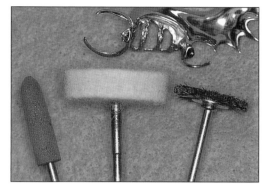

**Fig 11-34** Upon completion of the adjustment process, the framework is finished and polished with an array of rubber points, felt wheels, and brushes.

sions of a removable partial denture framework. In this manner, overcutting may be avoided.

In rare instances, the practitioner may choose to reshape the opposing tooth rather than perform additional adjustments on a removable partial denture framework. Reduction of opposing teeth should be avoided if possible. If this method is employed, the practitioner must ensure that the patient's natural occlusion remains stable with or without the prosthesis in position. While minor adjustments to the opposing teeth are permissible, a consistent pattern of adjustments usually indicates inadequate planning and insufficient preparation of abutments. These shortcomings should be avoided.

### Finishing and polishing ground surfaces

After the framework has been fitted to the supporting teeth and opposing occlusal surfaces, the corrected surfaces must be finished and polished. This is accomplished using mounted stones, as well as carborundum-impregnated wheels and points (Fig 11-34). The operator must be careful not to destroy the fit of removable partial denture components. An adequate thickness of metal must be preserved to minimize the likelihood of breakage during function.

An experienced practitioner should require 30 to 45 minutes for this appointment. A beginning practitioner may require 2 to 3 hours.

### ⌨ Next Appointment

Before dismissing the patient, the practitioner should determine what treatment will be provided at the next appointment. Treatment may follow several courses, including the following:

1. Corrected cast impression procedures. This appointment is necessary for patients requiring mandibular distal extension removable partial dentures, those requiring long-span maxillary distal extension removable partial dentures, and those requiring long-span anterior replacements.
2. Jaw relation records. This appointment is required for patients who do not need corrected cast impression procedures, yet do not have a sufficient number and distribution of teeth to permit accurate hand articulation of casts. Jaw relation records may be made at the framework try-in appointment if sufficient time is available.
3. Esthetic try-in. This appointment is required for patients who do not need corrected cast impression procedures or jaw relation records, but who will have anterior teeth replaced with denture teeth on a denture base.
4. Insertion. If none of the foregoing appointments are needed, the removable partial denture may be completed and inserted at the next appointment. When all the replacement teeth are reinforced

acrylic pontics or metal pontics, insertion may be accomplished during the framework-fitting appointment. If this is the case, home care instructions should be provided and an appropriate recall schedule should be established.

## ⊟ **Bibliography**

Kaiser DA, Wise HB. Fitting cast gold restorations with the aid of disclosing wax. J Prosthet Dent 1980;43:227–228.

Ostlund LE. Improving the marginal fit of cast restorations. J Am Acad Gold Foil Oper 1974;17:56–65.

Rudd KD, Dunn BW. Accurate removable partial dentures. J Prosthet Dent 1967;18:559–570.

Shillingburg HT Jr. Cast gold restorations. In: Clark JW (ed). Clinical Dentistry. New York: Harper & Row, 1976.

Stewart KL, Rudd KD. Stabilizing periodontally weakened teeth with removable partial dentures. J Prosthet Dent 1968;19:475–482.

# Special Impression Procedures for Tooth-Tissue–Supported Removable Partial Dentures

**Ronald G. Verrett,** DDS, MS, FACP

When occlusal forces are applied to a tooth-supported removable partial denture, they are directed through the rests and transmitted to the abutments (Fig 12-1). The edentulous ridges do not contribute to the support of the partial denture because the teeth absorb these forces before the forces can be transmitted to the tissues of the residual ridge. Since the denture base does not contribute to the support of the partial denture and the underlying mucosa and bone are not subjected to functional forces, a tooth-supported removable partial denture can be constructed on a master cast made from a single impression that records the teeth and soft tissues in their anatomic form.

When occlusal forces are applied to a tooth-tissue–supported removable partial denture, these forces must be equitably distributed to the abutments and the tissues of the ridge (Fig 12-2). This cannot be accomplished on a master cast made from a single impression. Instead, a dual impression technique is used in which a "corrected cast" is generated. The impression of the teeth is made with a material that captures the teeth in their anatomic positions. In contrast, the impression of the residual ridge must record the soft tissues in their functional form. Therefore, the impression of the residual ridge must (1) record and relate the tissues under uniform loading, (2) distribute the load over as large an area as possible, and (3) accurately delineate the peripheral extent of the denture base.

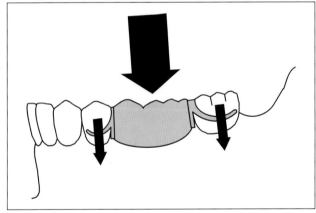

**Fig 12-1** Forces on a tooth-supported removable partial denture *(large arrow)* are directed through the rests and transmitted to the abutments *(small arrows).*

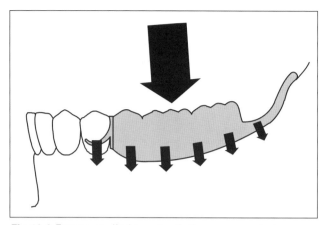

Fig 12-2 Forces applied to a tooth–tissue–supported removable partial denture *(large arrow)* must be equitably distributed to the abutments and the tissues of the residual ridge *(small arrows)*.

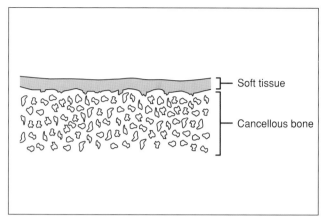

Fig 12-3 Cancellous bone displays an irregular surface that can irritate the overlying soft tissues when stress is applied.

## ▢ Factors Influencing Support of the Distal Extension Base

To determine the amount of pressure that must be applied to the soft tissues during a corrective impression procedure, the practitioner must consider a number of factors. Although these factors will be considered independently, one must remember that each factor influences the others.

### Quality of soft tissue covering edentulous ridge

The soft tissues covering the bony residual ridges are compressible to varying degrees. It is essential that this variability be recognized as treatment progresses. Not only may soft tissue displaceability vary from patient to patient, but significant differences may occur from site to site within the same patient. If the soft tissues of the edentulous ridge are thick and displaceable, less support for a denture base can be derived from that ridge. A firm, tightly attached mucosa displaying moderate thickness (2 to 3 mm) will offer the greatest support. If redundant soft tissues have accumulated, particularly over maxillary tuberosities, surgical removal may be indicated. Removal of redundant tissue not only minimizes vertical displacement of a denture base, but also improves resistance to lateral displacement.

### Type of bone in the denture-bearing area

Cancellous bone, as compared with cortical bone, is less able to resist vertical forces because its irregular surface acts as an irritant to the overlying soft tissue if vertical stress occurs (Fig 12-3). The result of the irritation is chronic inflammation, which often leads to oral discomfort and accelerated ridge resorption. Therefore, areas of cancellous bone should not be considered primary bearing areas. Instead, the practitioner should direct forces to dense cortical regions such as the buccal shelf.

### Design of the prosthesis

Knowledge of basic mechanical principles guides the management of functional forces in partially edentulous arches. Rotational forces passing through the most posterior clasp assemblies can be controlled using appropriate components. The most efficient method of controlling rotational movement is the use of one or more indirect retainers anterior to the fulcrum line (Fig 12-4). The indirect retainer is most often in the form of a rest attached to the major connector by a minor connector. If the distal extension denture is bilateral, one indirect retainer should be used on each side of the arch. If the distal extension base is unilateral, only one indirect retainer is needed. This indirect

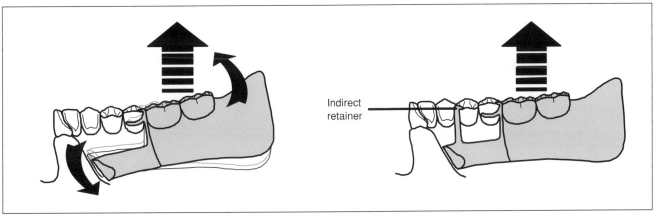

**Fig 12-4** An indirect retainer helps control rotation of a prosthesis *(small arrows)* and limits movement of a distal extension base away from the residual ridge *(large arrows).*

**Fig 12-5** Overextension of a denture base may cause rotation of the removable partial denture. This may result in torquing of the clasped abutments and orthodontic movement of teeth on the opposite side of the fulcrum line. In this instance, the indirect retainer has been omitted. This error permits uncontrolled rotation of the prosthesis *(large arrow).* Rotation may result in torquing of clasped abutments *(circular arrows)* and orthodontic movement of teeth anterior to the fulcrum line *(horizontal arrow).*

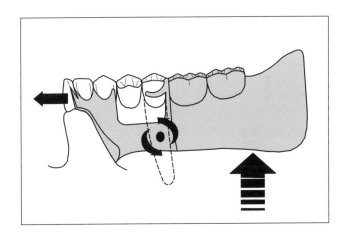

retainer is positioned anterior to the fulcrum line and on the opposite side of the arch from the distal extension ridge.

## Amount of tissue coverage of denture base

To counteract the tissueward component of a rotational force, each distal extension base must cover a relatively large surface area. The broader the coverage of the edentulous ridge, the greater the distribution of the load—and the smaller the force per unit area. All available space must be used without encroaching on movable tissues. Overextension of the denture base may cause irritation and ulceration of the soft tissues, as well as lifting or dislodging forces on the prosthesis. This may result in torquing of the clasped abutments and orthodontic movement of teeth anterior to the fulcrum line (Fig 12-5).

## Anatomy of the denture-bearing area

Occlusal forces must be directed to the portions of the ridge that are most capable of withstanding those forces. Therefore, the practitioner must understand the anatomic and structural characteristics of the maxillary and mandibular arches. For the sake of discussion, the maxillary and mandibular arches are addressed separately.

### Maxillary edentulous ridge

In the maxillary arch, few structures other than the crest of the ridge are capable of serving as primary stress-bearing areas. The buccal slope of the maxillary ridge is normally covered by a layer of cortical bone and can withstand a significant amount of stress. Unfortunately, the buccal slope of the maxillary arch is not oriented perpendicular to the vertical forces occur-

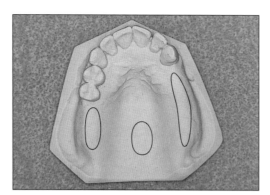

**Fig 12-6** In the maxillary arch, primary stress-bearing areas include the posterior ridge crests and horizontal portions of the hard palate *(circled regions)*.

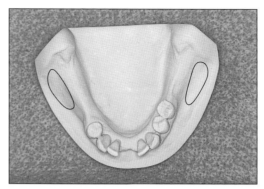

**Fig 12-7** In the mandibular arch, primary stress-bearing areas are limited to the buccal shelves *(circled regions)*.

ring against it, so it offers little resistance to them. The buccal slope does, however, resist lateral forces relatively well.

Some resistance to vertical displacement can be derived from the horizontal portion of the hard palate. Unfortunately, the tissues of the hard palate are relatively thin and incompressible. Therefore, the tissues of the hard palate are susceptible to irritation and ulceration.

Based upon the foregoing considerations, the majority of denture base support for a maxillary distal extension partial denture must come from the ridge crest (Fig 12-6). The mucosa covering the maxillary ridge crest is usually firm and capable of resisting occlusal forces. If the crestal mucosa is not firm and dense, it should be surgically corrected to provide an appropriate foundation for the prosthesis.

### Mandibular edentulous ridge

The crest of the mandibular ridge cannot be used as a primary stress-bearing area because it is composed of cancellous bone covered by soft tissues that are more susceptible to injury than are those in the maxillary arch. Fortunately, the dense cortical bone of the buccal shelf area makes an excellent stress-bearing site (Fig 12-7). The soft tissues covering the cortical bone in this region are usually firm and dense. The anatomy of the buccal shelf area is nearly perpendicular to the forces of occlusion, thereby allowing the region to tolerate the accompanying stresses. Resistance to horizontal forces is provided by the buccal and lingual slopes of the residual ridge.

### *Fit of denture base*

Each denture base must be made to fit the areas that can serve as primary stress-bearing regions. The rest of this chapter discusses how best to record these areas to take advantage of the anatomic features.

## ▭ Indications

In some mouths, soft tissue displacement is slight. As a result, the functional and anatomic contours of the ridge may be virtually identical.

The decision to use a dual impression technique may be determined using the following test: *(1)* Acrylic resin bases are added to the framework and *(2)* the framework is placed in the mouth and finger pressure is applied to the base or bases. If the base can be depressed enough that the indirect retainers or lingual plating lifts away from the teeth, a dual impression technique should be used. If, however, there is no discernible movement, consideration should be given to using a single impression technique. It should be noted that dispensing with the dual impression procedure eliminates the opportunity of establishing precise and functionally formed denture borders.

The dual impression technique is most often indicated for mandibular distal extension applications because only a limited ridge area can be used as a stress-bearing site. It is more difficult to obtain the proper peripheral extension of the mandibular denture base than it is to perform this same procedure for a maxillary denture base. This is primarily due to the mobility of the floor of the mouth.

The maxillary distal extension ridge is usually covered by a firm, well-attached mucosa or can be surgically prepared in that form. The stress-bearing area includes the crest and buccal slope of the ridge. Therefore, a dual impression does not often improve the stress distribution. The border definition is also much simpler and can be read from a single anatomic impression.

The other indication for a dual impression technique is a long-span anterior edentulous base (normally including at least the six anterior teeth), where the ridge must supply some support for the prosthesis. Improving the accuracy of the cast with a secondary impression and defining the peripheral extension of the anterior flange can be helpful in distributing forces that act against a weaker portion of the dental arch.

## ▱ Impression Methods

There are two categories of dual impression techniques. These categories may be defined as *physiologic impression techniques* and *selected pressure techniques*.

Physiologic impression techniques record the ridge portion of the cast in its functional form by placing an occlusal load on the impression tray during the impression procedure. Three physiologic impression procedures are presented in this chapter: the McLean-Hindels method; the functional reline method; and the fluid wax method.

Selected pressure impression techniques are intended to equalize the support between the abutments and the soft tissues and to direct forces to the portions of the ridge that are most capable of withstanding such forces. This is accomplished by relieving the tray in some areas while allowing the impression tray to contact the ridge in other areas. Areas where relief is provided are minimally displaced during impression procedures. In those areas where relief is not provided, greater soft tissue displacement occurs.

In both the fluid wax technique and the selected pressure technique, an impression of the edentulous ridge is made using an impression tray attached to the framework. The master cast is altered to accom-

modate the secondary impression, and a corrected cast is generated. For this reason, the technique is often referred to as a *corrected cast* or *altered cast* procedure. This procedure is more fully described in subsequent sections.

The terminology used in any discussion of impression-making procedures must be carefully selected. This discussion is no exception. An important distinction must be made between the terms *minimally displaced* and *excessively displaced*. Soft tissues are said to have been minimally displaced if insertion and wear of the prosthesis produces no adverse soft tissue response. Conversely, if the tissues demonstrate an inflammatory response with accompanying bone resorption, the tissues are said to have been excessively displaced. These terms will be used in subsequent discussions regarding impression procedures.

### McLean physiologic impression

The need for physiologic impressions was first proposed by McLean and others. They realized the need for recording the tissues of the residual ridge in a functional form while capturing the remaining teeth in the anatomic form. As a result, they developed a dual impression technique.

To accomplish their objectives, these practitioners constructed a custom tray on a diagnostic cast (Fig 12-8). A functional impression was made using this tray and a suitable impression material (Fig 12-9). A hydrocolloid "over-impression" was then made while maintaining the functional impression in its intended position (Fig 12-10). The greatest weakness of the technique was that practitioners could not produce the same functional displacement generated by occlusal forces.

In response to this shortcoming, Hindels and others developed modified impression trays for the second impression procedure. These trays had large holes in their posterior segments (Fig 12-11). As a result, the operator could apply finger pressure to the functional impression as the hydrocolloid impression was being made. The finished impression was a reproduction of the anatomic surface of the ridge and the surfaces of the teeth. The two were related to each other, however, as if masticating forces were taking place on the denture base.

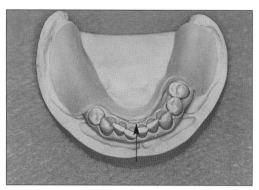

**Fig 12-8** The McLean technique employs a custom tray for distal extension areas. Notice that relief is provided between the anterior connector and the soft tissues *(arrow)*.

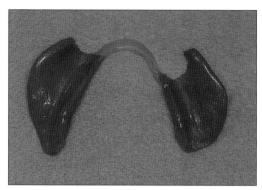

**Fig 12-9** A functional impression is completed using an appropriate impression material. The impression is removed from the oral cavity and examined. If acceptable, the functional impression is repositioned in the mouth.

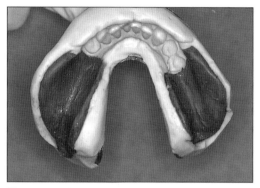

**Fig 12-10** An alginate "over-impression" is made while applying pressure to the previously completed functional impression. The resultant two-piece impression relates the functional form of the posterior ridges to the anatomic form of the remaining teeth.

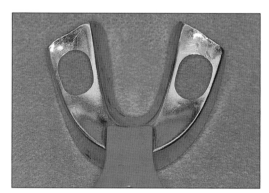

**Fig 12-11** Modification of a stock tray allows the practitioner to apply finger pressure to the functional impression tray.

Disadvantages of these techniques are closely related to direct retention. If the action of the retentive clasps is sufficient to maintain a denture base in its intended position, the tissues of the ridge will be in the functional form. This may result in compromised blood flow with adverse soft tissue reaction and resorption of the underlying bone.

If the action of the retentive clasps is not sufficient to maintain that functional relationship of the denture base to the soft tissues, the denture base will be occlusally positioned when the soft tissues are at rest. This results in premature contact of the artificial teeth, which may be objectionable to many patients.

## Functional reline method

Most methods of obtaining a physiologic impression for support of a distal extension denture base require accomplishment of the impression procedure before completion of the prosthesis. It is possible, however, to obtain equally effective results after the partial denture has been completed. The technique is referred to as a *functional reline method*, and it consists of adding a new surface to the intaglio of the denture base. The procedure may be accomplished before the insertion of the partial denture, or it may be done at a later date if the denture base no longer fits the ridge adequately.

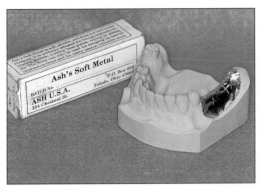

**Fig 12-12** A metal spacer may be placed on the dental cast to provide space for a functional reline.

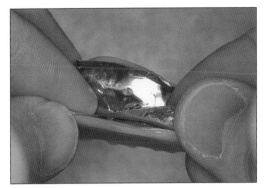

**Fig 12-13** After the denture base has been processed, the metal spacer is removed.

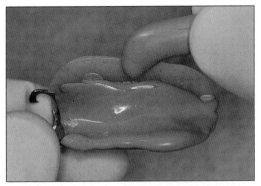

**Fig 12-14** Heated modeling plastic is carefully applied to the intaglio of the denture base.

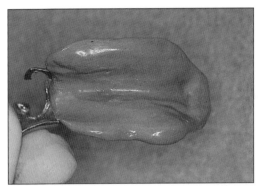

**Fig 12-15** The modeling plastic impression is completed.

Although the functional reline method has many advantages, it also presents many difficulties. The main problems are caused by failure to maintain the correct relationship between the framework and the abutment teeth during the impression procedure and failure to achieve accurate occlusal contact following the reline procedure.

The partial denture is constructed on a cast made from a single impression, usually irreversible hydrocolloid. This is an anatomic impression, and no attempt is made to alter it or produce a functional impression of the edentulous ridge.

To allow room for the impression material between the denture base and the ridge, space must be provided. One of the most accurate methods of ensuring uniform space for the impression material is to adapt a soft metal spacer (Ash's No. 7 metal, Ash USA, Toledo, OH) over the ridge on the cast before

processing the denture base. After processing, the metal is removed, leaving an even space between the base and the edentulous ridge (Figs 12-12 and 12-13).

The portion of the technique that introduces the greatest hazard is the reline impression procedure. The patient must keep the mouth partially open throughout the procedure to permit appropriate tissue control and the required visual assessment. Low-fusing modeling plastic is applied to the intaglio of the denture base, tempered in a water bath, and seated in the patient's mouth (Fig 12-14). This sequence must be repeated until an accurate impression of the edentulous ridge has been accomplished (Fig 12-15). The border extensions are determined by heating to the borders and guiding the placement of the cheek and tongue.

To provide space for the impression material, 1 mm of modeling plastic is removed from the intaglio surface (Fig 12-16). An impression is made with a free-

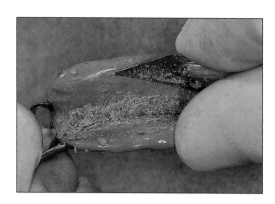

**Fig 12-16** Modeling plastic is removed from the ridge crest before the final impression is made.

flowing zinc oxide–eugenol paste or a light-bodied polysulfide rubber base.

In the functional reline procedure, as in all reline procedures, occlusal discrepancies must be corrected after the new denture base has been processed. Since the open-mouth impression technique must be used, it is impossible to maintain previously established occlusal contacts. If errors in occlusion are slight, the correction may be accomplished in the mouth. However, in a majority of cases, it will be necessary to remount the partial denture on an articulator to correct the occlusion. (The technique for remounting a partial denture to correct occlusal discrepancies is described in chapter 16.)

Although fraught with danger, the functional reline method can be used successfully.

## Corrected cast procedure

### Adding an impression tray

Preparation for the corrected cast impression appointment requires the addition of one or more impression trays. This should be accomplished only after the framework has been fitted to the teeth and soft tissues. A tray may then be added using a chemically-activated or light-activated resin.

Before adding the impression tray material, the master cast is carefully examined. Undercuts that would interfere with removal of the tray are blocked out using baseplate wax (Fig 12-17). An appropriate separating medium is then placed on the corresponding area of the cast (Fig 12-18), and the framework is completely seated (Fig 12-19). A chemically-activated or light-activated resin is adapted to the struts of the minor connector (Fig 12-20). The borders are

trimmed using a laboratory knife (Fig 12-21). Following polymerization, the denture base resin is trimmed and smoothed using laboratory burs and arbor bands (Fig 12-22). Care is taken to ensure that all borders are gently rounded. The tissue surface of the impression tray is not relieved at this time.

### Correcting peripheral extensions

The framework-tray assembly is fully seated in the mouth. It is important to note that from this point forward, each time the framework is seated on the cast or in the mouth, visual verification of complete seating *must* be made.

This description is primarily concerned with adjusting the extensions for a mandibular distal extension impression, but manipulating border tissues to arrive at the proper tray contour applies to any situation.

The buccal extension of the tray is observed as the cheek is moved downward, outward, and upward. As this movement is taking place, the edge of the tray should be 2 to 3 mm from the depth of the buccal vestibule.

Posteriorly, the mandibular tray should reach two thirds the height of the retromolar pad. This, too, must be determined by direct observation.

The distolingual length of the tray is assessed by directing the patient to place the tip of the tongue against the upper lip. The operator's fingers should rest lightly on the tray during this process. If the tray lifts, even slightly, during this movement, the distolingual length should be shortened.

The remainder of the lingual flange is evaluated by having the patient place the tip of the tongue into each cheek. This movement need not be forceful, but only enough to distend the cheek slightly. The opera-

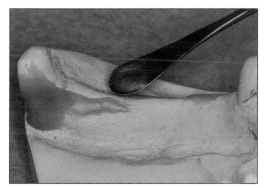

**Fig 12-17** Undercuts that would interfere with removal of the tray are eliminated using baseplate wax.

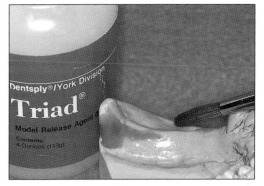

**Fig 12-18** An appropriate separating medium is applied to the cast.

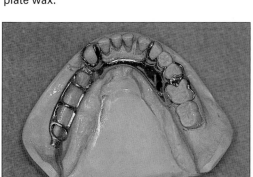

**Fig 12-19** The framework is seated on the cast.

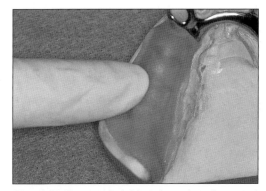

**Fig 12-20** Tray material is adapted to the metal struts and dental cast using finger pressure.

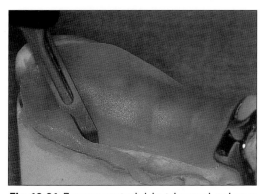

**Fig 12-21** Excess material is trimmed using a surgical scalpel or similar instrument.

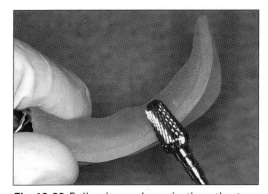

**Fig 12-22** Following polymerization, the tray material is smoothed using a laboratory bur.

tor's fingers are used to detect movement of the tray. Lifting of the mandibular left tray is usually produced when the tongue is placed in the right cheek, while lifting of the mandibular right tray is produced by a leftward movement of the tongue. The practitioner should assess these movements and make appropriate adjustments to the lingual flanges.

When the tray extensions are correct, moderate manipulation of the border tissues, including thrusting the tongue forward and into both cheeks, should not produce any movement of the tray. An overextended tray will cause a constant force to be placed on the abutment teeth as the border tissues attempt to unseat the denture.

## Border molding the impression tray

A mandibular distal extension tray may be border molded in two steps: *(1)* from the anterior extent of

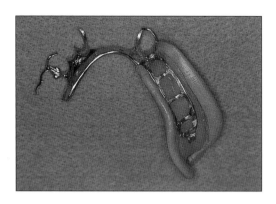

**Fig 12-23** Border molding using a low-fusing modeling plastic is completed.

the buccal flange to the most posterior extent of the tray and *(2)* on the lingual and distolingual flanges.

Border molding for a corrected cast is basically the same as that for a complete denture. Tissue manipulation is the same as that used in correcting the peripheral extensions of the tray. A low-fusing modeling plastic, green or gray stick, is used for the procedure. Results are illustrated in Fig 12-23.

When the border molding is complete, the tongue and other tissues should have freedom of motion without dislodging the tray.

### Relieving the tray and making the impression
When the acrylic resin tray material was adapted to the framework on the master cast, no relief was provided between the cast and the tray material. This permitted firm attachment of the tray to the latticework and provided optimum stability during border molding procedures.

At this stage, relief is provided to create room for the chosen impression material. The technique for the fluid wax functional impression differs from that of the selected pressure impression.

### Fluid wax functional impression
The fluid wax impression may be used to make a reline impression for an existing partial denture or to correct the edentulous ridge portion of a master cast.

The objectives of the technique are *(1)* to obtain maximum extension of the peripheral borders while not interfering with the function of movable border tissues, *(2)* to record the stress-bearing areas of the ridge in their functional form, and *(3)* to record non-pressure-bearing areas in their anatomic form. The

fluid wax impression is made using an open-mouth technique so that there is less danger of overdisplacement of the soft tissues by occlusal or vertical forces.

The term *fluid wax* is used to denote waxes that are firm at room temperature and have the ability to flow at mouth temperature. The most frequently used fluid waxes are Iowa wax, developed by Dr Earle S. Smith at the University of Iowa, and Korrecta Wax No. 4, developed by Drs O. C. and S. G. Applegate at the Universities of Michigan and Detroit, respectively. Korrecta Wax No. 4 (D-R Miner, Medford, OR) is slightly more fluid than Iowa wax (D-R Miner).

The use of fluid wax requires control of the critical factors of space and time. Space refers to the amount of relief provided between the impression tray and the edentulous ridge. The impression wax flows sluggishly, and a thin layer of wax will flow less readily than a thicker layer. One to two millimeters of relief is required between the tray and the tissues of the edentulous ridge. Each time the tray is introduced into the mouth, it must remain in place 5 to 7 minutes to allow the wax to flow and to prevent buildup of pressure under the tray with resulting distortion or displacement of the tissue.

The clinical technique for the use of fluid wax calls for a water bath maintained at 51°C to 54°C (125°F to 130°F), into which a container of the wax is placed (Fig 12-24). At this temperature the wax becomes fluid. The wax is painted onto the impression tray with a brush (Fig 12-25). The peripheral extension of the impression tray is critical. The borders must be short of all movable tissues, but this space should not be more than 2 mm because the fluid wax does not have sufficient strength to support itself beyond that dis-

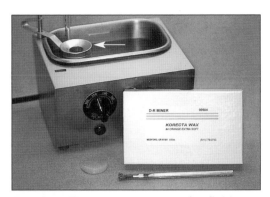

Fig 12-24 The armamentarium for fluid wax technique includes the wax itself, a stiff brush, a water bath, and a container for confining the wax *(arrow)*.

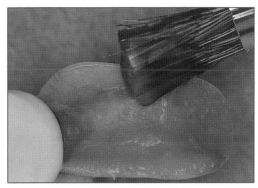

Fig 12-25 Fluid wax is painted onto the intaglio surface of a tray or denture base. Subsequently, the framework will be seated in the oral cavity.

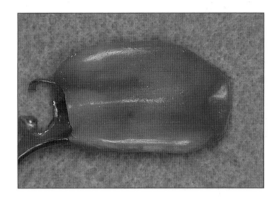

Fig 12-26 The completed impression shows evidence of proper extension and appropriate tissue contact.

tance. Inaccuracies will develop if the wax is extended beyond that length. Originally a harder wax, Korecta Wax No. 1, was used to support the softer No. 4 wax if extension beyond that length was needed. However, the No. 1 wax is no longer available.

The wax is painted on the surface of the tray to a depth slightly greater than the amount of relief provided. The tray is then seated in the mouth. The patient must hold the mouth half open for about 5 minutes. The tray is removed, and the wax is examined for evidence of tissue contact. Where tissue contact is present, the wax surface will be glossy. Where there is no contact, the surface will be dull. If needed, additional wax is painted on those areas not in contact with the tissue. The tray must remain in the mouth a minimum of 5 minutes after each addition of wax. The peripheral extensions are developed by tissue movements by the patient.

For the buccal and distobuccal extensions in a mandibular impression, the patient must employ a wide-open mouth position. This will activate the buccinator muscle and pterygomandibular raphe and produce the desired border anatomy. For the proper lingual extension for a mandibular impression, the patient must thrust the tongue into the cheek opposite the side of the arch being border molded. The distolingual extension is obtained by having the patient press the tongue against the lingual surfaces of the anterior teeth. These movements must be repeated a number of times once the impression has been in the mouth long enough for the wax to flow.

When the impression shows evidence of complete tissue contact and the anatomy of the limiting border structures has been established, the impression is positioned in the mouth for a final time. The impression should be left in the mouth for 12 minutes to ensure that the wax has completely flowed and released any pressure that may be present (Fig 12-26).

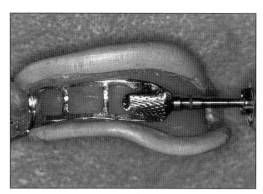

**Fig 12-27** The mandibular impression tray is selectively reduced at the ridge crest. This provides additional room for impression material and minimizes displacement of the soft tissues.

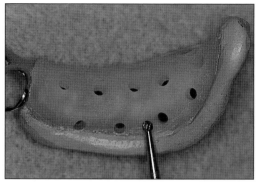

**Fig 12-28** Holes may be placed in the tray to further minimize the pressures generated during impression procedures.

The finished impression must be handled carefully and the new cast poured as soon as possible because the wax is fragile and subject to distortion.

The fluid wax impression technique can produce an accurate impression if the technique is properly executed. The procedure is time consuming, but if the time periods are not followed accurately, an impression with excessive tissue displacement will result.

### Selected pressure impression

The impression techniques presented to this point are included in the general category of physiologic impressions. They produce a generalized displacement of the mucosa. This displacement is intended to record the tissues as they would exist under functional occlusal loading.

The selected pressure impression attempts to direct more force to those portions of the ridge able to absorb stress and to protect the areas of the ridge least able to absorb stress. To accomplish this, the intaglio surface of the tray is selectively relieved (Fig 12-27).

For the mandibular posterior region, the crest of the ridge is not considered to be a pressure-bearing area. To minimize the pressure that will be placed on this area during the final impression, the intaglio surface of the tray is relieved down to the metal retention struts using a laboratory bur. The amount of relief is dependent upon the blockout and relief procedures performed during the laboratory phases of framework construction. This is usually about 1 mm, but may

vary depending upon removable partial denture design and laboratory philosophy.

The buccal shelf is the primary stress-bearing area in the mandibular arch. As a result, only slight relief is provided. Excess modeling plastic on the intaglio of the tray should be removed. The tissue contact area of the border molding should be scraped lightly with a knife.

The lingual slope of the mandibular residual ridge may provide a limited amount of vertical support, but principally it resists horizontal or rotational forces. The relief provided over the lingual slope should be the same as the relief provided over the buccal shelf. The impression should record these tissues in a slightly displaced form.

As the impression is made, the material over the crest of the ridge is not closely confined and will exert minimal tissueward force. This will result in minimal tissue displacement. The impression material over the buccal shelf, being somewhat more confined, will exert somewhat greater tissueward force, and a slightly greater amount of tissue displacement will occur.

The selected pressure impression technique results in a denture base that is closely adapted to, and in firm contact with, the tissues covering the buccal shelf area. In contrast, the crestal portion of the denture base is lightly adapted to the soft tissues, resulting in minimal force application.

In some patients, the soft tissues covering the ridge will be easily displaced. To obtain more relief and prevent excessive tissue displacement, holes may be drilled through the impression tray (Fig 12-28). These holes allow impression material to flow through the tray and dissipate pressure that might otherwise occur.

Several impression materials can be used to record the selected pressure impression. A more viscous impression material results in greater displacement of the soft tissues, while a less viscous impression material provides decreased tissue displacement. Overdisplacement of resilient tissues should be avoided because it may result in an inflammatory reaction beneath the denture base. Displaced tissues also have a tendency to rebound to their anatomic contours, resulting in occlusal displacement of the prosthesis and placing additional stresses on the abutments.

**Impression materials** A thorough understanding of impression materials and associated techniques is a critical factor in the decision-making process. A brief description of commonly used impression materials is provided for the reader's convenience.

*Zinc oxide–eugenol.* Zinc oxide–eugenol paste is an accurate impression material of intermediate viscosity. One of its main advantages is that it requires a minimal amount of time to set. The impression must be obtained in a single insertion, so correct placement of the framework is essential. Although some authorities state that defects in an impression can be corrected by small additions of a second mix, this is not good practice. It will usually result in uneven distribution of forces and incomplete seating of the framework.

Zinc oxide–eugenol paste is generally considered to be the impression material of choice if the edentulous ridge is free from gross undercuts. It is particularly effective when soft, flabby tissue is involved.

*Rubber base.* Polysulfide rubber base impression materials are excellent for use with the selected pressure impression technique. Polysulfide materials are only slightly more viscous than zinc oxide–eugenol paste, and this viscosity can be reduced by using a higher percentage of light-bodied material in the mix.

Slightly more time is required to make the impression because of the prolonged setting time. In addition, defects cannot be corrected by addition of a sec-

ond mix. If an impression is deemed inaccurate, the impression material should be stripped from the tray and the impression remade.

When using a polysulfide rubber base impression material, an adhesive should be applied to the tray to ensure that the impression material adheres to the acrylic resin and modeling plastic.

To help prevent the rubber base material from displacing soft tissues, several holes may be drilled through the tray over the crest of the ridge using a No. 6 or No. 8 round bur (see Fig 12-28). This decreases the probability that excess pressure will be developed. The holes will also help minimize air entrapment. This may be especially helpful when dealing with long edentulous spans.

Rubber base impression material is particularly appropriate for those patients displaying moderate to severe undercuts of the edentulous ridge.

**Impression technique** The area of the mouth that is to be involved in the impression is dried and isolated with gauze before the impression material is mixed. The preferred technique involves unfolding 4 x 4-inch gauze squares and placing them on the facial and lingual surfaces of the dental arch.

The chosen impression material is then mixed according to the manufacturer's directions and applied to the surface of the tray. Care should be taken to cover the peripheries of the tray with a thin layer of the impression material. Overloading the tray complicates the impression technique. The material should not be allowed to flow onto the internal surface of the minor connector or under occlusal rests.

Gauze pads are gently removed from the mouth, and the framework is completely seated. The buccal tissues are cleared by moving the cheek(s) apically, outward, and then occlusally. The patient is instructed to relax the tongue as the tray is being seated. Subsequently, the patient is told to protrude the tongue very slightly (the tip of the tongue should be just anterior to the incisal edges of the teeth).

The practitioner must verify that all rests and indirect retainers are completely seated while the impression material is still fluid. Pressure is applied to the occlusal rests as border molding movements are performed. Care is taken to avoid the application of vertical forces on impression trays. This may cause the

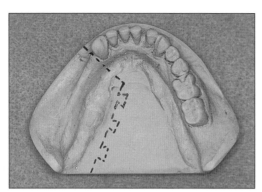

**Fig 12-29** The master cast must be modified in preparation for corrected cast procedures. The broken line indicates the proposed cast modifications for a unilateral corrected cast process.

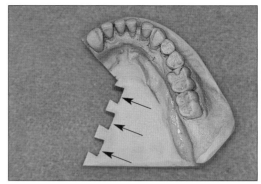

**Fig 12-30** The master cast following modification. Dovetails *(arrows)* have been prepared to permit mechanical interlocking of cast segments.

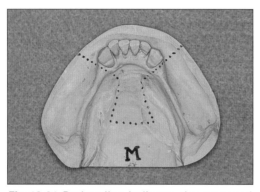

**Fig 12-31** Broken line indicates the proposed cast modifications for a bilateral corrected cast process.

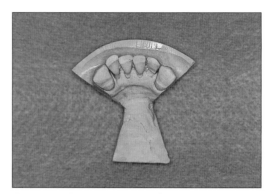

**Fig 12-32** The master cast following modification.

framework to rotate around the occlusal rests, lifting the indirect retainers from their rest seats and producing an inaccurate impression.

The patient's mouth must remain open with the tongue slightly protruded until the material reaches its final set. The tendency on the part of most patients is to allow the tongue to fall back in the mouth and the mouth to close partially. These actions will cause inaccuracies in the impression. Consequently, the operator must remind the patient of the correct position from time to time.

**Examining the impression** The impression must be thoroughly inspected and any cause for rejection carefully considered. Any impression exhibiting a void or underextension should be rejected. In addition, any evidence that the framework was not seated completely,

such as the presence of impression material beneath rests, is reason to remake the impression. If any doubt exists, the impression must not be accepted.

### Preparing the original cast and pouring a corrected cast

Figures 12-29 to 12-38 illustrate the procedure for producing a corrected cast in a mandibular distal extension application. These procedures can be applied to any other removable partial denture situation requiring a corrected cast impression technique.

### Length of appointment

An experienced clinician should complete the corrected cast impression in 20 to 30 minutes. A dental student usually will require about 2 hours.

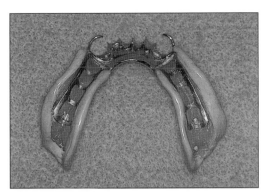

**Fig 12-33** Properly border molded impression tray.

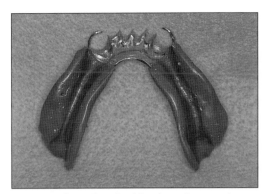

**Fig 12-34** Completed rubber base impression.

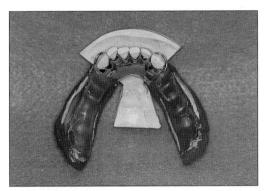

**Fig 12-35** Framework-impression assembly is properly seated on modified master cast. At this stage, the framework should be affixed to the modified master cast using modeling plastic. This minimizes the likelihood of displacement and distortion.

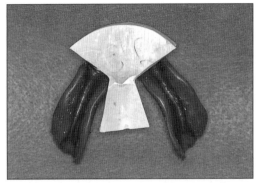

**Fig 12-36** The assembly is inverted in preparation for rimming and boxing procedures.

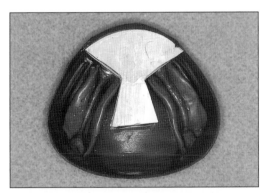

**Fig 12-37** Utility wax is used to rim the impression. The utility wax should be located 2 to 3 mm from impression borders and should extend peripherally 3 to 4 mm. Boxing wax is added to form a watertight vertical wall. When this has been accomplished, freshly mixed dental stone is introduced.

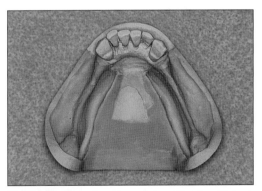

**Fig 12-38** After the stone has gained sufficient strength, the corrected cast is recovered and trimmed.

# ⊔ **Bibliography**

Applegate OC. Essentials of Removable Partial Denture Prosthesis, ed 2. Philadelphia: Saunders, 1960.

Applegate OC. An evaluation of the support for the removable partial denture. J Prosthet Dent 1960;10:112–123.

Applegate OC. The partial denture base. J Prosthet Dent 1955; 5:636–648.

Beckett LS. Partial denture. The rebasing of tissue borne saddles. Theory and practice. Aust Dent J 1971;16:340–346.

Craig RG. Dental Materials. St. Louis: Mosby, 1978.

Cummer WE. Impression in partial denture service. Dent Cosmos 1928;70:72,278.

DeVan MM. Basic principles of impression making. J Prosthet Dent 1952;2:26–35.

Everett GE. Impression taking with a fluid wax compound. J Aust Dent Soc 1922;2:294.

Hindels GW. Load distribution in extension saddle partial dentures. J Prosthet Dent 1952;2:92.

Hindels GW. Stress analysis in distal extension partial dentures. J Prosthet Dent 1957;7:197–205.

Holmes JB. Influence of impression procedures and occlusal loading on partial denture movement. J Prosthet Dent 1965; 15:474–481.

Leupold RJ. A comparative study of impression procedures for distal extension removable partial dentures. J Prosthet Dent 1966;16:708.

Leupold RJ, Kratochvil FJ. An altered cast procedure to improve tissue support for removable partial dentures. J Prosthet Dent 1965;15:672.

Lytle RB. Soft tissue displacement beneath removable partial and complete dentures. J Prosthet Dent 1962;12:34–43.

McCracken WL. A comparison of tooth-borne and tooth-tissue-borne removable partial dentures. J Prosthet Dent 1953;3: 375–381.

McLean DW. The partial denture as a vehicle for function. J Am Dent Assoc 1936;23:1271–1278.

Melty AC. Obtaining efficient soft tissue support for the denture base. J Am Dent Assoc 1958;56:679.

Rapuano JA. Single-tray dual-impression technique for distal extension partial dentures. J Prosthet Dent 1970;24:41–46.

Vahidi F. Vertical displacement of distal-extension ridges by different impression techniques. J Prosthet Dent 1978;40: 374–377.

Von Kramer R. A two-stage impression technique for distal-extension removable partial dentures. J Prosthet Dent 1988;60:199–201.

Walter JD. Composite impression procedures. J Prosthet Dent 1973;30:385–389.

Weinnann JP, Sicher H. Bone and Bones, ed 2. St Louis: Mosby, 1955.

Wilson JH. Partial dentures—Relining the saddle supported by the mucosa and alveolar bone. J Prosthet Dent 1953;3:807–813.

# Establishing Occlusal Relationships

The clinical appointment for accurately establishing a definitive jaw relation is often overlooked. This appointment is essential when the opposing casts cannot be accurately hand articulated or when the removable partial denture will be constructed at a position other than maximal intercuspal position. The appointment is usually needed following a corrected cast procedure, since the lack of posterior occlusion in Class I and Class II partially edentulous arches makes it impossible to accurately hand articulate the master casts.

The desired occlusal scheme for a removable partial denture may vary from that of a complete denture (bilaterally balanced occlusion) to that of a fixed partial denture (disclusion of the posterior teeth in eccentric jaw positions). The decision must be based upon a variety of factors, including the number and distribution of remaining teeth, the existing periodontal conditions, and the type of occlusion in the opposing arch.

The goal in developing an occlusal scheme for a removable partial denture is to establish and maintain a harmonious relationship with all oral structures and to provide a masticatory apparatus that is efficient and esthetically acceptable. In the case of a tooth-tissue–

supported removable partial denture, the practitioner must attempt to distribute forces to those structures capable of withstanding them.

Occlusal harmony must be present in centric relation, maximal intercuspal position, and all eccentric positions. Sustained deflective contact in any position will result in damage to the periodontium or the neuromuscular system that controls mandibular movement.

For practical purposes, occlusal relationships may be described in terms of vertical and horizontal components. Vertical and horizontal jaw relations are presented in the following sections.

## ⌑ Vertical Jaw Relation

Vertical dimension refers to a vertical measurement of the face between two arbitrary points. For convenience, one point is generally placed on a patient's nose and the other on the patient's chin.

Two very important vertical dimensions are recognized for each patient. They are described as the *physiologic rest dimension* (Fig 13-1) and the *occlusal vertical di-*

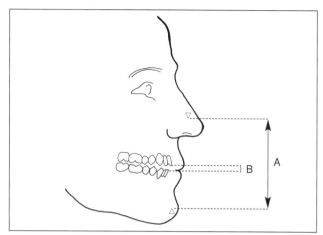

**Fig 13-1** Vertical dimension refers to a vertical measurement of the face between two arbitrary points *(triangles)*. The physiologic rest dimension (A) is determined when the patient is in an upright position and is completely at rest, with the maxillary and mandibular teeth slightly separated. The space between the maxillary and mandibular teeth is termed the *interocclusal rest space* (B).

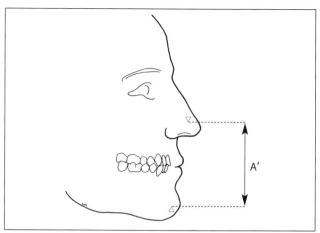

**Fig 13-2** When the patient brings the teeth into tight intercuspation, the interocclusal rest space is eliminated. The resultant nose-to-chin distance is termed the *occlusal vertical dimension* (A').

mension (Fig 13-2). The physiologic rest dimension is determined when the patient is in an upright position and is completely at rest. The mandibular position is produced by a muscular balance between the muscles of mastication, the postcervical muscle group, the infrahyoid muscle group, and the suprahyoid muscle group. At this position, the patient's maxillary and mandibular teeth should not be touching. The space between the maxillary and mandibular teeth is referred to as the *interocclusal rest space* (see Fig 13-1).

If the patient elevates the mandible from the rest position, the teeth will come into contact. The occlusal vertical dimension is then determined by measuring the vertical dimension while the patient's teeth are in maximal intercuspal position.

The physiologic rest dimension will always be greater than the occlusal vertical dimension. In most patients, the difference in these measurements will be 2 to 4 mm. This relationship was first studied by Dr M. E. Niswonger in 1934.[1] Niswonger measured the interocclusal rest space in 200 patients with natural teeth and found that 83% of the patients displayed a rest space of approximately 3 mm. Of the patients included in Niswonger's investigation, none displayed an interocclusal rest space less than 1 mm or greater than 6 mm.

## Altering the existing occlusal vertical dimension

For most patients requiring removable partial dentures, measurement of the occlusal vertical dimension is not necessary. If the remaining natural teeth appear normal in size, shape, and position, and these teeth display acceptable contact during closure, this vertical relationship should be considered the occlusal vertical dimension. Changing this dimension should be considered only if the patient displays signs and symptoms suggesting a significant decrease in vertical dimension. Signs and symptoms may include severe tooth wear, a markedly decreased nose-to-chin distance, or unexplained discomfort in the orofacial musculature (Figs 13-3 and 13-4).

The fact that the occlusal surfaces of the teeth have been worn excessively does not in itself warrant the assumption that the occlusal vertical dimension has been decreased. Under certain circumstances, continued eruption of the teeth can maintain the appropriate vertical dimension.

Another clinical sign that has often been misinterpreted is an extreme anterior vertical overlap in which the mandibular teeth actually strike the soft tissues of the palate. This condition may or may not indicate a de-

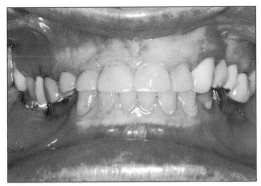

**Fig 13-3** A decrease in the occlusal vertical dimension may be accompanied by significant tooth wear, a noticeable decrease in the patient's nose-to-chin distance, or unexplained discomfort in the orofacial musculature. This patient displays signs of wear.

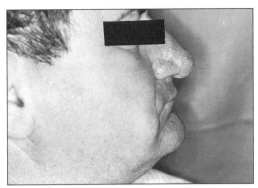

**Fig 13-4** A decrease in the nose-to-chin distance is often accompanied by pronounced folding at the commissures.

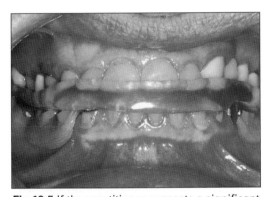

**Fig 13-5** If the practitioner suspects a significant decrease in the occlusal vertical dimension, a temporary increase should be considered. This increase should be accomplished using a temporary removable device in the form of an occlusal overlay.

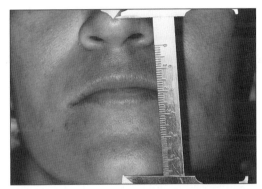

**Fig 13-6** The occlusal vertical dimension may be estimated by determining the patient's physiologic rest dimension and subtracting 2 to 3 mm. A number of measurements should be made in order to establish repeatable results.

crease in the occlusal vertical dimension. Therefore, no treatment should be instituted without more definite proof that a loss of vertical dimension has occurred.

Confirmation of a decrease in vertical dimension requires a history of physical discomfort related to overclosure, objective evidence of severe tooth wear or intrusion, and greater than 4 mm of interocclusal rest space. If these signs and symptoms are present, a temporary increase in the existing occlusal vertical dimension should be considered. This increase in interocclusal height should be accomplished using a temporary removable device in the form of an acrylic resin overlay (Fig 13-5).

The acrylic resin overlay, or occlusal device, must contact the remaining teeth in both arches in order to prevent supraeruption or intrusion of the teeth. Furthermore, the occlusal device must be worn 24 hours per

day, with the exception of removal for cleaning and maintenance. If the patient can tolerate the newly established occlusal vertical dimension for a period of 1 to 3 months, definitive correction may be instituted. Treatment must be planned so that all dimension-altering prostheses are inserted at the same time. Failure to place the prostheses in this manner can result in severe patient discomfort and failure of the occlusal rehabilitation.

## Establishing the occlusal vertical dimension

Only a small percentage of partial denture patients must have the occlusal vertical dimension established by measurement. This is accomplished by determining the physiologic rest dimension (Fig 13-6) and then subtracting 2 to 3 mm (the average interocclusal rest

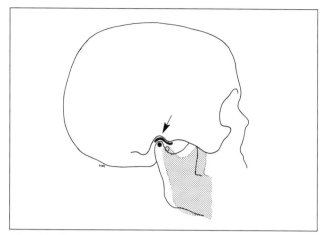

**Fig 13-7** Centric relation is the physiologic relationship of the mandible to the maxilla when both condyle-disc assemblies are stabilized against the posterior slopes of the articular eminences *(arrow)*. By definition, centric relation is a bone-to-bone relationship of the mandible to the maxilla. Remaining mandibular positions *(shading)* are anterior to centric relation.

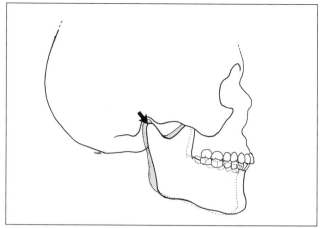

**Fig 13-8** Maximal intercuspal position represents the most complete interdigitation of the teeth. In most instances, the maximal intercuspal position *(arrow)* is anterior and inferior to centric relation *(shading, broken line)*. In the remaining instances, these positions are coincident.

space). The resultant measurement is the dimension at which the prosthesis should be constructed. The practitioner should keep in mind that this calculation is based on an average interocclusal space. Therefore, the occlusal vertical dimension should be evaluated before completion of the prosthesis.

## ☐ Horizontal Jaw Relation

Two horizontal relationships of the mandible to the maxilla must be considered in removable partial denture therapy. The first of these relationships is centric relation (Fig 13-7). As noted in chapter 1, centric relation is the physiologic relationship of the mandible to the maxilla when both condyles are properly related to their articular discs, and the condyle-disc assemblies are stabilized against the posterior slopes of the articular eminences. Centric relation is a bone-to-bone relation of the mandible to the maxilla; cuspal relationships of the teeth are not considered. The mandible can be returned to this position repeatedly, so it is considered a reference point in developing the occlusion for a patient.

The second horizontal relationship of the mandible to the maxilla is maximal intercuspal position. Maximal intercuspal position may be defined as the most complete interdigitation of the teeth independent of the condylar position (Fig 13-8). This is a tooth-to-tooth relationship; there is no mention of jaw position. This is not a terminal position of the mandible, but takes place somewhere within the borders of mandibular movement. It is a position of learned, conscious, habitual closure.

In more than 90% of all persons, centric relation and maximal intercuspal position do not coincide. When different, maximal intercuspal position will always be anterior to centric relation. The difference can range from tenths of a millimeter to 5 mm or more, but 1 to 2 mm is most frequent. Regardless of the position selected for development of an occlusal scheme, the practitioner must ensure harmony between these two positions. Patients should always have the ability to function in these two positions and the intervening space. Therefore, deflective contacts in either position must be avoided.

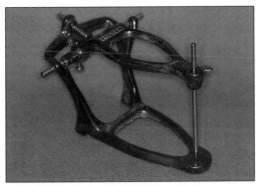

**Fig 13-9** The Foster articulator (Ray Foster Dental Equipment, Huntington Beach, CA) is an example of a nonadjustable instrument.

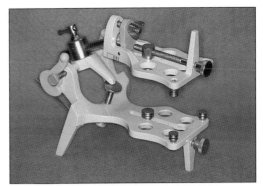

**Fig 13-10** The Gnatus articulator (Waterpik, Fort Collins, CO) is a nonadjustable instrument.

## ▢ Mounting the Dental Casts

At this stage, the practitioner must mount the dental casts in preparation for the arrangement of prosthetic teeth. Casts must be accurately related to the opening and closing axis of the chosen articulator and to one another. To accomplish these objectives, the practitioner must choose an appropriate articulator. In turn, the maxillary and mandibular casts must be properly mounted on the articulator.

Considerations for each procedure are presented in the following sections. Clinical procedures also are described.

### Choosing an articulator

Dental articulators are capable of performing a variety of movements. These movements may range from simple opening and closing around a fixed axis to complex movements that simulate mandibular motion. As a result, dental articulators have been classified using a number of systems.

The simplest and most understandable system for classification is based upon the adjustability of individual articulators. The system consists of three categories: nonadjustable, semiadjustable, and highly adjustable.

### Nonadjustable articulators

Nonadjustable articulators open and close around a fixed horizontal axis (Figs 13-9 and 13-10). The condylar element is normally attached to the upper member of the articulator and rotates in a groove or slot in the lower member of the articulator. A few representatives of this class have a fixed condylar path along which the condylar element can be moved to simulate lateral and protrusive jaw movement. The condylar path is set at a fixed angle and cannot be adjusted, so the instrument is still considered to be nonadjustable. Some of these instruments also may have incisal guide pins that rest on an inclined plate. Because the inclination of this plate is fixed, such instruments also are considered nonadjustable.

A nonadjustable articulator may be used in the fabrication of relatively simple removable partial dentures in which only a few posterior teeth are being replaced and canine disclusion exists. This class of articulator also may be used in specialized applications such as functionally generated path techniques.

The greatest requirement for a simple hinge articulator is that it be rigid. Flexure of the upper and lower members of the articulator or lateral movement of the joint between the two members can lead to significant errors in occlusion.

Nonadjustable articulators should be used rather sparingly.

### Semiadjustable articulators

Semiadjustable articulators represent the largest group in this classification system. All semiadjustable articulators have adjustable horizontal condylar paths, adjustable lateral condylar paths, and adjustable incisal guide tables (Figs 13-11 and 13-12). The range and accuracy of these adjustments may

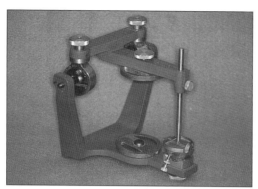

**Fig 13-11** The Hanau 158 (Waterpik) is classified as a semiadjustable articulator.

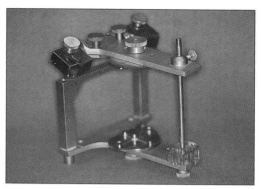

**Fig 13-12** The Whip-Mix articulator (Whip-Mix, Louisville, KY) is a semiadjustable instrument.

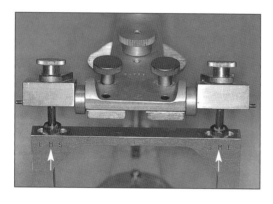

**Fig 13-13** The Whip-Mix articulator displays adjustable intercondylar distances *(arrows)*.

vary, but these articulators can be adjusted to follow the mandibular movements of a patient quite closely.

Certain instruments in this class display adjustable intercondylar distances (Fig 13-13). The condylar elements for these instruments may be moved medially or laterally to approximate the intercondylar distance of the patient. This adjustment controls the arcs scribed by the cusps of the teeth during mandibular movement. Proper adjustment permits more accurate placement of maxillary and mandibular cusps and minimizes cuspal interferences in eccentric movements.

It should not be inferred that the semiadjustable instruments are capable of following mandibular movements in their entirety. These articulators offer a close approximation of actual mandibular position, not a truly accurate one. These instruments are set principally from positional jaw relation records.

Hanau articulators are adjusted using a protrusive jaw relation record. The protrusive record enables the practitioner to determine the angle of the horizontal condylar path. The angle is determined by observing the fit of the casts into the protrusive record. The appropriate angle is the one that provides maximal cuspal contact with the record. The lateral condylar setting is then determined using the following formula:

$$L = \frac{H}{8} + 12$$

where *L* is the lateral condylar inclination in degrees and *H* is the horizontal condylar inclination in degrees as established by the protrusive jaw relation record.

The horizontal and lateral condylar guidances of Whip-Mix articulators are adjusted using lateral jaw relation records. The clinical component of this procedure is accomplished by introducing an appropriate recording medium and then guiding the patient into a lateral closure. The patient is maintained in this position until the recording medium reaches the desired consistency. The recording medium is then removed from the mouth and trimmed as necessary.

To receive the record and permit adjustment of the articulator, the practitioner loosens the set screws

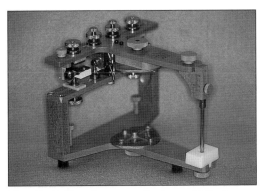

**Fig 13-14** The Stuart articulator (C.E. Stuart Gnathological Instruments, Ventura, CA) is classified as a highly adjustable instrument.

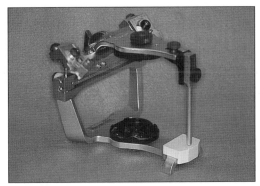

**Fig 13-15** The Denar D5A (Waterpik) also is a highly adjustable instrument.

to permit unrestricted movement of the horizontal and lateral condylar path elements. This procedure should be accomplished for the side opposite the mandibular movement. Therefore, if a right working movement was recorded, the condylar path elements on the left side should be permitted to move freely, and vice versa.

At this stage, the lateral record is positioned between the casts and the articulator is moved into the appropriate lateral position. The condylar path elements are then rotated into light contact with the condylar ball and locked into position. This procedure is then repeated for the opposite side. This procedure provides reasonable approximations for the pathways of mandibular movement.

Articulators may be further subdivided based upon configurations of their condylar elements. On some articulators, the condyles are attached to the lower member—just as in nature. These instruments are referred to as *arcon articulators*. The term was coined by Bergstrom and was derived from the words *articulation* and *condyle*. Other articulators display condyles that are part of the instrument's upper member. These articulators are referred to as *nonarcon articulators*.

The main advantage of an arcon articulator becomes apparent if one examines the relationship between a mounted maxillary cast and the element that establishes the horizontal condylar guidance. When using an arcon articulator, the relationship between the occlusal plane and the horizontal condylar guidance remains constant regardless of the opening or closure of the instrument. This is

identical to the situation observed in the human masticatory system.

When a nonarcon instrument is used, opening or closure of the instrument affects the relationship between the maxillary cast and the horizontal condylar guidance. As might be expected, these changes can affect occlusal factors and cause difficulties for the practitioner and dental laboratory technician alike. Consequently, an arcon articulator should be used whenever possible.

### Highly adjustable articulators

Highly adjustable articulators are capable of being adjusted to closely simulate mandibular motion. Representative instruments include the Stuart and Denar D5A instruments (Figs 13-14 and 13-15).

The use of a highly adjustable instrument requires accurate location of the transverse axis and some form of three-dimensional recording. In turn, the articulator must be adjusted to duplicate all recorded movements. This is a time- and labor-intensive process that requires a thorough understanding of the chosen instrumentation and meticulous attention to detail.

In considering the use of a highly adjustable articulator, the practitioner must consider the time required to accomplish associated diagnostic procedures, location of the transverse axis, development of the pantographic tracing, and programming of the articulator. These factors must be weighed against the potential advantages of using a more sophisticated instrument. As a general rule, unless the patient is to undergo a complete oral rehabilitation, the use of a highly ad-

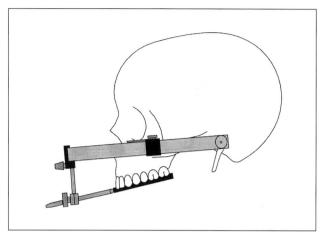

**Fig 13-16** Most arbitrary facebows are based upon the positions of the external auditory openings and a "point of reference." Orbitale is commonly used as a point of reference.

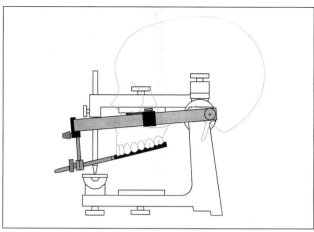

**Fig 13-17** A facebow record allows the practitioner to transfer the position of the maxillary cast to an articulator.

justable instrument is not indicated. The inherent stability of most removable partial dentures makes it possible to refine the occlusion intraorally and eliminates the need for highly adjustable instrumentation.

### Considerations in selecting an articulator

A practitioner should select the simplest instrument that meets the requirements of dental treatment. As the complexity of the articulator increases, so does the probability of making significant errors.

A simple hinge or a nonadjustable articulator is frequently indicated in the treatment of patients with Kennedy Class III partially edentulous arches. A semiadjustable instrument is most often indicated for Kennedy Class I, II, and IV arches. A highly adjustable instrument is usually limited to use in patients needing extensive occlusal rehabilitation.

### *Facebow transfer*

Following selection of an appropriate articulator, the practitioner must mount the maxillary and mandibular casts so they are properly related to the opening and closing axis of the instrument and to each other. The initial step in this procedure is accomplished using a caliper-like device termed a *facebow* (see chapter 6). The purpose of the facebow is to relate the maxillary cast to the opening and closing axis of the articulator. Consequently, the practitioner must select a facebow that is compatible with the chosen articulator.

In addition to placing the maxillary cast in the proper relationship to the opening and closing axis of the articulator, the facebow also can be used to place the maxillary cast in the proper relationship to the horizontal plane. This allows the practitioner and the dental laboratory technician to view the maxillary arch as it appears in the patient. This yields improved visualization, which is essential in the creation of esthetic prostheses.

To properly relate the maxillary cast to the horizontal plane, the practitioner must use a point of reference located anterior to the two condylar locations. The point that is most commonly used is orbitale, the lowest portion of the bony orbit. The two condylar locations and the lowest portion of the bony orbit approximate the Frankfort horizontal plane (orbitale to tragion). As a result, the relationship of the maxillary cast relative to the horizontal plane may be transferred to the articulator (Figs 13-16 and 13-17).

An additional advantage of the facebow transfer is its convenience. Although this aspect is often overlooked, the facebow supports the maxillary cast and allows the practitioner to accomplish the mounting process accurately and efficiently.

### *Jaw relation records and transfer*

There are many instances in which a maxillary cast and a mandibular cast can be accurately and repeatably articulated without the use of interocclusal records. In these instances, the mandibular cast may be properly

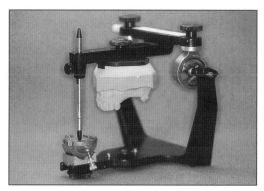

**Fig 13-18** Maxillary cast following completion of mounting procedures.

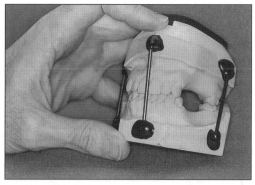

**Fig 13-19** The maxillary and mandibular casts are properly related. In turn, the casts are stabilized using modeling plastic and metal struts.

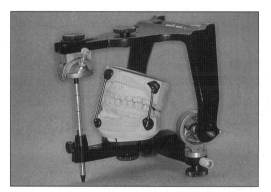

**Fig 13-20** The stabilized casts are returned to the articulator. The articulator is inverted to permit completion of the mounting process.

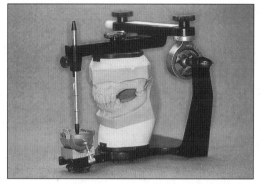

**Fig 13-21** Properly mounted maxillary and mandibular casts.

related to the mounted maxillary cast, stabilized using wire struts and modeling plastic, and attached to the lower member of the articulator (Figs 13-18 to 13-21).

In some applications, there may be an inadequate number or distribution of teeth to permit accurate hand articulation of the casts. As a result, interocclusal records must be used to record occlusal relationships. When this is the case, the fitted removable partial denture framework should be used as an integral portion of the record-making and cast-mounting processes. The framework provides a stable and accurate base on which to record the desired maxillomandibular relationship.

If this appointment follows the fabrication of a corrected cast, the framework and accompanying impression must be recovered. Before removing the framework from the corrected cast, the practitioner should carefully examine the relationship of the framework to the stone teeth. Care should be taken to ensure that the framework did not move as the corrected

cast was being poured. If any change in the position of the framework is noted, the corrected cast procedure should be repeated.

At this stage of the process, the resin tray that was used during the corrected cast impression procedure must be removed from the metal framework. This is accomplished by removing the impression material from the tray, then heating the tray material over a properly adjusted laboratory burner (Fig 13-22). The tray material is heated until it begins to smoke. It is then teased away from the framework using a plier or a hemostat (Fig 13-23).

### Making the record base

If the removable partial denture will be used to support a jaw relation record, an appropriate record base must first be constructed. A small, tooth-bounded record base may be constructed using hard baseplate wax. The baseplate wax must be heated and adapted to the resin-retaining components of the framework

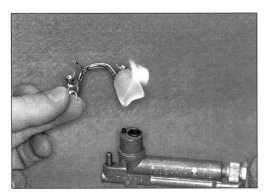

**Fig 13-22** A resin tray is heated to facilitate its removal from a removable partial denture framework.

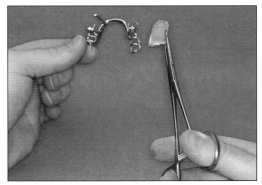

**Fig 13-23** After being heated, the resin is grasped using a hemostat. The tray is then removed from the framework.

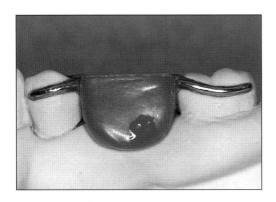

**Fig 13-24** A small, tooth-bounded record base may be constructed using hard baseplate wax.

(Fig 13-24). This type of record base usually will be strong enough to withstand the forces encountered during record-making and cast-mounting procedures. The greatest danger in using a wax record base is distortion. Therefore, a record base made from wax must not be stored for more than 1 hour or subjected to changes in temperature or humidity.

Larger record bases should always be constructed using rigid record base materials such as acrylic resins. Light-activated or chemically-activated resins may be used to construct these record bases. Each material has inherent advantages and disadvantages, but both display sufficient strength and accuracy to serve as record base materials.

Regardless of the material chosen for this purpose, soft tissue undercuts must be eliminated before beginning the resin adaptation process (Fig 13-25). Failure to eliminate soft tissue undercuts can result in irreparable damage to the master cast and must be avoided.

Upon completion of the blockout process, the cast is coated with an appropriate separating medium (Fig 13-26). The framework is then seated on the cast (Fig 13-27), and tray material is adapted over the resin-retaining components (Fig 13-28). Adaptation must be thorough enough to ensure firm attachment of the resin and to promote vertical stability of the framework. Following completion of the polymerization process, the borders of the resin are trimmed and smoothed to ensure patient comfort (Fig 13-29). The record base should not be polished.

### Attaching the occlusion rim

An occlusion rim is constructed by heating hard baseplate wax over a laboratory burner. The softened wax is then folded to create a moldable block of the desired size and shape (Fig 13-30). The wax block is centered over the record base and pressed into position (Fig 13-31). The wax should be approximately even with the fossae of the neighboring abutments. In distal extension applications, the height of the wax block should be approximately two thirds the height of the retromolar pad. The borders of the wax should be

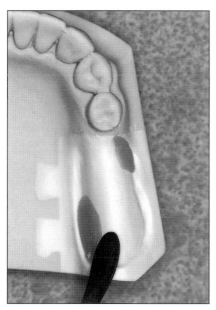

**Fig 13-25** Large record bases are constructed using rigid materials such as acrylic resins. To prevent damaging the dental cast, mechanical undercuts are eliminated using baseplate wax.

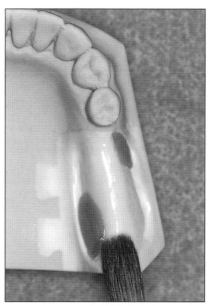

**Fig 13-26** The cast is coated with an appropriate separating medium.

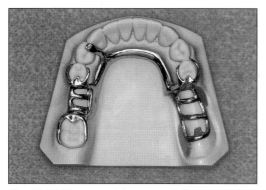

**Fig 13-27** The metal framework is returned to the master cast. The practitioner must ensure that the framework is fully seated.

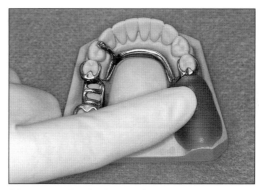

**Fig 13-28** Resin is carefully adapted to the struts of the minor connector.

**Fig 13-29** Following polymerization, the borders of the record base are trimmed and smoothed.

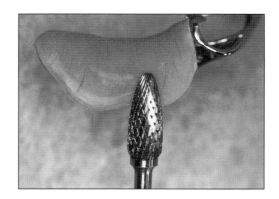

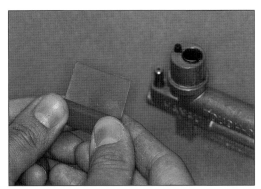

**Fig 13-30** After it has been softened over a laboratory burner, baseplate wax is folded to create a block of the desired size and shape.

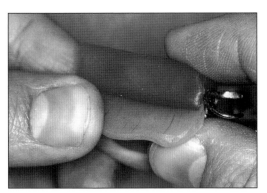

**Fig 13-31** The wax block is properly positioned.

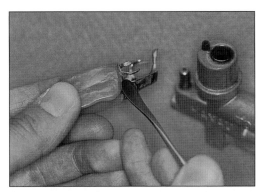

**Fig 13-32** Baseplate wax is sealed to the record base using a wax spatula.

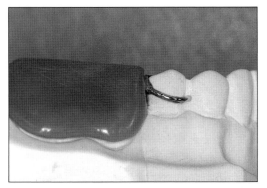

**Fig 13-33** The completed occlusion rim should display smooth, clean surfaces.

sealed to the underlying record base using a heated wax spatula (Fig 13-32). All contours should be well defined, and the wax should display a smooth, clean surface (Fig 13-33).

### Recording media

There is a wide variety of materials that can be used to record jaw relationships in removable partial denture applications. These include waxes, modeling plastics, accelerated dental stones, zinc oxide–eugenol impression pastes, polyethers, and polyvinylsiloxanes.

Waxes and modeling plastics are easy to use and display acceptable detail, but are susceptible to distortion. If these materials are used, articulator mountings must be completed within a few minutes of record-making procedures. If this is not accomplished, the accuracy of the mounting procedure can be adversely affected.

Accelerated dental stones and zinc oxide–eugenol impression pastes are extremely accurate, but can be

difficult to use in the oral cavity. While these materials are rigid and dimensionally stable, they are difficult to trim and are subject to fracture. Consequently, the use of these materials is declining.

Polyether and polyvinylsiloxane materials display extreme accuracy and are relatively easy to use in the oral cavity. Because these materials exhibit some compressibility, records should be relatively thin (< 2 mm). Polyether and polyvinylsiloxane registration materials can be trimmed with a surgical blade and are dimensionally stable for extended periods. Perhaps the greatest drawback associated with these materials is related to cost. Despite the increased expense, these materials are among the most commonly used recording media in contemporary dental practice.

### Clinical procedures

The framework with the record base and occlusion rim is properly positioned in the patient's mouth. The fit is evaluated to ensure that the assembly is fully seated.

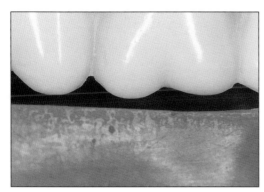

**Fig 13-34** Each occlusion rim is adjusted so that no contact occurs between its surface and the opposing occlusal surfaces. A space of approximately 1 mm should be evident.

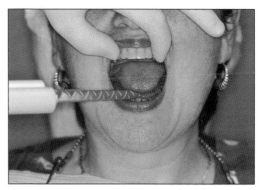

**Fig 13-35** The chosen recording medium is introduced into the oral cavity.

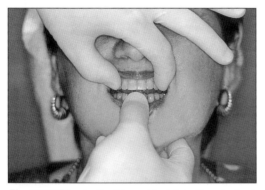

**Fig 13-36** The patient is guided into the desired closure.

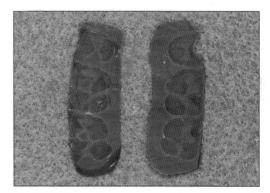

**Fig 13-37** Records are removed from the mouth and properly trimmed.

At this stage, the borders of the record base are adjusted to permit complete seating.

If the record is to be made at the centric relation position, the mandible is guided posteriorly and the patient is instructed to close to the desired occlusal vertical dimension. If the maximal intercuspal position is to be used, the patient is instructed to close into that position. Each occlusion rim is adjusted so that no contact occurs between its surface and the cusps of the opposing teeth. A space of approximately 1 mm should be visible (Fig 13-34).

In the event that opposing occlusion rims are to be used, one rim is adjusted to establish an ideal occlusal plane. The opposing rim is then adjusted to be approximately 1 mm short of contact. In most instances, the mandibular rim is used to establish the ideal occlusal plane. This is accomplished using the heights of remaining teeth anteriorly and two thirds the height of the retromolar pad posteriorly.

At this juncture, the practitioner should remove the framework from the mouth and prepare shallow V-shaped grooves on the wax surfaces. These grooves permit the removal and accurate replacement of records during record-making and cast-mounting procedures.

The entire assembly is then returned to the mouth in preparation for jaw relation procedures. The practitioner should explain the process to the patient and rehearse the procedures several times before the first record is made. An informed patient is generally more cooperative and more likely to perform the required movements in an accurate and timely manner.

The chosen recording material is prepared and introduced into the oral cavity (Fig 13-35). The patient is then guided into the desired closure and the recording medium is allowed to reach the appropriate consistency (Fig 13-36). The record is removed from the mouth and trimmed to the desired dimensions (Fig 13-37). If desired, additional records may be made at this time.

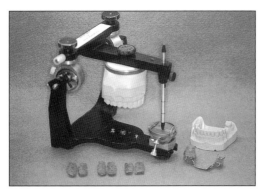

**Fig 13-38** The mounting procedure requires a properly mounted maxillary cast, a mandibular cast, one or more properly adjusted frameworks with occlusion rims, and accurate interocclusal records.

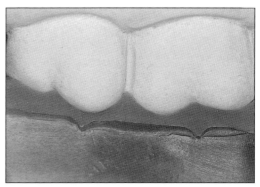

**Fig 13-39** The dental casts must accurately fit into the interocclusal records. This photograph shows accurate interdigitation on the right side.

The greatest cause of inaccurate jaw relation records is uncontrolled pressure. If any force is placed on a tissue-borne occlusion rim, the associated record base will depress the underlying soft tissues. This results in movement of the record base and an inaccurate jaw relation record. Therefore, if any portion of the wax occlusion rim shows through the recording medium, that portion of the occlusion rim should be reduced and the record should be remade.

If the jaw relation record is accurate, the mandibular cast may be mounted on the articulator.

### Mounting the mandibular cast

At this stage, the practitioner should have *(1)* an accurate maxillary cast that has been properly mounted on the chosen articulator, *(2)* an accurate mandibular cast, *(3)* one or more properly adjusted frameworks with the associated record bases and occlusion rims, and *(4)* accurate interocclusal records (Fig 13-38).

Before proceeding, each framework is returned to its master cast. The practitioner must ensure that each framework is completely seated and that the record bases and occlusion rims have not been damaged.

To complete the mounting process, the articulator is inverted and the interocclusal record is positioned on the occlusal surfaces of the maxillary cast. The cusps of the mandibular cast are settled into the corresponding

depressions on the interocclusal record (Fig 13-39). The practitioner should be certain that the record is not compressed or distorted during this procedure.

If the practitioner determines that the maxillary and mandibular casts accurately fit the record, the casts should be stabilized using metal struts and modeling plastic. This is accomplished by heating the modeling plastic over a properly adjusted flame and then placing the heated modeling plastic at three widely spaced areas on the maxillary and mandibular casts. Metal struts are gently pressed into the modeling plastic. Additional modeling plastic is then added to ensure that the struts are held firmly to the respective casts (Fig 13-40). The practitioner must maintain the appropriate spatial relationships until the modeling plastic cools and becomes rigid. The mounting procedure may then be completed with relative ease (Figs 13-41 and 13-42).

A brittle material such as modeling plastic should always be used to position bracing struts. If the relationship of the casts changes during the mounting process, the brittle material will separate from one or both casts, thereby alerting the practitioner to an inaccuracy. If this occurs, the orientation of the casts should be corrected and the mounting procedure reaccomplished.

A brittle material also simplifies the cleanup following completion of the mounting process. After the mounting stone has set, the modeling plastic and

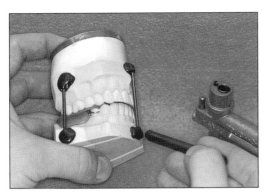

**Fig 13-40** The entire assembly is stabilized using metal struts and modeling plastic.

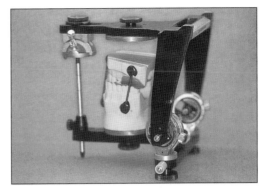

**Fig 13-41** The assembly is returned to the articulator. The articulator is inverted to facilitate completion of the mounting process.

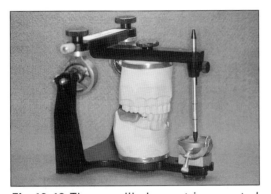

**Fig 13-42** The mandibular cast is mounted using a minimal-expansion dental stone. When the dental stone has hardened, the metal struts and modeling plastic are removed from the casts. Subsequently, the interocclusal records are removed.

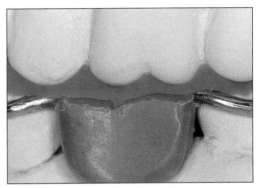

**Fig 13-43** Additional interocclusal records are used to assess the accuracy of the mounting. Here, accurate interdigitation is evident on the left side.

metal struts can be removed by grasping the struts and applying torquing forces.

Metal struts should be used in preference to wooden struts, which may undergo noticeable dimensional changes if they become wet during the mounting process. Metal struts may be made by cutting wire clothes hangers into 50-mm segments. These struts may be cleaned and used repeatedly.

Additional interocclusal records may be used to verify the accuracy of the mounting (Fig 13-43). Accuracy of the mounting should always be verified before prosthetic teeth are added to a removable partial denture framework.

## Factors Influencing the Development of Occlusion

Several factors influence the occlusal scheme for a removable partial denture patient. The interaction of these factors is crucial to restorative success and, therefore, must be understood by the practitioner.

During the early part of the twentieth century, an engineer by the name of Rudolph L. Hanau postulated nine laws of articulation.[2] These laws were intended to provide a basic understanding of balanced articulation. Of the nine factors originally proposed by Hanau, five factors emerged as critical elements in

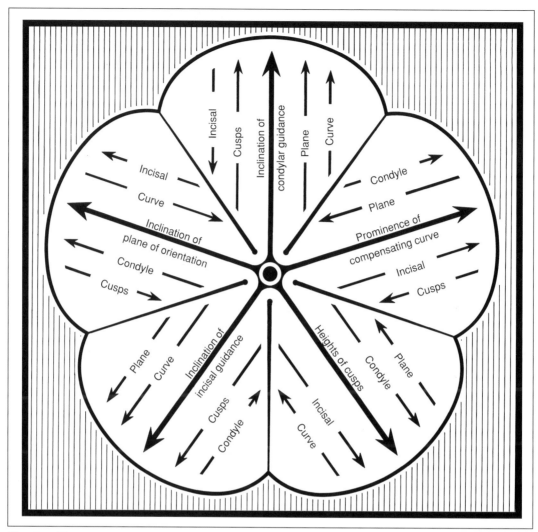

**Fig 13-44** The Hanau Quint consists of five elements. These elements display consistent relationships to one another. *Arrows* pointing away from the center indicate increasing values. *Arrows* pointing toward the center indicate decreasing values. (Courtesy of Teledyne Hanau/Waterpik Technologies.)

prosthodontic therapy. Collectively, these five factors became known as the Hanau Quint (Fig 13-44). The factors comprising the Hanau Quint include

1. The inclination of the condylar guidance (Fig 13-45)
2. The inclination of the plane of orientation (Fig 13-46)
3. The prominence of the compensating curve (Fig 13-47)
4. The inclination of the incisal guidance (Fig 13-48)
5. The heights of the cusps (Fig 13-49)

In complete denture prosthodontics, the condylar guidance is the only factor that cannot be altered.

The compensating curve, plane of orientation, incisal guidance, and heights of the cusps may be changed rather easily. The ability to alter four of the five factors makes it possible to develop a satisfactory occlusal scheme for a patient requiring complete dentures.

In a patient who requires a removable partial denture, the development of a satisfactory occlusal scheme can be more difficult. Due to the presence of natural teeth, many factors are predetermined. The presence of natural teeth often establishes the prominence of the compensating curve, the plane of orientation, the incisal guidance, and the heights of the cusps. Consequently, the remaining natural teeth usu-

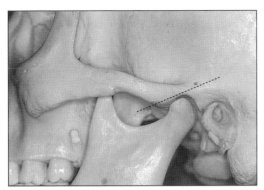

**Fig 13-45** Inclination of the condylar guidance *(broken line)*. This element is dependent upon the anatomy of the glenoid fossa.

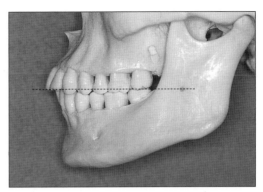

**Fig 13-46** Inclination of the plane of orientation *(broken line)*. This plane passes through the tips of the mandibular central incisors anteriorly and the mesiobuccal cusps of the mandibular second molars posteriorly. The angle is measured relative to the horizontal plane.

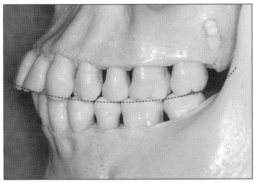

**Fig 13-47** Prominence of the compensating curve *(broken line)*. This is the relative curvature of the occlusal plane in an anteroposterior direction.

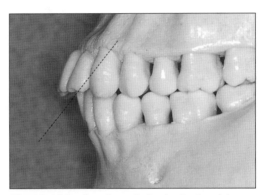

**Fig 13-48** Inclination of the incisal guidance *(broken line)*. This element is determined by the relationship of the mandibular anterior teeth to the lingual surfaces of the maxillary anterior teeth. This angle is measured relative to the horizontal plane.

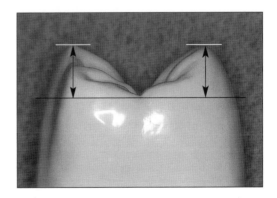

**Fig 13-49** Heights of the cusps *(arrows)*. Cusp height is the vertical distance from cusp base to cusp tip.

ally dictate the form and positions of the prosthetic teeth. The only exceptions occur *(1)* when the removable partial denture is opposed by a complete den-

ture and *(2)* when only anterior teeth remain in both arches and the incisal relationship does not interfere with establishment of the desired occlusal scheme.

# ☐ Arrangement of Prosthetic Teeth

Upon completion of the articulator mounting and a thorough assessment of the occlusal requirements, the practitioner should be able to perform or prescribe the proper arrangement of prosthetic teeth.

The various types of replacements are described in chapter 3. The considerations and techniques for tooth placement are presented in the following sections.

## Anterior teeth

As a general rule, the most difficult part of arranging anterior denture teeth is directly related to a loss of restorative space. Unless anterior teeth are replaced immediately following their extraction, the natural teeth adjacent to the space will either drift or tilt into the space. The drifting or tilting produces a noticeable decrease in the restorative space and forces the selection of one or more prosthetic teeth that are narrower than their natural counterparts. This will inevitably produce an artificial appearance in the patient's mouth (Fig 13-50). During the mouth preparation appointment, an attempt should have been made to regain the original width of the space by reshaping the proximal surfaces of the adjacent teeth (Fig 13-51). If the entire width cannot be recovered, consideration should be given to overlapping the artificial teeth so that a normal-sized tooth may be used to harmonize with the patient's face and remaining teeth.

Anterior denture teeth are generally supplied in sets of six and are available in a wide variety of sizes, shapes, and colors (Fig 13-52). Because of their availability, ease of adjustment, and surface wear characteristics, acrylic resin teeth are more commonly used than are porcelain teeth. While esthetically pleasing, porcelain teeth are relatively brittle and cause accelerated wear of opposing enamel, gold, and acrylic resin surfaces.

When selecting denture teeth, the practitioner should use the shade guide provided by the tooth manufacturer (Fig 13-53). Artificial teeth should be matched as closely as possible to the adjacent natural teeth or fixed restorations. The matching process should be accomplished using natural light and should be completed as quickly as possible. The first assessment usually will be the most accurate since the ability to discriminate between shades decreases rapidly as a result of eye fatigue.

Following shade selection, the practitioner must select the appropriate mold. Each mold exhibits a defined size and shape, as well as distinctive surface characteristics (eg, lobes and depressions). Consequently, mold selection must be approached with great care.

Mold selection is based upon two important factors. Perhaps the most important factor is related to the space that has been created by tooth loss. If a single anterior tooth is being replaced, the practitioner must consider not only the size of the individual edentulous space, but also the dimensions of the corresponding tooth on the opposite side of the arch. If multiple anterior teeth are being replaced, the practitioner must measure the entire restorative space. The resultant measurement should then be recorded to permit comparison with available molds.

Under certain circumstances, the practitioner may wish to estimate the sizes of the patient's natural maxillary central incisors. This may be accomplished using a technique popularized by Dr M. M. House. The House technique coordinates the width and length of each maxillary central incisor with the width and length of the patient's face. To estimate the width of one maxillary central incisor, the practitioner determines the patient's bizygomatic width and divides by 16 (Fig 13-54). For example, a patient with a bizygomatic width of 136 mm would have an estimated maxillary central incisor width of 8.5 mm. To estimate the length of the clinical crown, the practitioner measures the patient's chin-to-hairline distance and again divides by 16 (Fig 13-55). Hence, a patient with a chin-to-hairline distance of 163 mm would have an estimated maxillary central incisor length of 10.2 mm. The practitioner must remember that estimates are based on anatomic norms. Consequently, this technique may serve as a starting point for tooth selection, but may not satisfy all functional and esthetic requirements.

The second factor in mold selection is the overall form or shape of the teeth. For convenience, teeth are usually divided into four basic forms: square, tapering, square-tapering, and ovoid. The basic elements of this classification system are attributed to Dr J. Leon Williams. Williams observed that anterior teeth exhibit a relatively limited number of shapes, and that these

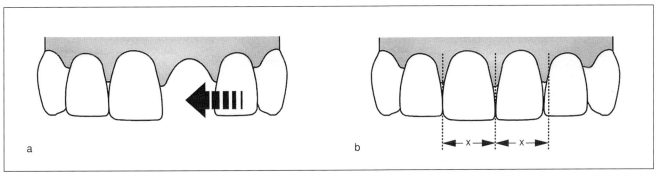

**Fig 13-50** *(a)* When an anterior tooth is lost, adjacent teeth often drift or tip into the space. *(b)* This produces a noticeable decrease in restorative space and forces the selection of a replacement that is too narrow.

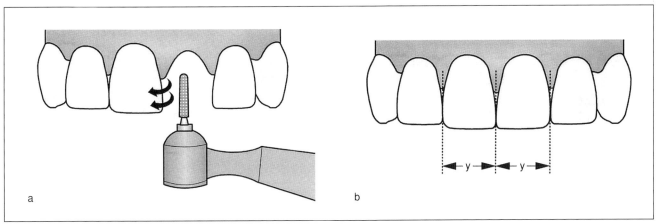

**Fig 13-51** *(a)* When space has been lost, reshaping of adjacent teeth is indicated. *(b)* This permits the practitioner to achieve an improved esthetic result.

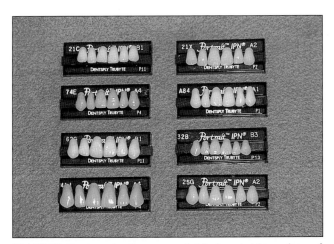

**Fig 13-52** Denture teeth are available in a wide variety of sizes, shapes, and colors.

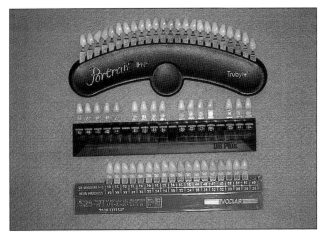

**Fig 13-53** When selecting denture teeth, the practitioner should use the shade guide provided by the tooth manufacturer.

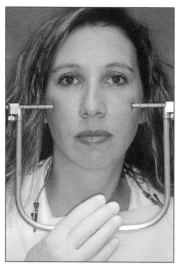

**Fig 13-54** The practitioner may estimate the width of a maxillary central incisor by determining the bizygomatic width and dividing it by 16.

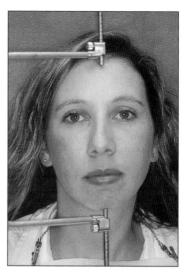

**Fig 13-55** The length of a maxillary central incisor may be estimated by determining the chin-to-hairline distance and dividing it by 16.

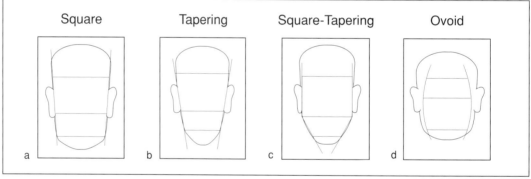

| Square | Tapering | Square-Tapering | Ovoid |
|--------|----------|-----------------|-------|
| a | b | c | d |

**Fig 13-56** The four most commonly observed facial forms are square *(a)*, tapering *(b)*, square-tapering *(c)*, and ovoid *(d)*.

shapes are closely related to facial form (Fig 13-56). Therefore, by determining the shape of a patient's face, the practitioner can determine the appropriate form for the anterior teeth.

At this stage, the practitioner can select the anterior teeth by combining the prescribed shade, dimensions, and tooth form. In turn, the anterior teeth may be arranged.

If one or more acrylic resin record bases were added to the framework, these bases must be removed before the teeth are arranged. This is accomplished by heating the acrylic resin over a properly adjusted burner and using a plier or a hemostat to tease the softened material away from the metal framework. Tinfoil is then applied to the cast in areas where denture bases are to be added. The tinfoil prevents adherence of wax to the stone cast and permits removal of the framework during the esthetic try-in stage. Following adaptation of the foil, baseplate wax is heated and adapted to the framework.

Denture teeth on a denture base generally provide the greatest latitude in tooth arrangement and permit the most esthetic results. This is particularly true when a patient has lost a large segment of the anterior ridge because of periodontal disease or trauma. In such a situation, the denture base may be built to provide the

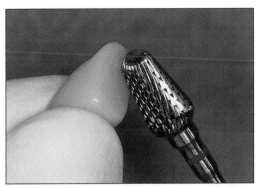

**Fig 13-57** In most instances, it will be necessary to reshape the ridge lap portion of an artificial tooth to position it over components of the framework.

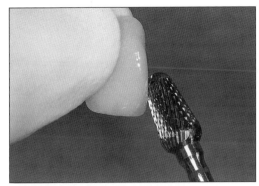

**Fig 13-58** Selective recontouring of axial and incisal surfaces permits improved adaptation and appearance.

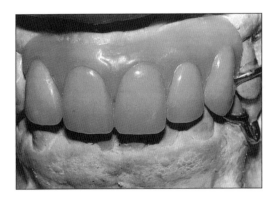

**Fig 13-59** Prosthetic teeth are arranged, and denture bases are contoured in preparation for the try-in appointment.

appropriate support and contour for the lips. If, on the other hand, the residual ridge is large and full, the denture teeth may be positioned directly against the ridge to avoid unnecessarily plumping the lips.

If the maxillary central incisors are missing, it is essential that these teeth be set first. This allows the practitioner to reestablish the maxillary midline in the center of the face. One of the most distracting errors in denture service occurs when the maxillary midline is not coincident with the facial midline. Another occurs when the midline deviates from the vertical. Therefore, the midline should be determined at the framework try-in appointment or the jaw relation appointment, and its position and orientation should be transferred to the master cast.

It will almost always be necessary to reshape the ridge lap portion of an artificial tooth to position it over the associated minor connector (Fig 13-57). The practitioner should be certain to maintain the collar or

neck of the tooth, since this segment is critical in the development of esthetics. Axial and incisal surfaces of the prosthetic teeth should be recontoured to improve adaptation and esthetics. Each denture tooth should be positioned as close to the location of the corresponding natural tooth as possible.

If an anterior denture tooth is to be positioned against a natural tooth, the proximal surface of the prosthetic tooth must be contoured to permit close adaptation (Fig 13-58). The incisal angles should be maintained to preserve the natural morphology of the crown.

The denture base flanges should be contoured and smoothed to provide a pleasing appearance. Excess wax should be removed from the cast and framework before the patient's arrival. The try-in appointment will be the first time the patient sees the prosthesis in its final form, and the first impression should be a pleasant one (Fig 13-59).

During the try-in appointment, the practitioner should seek feedback regarding tooth arrangement. Therefore, the patient should be encouraged to bring a family member or close friend to this appointment. Oftentimes, a patient is reluctant to provide feedback regarding arrangement of the anterior teeth. A family member or friend may be the dentist's best source of information regarding tooth arrangement and lip contour.

Final positioning and contouring of the teeth should be accomplished with the patient present.

## Posterior teeth

Posterior replacement teeth must not only fit into the available edentulous spaces, but also must be in harmony with the opposing occlusal surfaces. The dentist should not be overly concerned with replacing the exact number and type of teeth that are missing. For example, the edentulous space may have been occupied by a second premolar and first molar, but because of drifting of the remaining teeth, the most suitable replacement teeth may well be two premolars. Similarly, a space previously occupied by two premolars may present room for only one premolar. Consequently, the practitioner must always consider the most suitable combination of artificial teeth.

For the same reasons that acrylic resin denture teeth are usually selected in anterior applications, resin denture teeth are also indicated in posterior positions. Acrylic resin teeth can be altered rather easily. Axial and occlusal recontouring permits these teeth to be used in a wide variety of applications. Acrylic resin teeth also may oppose enamel, gold, and other resin surfaces without causing accelerated wear. In contrast, porcelain teeth are brittle, difficult to adjust, and cause significant abrasion of most opposing surfaces. Therefore, porcelain teeth are indicated only if they will oppose similar porcelain surfaces.

As noted for anterior teeth, shade selection should be accomplished using the shade guide provided by the manufacturer. To provide the best possible result, the posterior teeth should be matched as closely as possible to the adjacent teeth or fixed restorations.

The practitioner should then choose the appropriate mold for the tooth or teeth to be replaced. In a tooth-bounded application, tooth size is determined

by the length of the edentulous space. In a distal extension application, tooth size usually is determined by the sizes of the opposing teeth. When the removable partial denture is to be opposed by a complete denture, the practitioner measures from the distal surface of a natural canine to the incline of the ramus in the mandibular arch or the mesial aspect of the tuberosity in the maxillary arch (Fig 13-60). This distance normally ranges from 28 to 32 mm. As a result, manufacturers create posterior denture molds within the same range.

Before deciding upon a posterior mold, the practitioner also must consider the occlusogingival height for each replacement tooth. Most posterior molds are available in short, medium, and long embodiments. Denture teeth that are too tall often require a great deal of adjustment. In contrast, denture teeth that are too short may create significant esthetic problems. This is particularly true when a short artificial tooth is placed adjacent to a natural tooth with a relatively long clinical crown (Figs 13-61 and 13-62). To avoid these difficulties, the practitioner should consider a mold that is slightly longer than the remaining natural teeth.

The definitive choice for a posterior mold should be made by combining the shade, length, and occlusogingival height determined in the foregoing process. Subsequently, the posterior teeth should be arranged.

As a general rule, the practitioner should strive for a classic pattern of intercuspation between the maxillary and mandibular teeth. While this cannot always be accomplished, an effective, functional occlusion can usually be established.

One of the primary goals in establishing an effective occlusal scheme is to develop an acceptable pattern of maxillomandibular contacts. To do this, it is necessary to set the denture teeth at a height that is slightly greater than the proposed occlusal vertical dimension. The operator may then perform corrective grinding procedures, which (1) return the teeth to the proposed occlusal vertical dimension and (2) provide maximum planned contact between opposing occlusal surfaces.

To set the teeth at a slightly increased vertical dimension, the operator increases the incisal pin setting by 0.5 mm (Fig 13-63). This produces a slight increase in the distance between the upper and lower members of the articulator. The posterior teeth are then arranged (Fig 13-64). When this has been accom-

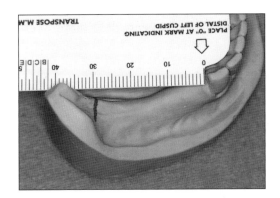

**Fig 13-60** Posterior denture teeth are often selected by measuring from the distal surface of the mandibular canine to the incline of the ramus. This distance is then compared with available molds.

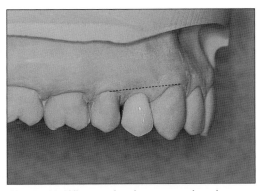

**Fig 13-61** When selecting posterior denture teeth, the practitioner must consider the occlusogingival height for each denture tooth. Denture teeth that are too short may create esthetic problems. In this instance, a short artificial tooth is positioned between teeth with relatively long clinical crowns.

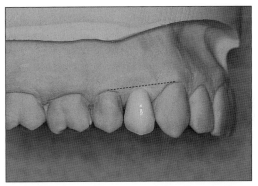

**Fig 13-62** To avoid esthetic difficulties, artificial teeth must harmonize with natural teeth. This denture tooth displays appropriate occlusogingival height.

plished, the incisal pin is returned to its original setting (Figs 13-65 and 13-66). The occlusal surfaces of the prosthetic teeth are then marked using articulating paper and adjusted using appropriate burs in a laboratory handpiece (Figs 13-67 and 13-68). Upon completion of this process, a suitable pattern of occlusal contact should be evident and the incisal pin should contact the incisal table (Figs 13-69 and 13-70). After verifying contact of the incisal pin and incisal table,

the practitioner marks the occlusal contacts once again. Occlusal grooves and sluiceways are then reestablished to improve masticatory efficiency (Fig 13-71). During this process, the practitioner must be certain to maintain the existing occlusal contacts. Failure to do this may result in alteration of occlusal contacts and an undesirable decrease in the occlusal vertical dimension.

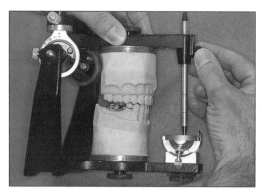

**Fig 13-63** To set the teeth at a slightly increased vertical dimension, the practitioner increases the incisal pin setting by 0.5 mm before arranging the denture teeth.

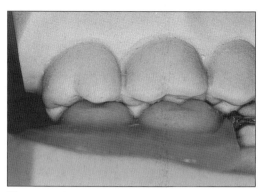

**Fig 13-64** Posterior teeth are arranged to provide maximum contact.

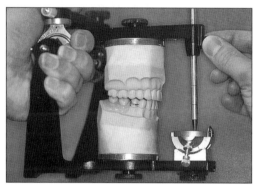

**Fig 13-65** Following placement of artificial teeth, the incisal pin is returned to its original setting.

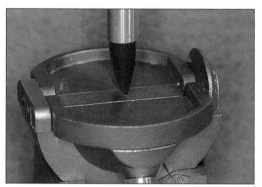

**Fig 13-66** When the articulator is closed, the incisal pin will be positioned above the incisal table.

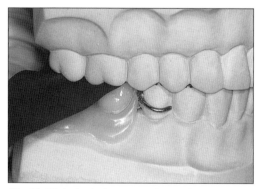

**Fig 13-67** Articulating paper is used to evaluate the occlusion.

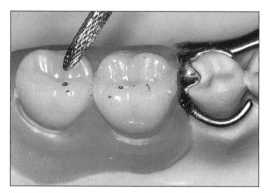

**Fig 13-68** The occlusion is adjusted by recontouring the occlusal surfaces of the artificial teeth.

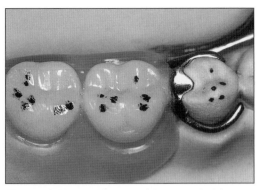

**Fig 13-69** The goal is to achieve a suitable pattern of occlusal contact at the established occlusal vertical dimension.

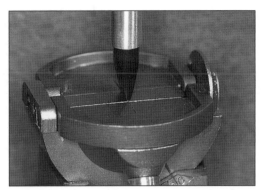

**Fig 13-70** The process is continued until the incisal pin is in contact with the incisal table.

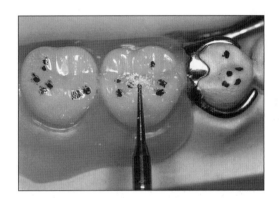

**Fig 13-71** Occlusal grooves and sluiceways are reestablished using a small round bur in a low-speed handpiece. Care is taken to avoid the established contacts (identified using articulating paper).

## Positioning a denture tooth adjacent to a clasp assembly

It is often difficult to properly position a denture tooth adjacent to a clasp assembly or a minor connector. Such a tooth must not only be adapted to function against the opposing occlusion, but also must be adapted to the clasp assembly, the minor connector, the residual ridge, and the resin-retaining components of the framework.

To minimize the amount of recontouring that must be done at any one time, tooth adaptation may be done in stages. During the first stage of this process, the practitioner removes the metal framework and fits the tooth to the residual ridge and the opposing occlusion (Figs 13-72 and 13-73). The denture tooth is reduced by grinding on the lingual and central portions of the ridge lap. The facial surface of the tooth is preserved to maintain crown length. The tooth is then positioned to provide the most ideal cusp-to-fossa relationship that is obtainable.

When the correct adaptation has been achieved, the framework is repositioned on the cast and the denture tooth is adjusted to accommodate the components. A simple method for identifying areas of the denture tooth that must be reshaped is shown in Figs 13-74 to 13-77. The purpose of this procedure is to ensure adequate room for acrylic resin, not to gain intimate contact between the denture tooth and the underlying struts. There must be a space of at least 1 mm between the ridge lap and the resin-retaining element if the resin is to exhibit sufficient strength.

At this stage, surfaces adjacent to proximal plates must be adjusted. This is accomplished using the technique illustrated in Figs 13-78 to 13-81. Unlike the ridge lap, the axial surface of the denture tooth should be tightly adapted to the surface of the metal.

When the denture tooth has been properly adjusted, hard baseplate wax may be used to secure the tooth in position. The remaining prosthetic teeth are adjusted and arranged in a similar manner. The oc-

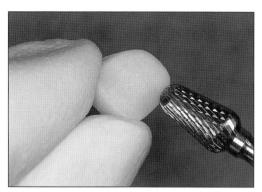

**Fig 13-72** During the initial stages of the tooth arrangement process, the practitioner fits each tooth to the corresponding ridge area of the master cast. In most instances, this requires adjustment of the ridge lap of each tooth. Care should be taken to avoid unnecessary reduction of the buccal surface.

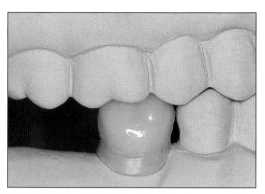

**Fig 13-73** Each tooth is fitted to the opposing occlusal surfaces.

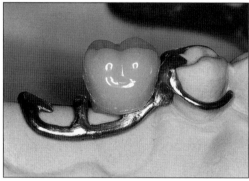

**Fig 13-74** The framework is then positioned on the master cast and each tooth is repositioned. Initially, resin-retaining components (ie, struts, meshwork, beads) may interfere with placement of artificial teeth. In this photograph, the occlusal surface of the molar is positioned above the occlusal plane.

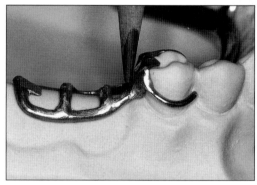

**Fig 13-75** Areas that interfere with tooth placement must be identified. To accomplish this, a light coating of graphite is placed on the resin-retaining components.

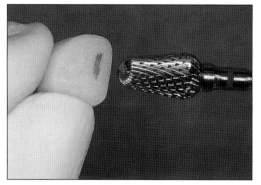

**Fig 13-76** Each denture tooth is then repositioned on the framework. Graphite is transferred to areas of interference. These areas are adjusted using appropriate rotary instruments.

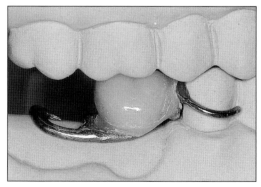

**Fig 13-77** The process is repeated until each denture tooth is properly positioned.

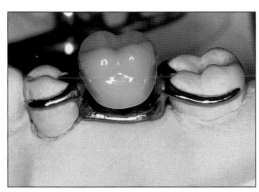

**Fig 13-78** Surfaces that are adjacent to proximal plates also must be adjusted. In this instance, proximal plates on both sides of the edentulous space interfere with tooth placement.

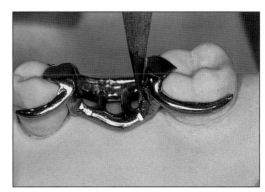

**Fig 13-79** A light coating of graphite is placed on the proximal plates.

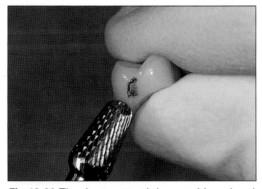

**Fig 13-80** The denture tooth is repositioned and subsequently removed. Graphite is transferred to areas of interference. Adjustment is performed using appropriate rotary instrumentation.

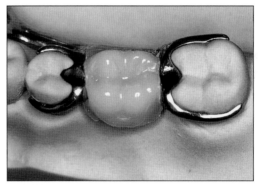

**Fig 13-81** Upon completion of the adjustment process, the denture tooth should fit tightly against the proximal plates.

clusal surfaces of the artificial teeth are positioned to provide the most favorable relationships to the opposing occlusal surfaces. Slight spacing between posterior teeth is sometimes necessary, but excessive spacing should be avoided. If excessive spacing is evident, the practitioner should consider using denture teeth with greater mesiodistal dimensions.

Following the correct placement of the artificial posterior teeth, the denture base is waxed to the desired contours. Subsequently, the incisal guide pin is returned to its correct vertical position and the teeth are adjusted to reestablish the proposed occlusal vertical dimension. If a semiadjustable or highly adjustable articulator is being used and has been properly programmed, articulation in lateral and protrusive movements also should be adjusted.

The desired occlusal contacts for artificial teeth for removable partial dentures vary according to the class of partially edentulous arch being treated. The following is a brief summary of the various occlusal schemes that may be used in removable partial denture therapy.

1. Simultaneous bilateral occlusal contact of opposing posterior teeth should be present when the patient is in maximal intercuspal position. Contact must occur between natural teeth, between natural and artificial teeth, and between artificial teeth. A prosthesis must not hold opposing natural teeth apart, or some form of destruction will occur.

2. For a tooth-borne removable partial denture, the occlusion should be similar to a harmonious natural dentition. In most patients, a mutually pro-

tected articulation is the goal. In a mutually protected articulation, the posterior teeth provide slight separation of the anterior teeth when the patient is in a maximal intercuspal position. As the mandible moves eccentrically, the posterior teeth separate because of contact of the anterior teeth. This is a normal occlusal scheme and should be retained when possible.

For some patients, a group function articulation may be required. In a group function articulation, lateral movement of the mandible results in numerous anterior and posterior contacts. These contacts are simultaneous and are characteristically limited to the working side. Group function articulation should not be used unless it was present before the loss of teeth and did not contribute to this loss.

3. For a removable partial denture opposing a complete denture, balanced articulation is desirable. Balanced articulation is the bilateral, simultaneous contact of anterior and posterior teeth in centric and eccentric positions. The inability to achieve bilateral balance may result in an unstable denture and destruction of the residual ridge.

4. In Class IV applications, it is desirable to have light contact with the opposing natural teeth in maximal intercuspal position. This prevents further eruption of the natural teeth and improves the stability of the dental arch. Eccentric occlusion must be developed so the prosthetic teeth are in harmony with the chosen occlusal scheme (ie, mutually protected articulation, group function articulation, or balanced articulation).

5. Artificial teeth should not be positioned on the upward incline of the mandibular ridge (as it ascends the mandibular ramus). Placement of forces in this region produces an inclined plane effect involving the intaglio surface of the prosthesis and the tissues of the mandibular ridge. This may result in movement of the prosthesis and the application of destructive forces to the remaining teeth and tissues.

## ☐ Length of Appointment

An experienced practitioner should be able to adjust the occlusion rim(s) and complete the required jaw relation records in about 45 minutes. A novice should allow 60 to 90 minutes for these procedures.

## ☐ References

1. Niswonger ME. The rest position of the mandible. J Am Dent Assoc 1934;21:1572–1582.
2. Hanau RL. Articulation defined, analyzed and formulated. J Am Dent Assoc 1926;13:1694–1709.

## ☐ Bibliography

Applegate OC. The partial denture base. J Prosthet Dent 1955;5:636–648.

Baraban DJ. Establishing centric relation and vertical dimension in occlusal rehabilitation. J Prosthet Dent 1962;12:1157–1165.

Beck HO. Choosing the articulator. J Am Dent Assoc 1962;64:468–475.

Beck HO. A clinical evaluation of the Arcon concept of articulation. J Prosthet Dent 1959;9:409–421.

Beck HO. Selection of an articulator and jaw registration. J Prosthet Dent 1960;10:878–886.

Beckett LS. Accurate occlusal relations in partial denture construction. J Prosthet Dent 1954;4:487–495.

Beyron HL. Occlusal relationship. Int Dent J 1952;2:467–496.

Block LS. Preparing and conditioning the patient for intermaxillary relations. J Prosthet Dent 1952;2:599–603.

Boos RH. Maxillomandibular relations: Occlusion and the temporomandibular joint. Dent Clin North Am 1962;6:19–35.

Borg I, Posselt U. Hinge axis registration: Experiments on the articulator. J Prosthet Dent 1958;8:35–40.

Boucher CO. Occlusion in prosthodontics. J Prosthet Dent 1953;3:633–656.

Brown SW. Disharmony between centric relation and centric occlusion as a factor in producing improper tooth wear and trauma. Dent Digest 1946;52:434–440.

Christensen PB. Accurate casts and positional relation records. J Prosthet Dent 1958;8:475–482.

Colman AJ. Occlusal requirements for removable partial dentures. J Prosthet Dent 1967;17:155–162.

Craddock FW. The accuracy and practical value of records and condyle path inclination. J Am Dent Assoc 1949;38:697–710.

D'Amico A. Functional occlusion of the natural teeth of man. J Prosthet Dent 1961;11:899–915.

Emmert JH. A method of registering occlusion in semiedentulous mouths. J Prosthet Dent 1958;8:94–99.

Fedi PF. Cardinal differences in occlusion of natural teeth and that of artificial teeth. J Am Dent Assoc 1962;62:482–483.

Fountain HW. Seating the condyles for centric relation records. J Prosthet Dent 1961;11:1050–1058.

Granger ER. The articulator and the patient. Dent Clin North Am 1960;4:527–539.

Hall WA. Variations in registering interarch transfers in removable partial denture construction. J Prosthet Dent 1973;30:548–553.

Hanau RL. Full Denture Prosthesis: Intraoral Technique, ed 4. Buffalo, NY: Thorner-Sidney, 1930.

Henderson D. Occlusion in removable partial prosthodontics. J Prosthet Dent 1972;27:151–159.

Hindels GW. Occlusion in removable partial denture prosthesis. Dent Clin North Am 1962;6:137–146.

Jaffe VN. The functionally generated path in full denture construction. J Prosthet Dent 1954;4:214–221.

Jeffreys FE, Platner RL. Occlusion in removable partial dentures. J Prosthet Dent 1960;10:912–920.

Koehne CL, Morrow RM. Construction of denture teeth with gold occlusal surfaces. J Prosthet Dent 1970;23:449–455.

Lucia VO. Centric relation: Theory and practice. J Prosthet Dent 1960;10:849–856.

Mann AW, Pankey LD. The P. M. philosophy of occlusal rehabilitation. Dent Clin North Am 1963;7:621–636.

McCollum BB. The mandibular hinge axis and a method of locating it. J Prosthet Dent 1960;10:428–435.

McCracken WL. Functional occlusion in removable partial construction. J Prosthet Dent 1958;8:955–963.

Mehta JD, Joglekar AP. Vertical jaw relation as a factor in partial dentures. J Prosthet Dent 1969;21:618–625.

Meyer FS. The generated path technique in reconstruction dentistry. I. J Prosthet Dent 1959;9:354–366.

Meyer FS. The generated path technique in reconstruction dentistry. II. J Prosthet Dent 1959;9:432–440.

Müller J, Götz G, Hörz W, Kraft E. Study of the accuracy of different recording materials. J Prosthet Dent 1990;63:41–46.

Nuttell EB. Establishing posterior functional occlusion for fixed partial dentures. J Am Dent Assoc 1963;66:341–348.

O'Leary TJ, Shanley DB, Drake RB. Tooth mobility in cuspid-protected and group-function occlusions. J Prosthet Dent 1972;27:21–25.

Ow RKK, Djeng SK, Ho CK. Orientation of the plane of occlusion. J Prosthet Dent 1966;64:31–36.

Peregrina A, Reisbick MH. Occlusal accuracy of casts made and articulated differently. J Prosthet Dent 1990;63:422–425.

Perry CK. Transfer base for removable partial dentures. J Prosthet Dent 1974;31:582–584.

Robinson MJ. Centric position. J Prosthet Dent 1951;1:384–386.

Roedema WH. Relationship between the width of the occlusal table and pressures under dentures during function. J Prosthet Dent 1976;36:24–34.

Schuyler CH. Factors contributing to traumatic occlusion. J Prosthet Dent 1961;11:708–715.

Schuyler CH. Fundamental principles in the correction of occlusal disharmony: Natural and artificial (grinding). J Am Dent Assoc 1935;22:1193–1202.

Sears VC. Occlusion: The common meeting ground in dentistry. J Prosthet Dent 1952;2:15–21.

Shanahan TEJ, Leff A. Interocclusal records. J Prosthet Dent 1960;10:842–848.

Silverman MM. Centric occlusion and jaw relation and fallacies of current concepts. J Prosthet Dent 1957;7:750–769.

Silverman MM. Determination of vertical dimension by phonetics. J Prosthet Dent 1956;6:465–471.

Stern N, Hatano Y, Kolling JN, Clayton JA. A graphic comparison of mandibular border movements generated by various articulators: Part I Methodology. J Prosthet Dent 1988;60:194–198.

Stuart CE. Accuracy in measuring functional dimension and relation in oral prosthesis. J Prosthet Dent 1959;9:220–236.

Teteruck WR, Lundeen HC. The accuracy of an ear face-bow. J Prosthet Dent 1966;16:1039–1046.

Thompson JR, Brodie AG. Factors in the position of the mandible. J Am Dent Assoc 1942;29:925–941.

Weinberg LA. An evaluation of basic articulators and their concepts, I and II. J Prosthet Dent 1963;13:662–663.

Weinberg LA. The transverse hinge axis: Real or imaginary. J Prosthet Dent 1959;9:775–787.

Wilson JH. The use of partial dentures in the restoration of occlusal standards. Aust Dent J 1956;1:93–101.

Woodward JD, Gattozzi JG. Simplified gold occlusal technique for removable restorations. J Prosthet Dent 1972;27:447–450.

# Try-In and Completion of the Partial Denture

## ☐ Indications for Clinical Appointment

The replacement of anterior teeth often represents an important event in the life of an individual. Many cultures place a great deal of emphasis upon physical appearance, and facial esthetics are central to this concept. Although many patients identify improved function as the primary reason for seeking treatment, a sense of vanity always remains. A patient may be dissatisfied with a prosthesis even if it meets all functional and biologic requirements. Therefore, if anterior teeth are to be replaced, an esthetic try-in is essential. A try-in appointment allows the patient to view the prosthesis and provide feedback. This appointment also allows the practitioner to evaluate the esthetic and phonetic characteristics of the prosthesis and to make appropriate changes in the arrangement of teeth.

An additional indication for the appointment is to verify the accuracy of jaw relation records made during the previous appointment. If there is any doubt regarding the accuracy of the articulator mounting, a try-in appointment should be scheduled.

## ☐ Esthetic Try-In

The patient should be seated in a treatment room that provides a quiet, relaxed atmosphere. This helps to alleviate the tension that may develop as the patient views the tooth arrangement for the first time.

The denture base need not be waxed to full contour, but it should be neat, clean, and resistant to tooth displacement (Figs 14-1 and 14-2). The practitioner should carefully insert the removable partial denture and tell the patient to avoid the application of biting forces. The patient may then be directed to close lightly to ensure that no interferences are present.

The patient should be encouraged to relax. When the patient is at ease, the teeth may be evaluated. It is better if the dentist examines the teeth before the patient has an opportunity to observe them This gives the practitioner an opportunity to correct noticeable discrepancies without upsetting the patient.

The dentist should evaluate the positions of anterior teeth and assess lip support (Fig 14-3). There is a tendency to position the artificial teeth lingual to the positions occupied by the natural teeth. If anterior teeth have been missing for 6 months or more, the pa-

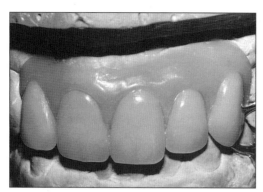

**Fig 14-1** The denture base is waxed to a neat anatomic appearance.

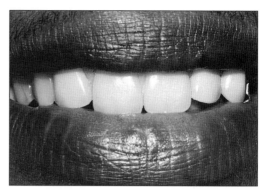

**Fig 14-2** With the exception of denture base coloration, the trial denture should have the same esthetic qualities as the completed prosthesis.

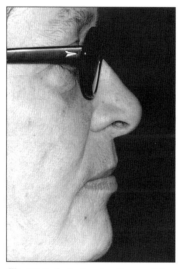

**Fig 14-3** Anterior teeth must be positioned to provide appropriate lip support.

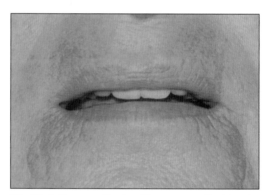

**Fig 14-4** For a patient with average lip length, the edges of the maxillary central incisors should be visible when the lips are relaxed.

tient may report a sensation of abnormal fullness at the upper lip. A short period of accommodation usually will eliminate this problem.

Tooth length should be carefully evaluated. If all anterior teeth are being replaced and the upper lip is of normal length, the edges of the central incisors should be visible when the lip is relaxed (Fig 14-4). When the lip is drawn upward (eg, in an exaggerated smile), the gingival contours of the denture base should be minimally evident (Fig 14-5).

If an anterior edentulous space has been decreased by drifting of the teeth, a decreased number of teeth should not be placed. This technique usually results in

an abnormal appearance. Instead, attempts should be made to rotate or overlap the denture teeth in order to achieve an acceptable esthetic result.

If the anterior edentulous space is relatively large, diastemata may be incorporated into the tooth arrangement (Fig 14-6). If this is to be accomplished, the patient should be informed of potential difficulties associated with interdental spacing. Spacing complicates oral hygiene procedures, increases the likelihood of food impaction, and may create difficulties with phonetics.

Attention should be paid to the horizontal and vertical overlap of the anterior teeth (Fig 14-7). If some

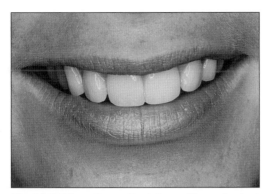

**Fig 14-5** When the patient is smiling, gingival contours of the denture may be visible. As the denture base becomes more evident, its contours and coloration become more important.

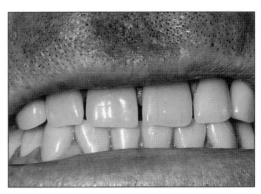

**Fig 14-6** Spacing between the anterior teeth may produce a more natural appearance, but also may affect oral hygiene and phonetics.

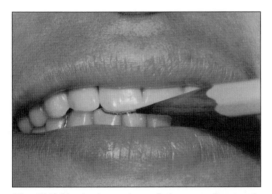

**Fig 14-7** Vertical overlap of the anterior teeth must be accompanied by sufficient horizontal overlap.

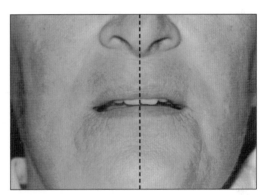

**Fig 14-8** The maxillary midline must be in harmony with the midline of the face.

natural anterior teeth remain, the overlap should be duplicated. If no natural teeth remain, care should be taken to avoid excessive vertical overlap without accompanying horizontal overlap. This could result in the application of undesirable forces to the artificial teeth and associated soft tissues.

Vertical alignment of the teeth also should be evaluated. A slight deviation from the vertical can produce an acceptable esthetic result, but a significant deviation can create esthetic difficulties. The practitioner should pay particular attention to the maxillary midline. This midline must be examined for its vertical alignment and for its midface position (Fig 14-8). Any

error in the position of the maxillary midline can be extremely distracting.

Verification of tooth shade should be accomplished during the evaluation process. The presence of natural teeth makes shade selection and patient acceptance a critical component of removable partial denture therapy. To ensure selection of an appropriate shade, the prosthesis should be viewed using a variety of light sources (eg, natural, fluorescent, and incandescent).

Once the technical and mechanical requirements are satisfied, the patient should be allowed to view the tooth arrangement and comment on the results. The patient should stand several feet from a wall mir-

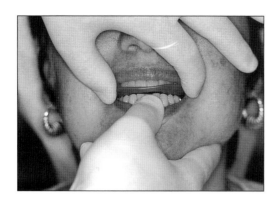

**Fig 14-9** The articulator mounting must be evaluated using additional jaw relation records.

ror to examine the teeth critically. The use of a hand mirror should be discouraged because the patient's attention will be focused on individual teeth and not on the overall effect of the prosthesis. The patient's remarks should be noted, and required changes should be made. Arrival at mutual acceptance by the patient and dentist frequently demands a high level of communicative skill combined with psychological insight.

Treatment should not proceed until patient approval has been gained. Many practitioners insist upon written approval by the patient. When uncertainty exists, a suitable entry should be placed in the record and signed by the patient.

## ⌨ Verification of Jaw Relation

The jaw relation only needs to be verified in limited instances:

1. If problems were encountered during jaw relation procedures and there is any doubt regarding the accuracy of the articulator mounting
2. If the partial denture is opposed by a complete denture
3. If all posterior teeth in both arches are being replaced
4. If there are no opposing natural teeth in contact and verification of the occlusal vertical dimension is necessary

A dentist should never complete a prosthesis without confidence in the accuracy of the jaw relation records and the articulator mounting. A considerable amount of unnecessary work can be avoided if the practitioner pays close attention to detail throughout these procedures.

To ensure accuracy, it is essential that the practitioner evaluate the mounting using additional jaw relation records (Fig 14-9). As a result, the importance of a facebow transfer becomes particularly evident at this stage of treatment. For a mounting to accept additional jaw relation records, the arc of rotation for the articulator must be the same as the arc of rotation for the patient's mandible. If this is not the case, the articulator may not accept a jaw relation record despite the fact that it is completely accurate (Figs 14-10 to 14-19).

In most instances, verification records are made at a slightly increased occlusal vertical dimension. This increase in occlusal vertical dimension will not create difficulties as long as *(1)* the maxillary cast is mounted in correct relation to the condylar elements of the articulator and *(2)* the mandible is in centric relation when jaw relation records are made. The mandible is capable of maintaining this nontranslating rotation over an arc of 10 to 20 mm (Fig 14-20). Hence, there will be no displacement of the condyle, and closure will be purely arcuate.

It is important to note that natural or artificial teeth must not be allowed to contact during the record-making process. Contact may result in deviation of the mandible and inaccuracy of the record.

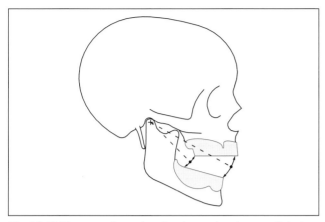

Fig 14-10 The arc of rotation for the patient's mandible is a critical factor in articulation.

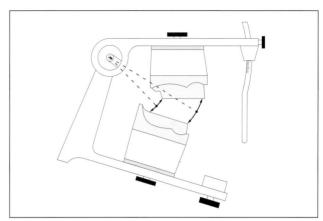

Fig 14-11 The arc of rotation for the articulator must reproduce the mandibular arc illustrated in Fig 14-10. Accurate occlusal contact on the articulator is expected only when *(1)* the maxillary cast is properly related to the articulator's axis (achieved using a facebow transfer) and *(2)* the mandibular cast is properly related to the maxillary cast (achieved using one or more jaw relation records).

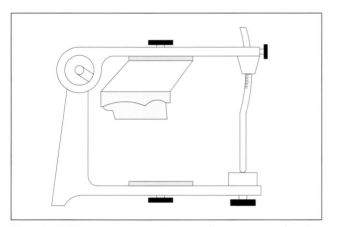

Fig 14-12 When mounted without a facebow transfer, the maxillary cast may be positioned too far posteriorly.

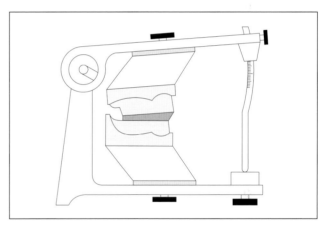

Fig 14-13 Subsequently, the articulator is opened so that a jaw relation record may be used to mount the mandibular cast.

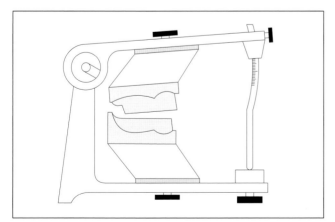

Fig 14-14 The jaw relation record is removed after the mandibular cast has been mounted.

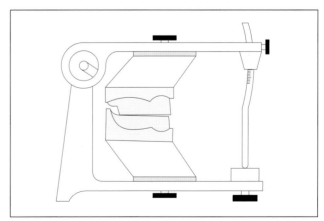

Fig 14-15 Closing the articulator results in posterior occlusal prematurity.

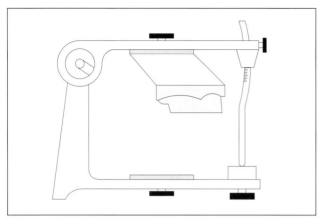

**Fig 14-16** When mounted without a facebow transfer, the maxillary cast also may be positioned too far anteriorly.

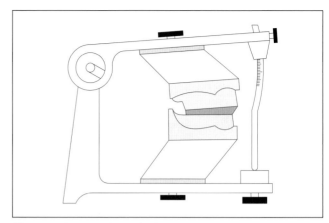

**Fig 14-17** In turn, the articulator is opened so that a jaw relation record may be used to mount the mandibular cast.

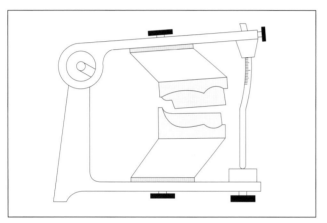

**Fig 14-18** The jaw relation record is removed after the mandibular cast has been mounted.

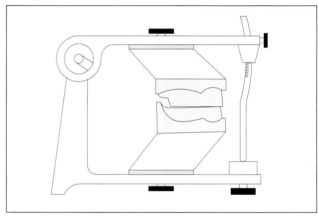

**Fig 14-19** Closing the articulator results in anterior occlusal prematurity.

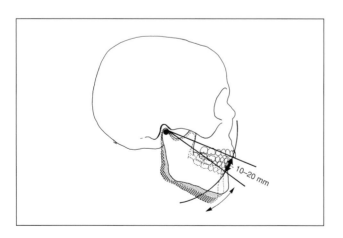

**Fig 14-20** The mandible is capable of pure rotational movements through an arc of 10 to 20 mm measured at the incisal edges.

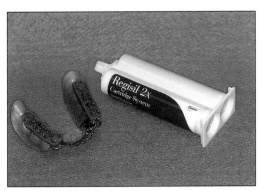

**Fig 14-21** Polyvinylsiloxane registration media are relatively easy to work with and exert minimal pressure.

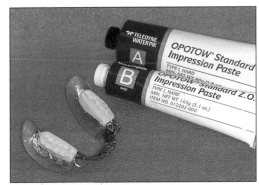

**Fig 14-22** Zinc oxide–eugenol registration media are extremely accurate, but are more difficult to use than other registration materials.

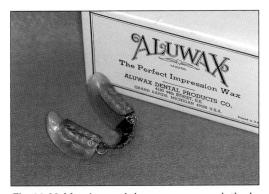

**Fig 14-23** Metal-containing waxes are relatively easy to use, but are susceptible to distortion.

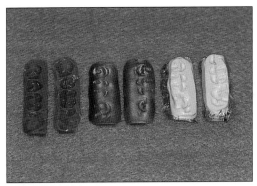

**Fig 14-24** Records made using polyvinylsiloxane *(left)*, metal-containing wax *(center)*, and zinc oxide–eugenol *(right)*.

## Materials

A recording medium must be as pressure-free as possible. Among the most suitable materials are the polyvinylsiloxanes (Fig 14-21) and zinc oxide–eugenol materials (Fig 14-22). These materials can be mixed and placed on the surfaces of the teeth with relative ease. Setting occurs in less than 1 minute in the oral cavity. Both materials are relatively rigid when set and display excellent dimensional stability.

A variety of waxes also may be used to make jaw relation records. One of the most commonly used materials is baseplate wax. To optimize results, the wax is heated in a temperature-controlled water bath at 60°C (140°F). Unfortunately, baseplate wax is diffi-

cult to soften uniformly and distorts rather easily. If baseplate wax is used as a recording medium, the mounting should be completed within 30 minutes of the recording process.

Waxes containing metal particles display improved uniformity in softening and hardening (Fig 14-23). Thermal conductivity of the metal permits the wax to be heated and cooled with greater consistency and control. Nevertheless, metal-containing waxes are susceptible to distortion, and the associated mounting should be completed within 30 minutes of the recording process.

Surface characteristics of polyvinylsiloxane, zinc oxide–eugenol, and metal-impregnated wax records are shown in Fig 14-24.

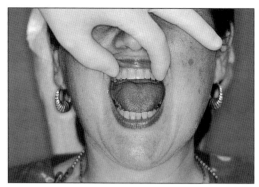

**Fig 14-25** The fingers of one hand are placed on the patient's maxillary arch. This placement provides improved visualization of the dental arches.

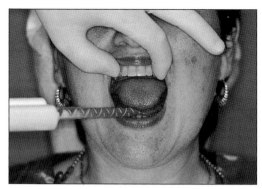

**Fig 14-26** Polyvinylsiloxane is expressed onto the mandibular occlusal surfaces.

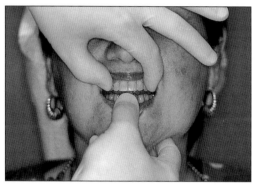

**Fig 14-27** The operator's dominant hand is properly positioned and used to guide mandibular closure.

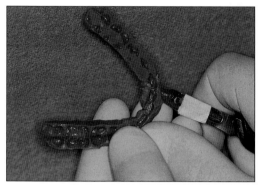

**Fig 14-28** The record is trimmed using a surgical scalpel.

## Clinical procedure

The patient should be seated, and the partial denture tried in the mouth. Visual observation of occlusal contacts should be used to determine whether gross errors are present. Necessary adjustments should be made. The patient should be permitted to wear the prosthesis for 3 to 5 minutes. During this time, the patient should be encouraged to speak. The practitioner should engage in conversation with the patient, using this opportunity to assess the phonetic and esthetic qualities of the prosthesis.

Normally, if two prostheses are being constructed, the recording medium is placed on the mandibular teeth for convenience. However, if the mandibular prosthesis does not provide a suitable platform, the recording medium may be placed on the maxillary prosthesis.

## Making a polyvinylsiloxane verification record

The method for making a polyvinylsiloxane verification record is nearly identical to the procedure described in chapter 6. The practitioner should rehearse the record-making procedure with the patient before placing the recording medium in the oral cavity. When this has been accomplished, the practitioner should begin the record-making process.

The patient is instructed to open the mouth moderately. The fingers of one hand are positioned to permit visualization of the dental arches (Fig 14-25). The polyvinylsiloxane registration material is mixed and introduced into the patient's mouth (Fig 14-26). The operator's remaining hand is then positioned on the facial surfaces of the mandibular anterior teeth, and the patient is guided into the prescribed closure (Fig

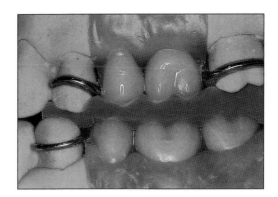

**Fig 14-29** Assessment of cast-to-record adaptation indicates acceptable fit.

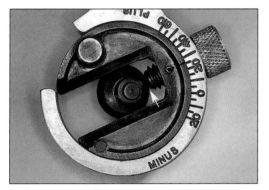

**Fig 14-30** This condylar element is fully seated in its housing. No space is evident between the condylar element and the posterior stop *(arrow)*.

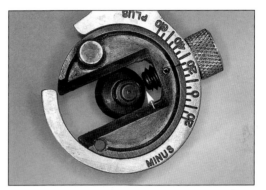

**Fig 14-31** This condylar element is not fully seated in its housing. Space is evident between the condylar element and the posterior stop *(arrow)*.

14-27). This position is maintained until the polyvinylsiloxane material has reached a suitable consistency.

When the recording medium has set, the patient is instructed to open the mouth. The record and removable partial denture (or dentures) are removed from the oral cavity. The record is carefully examined to determine its acceptability. There should be no signs of penetration through the record. If the record is acceptable, it is properly trimmed using a surgical scalpel (Fig 14-28). Additional records may be made in a similar manner.

### Verifying accuracy of an articulator mounting

There are a number of methods for determining the accuracy of an articulator mounting. The most commonly used methods include *(1)* assessment of cast-to-record

adaptation when the articulator is closed in a terminal hinge position (Fig 14-29) and *(2)* examination of the relationships between the condylar elements and condylar housings when the mounted casts are properly seated in a jaw relation record (Figs 14-30 and 14-31). The objective of the two techniques is the same—to determine the repeatability of closure. The major difference is the way in which the results are checked.

When using the first method, the articulator is placed in its terminal position (ie, the position at which the condylar elements are completely seated in their housings). In many instruments, the condylar elements may be locked into this terminal position using some form of governing device. A jaw relation record is placed on one cast, and the articulator is gently closed. During closure, the practitioner observes the relationships between the occlusal surfaces and the jaw relation record. The occlusal surfaces should follow an arcuate pathway into the record and should display excellent adaptation to the record (see Fig 14-29). The practitioner should never apply pressure to the articulator or casts because this will distort the record and provide an inaccurate result.

When using the second method, the condylar elements are unlocked and permitted to move freely within their condylar housings. A jaw relation record is placed on one cast, and the remaining cast is gently settled into this record. If the casts cannot be accurately positioned in the record, an inaccuracy exists, and the practitioner must determine the source of this inaccuracy. If the casts can be accurately positioned in the record, the practitioner must assess the relationship between the condylar elements and the condylar housings. Each condylar element should be located in its terminal position (see Fig 14-30). As previously noted, the practitioner should not apply undue pressure to the articulator or casts when evaluating the mounting.

If the original mounting is verified as correct, the practitioner may proceed. If the accuracy of the original mounting cannot be verified, another jaw relation record should be made and the mounting should be reevaluated. If this record fails to verify the original mounting, the practitioner should suspect an inaccuracy in the mounting and should remount the mandibular cast. The verification process should then be repeated. Completion of the prosthesis should not be considered until the practitioner has verified the accuracy of the mounting.

### Length of appointment

Depending on the difficulty encountered, the experienced practitioner should be able to complete the clinical procedures in 30 to 60 minutes. A dental student usually will require 1 to 2 hours.

## ☐ Laboratory Procedures for Completing the Removable Partial Denture

### Waxing denture base contours

Denture base contours should be completed in such a manner that they will enhance the retention and sta-

bility of a prosthesis. In general, the denture base contours for a removable partial denture should be nearly identical to those used for a complete denture. The primary differences are encountered when the operator waxes to and around exposed portions of the metal framework.

The importance of well-defined external and internal finish lines becomes obvious during the waxing process (Figs 14-32 and 14-33). If finish lines are not sharply defined, the metal-to-plastic joints will be difficult to establish and maintain. Acrylic resin should never be finished to a fine edge because it lacks strength and over a period of time will separate from the metal with resulting seepage of oral fluids and discoloration of the plastic in that area (Fig 14-34).

When waxing external finish lines, the wax should be left with sufficient bulk to allow for the loss of resin that will take place during the finishing and polishing phases. The height of the resin should never be below the height of the metal (Fig 14-35).

On metal parts lacking a finish line, such as the approach arm of vertical projection clasps, the wax should be left thick enough so that the resin will have sufficient bulk to avoid separation and seepage. Slightly roughening the metal that will be covered by resin may enhance mechanical retention of the resin.

Gingival contours should be esthetically pleasing and self-cleansing. Contours should reflect an appropriate amount of gingival recession. One of the most frequent errors in waxing is failure to keep the gingival contours of the prosthesis consistent with the gingival contours of the adjacent natural teeth (Figs 14-36 and 14-37). This is particularly critical for anterior and premolar teeth. Frush and Fisher have offered several rules for determining the height of the gingival contour at various positions.[1] For the central incisors, the gingival height should be slightly incisal to the high lip line. For the lateral incisors, it should be slightly incisal to the level established for the central incisors. At the canines, the level should be more apical than at either of the incisors. At the premolars, the gingival height should be slightly occlusal to the level established for the canines. From this point posteriorly, there should be a progression in which the clinical crowns appear slightly shorter.

A slight bulge should be waxed apical to the gingival margin of each posterior tooth. This bulge acts as a secondary food table to help control food flow (Fig

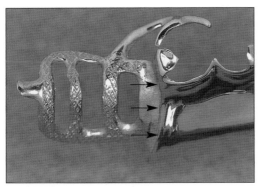

**Fig 14-32** Each external finish line should be sharply defined and should provide a slight mechanical undercut *(arrows)*.

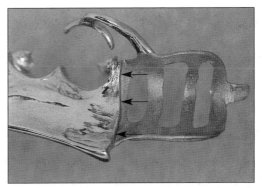

**Fig 14-33** Each internal finish line should provide a butt joint *(arrows)*.

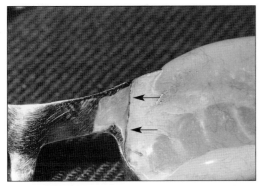

**Fig 14-34** Poorly developed finish lines may result in knifelike extensions of acrylic resin *(arrows)*. These extensions are susceptible to fracture.

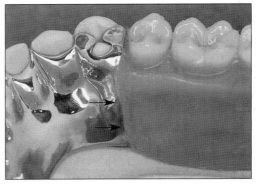

**Fig 14-35** When waxing denture base contours, wax is left slightly above the surface of the metal *(arrows)*. This provides for a slight loss of resin during finishing and polishing procedures.

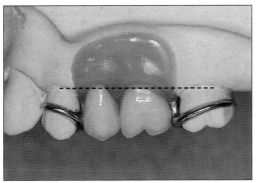

**Fig 14-36** The gingival contours of the artificial teeth should be consistent with those of the natural teeth. *Broken line* illustrates the consistency of the gingival architecture.

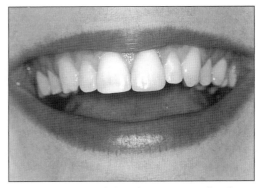

**Fig 14-37** The height of contour varies from central incisors to lateral incisors to canines.

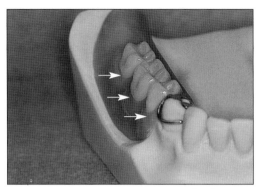

**Fig 14-38** A slight bulge or convexity *(arrows)* is waxed apical to the gingival margin of each posterior tooth. This convexity acts as a secondary food table to help control food flow.

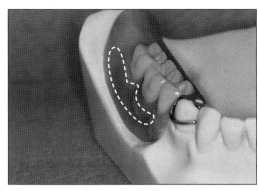

**Fig 14-39** A slight concavity *(outlined area)* should be provided between the gingival bulge and the periphery of the denture base.

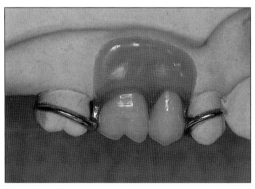

**Fig 14-40** For a tooth-supported segment, the denture base is waxed just short of the soft tissue reflection.

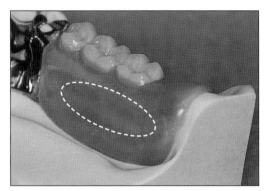

**Fig 14-41** A slight concavity *(outlined area)* is included on the posterior lingual flange of a mandibular denture base.

14-38). Between the gingival bulge and the periphery of the denture base, a slight concavity should be provided (Fig 14-39). The soft tissues of the cheek and fibers of the buccinator often fold into this area and help maintain the position of the prosthesis.

The width of the peripheral roll should be maintained if it were developed using a corrected cast impression. If a corrected cast impression was not made, the border should be approximately 2 mm thick. If the limits of the denture-bearing area are not obvious, it is better to overwax the denture base in both length and thickness (Fig 14-40). Final adjustments may be made at the insertion appointment.

A mandibular posterior denture base should be waxed with a distinct lingual concavity (Fig 14-41).

This permits the soft tissues of the floor of the mouth to rest in this area and provide increased resistance to displacement.

The exposed surfaces of the wax should be highly refined to minimize the necessity for finishing and polishing procedures. The possibility of damaging the framework is always present when cloth wheels are used on a bench lathe.

Two areas consistently require modification at the time of finishing and polishing. These are the distobuccal flanges of a maxillary denture base (to avoid interferences with the coronoid processes of the mandible) and the distolingual extension of the mandibular denture base (to provide additional room for tongue movement).

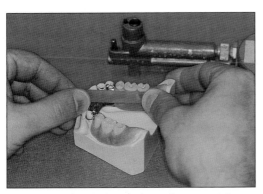

**Fig 14-42** After being softened over a laboratory burner, the baseplate wax is used to build the desired denture base contours.

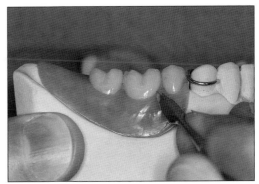

**Fig 14-43** Contours are refined with waxing instruments.

## Contouring a denture base

1. Make certain the artificial teeth are firmly waxed in position.
2. Soften small pieces of baseplate wax over a laboratory burner and mold them in position around the teeth and over the edentulous ridge (Fig 14-42). Make certain they are well adapted to exposed portions of the framework. This technique of forming the denture base has several advantages.
   - It decreases the time required for adding wax to the denture base.
   - The operator can exert more control than if the wax is melted and flowed onto denture base areas.
   - The wax may be more accurately positioned, thereby reducing the amount of carving that must be done.
   - This method results in reduced heat application and reduced tooth movement. If wax is melted and flowed onto the cast, the chances of tooth movement are significantly increased.
3. Ensure that a minimum thickness of 2 mm is established for denture bases. Peripheries should exhibit gently rounded margins.
4. Establish the borders of tooth-supported segments approximately 5 mm apical to the adjacent gingival margins. Final shaping may be accomplished at the insertion appointment.
5. Refine buccal and lingual flanges to ensure the presence of appropriate convexities and concavities.

6. Create gingival contours that are consistent with those of the adjacent natural teeth (Fig 14-43).
7. Finish and polish wax surfaces.
8. Evaluate the occlusion to ensure that none of the teeth have moved during waxing procedures. Correct tooth arrangement as necessary.

## Split-mold investing

The purpose of investing the master cast and partial denture in dental stone is to provide a smooth, dense mold. Following completion of the investment process, wax is eliminated from the mold, and acrylic resin is used to fill the resultant cavity. As the resin is processed, some dimensional changes in the resin occur. The prosthesis is then recovered from the mold, adjusted, and prepared for delivery.

The investment process begins with a "split-mold" investment procedure. As the name implies, the completed mold contains the master cast and metal framework in one portion of a denture flask. The artificial teeth are contained in the remaining portion of the denture flask. Although this method of investing requires special care, it provides excellent results and is commonly used in removable partial denture construction.

### Preparing flasks

Denture flasks must be kept in good condition. This may be accomplished using common sense and a minimal amount of maintenance. Assembled flasks should

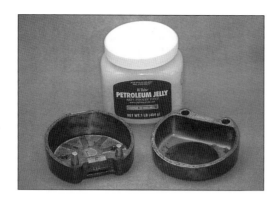

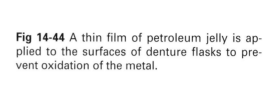

Fig 14-44 A thin film of petroleum jelly is applied to the surfaces of denture flasks to prevent oxidation of the metal.

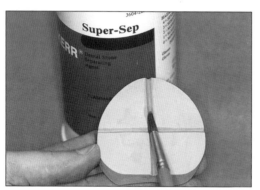

Fig 14-45 A gypsum separating medium is applied to the cast before beginning the investment process.

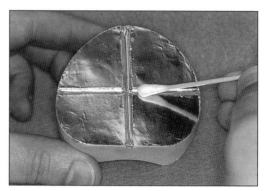

Fig 14-46 Tinfoil may be used in place of a liquid separating medium.

not rock when forces are applied. Unless there is solid metal-to-metal contact between flask components, the forces applied to compress the resin may not be appropriately distributed. This may result in processing difficulties. As a result, denture flasks should be checked before each use. Flasks displaying a noticeable rock should be replaced.

In addition to checking the flasks, a lubricant such as petroleum jelly should be applied periodically to the internal surfaces of each flask (Fig 14-44). This prevents oxidation, which can alter the fit of these components. A thin film of petroleum jelly also should be placed on the internal surfaces of a flask before beginning the investment process. This prevents pitting of the flask's surface and facilitates removal of the stone mold.

### First investment layer

The investment process for a removable partial denture consists of four major steps. The first step or "pour" is similar to that used in the complete denture investment process. The base of the master cast is ex-

amined for roughness, irregularities, and voids. Bubbles or voids are filled with baseplate wax, and the surface of the cast is painted with gypsum separating medium (Fig 14-45). Alternatively, tinfoil may be adapted to the base of the cast (Fig 14-46). It is important to note that lubricants such as petroleum jelly and silicone ointment should be avoided. These lubricants occupy space on the surface of a cast and permit movement of the cast within the mold. This may result in noticeable errors in the finished prosthesis.

The master cast with the partial denture in place is seated in the lower segment of the flask. It is important that there be at least 15 mm clearance between the occlusal surfaces of the teeth and the top of the flask's middle segment (Fig 14-47). This is one reason why it is important to control the thickness of the cast at the time it is poured and trimmed. If the cast is so thick that it must be trimmed to fit the flask, the indices on the base of the cast will be lost, and the cast cannot be remounted for the correction of processing errors.

A mix of Type III or IV dental stone is prepared and placed into the lower portion of the flask. The cast is

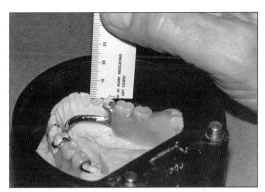

**Fig 14-47** There must be approximately 15 mm of clearance between the occlusal surfaces of the teeth and the top of the flask's middle segment.

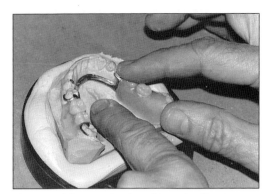

**Fig 14-48** The cast is placed into the first investment layer.

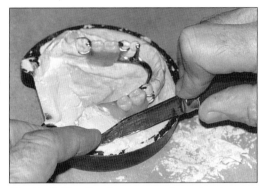

**Fig 14-49** The first investment layer is trimmed even with the land area of the cast and the edge of the flask's lower segment.

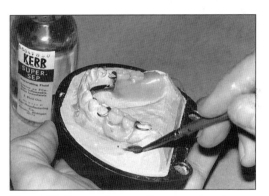

**Fig 14-50** Separating medium is painted onto the exposed stone surfaces.

**Fig 14-51** The flask is soaked in supernatant dental slurry.

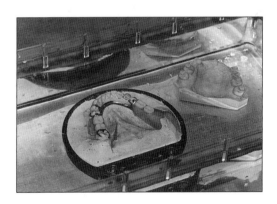

then settled into the flask and depressed until the land area of the cast is even with or slightly below the rim of the flask (Fig 14-48). The investing stone should be even with the land area of the cast and slightly above the rim of the flask. When the stone begins to harden, it is trimmed and smoothed with a sharp laboratory knife (Fig 14-49). Care must be taken to ensure that

the surface of the investing stone does not exhibit any mechanical undercuts.

After the final set of the first investment layer, a gypsum separating medium is painted onto all exposed stone surfaces (Fig 14-50). The flask is soaked in supernatant dental slurry before the second investment layer is added (Fig 14-51).

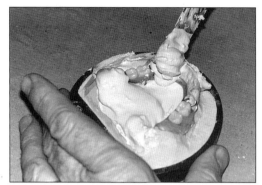

Fig 14-52 The second investment layer is added.

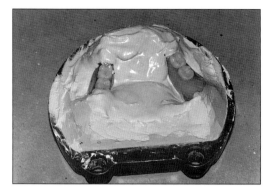

Fig 14-53 The second investment layer is formed to cover everything but the waxed denture bases and the artificial teeth.

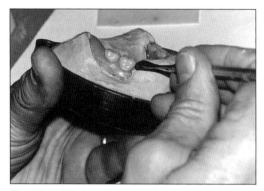

Fig 14-54 The second layer is trimmed to eliminate all undercuts and sharp projections.

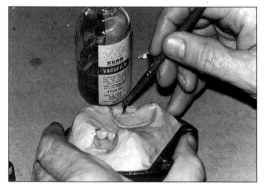

Fig 14-55 Denture base areas are painted with surface tension–reducing agent.

## Second investment layer

The second mix also is made using a Type III or IV dental stone. This layer is molded over the master cast and metal framework, covering everything but the waxed denture bases and the denture teeth (Figs 14-52 and 14-53). It is essential that no undercuts be present when the assembly is viewed from above. The second and third investment layers must separate cleanly following wax elimination. Any undercut in the second layer would prevent this and greatly complicate packing procedures.

There should be at least 7 mm of clearance between the upper surface of the second investment layer and the top of the flask. The outer edge of the second layer should end even with the rim of the lower half of the flask. When these requirements have been met, the operator should eliminate thin projections of stone that could fracture during the wax elimination process (Fig 14-54).

The more experienced dentist or technician can accomplish the purposes of the first and second layer in a single mix. The single mix, however, makes the deflasking procedure more difficult and hazardous.

After the second mix has set, exposed stone surfaces are painted with a gypsum separating medium and the assembly is soaked in supernatant dental slurry. A surface tension–reducing agent is brushed onto the surface of the wax to permit improved adaptation of the third investment layer (Fig 14-55).

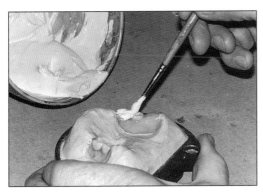

**Fig 14-56** After the second investment layer has been coated with separating medium and soaked in supernatant dental slurry, the third investment layer is added. A stiff brush is used to paint stone around the necks of the artificial teeth and over the surface of the wax.

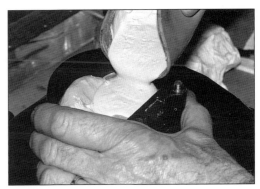

**Fig 14-57** The middle segment of the flask is positioned and dental stone is vibrated in the flask. The third investment layer should be 7 to 10 mm from the top of the flask.

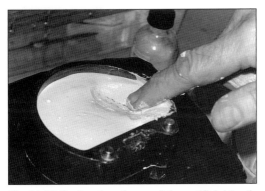

**Fig 14-58** Occlusal surfaces of the artificial teeth are exposed.

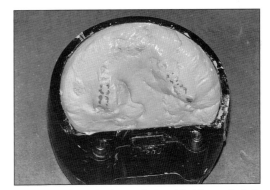

**Fig 14-59** The surface of the third layer is left slightly rough to hold the fourth investment layer in position.

## Third and fourth investment layers

A third mix of dental stone is prepared. The stone is painted onto the wax base and prosthetic teeth using a relatively stiff brush (Fig 14-56). Care is taken not to trap air bubbles around the necks of the teeth.

At this stage, the middle portion of the flask is positioned and the remaining stone is vibrated into the flask (Fig 14-57). The occlusal surfaces of the denture teeth are uncovered with the index finger, and the soft stone is shaped to form a concavity into which the final mix will be poured (Fig 14-58). The surface of the third layer is left slightly rough to hold the fourth layer in position (Fig 14-59). Exposed stone surfaces are painted with a gypsum separating medium and soaked in supernatant dental slurry (Figs 14-60 and 14-61).

The fourth investment layer is applied using a Type III or IV dental stone. The top of the flask is pressed into place immediately after introduction of the fourth investment layer (Fig 14-62). The flask is set aside for a minimum of 1 hour before the wax elimination process is begun.

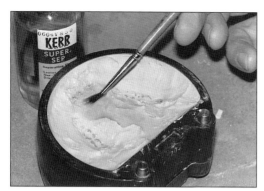

**Fig 14-60** The surface of the stone is painted with gypsum separating medium.

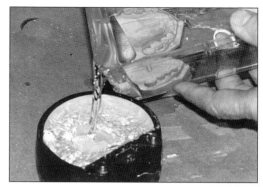

**Fig 14-61** Supernatant dental slurry is poured into the concavity to wet the stone.

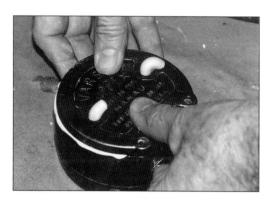

**Fig 14-62** The fourth investment layer is used to fill the remainder of the flask. The lid of the flask is pressed into place while the investing stone is still soft.

## Wax elimination

The flask is placed in boiling water for 5 minutes. At the end of this period, the flask is removed from the water and opened using a stiff, bladed instrument. The upper portion of the flask is lifted vertically (Fig 14-63), and the softened wax is removed from the mold (Fig 14-64). Remaining wax is flushed from the mold with boiling supernatant dental slurry (Fig 14-65). The mold is then cleaned with a soft brush and a detergent solution (Fig 14-66). Detergent is removed by flushing the mold with clean boiling water (Fig 14-67). Mold components are then placed vertically and allowed to drain for 3 to 5 minutes (Fig 14-68).

While the stone surfaces are still warm, alginate separating medium is applied to the mold (Figs 14-69 and 14-70). It is essential that a smooth and solid film of the material be applied to prevent the stone from adhering to the resin during processing. Nevertheless, care must be taken to ensure that separating medium is not painted onto the ridge lap areas of the artificial teeth, since this prevents chemical bonding of resin teeth to the denture base.

If the separating medium does not spread evenly on the stone surface or if it tends to "ball up" in certain areas, it should be suspected that wax elimination was not complete. If necessary, stone surfaces should be cleaned again.

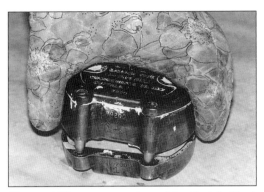

**Fig 14-63** The upper portion of the flask is lifted as vertically as possible to avoid fracturing the investment layers.

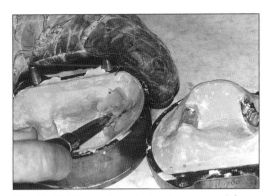

**Fig 14-64** The softened wax is removed from the mold.

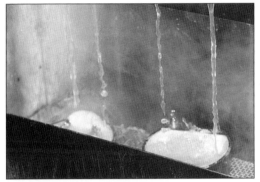

**Fig 14-65** The remainder of the wax is flushed from the mold with boiling supernatant dental slurry.

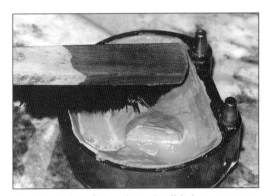

**Fig 14-66** A soft brush and mild detergent are used to clean wax residue from the mold.

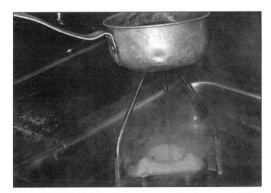

**Fig 14-67** Residual detergent is removed by flushing the mold with clean boiling water.

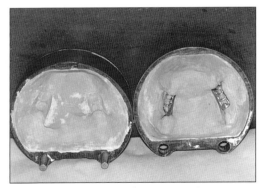

**Fig 14-68** Mold components are placed vertically so water may drain.

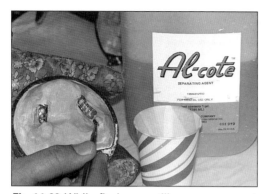

**Fig 14-69** While flasks are still warm, one coat of alginate separating medium is applied. The operator must ensure that separating medium is not applied to the ridge lap areas of the artificial teeth.

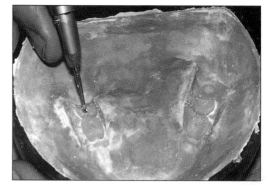

**Fig 14-70** Diatorics (retention features) are prepared in the denture teeth with a No. 6 round bur. Diatorics provide mechanical retention for the denture teeth. Subsequently, a second coat of alginate separating medium will be applied to the mold.

## Packing the acrylic resin denture base

If the operator chooses to characterize or stain a denture base, the coloration process should be accomplished before the bulk denture base resin is prepared. Resin stains are available in a variety of shades (Fig 14-71). The polymer (ie, powder) is sprinkled onto the appropriate surfaces of the mold (Fig 14-72). Monomer is then applied using a fine-tipped dropper (Fig 14-73). The amount of monomer is carefully controlled so the stain will not flow from its intended location. Upon completion of this process, the flask is closed to prevent evaporation of the monomer.

Before proceeding, the operator should evaluate the relationship between the metal framework and the master cast. This is particularly true when one or more extension bases exist. The operator must ensure that each cast stop is in contact with the surface of the master cast. Lack of contact may permit flexure of resin-retaining elements during resin-packing procedures. Flexure may produce noticeable inaccuracies in the completed removable partial denture. To prevent

this, a small amount of chemically activated resin should be sprinkled on or painted under the distal end of the latticework and allowed to set before the denture resin is packed (Fig 14-74).

At this stage, the denture base resin is introduced into the flask. The manufacturer's recommendations for mixing should be closely followed. In most instances, the polymer-monomer ratio will be 3:1 by volume. Components are carefully measured and placed in an appropriate mixing jar. The polymer and monomer are mixed for 30 seconds or until the polymer is thoroughly wet with monomer. The jar is tightly closed for 1 minute. The jar is then opened and the consistency of the resin is checked. This procedure is repeated every 30 seconds until the resin reaches a doughlike consistency. At this point, the resin should separate cleanly from the walls of the mixing jar (Fig 14-75). When pulled or drawn, the material should snap apart. Upon reaching this stage, the resin should be introduced into the mold. The packing process should be accomplished as quickly as possible.

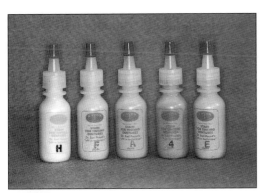

**Fig 14-71** Denture stains may be used to customize denture bases.

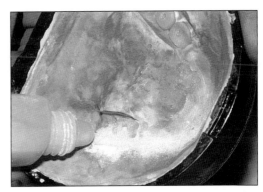

**Fig 14-72** A chosen stain is sprinkled onto the surface of the mold.

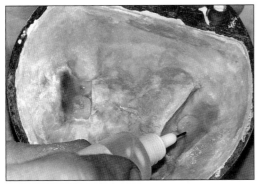

**Fig 14-73** Monomer is then applied using a fine-tipped dropper. Additional stains may be added as required.

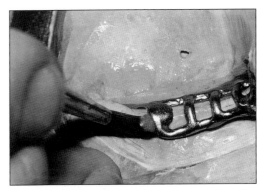

**Fig 14-74** The cast stop is not contacting the underlying cast. Therefore, chemically activated resin is added to prevent the minor connector from flexing during the packing process.

**Fig 14-75** When the consistency of the resin is correct, it will separate cleanly from the mixing jar. Notice that the operator is wearing plastic gloves.

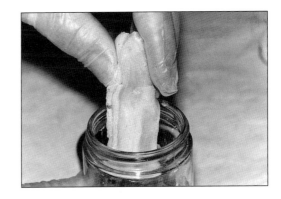

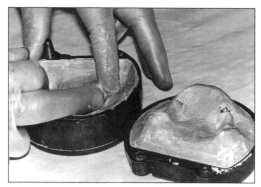

**Fig 14-76** Resin is pressed into and around the teeth in one portion of the flask.

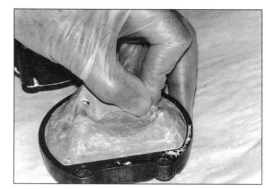

**Fig 14-77** Resin is placed in and around the framework in the remaining portion of the flask.

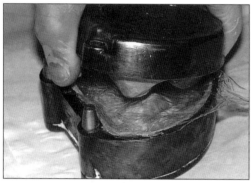

**Fig 14-78** A plastic sheet is placed between the portions of the flask, and the flask is closed.

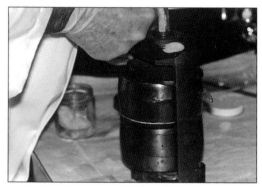

**Fig 14-79** The flask is placed into a flask carrier and pressure is applied. The resin is given sufficient time to flow.

It is important to note that the resin should not be handled with bare fingers during the mixing or packing phases. These resins may cause dermatologic responses that produce noticeable discomfort. As a result, disposable plastic gloves should be worn during mixing and packing procedures. If gloves are not available, the material should be handled between plastic sheets that will be used during the trial packing.

A split-packing technique is used for partial denture applications (Figs 14-76 to 14-84). If sufficient resin is used in each portion of the flask, there should be flash around all margins of the denture base in both sides of the flask. If flash is not present around all the margins, a small portion of resin is added to the deficient area before the next trial closure (see Fig 14-80). The flash is trimmed to the margin of the denture base using a small spatula or other dull instrument (see Fig 14-81). Care is taken not to "cut" the stone, since small pieces may become incorporated into the denture resin. The plastic sheet is replaced between the halves of the flask, and the trial closure repeated.

Trial packing is repeated until a minimal amount of flash is present. Under normal circumstances, at least three trial closures should be accomplished. Trial closures should be completed as rapidly as possible, while allowing the resin sufficient time to flow.

After final closure has been made, the flask is permitted to bench cure for 1 hour before processing is started.

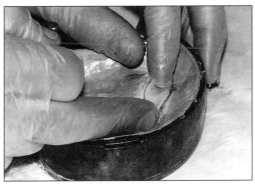

**Fig 14-80** The flask is opened and inspected. A small increment of resin is added to any deficient area. Subsequently, a plastic packing sheet will be placed, and another trial closure accomplished.

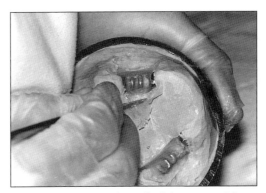

**Fig 14-81** Excess resin or flash is removed from the mold using a dull instrument.

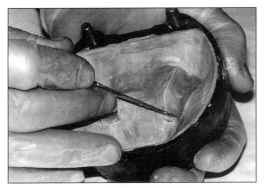

**Fig 14-82** After an additional closure, very little flash remains. Final closure can be made.

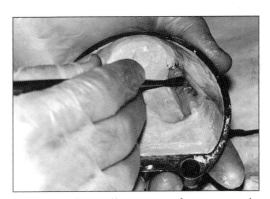

**Fig 14-83** A small amount of monomer is painted onto the exposed surfaces of the acrylic resin.

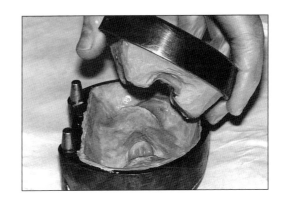

**Fig 14-84** The flask is closed without placing a plastic sheet. The flask will be placed in the flask carrier and pressure applied.

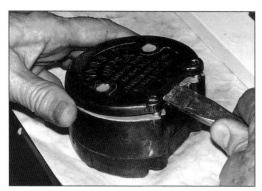

**Fig 14-85** The lid of the flask is removed by prying with a chisel.

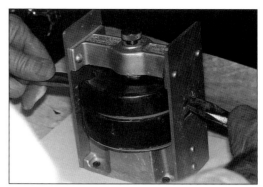

**Fig 14-86** A flask ejector is used to remove the remainder of the flask. The flask is positioned in the ejector. The top knob is turned down to contact the knockout plate. Chisels are inserted through the holes in the ejector and engage slots in the denture flask. Upward and downward forces are applied to the chisels to separate the flask from the mold.

## Processing the partial denture

After they have been bench cured for 1 hour, the flask and press are placed in a curing unit. If an electric unit is not available, the processing can be accomplished in any large metal container holding water. There must be enough water to completely cover the flask press to make certain that heat is being applied evenly.

Heat-activated acrylic resin is processed at 74°C (165°F). Lower temperatures will not activate the resin to produce the polymerization reaction, while higher temperatures will cause polymerization to proceed too rapidly and will bring about a rapid elevation of the internal temperature of the resin. This rapid rise in temperature may result in boiling of the monomer, which is one cause of porosity in denture base resins.

### Long-cure cycle

There are two common heating schedules used in the polymerization of heat-activated resins. The first is termed a *long cure*. It involves placement of a denture flask and carrier into a curing unit filled with room-temperature water. The water temperature is raised slowly to reach 74°C (165°F) in 1 hour. This temperature is maintained for an additional 7 hours. At the end of this period, the water is brought to a boil and maintained for an additional 30 minutes.

This curing cycle is the safest and should normally be used. If a suitable curing unit is available, the processing is usually accomplished at night and the denture is ready for deflasking the following morning. If deflasking cannot be done immediately after processing, the investment should not be allowed to dry. The flask should be kept covered with room-temperature water until deflasking can be accomplished.

### Short-cure cycle

A second heating schedule is termed the *short cure*. The short cure also involves placing a denture flask and carrier into a curing unit filled with room-temperature water. The water temperature is then raised to 74°C (165°F) in 1 hour. This temperature is maintained for 90 minutes. The water is then brought to a boil and maintained at this temperature for 30 minutes.

This procedure involves a certain element of risk, usually in the form of incomplete polymerization or increased porosity of the denture base.

## Deflasking the partial denture

Recovery of a prosthesis from the denture flask requires thought and patience. The stone mold is first removed from the flask itself. In turn, the layers of investment are carefully removed. Recommended deflasking procedures are illustrated in Figs 14-85 to 14-97.

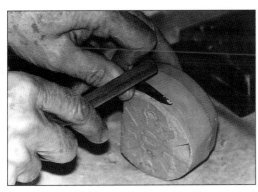

**Fig 14-87** A knife is positioned at the junction of the third and fourth investment layers. A light tap is used to remove the fourth investment layer.

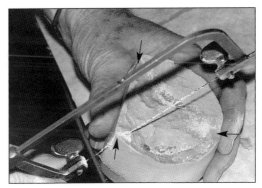

**Fig 14-88** A die saw is used to make three cuts *(arrows)*. The anterior cut must be deep enough to provide a purchase point, but not so deep as to damage the master cast or removable partial denture. Posterior cuts should reach but not damage the master cast.

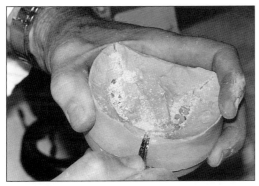

**Fig 14-89** A knife blade is inserted into the anterior cut and a twisting force is applied.

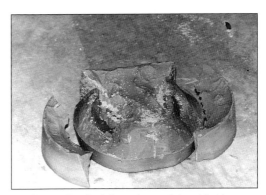

**Fig 14-90** The facial portions of the third investment layer separate cleanly.

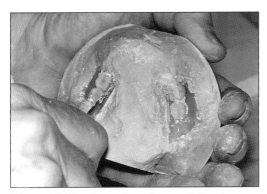

**Fig 14-91** The lingual surfaces of the denture teeth are exposed using a laboratory knife.

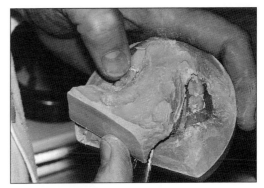

**Fig 14-92** The lingual portion of the third investment layer is teased away from the remainder of the assembly.

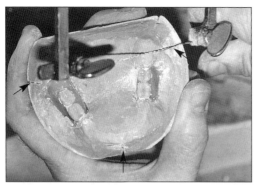

**Fig 14-93** The die saw is used to make three cuts in the second investment layer *(arrows)*.

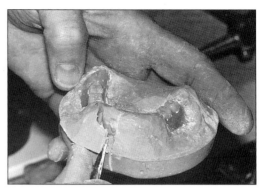

**Fig 14-94** A knife blade is inserted into the anterior saw cut and twisted to remove the sides of the second layer.

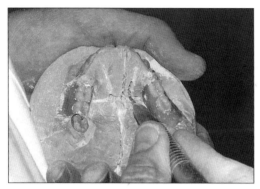

**Fig 14-95** A fissure bur in a low-speed handpiece is used to section the remainder of the second layer. Care is taken not to damage removable partial denture components.

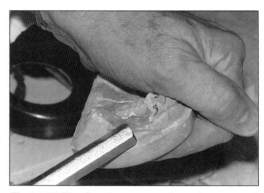

**Fig 14-96** The first investment layer is removed by tapping with a chisel.

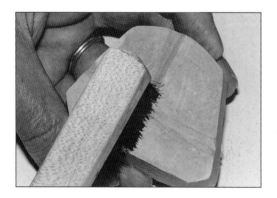

**Fig 14-97** Particles of investment are cleaned from the base of the cast.

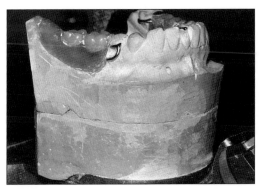

**Fig 14-98** The cast is repositioned on the articulator.

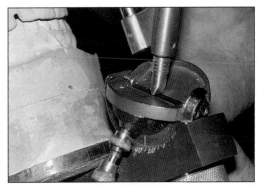

**Fig 14-99** The amount of pin opening indicates the amount of change that has occurred during processing.

## Correcting processing errors

Before the partial denture is removed from the cast, it must be remounted on the articulator for correction of changes that may have occurred as a result of processing. These changes generally affect the occlusion and may be significant. Many practitioners believe that processing errors can be corrected intraorally. This may be true when the prosthesis is entirely tooth supported and few teeth are being replaced. Unfortunately, as the prosthesis becomes more extensive, the adjustment process becomes increasingly difficult. Correction may involve excessive chair time and may not produce an acceptable result.

To correct the processing error, the master cast (with the partial denture in place) is properly positioned on the articulator (Fig 14-98). The fit of the base to the mounting stone is closely examined. Even a small error in adaptation can result in a significant error in adjustment. If adaptation is acceptable, the master cast is sealed to the mounting stone with modeling plastic or sticky wax.

The articulator is closed, and the size of the opening between the incisal guide pin and the incisal table is observed (Fig 14-99). If there is 1 mm or less of pin opening, the technique used in investing and processing was acceptable. If more than 1 mm of pin opening is present, some errors occurred during the investment procedure. If an excessive amount of pin opening occurs, the anatomy of the teeth may be de-

stroyed in reestablishing the proper occlusal relationship.

The condylar controls of the articulator are locked into the terminal hinge position. Occlusal discrepancies are located by positioning a piece of articulating paper between the mounted casts and gently tapping the casts together (Fig 14-100). Corrective grinding procedures are performed using appropriate burs in a low-speed handpiece. The occlusion is adjusted so that opposing teeth are returned to equal contact (Fig 14-101). At this point, the incisal pin should be in contact with the incisal table (Fig 14-102).

The occlusal surfaces of the teeth should be reshaped to provide inclines, grooves, and escapeways or sluiceways (Fig 14-103). At this stage, the anatomy of the occlusal surfaces of the artificial teeth should resemble the anatomy of the remaining natural teeth, particularly as far as cusp height is concerned. Any disparity between the natural and artificial teeth will result in a lack of occlusal harmony. Thin tissue paper is used to check contact between opposing teeth (Fig 14-104). There should be equal resistance between opposing teeth.

When the occlusal vertical dimension has been restored, eccentric (ie, right working, left working, protrusive) relationships of the teeth should be studied. Required adjustments should be made. Nonworking contacts in particular must be carefully checked and, if present, eliminated by selective grinding of the artificial teeth. The prosthesis should now be ready for decasting (Fig 14-105).

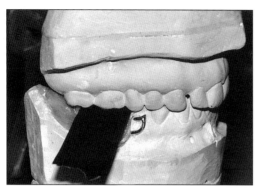

**Fig 14-100** Articulating paper is used to locate interferences.

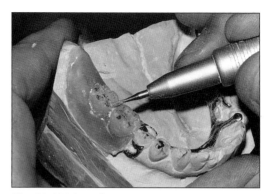

**Fig 14-101** Interferences are corrected using carbide burs in a low-speed handpiece.

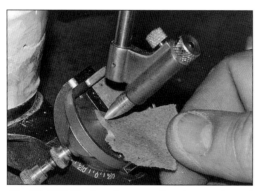

**Fig 14-102** Occlusal correction is continued until the incisal pin contacts the incisal table.

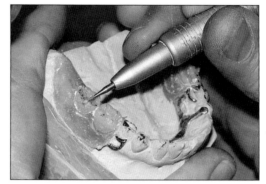

**Fig 14-103** Occlusal anatomy is restored to the denture teeth. Notice that articulating paper marks have been left in position. This permits the operator to reestablish anatomy without eliminating occlusal contacts.

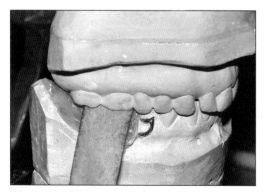

**Fig 14-104** Tissue paper is used to assess the consistency of contact. Here, the tissue paper is held firmly between the mandibular prosthesis and the maxillary cast. This should be repeated with the tissue paper held firmly between the stone teeth of the maxillary and mandibular casts.

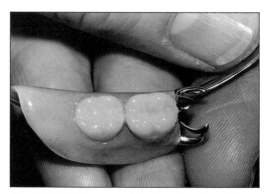

**Fig 14-105** The completed occlusal surfaces must have a sharp, functional anatomy.

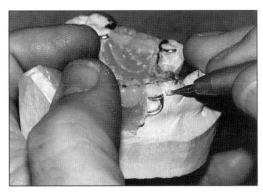

**Fig 14-106** Abutments are cut from the master cast using a fissure bur in a low-speed handpiece.

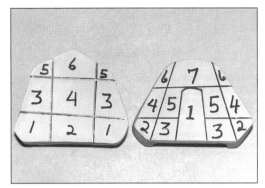

**Fig 14-107** To remove the processed denture from the master cast, it is often necessary to section the cast. The sequence for sectioning cuts is shown on the base of the maxillary cast *(left)* and mandibular cast *(right)*.

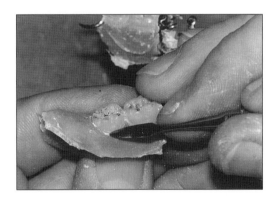

**Fig 14-108** Small hand instruments are used to remove stone particles from around the teeth.

## Decasting the partial denture

After processing errors have been corrected, the master cast is no longer of any value. Abutments are cut from the master cast using a fissure bur in a straight handpiece (Fig 14-106). Care must be taken not to scratch or cut the metal or resin of the denture. Generally, when the abutments have been removed, the partial denture can be carefully teased from the remainder of the cast. If undercuts are present, the master cast must be sectioned and removed piece by piece. Sectioning is accomplished using a plaster saw or a fissure bur in a straight handpiece. Sections are removed starting at the perimeter of the cast and proceeding inward (Fig 14-107).

When the partial denture has been recovered, particles of investment are removed from around the teeth and from the resin-to-metal joints. This is best accomplished with small hand instruments (Fig 14-108).

## Finishing and polishing the partial denture

There are three areas of primary concern during finishing and polishing procedures. They are *(1)* the cameo or external surfaces of the denture base, *(2)* the periphery or borders of the denture base, and *(3)* resin-metal and resin–artificial tooth interfaces.

The use of pumice to reduce the scratches or defects in the surface of acrylic resin must be performed with great care. Pumice can rapidly reduce the surface of resin. Coarse pumice has little or no indication in the finishing process. If the surface is so rough that coarse pumice is needed to correct the irregularities, the waxing technique should be reviewed and refined.

The rationale for polishing is to make little scratches out of big scratches. This progression should always be kept in mind. The fineness of the polishing instrument increases as the polishing process progresses. The final polish is always attained with the finest abrasive available.

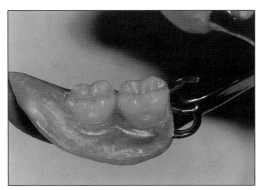

**Fig 14-109** The secondary food table and facial concavity must be maintained in the completed prosthesis. If waxing, investment, and packing procedures were properly performed, these areas should require only minimal finishing and polishing.

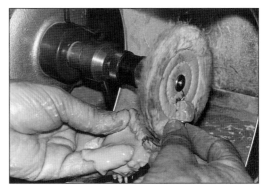

**Fig 14-110** Acrylic resin borders are smoothed using flour of pumice on a wet cloth wheel.

## External surfaces

The external surfaces of the denture base should have been developed in the waxing phase to the point that only minimum finishing will be required. The gingival bulge apical to the artificial teeth should be maintained (Fig 14-109). It will act as a secondary food table, enabling the cheeks to be a more positive factor in denture retention. Concavities on the facial and lingual surfaces of a mandibular denture provide space for the buccal tissues and tongue to assist in retention of the prosthesis.

If the waxing was done correctly, the use of laboratory burs should not be necessary. The lingual flanges may be brought to a high polish using flour of pumice on a wet cloth wheel (Fig 14-110). Proper preparation of the cloth wheel, as demonstrated in Figs 14-111 to 14-113, is essential if this process is to be successful. The use of a resin-polishing compound on a dry cloth wheel should produce a high gloss to the resin surface.

The facial surface of the denture base, particularly the anterior flange, should not be brought to a high polish, but should be smoothed. A high finish on the facial surface can produce an artificial appearance. Light stippling on the facial surface with an off-center round bur followed by light buffing with fine pumice produces an eggshell finish that does not reflect light and appears more natural (Figs 14-114 and 14-115).

## Periphery or borders of the denture base

Ideally, denture bases should be extended to the maximum length available to provide optimal support and stability. For a mandibular distal extension partial denture, the length and thickness of the extension are established by the corrected cast impression. As the impression is boxed, the length and width of the border are maintained. The resultant denture base reflects the dimensions created during impression procedures. To finish these borders, the operator removes the flash resulting from the packing procedures and smooths the denture base using flour of pumice on a wet rag wheel.

For borders that are not determined by a corrected cast impression, the length and thickness must be maintained until clinical placement can be accomplished. At this point, the borders may be adjusted.

As previously mentioned, two areas of partial dentures must be thinned prior to denture placement. These are the distobuccal extension of a maxillary denture base and the distolingual extension of a mandibular denture base. The procedures for thinning these areas are shown in Figs 14-116 and 14-117. The resultant borders should be 1.5 to 2.0 mm thick. Other borders should be 2 to 3 mm thick and should be gently rounded (Fig 14-118). A sharp border can be irritating to the adjacent soft tissues. Sustained irritation of these tissues can result in the development of a denture epulis (ie, epulis fissuratum).

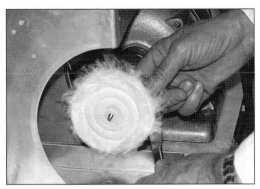

**Fig 14-111** A new cloth wheel is prepared for use by running the wheel against the dull blade of a laboratory spatula. This loosens the fibers of the wheel.

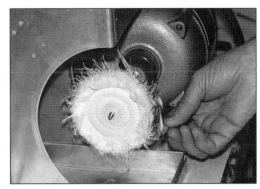

**Fig 14-112** The loosened fibers are then removed using a match or lighter.

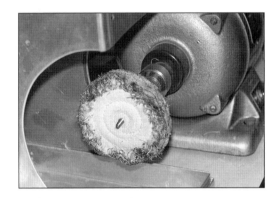

**Fig 14-113** The prepared cloth wheel has a smooth, soft surface.

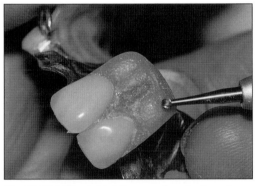

**Fig 14-114** The labial flange of a denture base may be stippled using an off-center round bur.

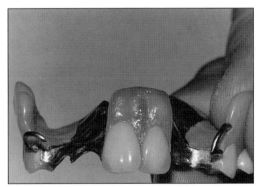

**Fig 14-115** Stippling creates a slightly irregular surface that reflects light more naturally.

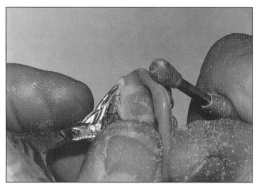

**Fig 14-116** The distobuccal extension of a maxillary distal extension prosthesis must be thinned to permit movement of the coronoid process of the mandible.

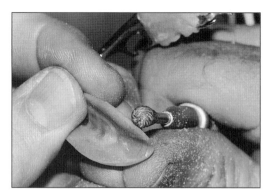

**Fig 14-117** The distolingual surface of a mandibular distal extension prosthesis is thinned to avoid crowding and irritation of the tongue.

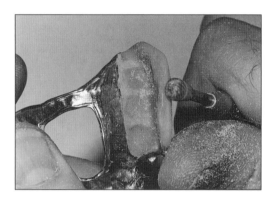

**Fig 14-118** Other acrylic resin borders should be 2 to 3 mm wide and gently rounded.

The borders are finished by removing any flash with laboratory burs in a low-speed handpiece. Smoothing is accomplished using flour of pumice on a wet cloth wheel. Polishing is performed using a buffing compound on a soft, dry cloth wheel.

### Resin-metal and resin–artificial tooth interfaces

Resin-to-metal junctions at the internal finish lines should not be polished. If any flash is present, it is removed and the junction smoothed.

The acrylic resin at the external finish line is trimmed, but left slightly above the level of the metal (Fig 14-119). This slight elevation is removed during the final polishing. The goal in this polishing procedure is to ensure an even, flowing surface from resin to metal. Any deviation from the surface of the resin to the metal may be annoying to the patient's tongue.

Finishing the gingival contours is particularly challenging. Attempts to smooth the resin–artificial tooth interfaces often result in destruction of the desired denture base contours and flattening of artificial tooth surfaces. As a result, the gingival margins are gently cleaned using an explorer. Flour of pumice and a soft brush wheel in a low-speed handpiece are then used to polish the areas around the artificial teeth (Fig 14-120).

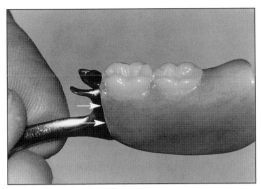

**Fig 14-119** Acrylic resin at external finish lines is left slightly above the level of the metal (*arrows*). This slight elevation will be removed during final polishing procedures.

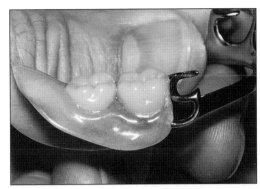

**Fig 14-120** The areas around the artificial teeth have been polished using flour of pumice and a soft brush wheel.

**Fig 14-121** The completed prosthesis should be smooth and free from defects.

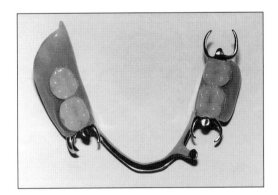

If polishing procedures are to be performed using a dental lathe, special care must be used. It is very easy for a clasp or other component to become entangled in the polishing wheel, particularly a cloth wheel. It is possible to distort a clasp arm, but, more importantly, it is possible that the denture can be thrown with considerable force against the lathe pan (or the operator). This can distort the major connector or fracture the denture base. The operator would be wise to line the lathe pan with soft towels or to keep the pan filled with wet pumice to cushion the shock should the partial denture be thrown from the polishing wheel.

After the polishing procedures are complete, the partial denture is washed with soap and water and a soft brush. If difficulty is encountered in removing remnants of polishing compound from the partial denture, it may be placed in an ultrasonic cleaner for a few minutes.

Upon completion of the foregoing procedures, the partial denture is carefully inspected to be certain that all scratches and defects have been removed (Fig 14-121). In turn, the partial denture is disinfected and stored in water.

## ☐ **Reference**

1. Frush JO, Fisher RD. Introduction to dentogenic restoration. J Prosthet Dent 1955;5:568–595.

## ☐ **Bibliography**

Bolouri A, Hilger TC, Gowrylok MD. Modified flasking technique for removable partial dentures. J Prosthet Dent 1975;34:221–223.

Clark EB. Tooth color selection. J Am Dent Assoc 1933;20:1065–1073.

Culpepper WD. A comparative study of shade matching procedures. J Prosthet Dent 1970;24:166–173.

DeVan MM. The appearance phase of denture construction. Dent Clin North Am 1957;1:255–268.

Grunewald AH, Paffenbarger GC, Dickson G. The effect of molding processes on some properties of denture resins. J Am Dent Assoc 1952;44:269–284.

Hughes GA. Facial types and tooth arrangement. J Prosthet Dent 1951;1:82–95.

Johnson HB. Technique for packing and staining complete or partial denture bases. J Prosthet Dent 1956;6:154–159.

Krajicek DD. Natural appearance for the individual denture patient. J Prosthet Dent 1960;10:205–214.

Lowe RD, Kydd WL, Smith DE. Swallowing and resting forces related to lingual flange thickness in removable partial dentures. J Prosthet Dent 1970;23:279–288.

Peyton FA, Anthony DH. Evaluation of dentures processed by different techniques. J Prosthet Dent 1963;13:269–281.

Pound E. Applying harmony in selecting and arranging teeth. Dent Clin North Am 1962;6:241–258.

Scandrett FR, Hanson JG, Unsicker RL. Layered silicone rubber technique for flasking removable partial dentures. J Prosthet Dent 1978;40:349–350.

Smith RH. Rapid removable partial denture processing with a cold-curing acrylic resin. J Prosthet Dent 1972;28:442–444.

Sproull RC. Color matching in dentistry, part I: The three dimensional nature of color. J Prosthet Dent 1973;29:416–424.

Tillman EJ. Molding and staining acrylic resin anterior teeth. J Prosthet Dent 1955;5:497–507.

Van Victor A. The mold guide cast—Its significance in denture esthetics. J Prosthet Dent 1953;3:165–177.

Vig RG. The denture look. J Prosthet Dent 1961;11:9–15.

Young HA. Denture esthetics. J Prosthet Dent 1956;6:748–755.

# Delivering the Removable Partial Denture

During the many clinical appointments required to fabricate a removable partial denture, the practitioner should educate the patient about the goals and benefits of the therapy. The patient should understand that the principal goal of prosthodontic therapy is not merely the replacement of missing teeth, but preservation of the remaining dentoalveolar structures. If these conditions are met, the practitioner and the patient can expect a reasonably good long-term prognosis for therapy.

Many patients will require a period of psychological and physical adjustment immediately following the insertion of a new removable partial denture. Patients must be mentally prepared for the realities of removable partial denture therapy. Even a short period of unexpected discomfort following insertion of a new removable partial denture may prevent long-term patient acceptance of the prosthesis. A significant percentage of unsuccessful removable partial denture therapies can be attributed to a lack of mental preparation preceding delivery of a removable partial denture.

Objectives of the insertion appointment are *(1)* to evaluate and correct the fit of the denture base, *(2)* to correct the occlusion, and *(3)* to adjust the retentive clasps. Additionally, the practitioner should provide verbal and written instructions regarding appropriate oral hygiene, removable partial denture hygiene, and the need for future evaluation and maintenance.

The first three objectives should be completed in order. The occlusion should not be evaluated until the denture base has been adjusted to fit the edentulous ridge and surrounding tissues. Adjustment of retentive clasps should not be considered until occlusal adjustments have been finalized.

## ❏ Fit of Denture Base

Despite the best efforts of clinical and laboratory personnel, the addition of one or more denture bases generally results in some form of misfit. Denture bases often display heavy contact with the lateral walls of the ridge and little or no contact with the ridge crest. This pattern of tissue contact results from the predictable distortion that occurs during polymerization of heat-activated denture base resins. Chemically-activated resins display slightly less distortion and

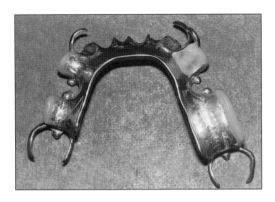

**Fig 15-1** Cast metal bases are adjusted at the framework try-in appointment. It should not be necessary to adjust cast bases during the delivery appointment.

therefore require less adjustment during the insertion appointment. Cast metal bases are not subject to the difficulties associated with polymerization shrinkage and usually do not require adjustment during the insertion appointment (Fig 15-1). Any correction to a cast metal base should have been performed at the framework try-in appointment.

## Pressure indicator paste

A disclosing medium with appropriate physical characteristics must be used to evaluate the fit of individual denture bases. Disclosing wax cannot be used for this purpose because it is resistant to displacement by the soft tissues. Aerosol sprays are equally ineffective and are messy when used in the oral cavity. Consequently, the practitioner must explore other options.

Currently, there are a variety of pastes that may be used in denture base evaluation. These materials, known as *pressure indicator pastes* (Fig 15-2), consist principally of zinc oxide powder combined with a medium-consistency vegetable fat or shortening. Other ingredients are added to improve the flavor and consistency of the paste.

A pressure indicator paste may also be prepared in the dental office. A simple recipe has been reported in the literature.[1,2] Equal volumes of zinc oxide powder (zinc oxide USP, Sultan Chemists, Englewood, NJ) and vegetable shortening (Crisco, Procter and Gamble, Cincinnati, OH) are thoroughly blended together in a kitchen mixer. The paste is then placed in a sealed stock container and stored for 24 hours. Small por-

tions can be removed from the stock container and placed in individual jars for use in the clinic. This method of producing and storing pressure indicator paste is inexpensive and convenient. The relative amounts of zinc oxide powder and vegetable shortening can be varied slightly to alter the viscosity of the paste to the preference of the dentist.

The consistency of pressure indicator paste should permit application of a thin layer to the intaglio surface of the denture base with a stiff brush. The brush can be used to place a distinct stroke pattern in the paste. The removable partial denture is then inserted, firmly seated, removed, and carefully inspected. Where no contact between the denture base and the soft tissues has occurred, the brush strokes will remain in place (Fig 15-3). Where moderate contact has occurred, the brush stroke pattern will be indistinct or obliterated (Fig 15-4). Where heavy contact has occurred, the pink denture base material will clearly show through the white paste (Fig 15-5). Areas of heavy contact should be relieved using appropriate rotary instruments.

A word of caution is in order. The use of pressure indicator paste to disclose areas requiring adjustment can help prevent the unnecessary discomfort caused by an ill-fitting prosthesis. However, unnecessary, random, or ill-advised adjustment of the removable partial denture may result in an inadequate fit and require that the new prosthesis be relined. This may discourage the patient, who generally expects prolonged, trouble-free service from the prosthesis. Experience is necessary to differentiate between marks that indicate

**Fig 15-2** Pressure indicator paste is commonly used for assessment of denture base adaptation.

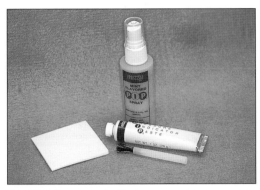

**Fig 15-3** Pressure indicator paste is applied so that brush strokes are evident. The prosthesis is then placed and removed. Where no contact between the denture base and the soft tissue has occurred, the brush strokes remain in place.

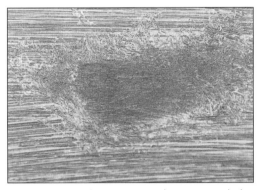

**Fig 15-4** Where moderate contact has occurred, brush strokes appear indistinct.

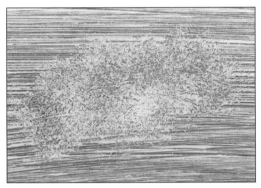

**Fig 15-5** Where heavy contact has occurred, the denture base material clearly shows through the pressure indicator paste.

normal contact with soft tissues and those that indicate excessive contact. Until sufficient clinical experience has been gained, the beginning practitioner should err on the side of conservative adjustment.

### Clinical use

Insertion of a new removable partial denture should not be attempted until a thin layer of pressure indicator paste has been carefully painted on the intaglio surfaces. It is often difficult to identify subtle undercuts in the supporting tissues. Seating the removable partial denture over these undercuts may produce pain or even lacerate the soft tissues. Without pressure indicator paste on the tissue surface of the prosthesis, identification of the offending undercut is impossible and the patient will be required to endure a second placement of the denture with pressure indicator

paste—although this time with considerable apprehension.

Clinically, the intaglio of the denture base is completely dried. A thin coat of pressure indicator paste is painted onto this surface. The prosthesis is then inserted using gentle pressure. If resistance is encountered, the prosthesis should be removed and the pressure indicator paste examined. Since the metal was adjusted to fit at the framework try-in appointment, resistance to insertion at this stage probably is due to contact between the denture base and the residual ridge. The pressure indicator paste over areas of interference will be displaced from the denture base. Relief is provided by subtle adjustment with acrylic resin rotary cutting instruments (Fig 15-6).

As previously noted, it is good practice to relieve the acrylic resin a little at a time, rather than perform-

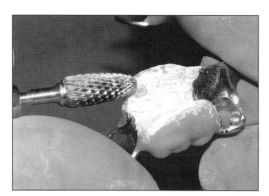

**Fig 15-6** The practitioner relieves pressure spots using a laboratory bur in a low-speed handpiece.

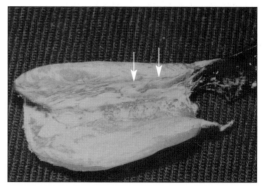

**Fig 15-7** The mylohyoid area of the mandibular ridge *(arrows)* is particularly sensitive to pressure.

ing overly aggressive adjustments and losing all tissue contact. After each adjustment, the pressure indicator paste and grinding debris should be removed and fresh paste applied. This procedure should be repeated until the removable partial denture can be completely seated without encountering unnecessary resistance or causing patient discomfort.

Areas of heavy contact are frequently located over bony prominences such as the maxillary tuberosity regions. Perhaps the most difficult area to correct, and one of the most sensitive to pressure, is the lingual surface of the mandibular edentulous ridge in the mylohyoid region (Fig 15-7). Careful examination and adjustment of the fit in this area is essential.

### Modifying the peripheral denture base extensions

Extension of acrylic resin denture flanges plays an important role in the support and stability of a removable partial denture. Maximum flange extension, within physiologically tolerable limits, provides optimal support and stability for the prosthesis. Extension of denture flanges into the facial vestibules and lingual sulci enhances resistance to horizontal displacement. Therefore, acrylic resin denture base flanges should not be arbitrarily reduced. Rather, they should be critically evaluated and adjusted only when physiologic limits have been exceeded.

For extension base removable partial dentures, proposed borders should be established during cor-

rected cast impression procedures. Visual and digital evaluation of the resin flanges should be performed during the insertion appointment (Fig 15-8). For purposes of examination, the buccal tissues should be held between the thumb and index finger and moved apically, laterally, and then occlusally. Soft tissue movement adjacent to each denture flange should be noted. Restriction of soft tissue movement can lead to irritation. Overextension of the borders also may result in the application of dislodging forces by the movable soft tissues. Therefore, while maximum tissue coverage is essential to support and stability, it is equally important to avoid overextension of denture borders.

Mandibular lingual and distolingual flange lengths may be evaluated using physiologic movements of the tongue and floor of the mouth. Clinical evaluation is accomplished by placing an index finger on the occlusal surfaces of the denture teeth on one side of the patient's mouth. The patient is then instructed to extend the tongue straight forward and then into the cheek on the opposite side of the mouth. If lingual or distolingual flanges are overextended, the denture base will lift away from the supporting tissues. This displacement is readily identified by pressure against the operator's index finger, allowing necessary flange adjustments to be made (Fig 15-9).

Disclosing wax can be placed on denture base flanges to help identify areas of overextension (Figs 15-10 to 15-12). Unfortunately, the flow characteristics of disclosing wax are not well suited to this application. Mixing petroleum jelly with the disclosing wax

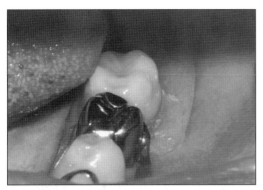

**Fig 15-8** Visual and digital examination of denture base flanges is performed at the time of placement. Overextension of the denture bases may lead to irritation of the soft tissues or displacement of the removable partial denture.

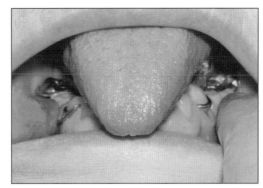

**Fig 15-9** Extension of a mandibular lingual flange is evaluated by placing the index fingers on the occlusal surfaces of the prosthetic teeth and having the patient protrude the tongue. The prosthesis will lift if it is overextended.

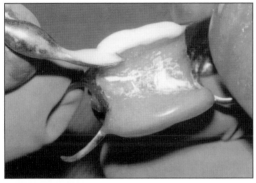

**Fig 15-10** Disclosing wax may be applied to acrylic resin borders to help identify areas of overextension.

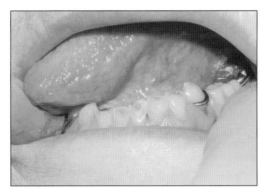

**Fig 15-11** The removable partial denture is carefully inserted, and the patient is told to move the tongue into the opposite cheek.

**Fig 15-12** Areas of overextension are identified, and borders are adjusted.

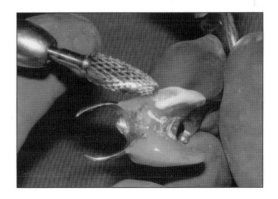

improves the flow characteristics of the disclosing material.[3] This mixture is more reliable when used routinely to disclose regions of flange overextension.

Corrected cast procedures are not usually accomplished for maxillary extension base removable partial dentures. To clinically evaluate denture base flange extension, direct visual examination is the method of choice. Tissues of the cheek are moved apically, outward, and occlusally. In turn, these tissues are moved anteroposteriorly. As the tissues are being manipu-

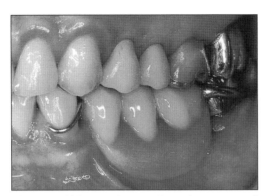

Fig 15-13 When a denture base is supported entirely by natural teeth, maximum extension of the denture base is not necessary.

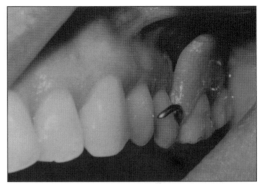

Fig 15-14 Thick leading edges of posterior denture base flanges are esthetically unattractive. These edges should be thinned to provide improved esthetics.

lated, the practitioner watches the soft tissues adjacent to the denture base. Tissue movement should not be restricted by a denture base, nor should it cause the prosthesis to be dislodged. The use of the disclosing wax, or a mixture of disclosing wax and petroleum jelly, may be helpful in identifying areas that require adjustment.

When a denture base is supported entirely by natural teeth, maximum extension of the denture base is normally not indicated (Fig 15-13). Since support and stability of the prosthesis are provided by the associated abutments, the denture base flange must extend only far enough to achieve positive soft tissue contact. This positive tissue contact is intended to prohibit the accumulation of food beneath the denture base.

In general, posterior denture base flanges should be at least 2 mm thick and should display rounded borders. Flanges should be slightly thinner at the distolingual aspects of mandibular extension base removable partial dentures and distofacial aspects of maxillary extension base removable partial dentures. Decreased flange thickness in these areas provides additional tongue space in the mandibular arch and freedom of movement for the coronoid processes in the maxillary arch. The leading edges of maxillary and mandibular posterior denture base flanges also should be thinned. This helps to disguise the presence of the flange when the patient is viewed from the front during normal conversation and while smiling. Thick leading edges of posterior denture base flanges are often esthetically unattractive (Fig 15-14).

## Contouring the anterior denture base flange

When designing a denture base for the anterior portion of the mouth, consideration must be given to the esthetic requirements of the patient. Slight overextension or overcontouring of the labial flange may cause an otherwise successful prosthesis to be a dismal esthetic failure.

Nearly all maxillary anterior edentulous ridges present undercuts relative to the removable partial denture's path of insertion. During removable partial denture construction, acrylic resin is usually processed into these undercuts. This presents a dilemma for the practitioner. In a practical sense, the only components of a removable partial denture permitted to contact oral tissues in areas of undercut are the termini of the retentive clasps. In reality, the displaceability of oral soft tissues permits many denture bases to enter limited soft tissue undercuts. Therefore, careful consideration must be given to denture base flange extensions and contours in areas of edentulous ridge undercuts.

The first step in anterior denture base adjustment is the application of pressure indicator paste to the intaglio surface of the resin (Fig 15-15). The removable partial denture is then positioned in the mouth and seated with gentle pressure. As resistance to the seating of the labial denture base flange is encountered, the partial denture is removed. Careful evaluation of the pressure indicator paste often will reveal excessive tis-

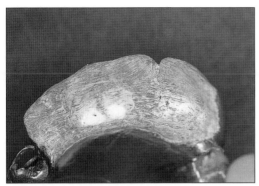

**Fig 15-15** Pressure indicator paste is applied to the intaglio of the denture base.

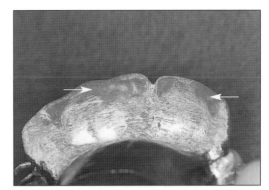

**Fig 15-16** Excessive contact is evident at the border of the denture base *(arrows)*.

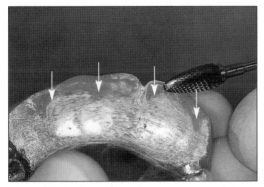

**Fig 15-17** Vertical reduction of the denture base *(arrows)* is accomplished.

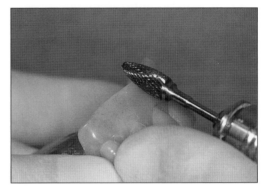

**Fig 15-18** Borders are beveled to permit a smooth transition from the denture base to the oral soft tissues.

sue contact along the border of the denture base (Fig 15-16). Correction of this interference involves vertical reduction of the flange length to the point of contact with the edentulous ridge (Fig 15-17). Following adjustment, the pressure indicator paste and grinding residue are wiped from all denture surfaces and fresh paste is applied. This procedure is repeated until the removable partial denture can be completely seated without encountering resistance, producing blanching of the soft tissues, or causing patient discomfort.

Once the anterior denture base flange has been adjusted to permit complete seating of the prosthesis, the superior and lateral margins of the flange are beveled to produce thin borders (Fig 15-18). This will permit a smooth transition from the denture base to the soft tissues, thereby producing a natural and esthetic effect.

## ☐ Correcting Occlusal Contacts

Correction of occlusal contacts must not be initiated until the removable partial denture can be completely and comfortably seated in the patient's mouth. Attempting to correct occlusal errors before establishing adequate fit of the denture base is inappropriate.

Occlusal contacts that exist when the removable partial denture is out of the mouth must also exist when the prosthesis is in place. The removable partial denture should not interfere with the mandible attaining the prescribed occlusal vertical dimension, nor with required guidance during eccentric mandibular movements.

If metallic components were properly adjusted during the framework try-in, occlusal interferences that occur during the insertion appointment should be limited to the prosthetic teeth. The procedures used to evaluate and correct these occlusal errors are similar to those used during the framework try-in appointment. Use of a systematic and logical sequence for correcting occlusal errors at the insertion appointment will not only save valuable chair time, but will also reduce the possibility of inappropriate occlusal adjustment.

The goals of occlusal evaluation and correction during the insertion appointment are *(1)* maintenance of existing natural tooth contacts and *(2)* establishment of occlusal harmony in all centric and eccentric positions. Failure to achieve these goals may result in the patient's inability to wear a new removable partial denture.

From a practical standpoint, the clinical techniques used to evaluate occlusal errors may be classified as either intraoral or extraoral procedures. The choice of procedure is primarily determined by the stability and support of the removable partial denture in the patient's mouth. A fairly large percentage of new removable partial dentures may be evaluated using an intraoral approach. However, for those patients in whom denture stability and support are compromised, use of the extraoral (or remount) procedure is most appropriate. The latter group includes patients with *(1)* removable partial dentures displaying long extension bases, *(2)* extension base removable partial dentures covering extremely mobile soft tissues, and *(3)* removable partial dentures opposed by conventional complete dentures. For clinical situations in which compromised stability and support make occlusal evaluation challenging, remounting the denture or dentures on an appropriate articulator will permit more accurate occlusal evaluation and adjustment.

### Intraoral detection and correction of occlusal discrepancies

The use of articulating paper or articulating film to disclose occlusal contacts makes intraoral evaluation of removable partial dentures possible. The development of ultrathin (8-μm) articulating films has all but eliminated false occlusal markings and simplified evaluation procedures. In addition, shim stock may be used to physically verify the presence and location of occlusal contacts (Figs 15-19 to 15-23).

In a clinical setting, occlusal interferences are identified using an appropriate articulating film. Careful adjustment of the prosthetic teeth is then accomplished

using a multifluted bur and a low-speed handpiece. It is recommended that occlusal corrections be accomplished outside of the oral cavity. The noise and vibration produced by a dental handpiece and bur are often magnified by a removable partial denture framework and can produce moderate discomfort for the patient.

The process of marking and adjusting occlusal surfaces is continued until contact between opposing natural teeth has been restored. At the same time, denture teeth should display firm occlusal contact.

Occlusal adjustment must not destroy the intended anatomy of the denture teeth. Careful adjustment and meticulous reshaping of altered occlusal surfaces are often necessary to optimize masticatory efficiency (Fig 15-24). Articulating film marks identifying the desired occlusal contacts should be preserved during the reshaping process. This allows the practitioner to maintain the desired occlusion while placing sluiceways and supplemental grooves. These anatomic features facilitate the escape of food particles and promote chewing efficiency.

### Occlusal correction using remount procedures

Identifying and correcting occlusal errors directly in the mouth is a reliable and accurate method. Unfortunately, intraoral methods cannot be used in all circumstances. Removable partial dentures exhibiting long extension bases or those supported by excessively mobile tissues may be difficult to evaluate because of significant functional movement. If a conventional complete denture opposes a removable partial denture, rules governing occlusal adjustment of complete dentures must be followed. If intraoral correction is attempted under the aforementioned circumstances, the soft tissues are likely to distort, producing inaccurate occlusal markings and unreliable occlusal results. Soft tissue distortion and denture base movement represent even greater problems during the evaluation of eccentric occlusal contacts. Under these conditions, the adjustment of erroneous articulator film markings is more likely to result in occlusal instability rather than occlusal correction.

Extraoral correction represents an alternative to intraoral procedures. When using the extraoral technique, the removable restoration or restorations are

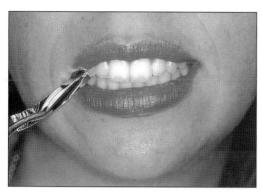

**Fig 15-19** Shim stock is used to identify contacts before placement of the removable partial denture. The shim stock is tightly held at the right first premolar region.

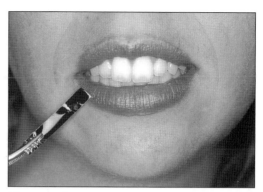

**Fig 15-20** Contacts are reevaluated with the removable partial denture in position. The introduction of the prosthesis prevents shim stock from being held at the right first premolar region.

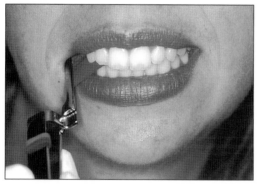

**Fig 15-21** Articulating paper is used to identify occlusal interferences.

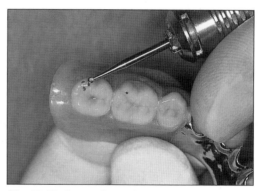

**Fig 15-22** Corrective grinding procedures are performed.

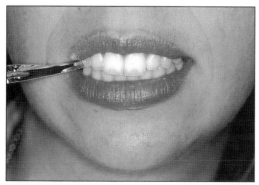

**Fig 15-23** The removable partial denture is repositioned and the occlusion is evaluated using shim stock. Firm contact is reestablished at the right first premolar region.

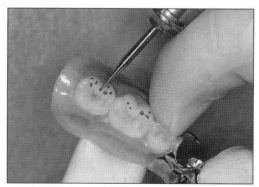

**Fig 15-24** Occlusal surfaces are reshaped to optimize masticatory efficiency.

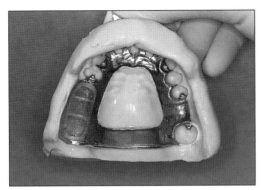

**Fig 15-25** A "pick-up" impression is made with the removable partial denture in the mouth. In most instances, the removable partial denture will remain in the impression when it is removed from the mouth.

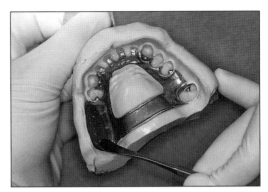

**Fig 15-26** Undercuts are blocked out using clay. Wet paper towels, wet facial tissues, or wax also may be used.

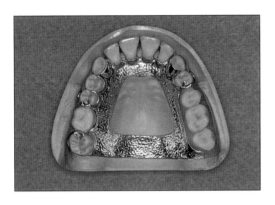

**Fig 15-27** A cast is then poured, recovered, and trimmed in preparation for mounting procedures.

mounted on a dental articulator using a facebow transfer and interocclusal records. Occlusal contacts are then marked, evaluated, and adjusted in the dry, well-illuminated environment of the dental laboratory.

To remount removable partial dentures in an articulator, it is necessary to secure casts of both the dental arch restored by the removable partial denture and the opposing arch. An irreversible hydrocolloid impression is made with the removable partial denture completely seated in the patient's mouth. In most instances, the prosthesis will remain in the impression when the impression is removed from the mouth (Fig 15-25). If the prosthesis remains in the mouth, it must be retrieved and carefully repositioned in the impression. Undercuts within the removable partial denture are then blocked out using baseplate wax, clay, wet paper towels, or wet facial tissues (Fig 15-26). Dental stone is mixed and vibrated into the impression. When the dental stone has

hardened, the cast is recovered and trimmed in preparation for mounting procedures (Fig 15-27).

A cast of the opposing dentition must also be fabricated. If the opposing arch is restored with a conventional complete denture, the denture itself may be remounted on the articulator. If this is not the case, an alginate impression of the arch is made and a cast is generated.

At this stage of the procedure, the maxillary cast is mounted on the articulator using a facebow record. The mandibular cast is mounted using jaw relation records. Before continuing, the accuracy of the mounting is verified using additional jaw relation records. Upon completion of the verification process, occlusal evaluation and correction procedures are initiated.

The techniques and goals used in extraoral correction procedures are similar to those described for the intraoral method. The adjustment of denture teeth is continued until simultaneous contact of opposing occlusal surfaces has been achieved. In turn, eccentric occlusion is adjusted.

After the occlusion of the removable partial denture has been refined on the articulator, appropriate occlusal anatomy is restored using fine burs and a low-speed handpiece.

## Adjusting Retentive Clasps

Up to this point in the denture insertion appointment, there has been no need to consider the amount of retention supplied by the direct retainers. Now that the removable partial denture has been adjusted to fit the supporting tissues and the occlusion has been corrected, the practitioner's attention may be turned to the retentive characteristics of the clasp assemblies. It is important to realize that, in most instances, no adjustment of the direct retainers is indicated during the insertion appointment. However, when clasp adjustment is necessary, the goals are to limit unnecessary force application to the abutments and assure that sufficient removable partial denture retention is provided.

Over the years, chromium-based casting alloys (Ni-Cr and Co-Cr) have developed the reputation for being difficult to adjust. For the most part, this reputation is based on poor handling rather than any inadequacies in the respective alloys.

When examining the physical characteristics of denture base alloys, the practitioner should pay particular attention to elongation. Elongation is a measure of ductility or brittleness of an alloy. Specifically, elongation represents the degree of plastic deformation that an alloy can undergo before it fractures. Ultimate tensile strength is the maximum stress that a material can withstand before failure. The combined effect of elongation and ultimate tensile strength is an indication of toughness of the material. Chromium-based alloys are relatively tough—that is, they possess high ultimate tensile strengths and favorable elongation characteristics. As a result, clasps made from these alloys are relatively resistant to fracture and can withstand moderate bending adjustments if properly managed.

Fracture of chromium-based clasps during adjustment is most often related to excessive or repeated bending at one location. Clasps should be adjusted in small increments and frequently checked to determine if the desired results have been achieved. Excessively bending a clasp in one direction only to have to rebend the clasp toward its original position will lead to accelerated fatigue and failure of the clasp. As a result, excessive bending must be avoided.

### Types of pliers

Various pliers are available for bending dental wires and clasps. In the practice of removable partial prosthodontics, two pliers are generally sufficient. These are the No. 139, or "bird-beak" plier, and the No. 200, or "three-prong" plier (Fig 15-28).

Proper technique for adjusting a clasp involves holding the clasp stationary between the beaks of a No. 139 plier and applying a bending force with the fingers of the opposite hand (Fig 15-29). This results in a gentle curvature of the clasp arm and minimizes the likelihood of clasp fracture.

Clasp adjustment may also be performed using a No. 200 plier. This is accomplished by engaging the clasp arm with the beaks of the plier and gently squeezing the handles until the desired bend has been achieved (Fig 15-30). Specific applications are described in the following sections.

### Adjusting wrought-wire clasps

Of all forms of clasp arms, wrought-wire clasp arms most commonly require adjustment. This is partially due to early distortion of clasps resulting from inappropriate design and application. All too often wrought-wire clasps are placed into excessive undercuts. As a result, the yield strength of the wrought metal is exceeded, and permanent deformation or fracture results.

Another factor that may contribute to early distortion and failure of a wrought-wire clasp is the technique used by the patient to remove the prosthesis. A patient who has not been taught the correct way to remove a partial denture may place a fingernail under the wrought-wire arm and force the clasp over the abutment's height of contour. This leads to significant distortion of the wrought-wire clasp arm and necessitates clasp adjustment.

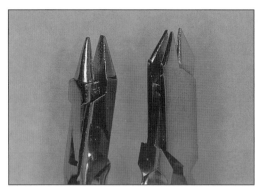

**Fig 15-28** A No. 139 plier *(left)* and a No. 200 plier *(right)*.

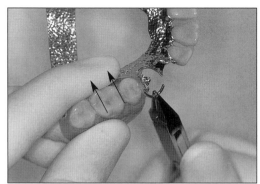

**Fig 15-29** Adjustment is performed by holding the clasp between the beaks of a No. 139 plier and applying a bending force with the fingers of the opposite hand. (*Arrows* denote direction of force.)

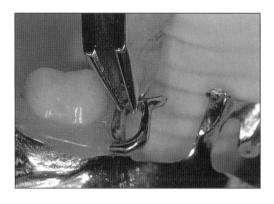

**Fig 15-30** A No. 200 plier has three distinct prongs. To use this plier, the operator engages the clasp and gently squeezes the handles until the desired bend is achieved.

The recommended method for adjusting a wrought-wire clasp is illustrated in Figs 15-31 and 15-32. If inadequate retention exists once tooth-clasp contact has been reestablished, it is likely that the clasp terminus is engaging an insufficient undercut. To correct this problem, the round beak of the No. 139 plier is placed near the mesiodistal center of the clasp. Gentle force is applied to move the clasp terminus in an apical direction (Fig 15-33). When this has been accomplished, the procedures illustrated in Figs 15-31 and 15-32 are performed to ensure readaptation of the clasp arm to the tooth surface.

Small bends made by twisting or rotating the plier should be avoided because they tend to nick or mar the smooth surface of the wrought clasp. Defects in the wire serve to concentrate stresses and reduce the strength of the wire. Any damage to the surface of the wire should be smoothed before the partial denture is delivered to the patient (Fig 15-34). The smoothing is best accomplished by carborundum-containing rubber points or wheels. Thinning the clasp by excessive polishing must be avoided.

### Adjusting half-round, cast circumferential clasps

Adjustments to a half-round, cast circumferential clasp should only be accomplished in a plane perpendicular to the flat surface of the clasp. Adjustments may be made by bending the clasp toward or away from the abutment surface. Attempts to bend a half-round, cast circumferential clasp in any other plane or direction will result in distortion of the clasp's functional form and alteration of the clasp's intended

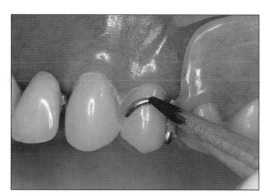

**Fig 15-31** The point at which a wrought-wire clasp loses contact with the tooth is marked using a pencil.

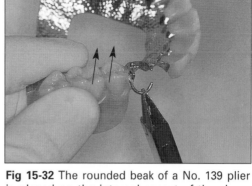

**Fig 15-32** The rounded beak of a No. 139 plier is placed on the internal aspect of the clasp, and the plier is aligned with the pencil mark. Pressure is applied to the removable partial denture using the fingers of the opposite hand. (*Arrows* denote direction of force.)

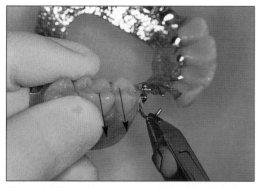

**Fig 15-33** To position a wrought-wire clasp in a slightly greater undercut, the rounded beak of a No. 139 plier is placed at 90 degrees to the long axis of the abutment. Pressure is applied to the removable partial denture using the fingers of the opposite hand. (*Arrows* denote direction of force.) The procedures illustrated in Figs 15-31 and 15-32 are then performed to ensure readaptation of the clasp arm to the tooth surface.

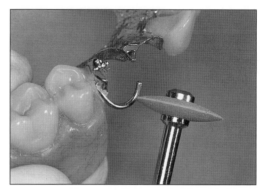

**Fig 15-34** Any irregularities on the surface of the clasp arm should be smoothed. This is best accomplished using a carborundum-impregnated rubber point or wheel.

performance. For this reason, if the retentive terminus of the clasp is located in an improper undercut, reconstruction of the framework is indicated.

Only the No. 139 plier should be used when adjusting a half-round, cast circumferential clasp. The proper technique for adjusting this clasp is similar to that described for a wrought-wire clasp. The first objective is to determine at what point along the clasp arm the adjustment should be made. If the clasp is not retentive and requires adjustment toward the abutment surface, careful intraoral evaluation of the clasp must be made. The point at which the clasp

loses contact with the tooth surface is marked to identify the location of the required adjustment. The adjustment is made by properly positioning the No. 139 plier and applying pressure with the opposite hand (Figs 15-35 to 15-37).

If it is necessary to reduce the amount of retention by bending the clasp away from the tooth, the adjustment is made at the junction of the middle and terminal thirds of the clasp. Force should be applied in a slow, controlled manner to avoid excessively bending the clasp arm.

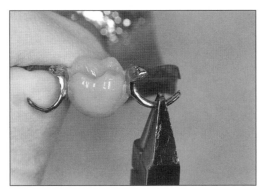

**Fig 15-35** The rounded beak of a No. 139 plier is placed against the flat internal surface of a half-round, cast circumferential clasp.

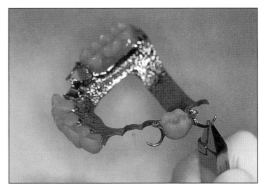

**Fig 15-36** All support is released to allow proper alignment of the plier and the clasp.

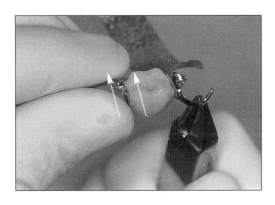

**Fig 15-37** Gentle pressure is applied to the removable partial denture using the fingers of the opposite hand. (*Arrows* denote direction of force.)

## Adjusting cast infrabulge clasps

Cast infrabulge clasps have half-round, cross-sectional forms. Therefore, like a cast circumferential clasp, adjustment of an infrabulge clasp can only be accomplished in a plane perpendicular to the flat surface of the clasp. This means that the clasp must be adjusted directly toward the abutment or directly away from the abutment.

A costly error that is commonly made while adjusting a T-clasp is application of a bending torque to the vertical approach arm in an attempt to move the retentive terminus toward the abutment surface. This will disrupt the consistent cross-sectional form of the vertical approach arm and compromise the intended function of the clasp.

If the retentive terminus of a T-clasp, or a modified T-clasp, requires adjustment to increase retention, a No. 200 plier should be used (Fig 15-38). This is the

only indication for use of this plier when adjusting removable partial denture clasps. When this adjustment is made, no twisting or bending force is applied to the plier. The prongs of the plier are positioned as close to the retentive terminus as possible. The single-prong portion of the plier is in contact with the clasp's inner, flat surface while the two-prong portion contacts the outer surface of the clasp. Closing the plier with slow, gradual force bends the retentive terminus toward the abutment surface. Extreme care must be taken when making this adjustment. The No. 200 plier is a very efficient wire-bending tool and can easily produce excessive bending. Subtle adjustment followed by intraoral reevaluation is indicated.

Often an infrabulge clasp lacks retention because of movement of the entire clasp away from the tooth surface (ie, deformation is located within the horizontal approach arm and results in the entire clasp arcing facially). Deformation of the clasp in this manner may

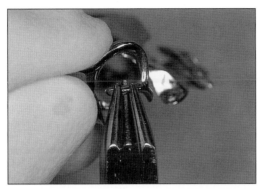

**Fig 15-38** The retentive terminus of a cast infrabulge clasp is adjusted using a No. 200 plier. This is accomplished by placing the single-prong portion of the plier in contact with the clasp's flat, inner surface. The handles of the plier are than squeezed until the desired bend is achieved.

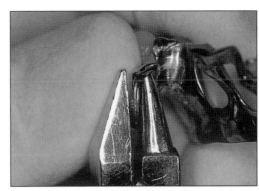

**Fig 15-39** The vertical projection arm of an infrabulge clasp is grasped in the beaks of a No. 139 plier. Notice that the rounded beak is positioned against the internal surface of the vertical projection arm.

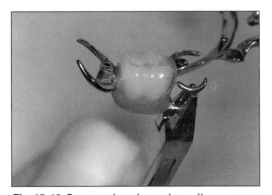

**Fig 15-40** Support is released to allow proper alignment and to prevent twisting bends within the vertical projection arm.

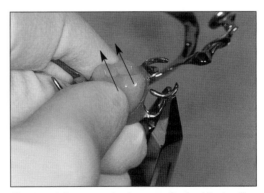

**Fig 15-41** Pressure is then applied with the fingers of the opposite hand. (*Arrows* denote direction of force.) The bend occurs in the horizontal portion of the clasp arm.

be caused by mishandling in the laboratory, the result of an accident, improper manipulation by the patient, or structural fatigue related to long-term service. To correct this problem, the vertical projection arm of the clasp is grasped in the beaks on a No. 139 plier (Figs 15-39 and 15-40). With a firm grasp of the removable partial denture, the entire vertical projection portion of the clasp is moved medially (Fig 15-41). This technique produces a bend in the horizontal projection of the clasp's approach arm. Subtle adjustment should be followed by intraoral reevaluation.

## Patient Instructions

### Oral hygiene

Providing the patient with appropriate oral hygiene instructions is extremely important. The patient must understand that meticulous home care is a prerequisite to removable partial denture success. Inadequate home care will hasten the destruction of the remaining teeth.

Though provided earlier in the therapy, instructions regarding the care and maintenance of the re-

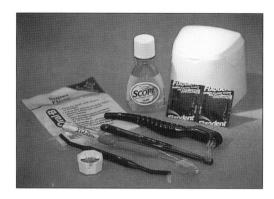

**Fig 15-42** Home care is discussed with the patient. Appropriate materials and methods are demonstrated.

maining natural teeth and oral soft tissues must now be reviewed. Proper brushing techniques and the use of dental floss as a routine part of the patient's home care should be emphasized (Fig 15-42). The patient must accept the need for periodic dental evaluation of oral tissues and dental prostheses. The interval between successive examinations will vary depending on the oral conditions and type of prosthesis, but should not exceed 1 year.

Use of plaque-disclosing tablets is an excellent way to communicate the need for meticulous attention to oral hygiene. Areas that are susceptible to plaque accumulation are readily visualized. The patient should be instructed to chew the disclosing tablets with the partial denture in the mouth. The denture can then be removed and examined for areas of plaque accumulation. Although accumulation on the removable partial denture will not be evident at the insertion appointment, the disclosing tablet technique should be demonstrated so the patient can periodically check the effectiveness of home care efforts.

Appropriate methods for denture hygiene should be demonstrated. Emphasis should be given to physically brushing the denture on a daily basis, rather than relying on a cleaning or soaking agent to remove debris. The use of common toothpastes should be avoided since these pastes often contain abrasive particles. Scouring powders and abrasive household cleaners should also be avoided because of their potential for damaging both acrylic resin and metal components of a removable partial denture. The patient must understand that the denture should never be brushed while in the mouth. Instead, the prosthesis should be removed to permit access to all surfaces.

The patient should also be instructed to clean the denture over a partially filled basin of water so that if the denture is dropped, little harm will be done.

The patient should be cautioned against using any cleansing solution containing chlorine. A popular and effective solution for cleaning acrylic resin complete dentures is a mixture of Clorox, Calgon, and water. However, if a chromium-based metal framework is soaked in this solution, the chlorine will irreparably damage the metal.

The patient should also be instructed to remove the prosthesis (or prostheses) before going to bed at night. The soft tissues covered by the denture bases and the major connectors must be given the opportunity to recover from constant mechanical stresses applied when the prosthesis is in place. While in place, the removable partial denture prohibits the beneficial bathing effects of saliva, which flush food and bacterial debris from the hard and soft supporting tissues. The risk of enamel decalcification and soft tissue inflammation is greatly increased when the prosthesis is worn for long periods of time.

If a patient has only a few remaining natural teeth and has a history of bruxism, less damage may be done to the remaining natural teeth if the denture is worn at night. If nighttime denture wear is necessary, the patient must identify several hours each day when the prosthesis can be removed from the mouth.

The patient should also be told to store the prosthesis in water when it is not in the oral cavity. Failure to do this may result in drying, cracking, and warpage of acrylic resin components. This is extremely damaging to the prosthesis and may necessitate repair or refabrication.

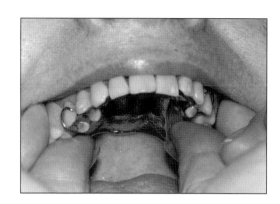

**Fig 15-43** A patient must avoid distortion of wrought-wire clasps. When wrought-wire clasps are present, the patient should grasp acrylic resin denture bases on each side of the arch and carefully withdraw the removable partial denture from the mouth.

## Prosthesis placement and removal

Teaching the patient how to insert and remove a dental prosthesis is essential. The patient's ability to adequately manage this task depends to some extent on his or her manual dexterity, muscular coordination, visual acuity, and physical condition. Additionally, design of the removable partial denture, the number and position of direct retainers, and the total amount of retentive force affect the ease with which the prosthesis can be removed from the mouth.

Insertion of a removable partial denture is generally less of a problem than is denture removal. The patient should be positioned in front of a wall-mounted mirror while the dentist inserts the prosthesis. It is important that the patient understand the need to properly align the removable partial denture over the abutments before applying seating pressure. The patient should be cautioned about trapping soft tissues of the cheeks, lips, or tongue between a clasp and its abutment. The amount of force needed to seat the prosthesis should be demonstrated, and the patient warned that if excessive pressure is required, alignment of the denture is probably incorrect. Seating the denture with biting pressure should be discouraged because damage to the denture, natural teeth, or soft tissues can easily result.

After the patient has observed insertion of the removable partial denture, its removal also should be demonstrated. The most convenient method for engaging the prosthesis is to position a fingernail or thumbnail apical to a facial clasp arm on each side of the dental arch and to move the clasp occlusally. This method is acceptable when cast circumferential clasps are readily available. However, if only wrought-wire clasps are available, this technique should be avoided. Wrought-wire clasps are easily distorted using this technique. When wrought-wire clasps are present, the patient should grasp the acrylic resin denture bases on each side of the arch and carefully withdraw the removable partial denture from the mouth (Fig 15-43).

For a prosthesis that incorporates one or more infrabulge clasps, positioning a fingernail apical to the approach arm and forcing the clasp occlusally is not an acceptable method of removal. This technique may lead to laceration of the adjacent soft tissues by the patient's fingernail. Additionally, this approach tends to force the retentive terminus of the clasp toward the abutment, making removal of the prosthesis even more difficult. The best method of removing a denture of this design is to engage the nonretentive portion of the T-clasp and apply occlusal pressure. The denture will disengage easily.

Before being excused from the office, the patient should be asked to demonstrate the proper methods of removable partial denture insertion and removal for the dentist.

## Written instructions

It is impractical to expect that patients will remember all of the instructions provided at the insertion appointment. Providing the patient with written instructions will permit the patient an opportunity to review the instructions at home. Written instructions may be in the form of personally generated handouts or professionally developed pamphlets. The American Dental Association provides very useful patient information materials describing wear and care of removable partial dentures.

## ⌑ Length of the Insertion Appointment

The experienced practitioner should be able to accomplish all necessary procedures for the insertion appointment in 30 to 45 minutes. The dental student may require 3 to 4 hours.

## ⌑ Postinsertion Appointment

Postinsertion difficulties should be expected by both the dentist and the patient. The types of difficulties encountered and methods of managing them are discussed in chapter 16. It is important that the practitioner address expected common complications at the insertion appointment so the patient is not alarmed by their occurrence. The patient must also be informed that sore teeth or painful soft tissue areas are not an integral part of removable partial denture therapy. These complications must be managed in a timely manner at scheduled postinsertion appointments.

Attention to detail during the fitting and insertion appointments will minimize, but not eliminate, all possible complications of removable partial denture therapy. Therefore, the patient should return to the office within 24 hours of partial denture insertion. This period is sufficient to allow detection of initial signs of most postinsertion complications. The procedures used to detect and interpret the onset of postinsertion difficulties are discussed in the next chapter.

## ⌑ References

1. Gronas DG. Preparation of pressure-indicator paste. J Prosthet Dent 1977;37:92–94.
2. Kuebker WA. Denture problems: Causes, diagnostic procedures, and clinical treatment. I. Retention problems. Quintessence Int 1984;15:1031–1044.
3. Phoenix RD, DeFreest CF. An effective technique for denture border evaluation. J Prosthodont 1997;6:215–217.

## ⌑ Bibliography

Backenstose WM, Wells JG. Side effects of immersion-type cleansers on metal components of dentures. J Prosthet Dent 1977;37:615–621.

Bauman R. Minimizing postinsertion problems: A procedure for removable partial denture placement. J Prosthet Dent 1979;42:381–385.

Brudvik JS, Wormley JH. Construction techniques for wrought-wire retentive clasp arms as related to clasp flexibility. J Prosthet Dent 1973;30:769–774.

Connor JN, Schoenfeld CM, Taylor RL. An evaluation of an enzyme denture cleanser. J Prosthet Dent 1977;37:147–157.

Firtell DN, Arnett WS, Holmes JB. Pressure indicators for removable prosthodontics. J Prosthet Dent 1985;54:226–229.

Fisher AA. Allergic sensitization of skin and oral mucosa to acrylic resin denture materials. J Prosthet Dent 1956;6:593–602.

Hanau RL. Full Denture Prosthesis, ed 4. Buffalo, NY: Thorner Sidney, 1930.

Jankelson BH. Adjustment of dentures at time of insertion and alterations to compensate for tissue changes. J Am Dent Assoc 1962;64:521–531.

Kirk GA. Convenient use of pressure indicating paste. J Prosthet Dent 1985;53:288.

Kuebker WA. Denture problems: Causes, diagnostic procedures, and clinical treatment. II. Patient discomfort problems. Quintessence Int 1984;15:1131–1141.

Kuebker WA. Denture problems: Causes, diagnostic procedures, and clinical treatment. III/IV. Gagging problems and speech problems. Quintessence Int 1984;15:1231–1238.

Levin B. Adjustments and improvement of border seal. In: Impressions for Complete Dentures. Chicago: Quintessence, 1984:159–191.

Lutes MR, Henderson D, Ellinger CW, et al. Denture modification during adjustment phase of complete denture service. J Prosthet Dent 1972;28:572–579.

Lytle RB. Complete denture construction based on a study of the deformation of the underlying soft tissues. J Prosthet Dent 1959;9:539.

Lytle RB. Soft tissue displacement beneath removable partial and complete dentures. J Prosthet Dent 1962;12:34.

Maison WG. Instructions to denture patients. J Prosthet Dent 1959;9:825–831.

Means CR, Flenniken IE. Gagging—A problem in prosthetic dentistry. J Prosthet Dent 1970;23:614–620.

Mehringer EJ. The saliva as it is related to the wearing of dentures. J Prosthet Dent 1954;4:312–318.

Morden JFC, Lammie GA, Osborne J. Effect of various cleaning solutions on chrome-cobalt alloys. Dent Pract Dent Rec 1956;6:304–310.

Myers HM, Krol AJ. Effectiveness of a sonification denture cleaning program. J Prosthet Dent 1974;32:613–618.

Neill DJ. A study of materials and methods employed in cleaning dentures. Br Dent J 1968;124:107–115.

Plainfield S. Communication distortion: The language of patients and practitioners of dentistry. J Prosthet Dent 1969;22:11–19.

Rodegerts CR. The relationship of pressure spots in complete denture impression with mucosal irritations. J Prosthet Dent 1964;14:1040.

Rothman R. Phonetic considerations in denture prosthesis. J Prosthet Dent 1961;11:214–233.

Stevenson-Moore P, Daly CH, Smith DE. Indicator pastes: Their behavior and use. J Prosthet Dent 1979;41:258–265.

Tautin FS. Should dentures be worn continuously? J Prosthet Dent 1978;39:372–374.

Wagner AG. Instructions for the use and care of removable partial dentures. J Prosthet Dent 1971;26:477–479.

Wagner AG. Maintenance of the partially edentulous mouth and care of the denture. Dent Clin North Am 1973;17:755–768.

Woelfel JB, Paffenbarger GC. Pressure indicator paste patterns in duplicate denture made by different processing techniques for the same patient. J Am Dent Assoc 1965;70:339.

Woelfel JB, Paffenbarger GC, Sweeney WT. Dimensional changes occurring in dentures during processing. J Am Dent Assoc 1960;61:413–430.

# Postinsertion Observations

The patient should be seen within 24 hours after the insertion of any removable prosthesis. Often, irritation produced by the denture will not yet be felt by the patient, but it can be detected by the dentist. If potential difficulties are detected and corrected in their early stages, the patient may never be subjected to the pain and discomfort that might otherwise occur.

After the patient has been seated and before the mouth examination is begun, the patient should be questioned regarding whether there are specific problems and, if so, the exact nature of these problems. The patient should be reassured that most problems can be solved rapidly and simply. Even if there are no complaints, the mouth should be examined carefully with the prosthesis in and out of the mouth.

Complaints normally fall into three main categories: *(1)* pain or discomfort arising from the hard and soft tissues of the edentulous ridge; *(2)* soreness of one or more teeth; and *(3)* miscellaneous items such as instability of the prosthesis, tongue and cheek biting, and difficulties with speech and/or eating. Each of these groups is addressed in the following sections.

## ▣ Soft Tissue Irritation

### *Laceration or ulceration*

Laceration or ulceration of the soft tissues surrounding the denture base is generally produced by an overextended denture base (Fig 16-1). The patient may not be aware of the problem or may complain of soreness or irritation. In any event, careful examination of the border tissues should be made. Any area displaying increased redness or translucency should arouse suspicion of overextension. The translucent appearance becomes evident just before actual ulceration occurs (Fig 16-2). It may or may not be accompanied by noticeable discomfort.

The degree of overextension of the denture base usually can be determined by visual examination. With the prosthesis in position, the buccal tissues should be manipulated in downward, outward, upward, and anteroposterior directions. If the denture border is overextended, movement of the border tissues will be impeded. If interference with movement and a change in soft tissue color are evident, the denture flange must be reduced.

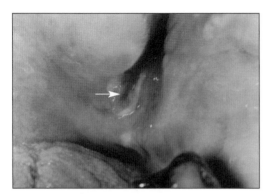

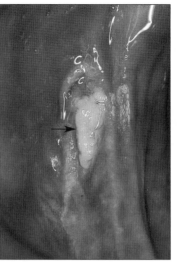

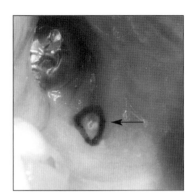

**Fig 16-1** A slight change in the color of the soft tissues often indicates irritation. This lesion *(arrow)* was produced by an overextended denture base.

**Fig 16-2** A translucent or whitish appearance *(arrow)* may be present at the border of an overextended denture base. Such a lesion usually precedes ulceration.

**Fig 16-3** An area of soft tissue irritation is circled *(arrow)* using an indelible pencil.

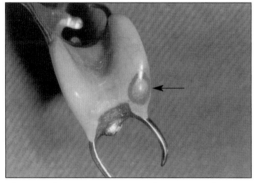

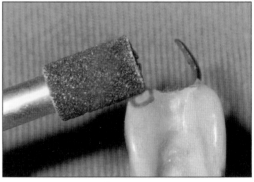

**Fig 16-4** The removable partial denture is completely seated in the mouth, and indelible pencil is transferred to the corresponding area of the denture base *(arrow)*.

**Fig 16-5** The area of the denture base responsible for soft tissue irritation is adjusted using an arbor band or laboratory bur in a low-speed handpiece.

Overextension of the denture base on the lingual aspect of the mandibular edentulous ridge may be identified and confirmed by manipulation of the patient's tongue. A forward or lateral thrust of the tongue usually will disclose the location of the overextension.

Another method for determining denture base overextension is through the use of disclosing wax as described in chapter 15 and illustrated in Figs 15-9 to 15-12. Nevertheless, this technique must be used with caution. It is normally used to verify or to isolate an area that is under suspicion following visual observation.

The use of pressure indicator paste for the purpose of locating areas of border overextension is generally not indicated. Due to its softness, pressure indicator paste is easily displaced and, therefore, is not reliable.

A dependable method for identifying an overextension is through the use of an indelible pencil. The area in question is dried with gauze and marked with the indelible pencil (Fig 16-3). The prosthesis is placed, and the border tissues activated. Immediately thereafter, the removable partial denture is removed and examined. The area requiring relief will be outlined by the transfer of the indelible ink to the acrylic resin border (Fig 16-4).

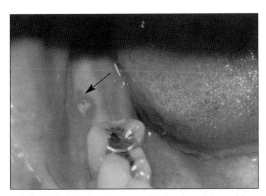

**Fig 16-6** A localized area of irritation *(arrow)* beneath a denture base.

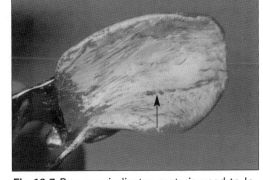

**Fig 16-7** Pressure indicator paste is used to locate the area of the denture base that is causing irritation *(arrow).*

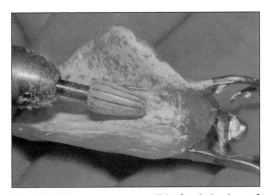

**Fig 16-8** The area responsible for irritation of the soft tissues is adjusted using a laboratory bur in a low-speed handpiece.

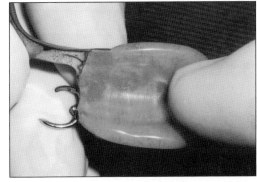

**Fig 16-9** Feeling the intaglio surface of a denture base often discloses irregularities that must be eliminated.

Border overextension is best corrected with a laboratory bur or an arbor band (Fig 16-5). The flange must be rounded as it is being shortened. The tendency is to over-relieve these areas, so it is best to err on the side of conservatism rather than to overcut the denture base. Any soreness at the time of adjustment will generally remain for at least 24 hours. Healing can be hastened if the patient uses a warm saline mouthwash (half a teaspoon of salt in a 6-ounce glass of water) at least every 4 hours. The patient should take a mouthful of the solution and hold it until the temperature of the solution drops. This procedure is repeated until the 6 ounces are finished.

The use of topical anesthetics should not be encouraged because they tend to mask the problem. If the patient is seen within 24 hours, discomfort should not be severe enough to require this type of medication. If more time has elapsed and pain is sufficient to warrant the local application of topical medication, the prosthesis should not be worn until the pain has

been controlled. At that time, adjustment of the prosthesis should be accomplished.

## Erythema

Redness, or erythema, of the soft tissues is generally caused either by roughness of the denture base or by a slight rubbing movement of the denture base against the soft tissues (Fig 16-6). Roughness of the denture base can be corrected simply by using pressure indicator paste to reveal the area of roughness (Fig 16-7) and relieving the acrylic resin with a laboratory bur in a low-speed handpiece (Fig 16-8). After the adjustment is made, another trial with pressure indicator paste should be made to verify that the pressure has been relieved.

An excellent method of identifying irregularities on the intaglio surface is to pass a fingertip or gauze pad over the tissue surface of the resin (Fig 16-9). Irregularities may be readily identified using the sensitivity

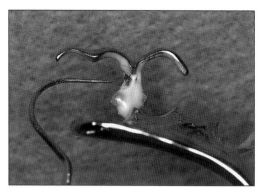

**Fig 16-10** Disclosing wax is displaced from an area that is causing pressure.

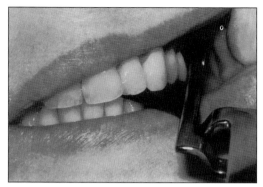

**Fig 16-11** Articulating paper is used to identify areas of occlusal interference.

of the fingertip or by observing "snagging" of the gauze.

The second factor that may produce redness of the soft tissues underlying a denture base is the presence of occlusal discrepancies or prematurities. This lack of occlusal harmony is the greatest factor in prosthesis-related discomfort. Therefore, a great deal of emphasis must be placed upon occlusal factors in those patients who are having difficulty adjusting to removable prostheses. The technique for correcting occlusal disharmonies will be discussed in the following section.

## ⌨ Irritation to Teeth

When soft tissue irritation has been eliminated, the practitioner should evaluate all teeth that are in contact with the prosthesis. With the prosthesis out of the mouth, mesial, distal, buccal, and lingual pressure should be applied to the remaining natural teeth. Pressure can best be applied using the index fingers of each hand. If the prosthesis has exerted undesirable forces on one or more teeth, a painful response will result.

If the postinsertion appointment is accomplished within 24 hours of placement, the patient may not be aware of discomfort until finger pressure is applied. If a longer time has elapsed, the tooth or teeth may be so painful that the patient has difficulty tolerating such pressure. In these instances, the patient must leave the removable partial denture out of the mouth until the discomfort subsides. Then he or she must re-

port to the practitioner's office for reevaluation and adjustment of the prosthesis.

The use of disclosing wax is usually sufficient to pinpoint the area(s) that must be adjusted to prevent traumatic tooth movement. Disclosing wax is applied to the metal or resin that contacts the tooth, and the partial denture is fully seated in the mouth. When the denture is removed, the area that is causing the pressure will appear as a show-through in the disclosing wax (Fig 16-10). Areas of show-through can be relieved rather easily using a multifluted finishing bur in a high-speed handpiece.

If it can be demonstrated that the soreness or pain is not caused by pressure from the partial denture, then the most logical reason for pain is occlusal trauma. Failure to produce an area of show-through in the disclosing wax is reason enough to assume that the pain is being produced by occlusal stress and not by lateral pressure from the metal or resin of the prosthesis.

One of the most common causes of discomfort for a removable partial denture patient is occlusal interference between a natural tooth in one arch and the metal of the prosthesis in the opposite arch. The actual tooth-to-metal contact may appear minor and may be difficult to isolate, yet the resulting discomfort can be extremely aggravating. Articulating paper is commonly used to locate the portion of the partial denture causing the interference (Fig 16-11). The patient is instructed to tap the teeth together with the articulating paper in position. The patient is then in-

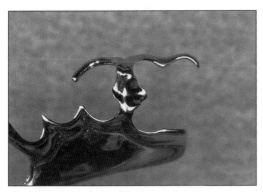

**Fig 16-12** It is often difficult to identify articulating paper marks on highly polished metal.

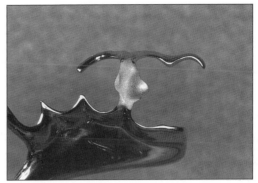

**Fig 16-13** If articulating paper marks are difficult to identify, the surface of the metal may be roughened using a fine stone or airborne particle abrasion system.

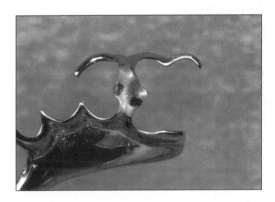

**Fig 16-14** Articulating paper marks are readily identified on a roughened surface.

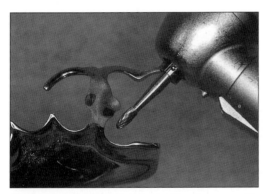

**Fig 16-15** Adjustments are made using a multifluted bur in a high-speed handpiece.

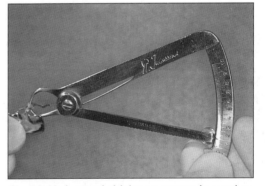

**Fig 16-16** A metal thickness gauge is used to evaluate the thickness of removable partial denture components. Rests and clasps must be at least 1 mm thick.

structed to move the mandible to both sides and protrusively. The prosthesis is then removed from the mouth and carefully examined.

Contacts on the metal of the framework should be identified (Figs 16-12 to 16-14) and subsequently corrected using a multifluted carbide bur in a high-speed handpiece (Fig 16-15). Care must be taken not to thin the metal excessively, particularly in critical areas such as occlusal rests and retentive clasps (Fig 16-16). Embrasure clasps are particularly troublesome in this regard. Reduction of opposing cusps may have to be accomplished to prevent unwarranted thinning of critical areas, but reduction of enamel surfaces at this stage of treatment is not the method of choice and indicates serious shortcomings in treatment planning, survey, and design.

## ⌨ Miscellaneous Complaints

### Gagging

Gagging is not often a complaint of patients wearing a removable partial denture. If gagging is coincident with the insertion of a removable partial denture, it is likely that the difficulty is physical rather than psychological. As a result, the adaptation and design of the prosthesis must be carefully examined.

Gagging frequently is caused by poor adaptation of a maxillary removable partial denture to the tissues of the hard palate. In most instances, this may be traced to faulty impression technique. Failure to modify a stock tray before making a maxillary master impression allows the impression material to slump before the final set occurs. This yields an inaccurate cast and results in a major connector that stands away from the hard palate. Saliva may accumulate in this space and cause the patient to gag. If the posterior portion of the prosthesis is constructed of acrylic resin, this problem may be addressed by relining the removable partial denture. Unfortunately, this is rarely the case. Most major connectors are made of cast metal and cannot be relined with acceptable results. In these instances, the prosthesis will have to be remade.

If the removable partial denture displays acceptable adaptation to the hard palate, the practitioner should determine whether the removable partial denture is overextended posteriorly. This is accomplished by removing the prosthesis from the mouth and using an indelible pencil to mark its posterior border (Fig 16-17). The removable partial denture is then returned to the mouth and completely seated (Fig 16-18), transferring the position of the posterior border to the patient's palatal tissues (Fig 16-19). The removable partial denture is then removed and the patient is instructed to say "ahh." If any vibration of the palatal soft tissues takes place anterior to the line, it is likely that the pos-

terior border of the prosthesis has been extended too far posteriorly. This type of overextension must be corrected by trimming the posterior border of the major connector (Figs 16-20 and 16-21) or remaking the removable partial denture.

Gagging following the insertion of a mandibular removable partial denture may be caused by an alteration of the occlusal vertical dimension. It was originally believed that only a decrease in the proper occlusal vertical dimension would stimulate gagging (caused primarily by crowding of the tongue and adjacent soft tissues). However, an investigation by Krol indicated that an increase in the occlusal vertical dimension with concomitant elimination of the freeway space also is capable of producing a prolonged gagging reaction.[1] The exact mechanism is not well understood, but is probably caused by spasm of the levator and tensor muscles of the velum palatinum. Correction of this difficulty requires reestablishment of the proper occlusal vertical dimension.

Another potential cause of gagging is the overextension, both in length and bulk, of the denture base flanges of a mandibular Class I removable partial denture. The overextension reduces the available tongue space and produces involuntary retching or nausea. To correct this problem, the posterior lingual borders should be thinned and shortened.

### Problems with phonetics

Phonetic problems are not commonly encountered in conjunction with removable partial denture service. Problems that do arise are usually associated with the improper placement of prosthetic maxillary anterior teeth or changes in the contour of the anterior palate.

The positions of artificial maxillary and mandibular premolar teeth also may create problems with phonetics (Figs 16-22 and 16-23). If the premolars are positioned too far lingually, the action of the tongue may be impeded and speech may be affected. If these teeth are positioned too far facially, air may escape between the tongue and teeth and a whistling or slurring of the speech may occur. If the latter error is present, soft utility wax adapted to the lingual surfaces of the premolar teeth should decrease the escape of air and the whistling or slurring effect.

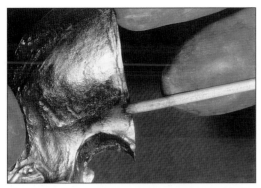

**Fig 16-17** An indelible pencil is used to mark the posterior border of a metal major connector.

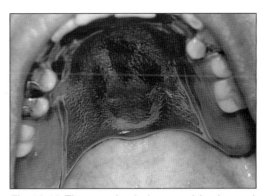

**Fig 16-18** The prosthesis is seated in the oral cavity.

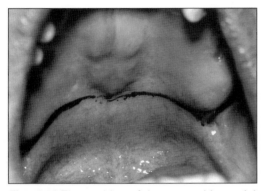

**Fig 16-19** The position of the removable partial denture's posterior border is transferred to the palatal tissues, and placement of the posterior border is evaluated.

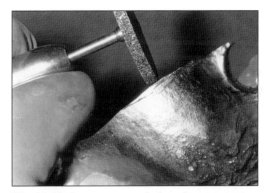

**Fig 16-20** An overextended major connector may be shortened using a heatless stone in a low-speed handpiece or dental laboratory engine.

**Fig 16-21** The bead line that prevents food from collecting between the major connector and the palatal tissues has been lost as a result of adjustment. This may necessitate remaking the removable partial denture.

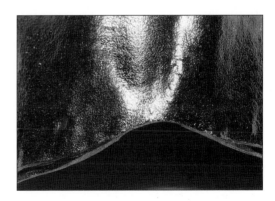

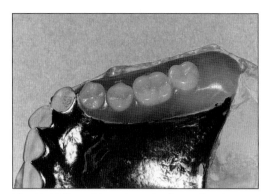

**Fig 16-22** If positioned too far lingually, the artificial premolars may interfere with speech.

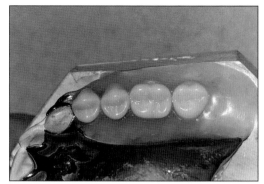

**Fig 16-23** Correcting prosthetic tooth placement will correct phonetic difficulties.

For other speech problems, the patient should be given a reasonable time (1 to 2 weeks) to adapt to the sensation and presence of the artificial teeth and to overcome the problem of articulation. Reading aloud is one of the best methods of adapting to a new removable partial denture. If the patient fails to adapt to the denture, repositioning of the anterior teeth will have to be accomplished and consideration given to altering the contour of the palatal major connector.

### Cheek or tongue biting

Cheek biting is usually caused by insufficient horizontal overlap of the maxillary and mandibular posterior teeth (Fig 16-24). Another contributing factor is the long-term absence of posterior teeth. In this situation, the buccinator muscle may sag into the space created by the missing teeth. This medial posture of the buccinator may lead to cheek biting. In most cases, the muscle will regain its normal tone following prosthesis insertion, and cheek biting will cease.

If the artificial teeth have been correctly positioned in a buccolingual direction, the practitioner may round the buccal cusps of the mandibular posterior teeth to control cheek biting (Fig 16-25). This rounding should move the buccal cusps slightly lingual, thereby creating a greater horizontal overlap.

Tongue biting frequently means that the artificial teeth have been positioned too far lingually and the tongue space has been decreased. The first attempt at

correcting this condition should be recontouring the lingual surfaces of the mandibular posterior teeth by gently rounding or "rolling" the lingual cusps of the teeth. It should be remembered that reducing the cusps of the teeth will also reduce the overall efficiency of the teeth. If tongue biting continues after the teeth have been reshaped, the artificial teeth will have to be removed and reset.

If the mandibular posterior teeth have been missing for a long time, the tongue will lose its tone and will broaden to fill the space once occupied by the teeth (Fig 16-26). When the partial denture is placed, the tongue will regain its normal contour. The process should be explained to the patient to improve understanding.

### Difficulty in chewing

Most patients who have trouble chewing with removable partial dentures have been missing teeth for several years. These patients have lost the neuromuscular skills required to incise and grind food. Such patients should be informed that it will take some time to relearn this process. The length of time will depend to some extent on the patient's innate neuromuscular coordination and determination, as well as the length of time that the patient was without teeth. To prevent the patient from becoming discouraged, reassurance should be given that the chewing pattern will eventually be reestablished. The patient should also be advised to

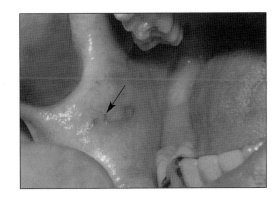

**Fig 16-24** Cheek biting results in linear ulceration of the buccal mucosa *(arrow)*.

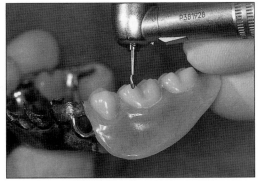

**Fig 16-25** Cheek biting may be minimized by rounding the mandibular buccal cusps.

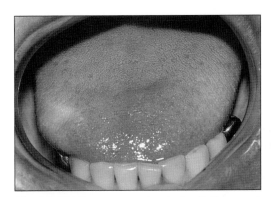

**Fig 16-26** The tongue tends to flatten and broaden when it is not confined by posterior teeth or appropriate prostheses.

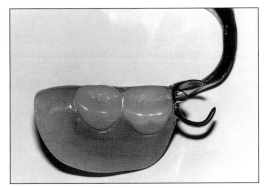

**Fig 16-27** The surfaces of acrylic resin teeth may become flattened and inefficient because of poor polishing technique or prolonged wear.

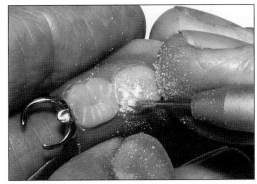

**Fig 16-28** Additional grooves and sluiceways improve masticatory efficiency.

avoid extremely tough, stringy, or sticky food during the early period of adjustment. Attempting to eat such foods will only add to the patient's discouragement.

It is also wise to examine the occlusal surfaces of the artificial teeth. If the occlusal anatomy of acrylic resin is not adequate, the tooth will be inefficient (Fig 16-27). Additional sluiceways and grooves should be added to the occlusal surface to increase the cutting efficiency (Fig 16-28).

## *Instability of a removable partial denture*

The most common causes of instability in a removable partial denture are fatigue and mishandling of retentive clasps. In many cases, this necessitates adjustment of one or more retentive clasps. The techniques described in chapter 15 are often needed to increase retention. If clasp adjustment does not produce the desired results, the prosthesis may have to be remade.

## ◻ Subsequent Adjustments

Occasionally, a single postinsertion adjustment will suffice, but more frequently two or three additional adjustments may be required. Some patients lack confidence in removable partial dentures or their ability to wear removable partial dentures. These patients should be seen for one or two additional appointments and should be reassured that they will overcome their problems and adjust to the prosthesis or prostheses.

A grave mistake is made by the practitioner who classifies these patients as chronic complainers and avoids continuing to work with them on postinsertion adjustments. Many dental prostheses have failed because of a practitioner's reluctance to provide adequate postinsertion care.

## ◻ Remount Procedures

A small percentage of patients present with multiple postinsertion complaints, all requiring adjustments. For these patients, clinical remount procedures may be indicated. Clinical remount procedures generally are completed using semiadjustable articulators and often reveal small discrepancies that were not evident in the mouth. The recommended technique is described in chapter 15.

## ◻ Patient Instruction

Instructions given to the patient at the insertion appointment should be reinforced at the time of each adjustment. The patient's mouth should be examined to observe the quality of home care. The use of disclosing tablets may be helpful in demonstrating problem areas where special care must be taken. The patient should also be questioned about any problems encountered when inserting or withdrawing the partial denture, and the technique to insert and remove the prosthesis should be reviewed.

Before being dismissed, the patient should be reminded of the importance of frequent maintenance checks by the dentist. Maintenance visits should be scheduled every 3 to 6 months. Seldom, if ever, should more than 12 months elapse between appointments. The frequency of these checks will depend, in part, on the condition of the patient's remaining dentition. If the remaining teeth are periodontally involved or the oral hygiene is questionable, maintenance visits should be more frequent.

The insertion of a removable partial denture, or any prosthesis, does not relieve the dentist of the responsibility of providing adequate maintenance for the patient.

## ◻ Length of Appointment

This appointment should be accomplished by an experienced practitioner in 30 to 45 minutes. A dental student will normally require 60 to 90 minutes.

## ◻ Reference

1. Krol AJ. A new approach to the gagging problem. J Prosthet Dent 1963;13:611–616.

## ◻ Bibliography

Bauman R. Inflammatory papillary hyperplasia and home-care instructions to denture patients. J Prosthet Dent 1977;37:608–609.

Brill N, Schübeler S, Tryde G. Aspects of occlusal sense in natural and artificial teeth. J Prosthet Dent 1962;12:123–128.

Cavalaris CJ. Pathologic considerations associated with partial dentures. Dent Clin North Am 1973;17:585–600.

Derry A, Bertram U. A clinical survey of removable partial dentures after 2 years usage. Acta Odontol Scand 1970;28:581–598.

Federation of Prosthodontic Organizations. Guidelines for evaluation of completed prosthodontic treatment for removable partial dentures. J Prosthet Dent 1972;27:326–328.

Immekus JE, Aramany M. Adverse effects of resilient denture liners in overlay dentures. J Prosthet Dent 1974;32:178-181.

MacCallum M, Stafford GD, MacCulloch WT, Combe EC. Which cleanser? A report on a survey of denture cleansing routine and the development of a new denture cleanser. Dent Pract Dent Rec 1968;19(3):83-89.

Maison WG. Instructions to denture patients. J Prosthet Dent 1959;9:825-831.

Miller EL. Clinical management of denture-induced inflammations. J Prosthet Dent 1977;38:362-365.

Newton AV. Denture sore mouth. Br Dent J 1962;112:357-360.

Ramsey WO. The relation of emotional factors to prosthodontic service. J Prosthet Dent 1970;23:4-10.

Rothman R. Phonetic considerations in denture prosthesis. J Prosthet Dent 1961;11:214-223.

Savage RD, MacGregor AR. Behavior therapy in prosthodontics. J Prosthet Dent 1970;24:126-132.

Schabel RW. Dentist-patient communication—A major factor in treatment prognosis. J Prosthet Dent 1969;21:3-5.

Schabel RW. The psychology of aging. J Prosthet Dent 1972;27:569-573.

Schole ML. Management of the gagging patient. J Prosthet Dent 1959;9:578-583.

Sharp GS. The etiology and treatment of the sore mouth. J Prosthet Dent 1966;16:855-860.

Sharp GS. Treatment of low tolerance to dentures. J Prosthet Dent 1960;10:47-52.

Wagner AG. Maintenance of the partially edentulous mouth and care of the denture. Dent Clin North Am 1973;17:755-768.

Webb CS. Gagging: A method for positive control. Dent Surv 1967;42:54-56.

Young HA. Factors contributing to success in prosthodontic practice. J Prosthet Dent 1955;5:354-360.

# Maintenance and Repair of Removable Partial Dentures

**James S. Brudvik,** DDS, FACP

Removable partial dentures require a level of maintenance that far exceeds that of fixed restorations. Because removable partial denture wearers are encouraged to keep their dentures out of the mouth for a significant portion of the day, there is increased potential for distortion and damage. In addition, tooth-tissue–supported removable partial dentures have a special need for maintenance, particularly relining and rebasing. When these prostheses lose soft tissue support and begin to move more freely, there is tremendous potential for damage to the abutments and soft tissues.

Relining is the most basic of the partial denture maintenance techniques. It involves adding new denture base material to the existing resin to make up for loss of tissue contact caused by resorption of the alveolar ridge. The addition may be performed in a dental laboratory, or it may be accomplished in the patient's mouth using specially formulated resins. Both techniques have advantages, but the physical characteristics of laboratory resins make the laboratory reline the method of choice in most instances.

Rebasing is a laboratory technique in which the bulk of the denture base is removed and replaced using new resin. This approach results in a base of uniform quality, but is technically complicated by the fact that the retentive meshwork is buried within the denture base—often without sufficient relief beneath the mesh to allow for adequate bulk of new resin.

When both the denture base and the denture teeth are involved in a maintenance or repair situation, the partial denture may need to be stripped of both teeth and denture base and reconstructed.

## ☐ Relining

To determine if a removable partial denture is in need of relining, some visual reference to the loss of supporting tissue must be established. Perhaps the easiest means of evaluating the space under the denture base is to place a thin mix of alginate (irreversible hydrocolloid) in the denture base area, seat the partial denture in the mouth, and maintain its position until the alginate sets. The denture can then be removed from the mouth, the thickness of the alginate measured, and an informed clinical judgment made (Fig 17-1). The alginate must be mixed with an increased water-powder

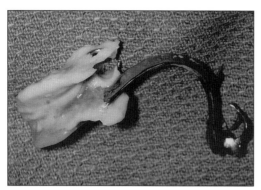

Fig 17-1 A thin mix of alginate impression material may be used to evaluate the fit of a denture base to the underlying soft tissues. In this instance, there is a bulk of alginate impression material at the buccal shelf area and at the crest of the ridge. A reline is indicated.

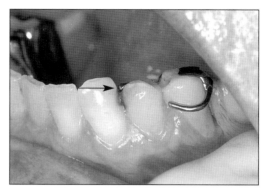

Fig 17-2 In a passive state, the indirect retainer on the mesial surface of the mandibular left first premolar is completely seated *(arrow)*.

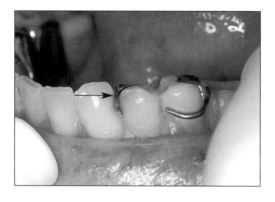

Fig 17-3 When pressure is applied to the distal extension base, the indirect retainer on the mandibular left first premolar is unseated *(arrow)*. This may indicate the need for a reline.

ratio to ensure minimal tissue displacement. One scoop of alginate powder mixed with two measures of hot water will provide a mix that is thin enough to not displace soft tissues and yet set quickly. The alginate separates easily and cleanly from the denture after the evaluation is made.

It is also possible to evaluate the loss of support on distal extension partial dentures by applying a seating force on the most posterior aspect of the denture base and observing an anterior indirect retainer. If significant changes have occurred, the indirect retainer will lift from its rest seat (Figs 17-2 and 17-3). The amount of space under the indirect retainer is an indicator of the amount of space to be found under the denture base. Some clinical judgment is essential here because the length of the distal extension base affects the amount of movement, as does the distance from the indirect retainer to the fulcrum line.

If at least 2 mm of alginate is present under the denture base or if the indirect retainer lifts 2 mm or more, the patient can be considered a candidate for a reline or rebase.

### Impression technique

For a removable partial denture reline to be successful, the denture base must extend to cover the available denture-bearing area. The impression material cannot be expected to extend beyond the support of the denture base. Consequently, if the existing denture is short of ideal coverage, a rebase should be used instead of a reline.

A resin denture base is prepared for a reline impression by removing a uniform amount of denture resin from the intaglio of the denture base. This process is often limited by the amount of resin under the resin-

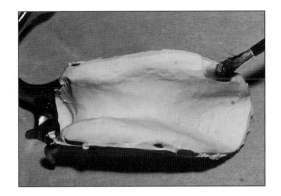

**Fig 17-4** A small brush is used to add mouth-temperature wax to correct an impression. The impression is then returned to the mouth for a period of 12 minutes.

retaining components (eg, struts, meshwork). The resin should be removed for two important reasons. First, space must be created so the impression material will not apply undue pressure to the underlying soft tissues. Second, the surface of the existing resin must be removed to eliminate potential contaminants and ensure a suitable bonding surface.

The more displaceable the tissues in the denture base area, the greater the space required for impression material. The choice of impression material depends on the characteristics of the tissues to be impressed. Mobile tissue on the crest of the ridge is a good indication to use a free-flowing, zinc oxide–eugenol impression material. Polysulfide rubber bases, polyethers, polyvinylsiloxanes, and mouth-temperature waxes may be used with confidence on dense, firm tissues. Tissue-conditioning materials also may be used as impression materials, although they offer no particular advantage and can easily distort the associated soft tissues.

The most critical step in the reline procedure is the maintenance of the tooth-framework relationship during the set of the impression material. Under no circumstances should the patient be allowed to bring the teeth into contact during the impression-making procedure. Rather, the dentist must hold the framework against the abutments until the impression material is to be removed from the mouth. In this way, soft tissue support will be in harmony with the tooth-framework relationship. This is the only way to ensure routine success of reline procedures.

When zinc oxide–eugenol impression materials are used, the clinician must remove any excess material that extrudes into tooth undercut areas or around active clasp arms. This is easily accomplished using an explorer or similar dental instrument in the hand that is not being used to maintain the tooth-framework relationship.

Small defects in the impression can usually be corrected with mouth-temperature wax. Thin extensions of impression material beyond the denture border should be removed as soon as the impression is removed from the mouth. Rough edges created by the removal of extraneous material can be covered with a thin coat of mouth-temperature wax and the reline impression reinserted in the mouth (Fig 17-4). At this time, the practitioner should attempt to rock the framework around its fulcrum to ensure that the desired support has been restored.

## Laboratory technique

The completed partial denture reline impression is presented to the laboratory for processing. At this stage, the removable partial denture must be introduced into a conventional denture flask. The framework and the stone teeth of the master cast are covered using a plaster-stone mixture. In reline investing, only the impression area (the stone replica of the edentulous ridge) remains with the first half of the flask (Fig 17-5). The entire partial denture is included in the second half of the flask. This makes complete flask closure before processing absolutely critical. An error here will result in the entire removable partial denture being held up by the denture base. In conventional construction, the failure to complete flask closure will result only in a prematurity on the denture teeth.

Depending on the instructions of the resin manufacturer, the partial denture can be flasked in dental

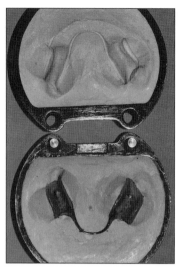

**Fig 17-5** The prosthesis to be relined is located in one part of the flask, while the replica of the edentulous ridge is found in the remaining part of the flask.

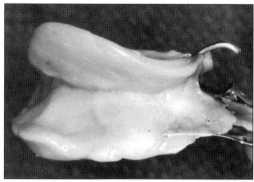

**Fig 17-6** When performing a chairside reline, the manufacturer's recommendations must be followed. Resin extending beyond the internal finish line must be removed while the resin is in a doughlike state.

stone. The flask can be warmed to facilitate the separation of zinc oxide–eugenol impression material or a mouth-temperature wax. Polysulfide rubber base, polyether, and polyvinylsiloxane impression materials can be separated immediately after the flasking stone is set without the need for heat.

In turn, the denture base area is completely cleared of impression material with laboratory burs and a laboratory engine. Separating material is applied to the cast in standard fashion. Resin is mixed according to the manufacturer's directions and placed in the flask. Again, complete closure of the flask is essential.

The relined impression also can be mounted on a duplicating device. This device is commonly used for complete denture reline procedures. Again, the entire partial denture must be in the top half of the mounting. The impression material is removed as in the flasked reline. Chemically activated resin is used with this device.

In either technique, once the resin is completely polymerized, the deflasking begins. This step is fraught with the potential for damaging the partial denture. Clasp arms, in particular, may be easily distorted as a result of careless deflasking. The final deflasking should be done with a shell blaster to avoid harming metal components.

The relined partial denture is shaped and polished using conventional techniques.

## Intraoral reline

There are commercially available, chemically activated resins that are intended to be used in the mouth. Intraoral relines are inferior to laboratory relines, but there are indications for their use in temporary applications. Preparation of the denture base is the same as for a laboratory reline. The mouth-curing resin must be mixed according to the manufacturer's directions, but special care must be taken to sift the polymer into the monomer without trapping air in the mixture. Spatulation of the resin is not critical when the material is to be packed under pressure, but when the resin is used as both a relatively free-flowing impression and the final base, any air trapped in the mix will inevitably result in a porous surface.

The denture base is prepared by covering the external surface with adhesive tape. The tape prevents resin from adhering to the cameo surface of the denture base and the denture teeth. The intaglio is wetted with monomer and resin is applied with a small spatula. Again, care must be taken not to trap air in the resin.

The partial denture is now placed in the mouth and held in proper relation by the clinician. At the time specified by the manufacturer, the denture is removed and any excess trimmed to the original border with sharp, curved scissors (Fig 17-6). The patient

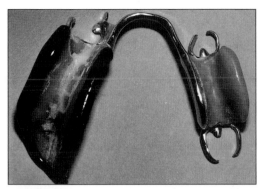

**Fig 17-7** The distal extension base has been relieved almost to the resin-retaining elements. The borders have been reestablished using modeling plastic.

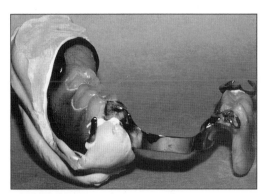

**Fig 17-8** A sectional cast is poured against a rebase impression.

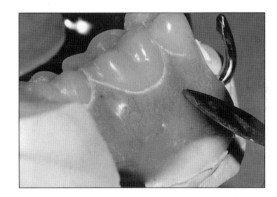

**Fig 17-9** Desired contours are reestablished using baseplate wax.

rinses the mouth with cold water to eliminate the taste of free monomer. The denture is then reseated while the resin is still moldable and held in place until the directions indicate that the denture should be removed and placed in a pressure pot for final polymerization.

The resin used in this type of reline will completely polymerize 12 to 15 minutes after the start of the mix. When the resin is set, it can be finished in the conventional manner. It can be expected that intraoral reline material will be porous and that it will lack color stability. Nevertheless, the procedure is quick and will provide an improved relationship between the denture base and the soft tissues.

## ⌨ Rebasing

Rebasing procedures are used to replace most, if not all, of a denture base. Rebasing is indicated when the denture bases do not extend to cover all of the denture-bearing tissues. It is also used when a denture base has fractured or has become irreparably discolored.

The denture resin is relieved and shortened to allow room for readaptation of the borders with modeling plastic. The modeling plastic is added in small increments and extended to cover the entire denture-bearing area (Fig 17-7). When the border molding is complete, the base is covered with a suitable impression material and the final impression made. During this procedure, the practitioner must ensure that the framework is properly related to the teeth.

It is best to pour a cast against the impression after it has been corrected for defects. The cast should involve only the edentulous ridge area and not the remainder of the framework (Fig 17-8). New peripheries can be blended into the polished surfaces of the denture base by adding small amounts of baseplate wax (Fig 17-9). This procedure provides an improved contour to the processed rebase and reduces finishing time.

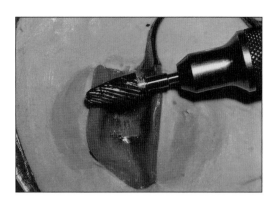

**Fig 17-10** Preparation for rebase requires that most of the existing denture base be eliminated. This is accomplished using a large laboratory bur in a low-speed handpiece or dental laboratory engine.

The rebase impression is flasked as described for the reline procedure. The entire partial denture remains in the second half of the flask. Because wax and modeling plastic are involved in this impression, the flask should be subjected to a brief boil-out procedure to soften these materials and facilitate separation of the flask. When the flask is opened and all traces of impression materials and wax removed, the remaining denture resin can be ground away to allow the majority of the finished rebase to be constructed using new resin (Fig 17-10). This resin removal must stop short of the denture teeth. Where anterior teeth are involved, the junction of the new resin and the existing denture base should be kept in an area that will not be visible when the patient smiles because there will often be a faint line at this junction.

Packing procedures are absolutely critical to success. Incomplete flask closure will provide a product that is unusable. Careful trial packing and attention to detail will eliminate potential problems.

The recovery of the processed rebase or reline from the flask presents another possible problem area. Because the entire framework is enveloped in the second half of the flasking, the potential for damaging or distorting the frame, and especially the clasp arms, is great. Investing the second portion in two stages can simplify this procedure. The first stage will consist of stone just covering the framework and extending up to the occlusal or incisal surfaces of the denture teeth. When this is set, it is painted with separating medium, and the flasking is completed with a stone core. Recovery now consists of removing the stone core and carefully removing the thin stone covering with a laboratory knife. This removal should be for bulk reduction

only, and final stone removal should be performed using a shell blaster.

Attention to detail will greatly reduce deflasking and finishing time. The interface of new and old resin often presents a line of demarcation. This is more an esthetic irritant than a structural flaw. Despite the utmost attention to detail, it may still occur. Shaping the borders of the old resin to a 90-degree angle to the external surface greatly reduces the chances of having an observable line. When the new resin does not meet the old resin at right angles, a thin flash of resin will be present. This usually results in a prominent line that may be esthetically objectionable. Where appearance is not an issue, the junction should be rounded to reduce stress concentration and increase strength.

## ▱ Reconstruction

If the denture base is destroyed or severely compromised, but the framework still demonstrates a clinically acceptable fit, the partial denture can be reconstructed by completely removing all resin and denture teeth. This is done by heating the resin from the tissue side while holding the framework in cotton forceps or a hemostat (Fig 17-11). The resin will soften or even ignite and can then be pried from the retentive meshwork. Subsequently, airborne particle abrasion may be used to remove any residue from the framework, which can then be repolished in a conventional manner.

Following resin removal, the framework is seated in the mouth and an alginate impression made over it (Fig 17-12). The framework must be removed from the mouth by the impression. If it separates from the algi-

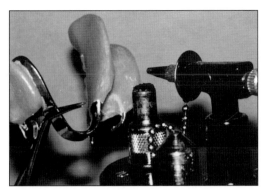

**Fig 17-11** Denture bases are burned away from the underlying framework before the reconstruction process is initiated.

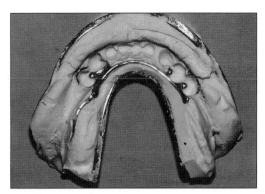

**Fig 17-12** An alginate impression is used to "pick up" the removable partial denture framework.

**Fig 17-13** The framework is gently removed from the cast. Care is used to avoid bending removable partial denture components.

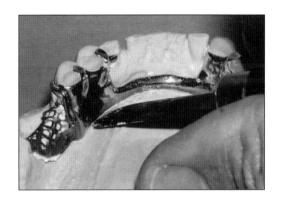

nate impression and remains in the mouth, the retentive clasp arms must be carefully adjusted to reduce retention, and the impression remade. When this has been accomplished, the impression is poured in dental stone and allowed to completely set before any attempt to recover the cast is made.

After the impression is separated from the cast and the cast trimmed in the standard fashion, the framework is carefully separated from the stone cast by prying it along the inferior border of the major connector (Fig 17-13). Force must not be applied to the retentive clasp arms since distortion is possible in these areas. In some instances, portions of the stone teeth will fracture during removal. If this occurs, the teeth can be attached to the cast with cyanoacrylate adhesive without influencing the result. With the framework successfully removed from the cast, an analysis of the edentulous areas can be made. If a corrected cast impression is indicated, a tray can be attached and the impression made in the usual manner. If no further

impression is indicated, the partial denture can be completed as if it were a routine construction.

## ⌑ Repairs

### *Denture base and artificial tooth repairs*

#### Impressions for denture base repairs

There will be occasions when a section of denture base is fractured from the remainder of the removable partial denture (Fig 17-14). If the section is available and can be accurately positioned on the fracture site, repair is a simple matter. Normally, the clinician holds the sections together in the desired relationship while an assistant places small amounts of sticky wax along the fracture line (Fig 17-15). Dental stone is poured against the tissue side of the denture base to preserve the relationship (Fig 17-16). When the stone has set, the denture is removed and cleansed of wax. At this

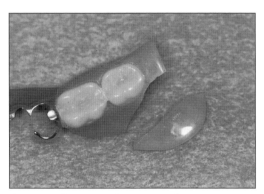

**Fig 17-14** Fractured distal extension base.

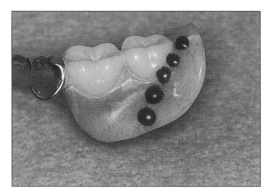

**Fig 17-15** The pieces of the denture base are positively related and luted together using sticky wax.

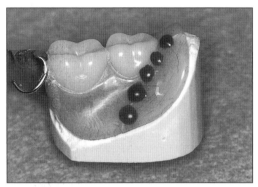

**Fig 17-16** A matrix is poured using dental stone. The matrix preserves the relationship of the denture base fragments.

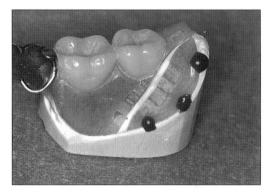

**Fig 17-17** The fracture line is opened using a laboratory bur in a dental laboratory engine, and dovetails are prepared to provide mechanical retention.

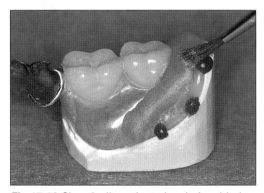

**Fig 17-18** Chemically activated resin is added to the prepared fracture line. The resin is slightly overbuilt to compensate for polymerization shrinkage.

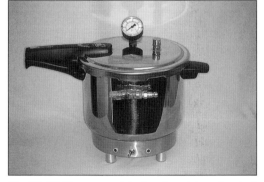

**Fig 17-19** The assembly is placed in a heated pressure pot to complete the polymerization cycle.

stage, the fracture line is opened and dovetailed. The cast is then painted with an alginate separating medium, and the parts are luted in position using sticky wax or modeling plastic (Fig 17-17). Chemically activated resin is added to the prepared fracture line (Fig 17-18), and the assembly is placed in a heated pressure pot to complete the polymerization cycle (Fig 17-19). The prosthesis is then retrieved, and the excess resin is removed (Fig 17-20). In turn, the denture base is finished and polished (Fig 17-21).

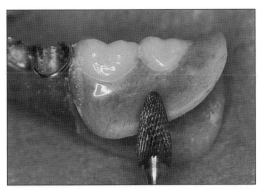

**Fig 17-20** Excess repair resin is removed using appropriate rotary instrumentation.

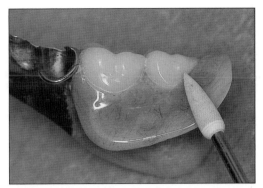

**Fig 17-21** The denture base is finished and polished.

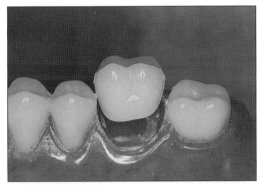

**Fig 17-22** Displacement of one or more prosthetic teeth sometimes occurs.

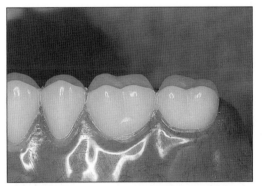

**Fig 17-23** If possible, the displaced tooth is repositioned in the denture base.

If a small segment is missing, it may be sufficient to simply adapt modeling plastic to the denture base and reconstruct that area in the mouth. The modeling plastic is added to the denture base with dry heat so it will stick to the base. It is molded by hand to approximate the soft tissue contours, flamed, tempered in the water bath, and seated in the mouth. The plastic will need to be refined by scraping and reheating one or two times to achieve an impression that does not displace the soft tissues. If the defect is large, it is advisable to first approximate the contour with modeling plastic and then make a "wash" impression. The remainder of the repair is done as a rebase, as previously described.

## Replacement of denture teeth

The replacement of a broken or missing denture tooth is a relatively simple laboratory procedure requiring only an accurate opposing cast and a jaw relation record. If the repair involves the replacement of a tooth with no fracture or loss of associated denture base, a tooth of the same mold and shade is selected and fitted into the existing space (Figs 17-22 and 17-23). An occlusal matrix is then fabricated to permit stabilization of the displaced tooth during repair procedures (Fig 17-24). The matrix is removed and inspected to ensure completeness. One or more diatorics are placed in the ridge lap area of the prosthetic tooth, and the tooth is affixed to the matrix using sticky wax (Fig 17-25). The lingual surface of the denture base is carefully prepared to provide access for the placement of repair material. The ridge lap area of the denture base is relieved to permit placement of at least 2 mm of repair resin beneath the prosthetic tooth. Subsequently, the occlusal matrix and denture tooth are repositioned on the prosthesis (Fig 17-26).

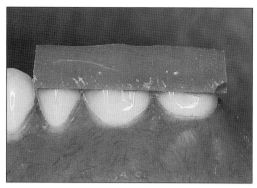

**Fig 17-24** A matrix is fabricated, in this case, using a rigid polyvinylsiloxane registration medium. Accelerated dental stone also may be used.

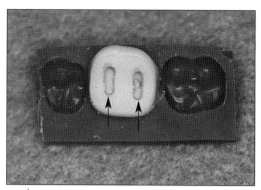

**Fig 17-25** Diatorics *(arrows)* are prepared in the ridge lap portion of the tooth to provide mechanical retention, and the denture tooth is affixed to the matrix using sticky wax.

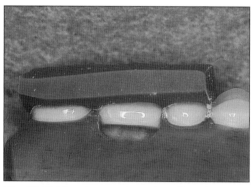

**Fig 17-26** The denture base is relieved to permit the placement of at least 2 mm of repair resin beneath the prosthetic tooth. In turn, the occlusal matrix and denture tooth are repositioned on the prosthesis.

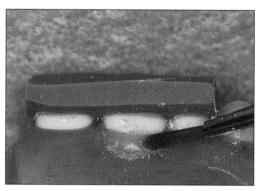

**Fig 17-27** Chemically activated repair resin is placed into the prepared space using a small brush. The resin is slightly overbuilt to account for polymerization shrinkage.

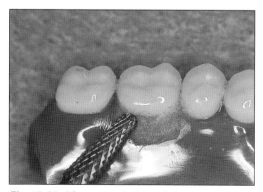

**Fig 17-28** After completion of the polymerization cycle in a heated pressure pot, excess resin is removed from the denture base using a laboratory bur.

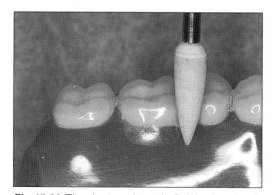

**Fig 17-29** The denture base is finished and polished.

At this stage, chemically activated repair resin is introduced into the prepared space (Fig 17-27). The resin is slightly overbuilt to account for polymerization shrinkage. The removable partial denture is then placed in a heated pressure pot to complete the polymerization cycle (see Fig 17-19).

Following completion of the polymerization process, the removable partial denture is retrieved and excess resin is removed from the surface of the denture base (Fig 17-28). The denture base is then finished and polished using conventional materials and techniques (Fig 17-29).

## ▣ Bibliography

Barrett DA, Pilling LO. The restoration of carious clasp-bearing teeth. J Prosthet Dent 1965;15:309–311.

Bates JF. Studies related to the fracture of partial dentures. Br Dent J 1966;120:79–83.

Beckett LS. Partial denture. The rebasing of tissue borne saddles: Theory and practice. Aust Dent J 1971;16:340–346.

Blatterfein L. Rebasing procedures for removable partial dentures. J Prosthet Dent 1958;8:441–467.

Breithart AR. Converting a tooth-supported denture to a distal extension removable partial denture. J Prosthet Dent 1967;18:233.

Brudvik JS, Fisher WT, Chandler HT. Repairs of metal parts of removable partial dentures. J Prosthet Dent 1972;28:205–208.

Ewing JE. The construction of accurate full crown restorations for an existing clasp by using a direct metal pattern technique. J Prosthet Dent 1965;15:889–899.

Goldberg AT, Jones RD. Constructing cast crowns to fit existing removable partial denture clasps. J Prosthet Dent 1976;36:382–386.

Kelly E. Unbending the bent lingual bar. J Prosthet Dent 1971;25:668–669.

Lewis AJ. Failure of removable partial denture casting during service. J Prosthet Dent 1978;39:147–149.

McCartney JW. Occlusal reconstruction and rebase procedure for distal extension removable partial dentures. J Prosthet Dent 1980;43:695–698.

Reynolds JM. Crown construction for abutments of existing removable partial dentures. J Am Dent Assoc 1964;69:423–426.

Scott J, Bates JF. The relining of partial dentures involving precision attachments. J Prosthet Dent 1972;23:325–333.

Stamps JT, Tanquist RA. Restoration of removable partial denture rest seats using dental amalgam. J Prosthet Dent 1979;41:224–227.

Steffel VL. Relining removable partial dentures for fit and function. J Prosthet Dent 1954;4:496–509.

Teppo KW, Smith FW. A method of immediate clasp repair. J Prosthet Dent 1975;30:77–80.

Wamick ME. Cast crown restoration of a badly involved abutment to fit an existing removable partial denture. Dent Clin North Am 1970;14:631–644.

Wilson JH. Partial dentures—Rebasing the saddle supported by the mucosa and alveolar bone. Aust Dent J 1952;24:185–188.

Wilson JH. Partial dentures—Relining the saddle supported by the mucosa and alveolar bone. J Prosthet Dent 1953;3:807–813.

# Interim, Transitional, and Treatment Prostheses

There are three basic types of temporary removable partial dentures. They are termed *interim, transitional,* and *treatment partial dentures* based upon their individual uses. An overview of these prostheses is provided in the following sections.

## ☐ Interim Partial Dentures

### Indications

Interim partial dentures are indicated when age, health, or lack of time precludes more definitive treatment. Interim removable partial dentures are often used in young patients who have lost one or more teeth as a result of trauma (Fig 18-1). In these instances, the large pulp chambers of adjacent teeth make tooth preparation hazardous at best (Fig 18-2). Risking mechanical exposure of the pulpal tissues is not warranted. Therefore, fixed partial dentures are often contraindicated. However, edentulous spaces should not be allowed to remain untreated, or a lifetime of difficulties may result. In some instances, the edentulous spaces may be maintained using ortho-

dontic bands and wires. Unfortunately, the teeth are often short, and maintaining the positions of these bands and wires may be difficult. Construction of an interim removable partial denture can solve space maintenance problems while restoring adequate occlusal function (Fig 18-3). With the proper instructions on home care and regular follow-up examinations, a young patient can be successfully treated using one or more interim partial dentures. Then, when the teeth and orofacial structures have matured, a more definitive therapy may be instituted.

Interim removable partial dentures also may be indicated for elderly patients whose health contraindicates the lengthy and physically trying appointments often associated with fixed partial denture construction. For these patients, the simple clinical procedures required to construct and insert interim partial dentures usually can be well tolerated.

Patients will often seek treatment following the unexpected loss of one or more teeth with a business trip or other important engagement in the near future. In many instances, the available time will not permit definitive care. In these cases, the construction of interim removable partial dentures may be indicated. It is far

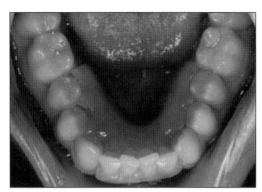

**Fig 18-1** A mandibular interim partial denture in a 12-year-old patient. Clasps are not needed for retention.

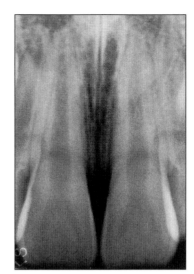

**Fig 18-2** The large pulp chambers in young patients often contraindicate preparation for fixed partial dentures.

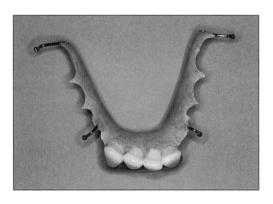

**Fig 18-3** An interim removable partial denture may be used until definitive treatment can be completed.

better to provide an interim replacement than to rush care and risk a mediocre result.

## Clinical procedures

After the teeth have been cleaned, maxillary and mandibular alginate impressions are made. Impressions should capture the peripheral rolls and should accurately record the remaining teeth and soft tissues. Casts should then be generated using a Type III or IV dental stone and two-stage pouring technique (see chapter 5).

If the casts can be unmistakably hand articulated, a jaw relation record will not be necessary. It is rare for an interim removable partial denture to be constructed at any position other than maximum intercuspation. If a jaw relation record is needed, the asso-

ciated record base must be made on the master cast (Fig 18-4). A light-activated or chemically-activated record base is suitable for this purpose.

The shade of the remaining teeth must be determined using an appropriate shade guide (Fig 18-5). The shapes and sizes of the artificial teeth can be determined based upon information derived from the master cast.

## Laboratory procedures

Most temporary removable partial dentures have acrylic resin denture bases and acrylic resin artificial teeth. When it is known that a patient must wear an interim denture for a prolonged time, such as in the case of a preadolescent patient, the practitioner must consider using a cast metal denture base (Fig 18-6).

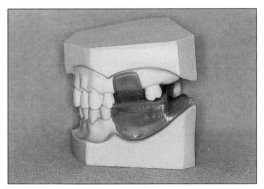

**Fig 18-4** Master casts must be mounted using accurate jaw relation records.

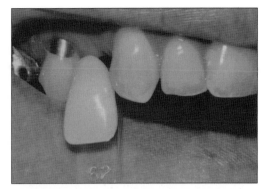

**Fig 18-5** The shade of adjacent teeth is determined using an appropriate shade guide.

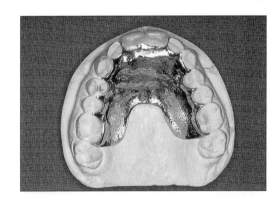

**Fig 18-6** If the interim prosthesis is to be worn for an extended period, a cast metal base should be considered.

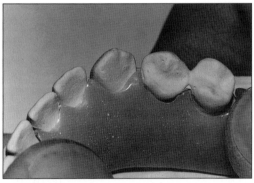

**Fig 18-7** An acrylic resin base that extends into interproximal areas provides retention for the prosthesis.

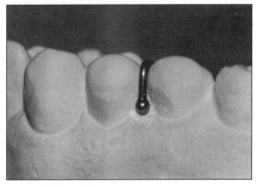

**Fig 18-8** A ball clasp crosses the marginal ridges of adjacent teeth and engages an interproximal undercut on the facial surface of one or both teeth.

The fit of a cast metal denture base undoubtedly will be more accurate, and oral hygiene will be simplified.

Retentive clasps are optional for interim partial dentures. It is possible for the acrylic resin contacting the lingual surfaces of the remaining teeth to project into slight interproximal undercuts and provide retention for the prosthesis (Fig 18-7).

When retentive clasps are desired, a surveyor must be used to locate retentive undercuts. If undercuts are not present for conventional clasps, ball clasps may be used. A ball clasp consists of a ball of solder on the end of a piece of wrought wire. The wire crosses the marginal ridges of adjacent teeth, and the ball engages the associated interproximal space (Fig 18-8).

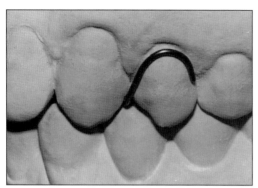

**Fig 18-9** Wrought-wire clasps may be used for retention, but sufficient occlusal space must be present.

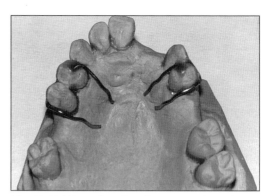

**Fig 18-10** Wrought-wire clasps are shaped and affixed to the cast using sticky wax.

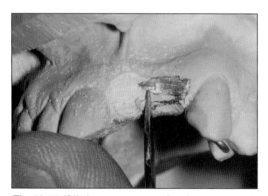

**Fig 18-11** If little or no resorption has occurred, the crest and labial surface of the cast are lightly scraped.

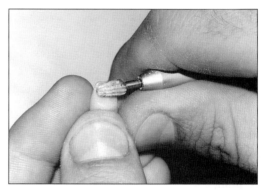

**Fig 18-12** The ridge lap of the artificial tooth is contoured to fit the cast.

This clasp can provide adequate retention without an untoward display of metal.

Wrought wire is commonly used for retentive clasps in temporary removable partial denture applications. The wrought wire should be of lighter gauge than that used for a conventional removable partial denture—20 gauge usually is adequate.

When wrought-wire retentive clasps are designed, particular attention must be given to occlusal clearance (Fig 18-9). Retentive clasps should be attached to the prosthesis by embedding the non-retentive portions of individual clasps in the denture base. After the retentive portion of each clasp is formed, the remainder of the clasp is coiled upon itself and bent so that as it rests in its ultimate position on the cast, the coiled portion of the wire will be slightly out of contact with the lingual or palatal surface of the cast. This will allow the acrylic resin of the denture base to flow completely around the wrought wire and lock it securely in place.

The retentive clasps are the first components of the interim partial denture to be formed. After being formed, they are attached to the associated tooth surfaces using sticky wax (Fig 18-10).

The next components to be selected and shaped are the artificial teeth (Figs 18-11 and 18-12). If little or no resorption of the edentulous ridge has taken place, the neck of a lone-standing replacement may be butted directly to the cast with no labial flange. To ensure intimate contact with the mucosa in the mouth, the crest and labial portion of the edentulous ridge should be scraped slightly. This will guarantee intimate contact between the ridge lap portion of the replacement tooth and the underlying soft tissues. This area of the prosthesis must be adjusted at the time of delivery to ensure that excessive pressure is not present. In the event that resorption of the edentulous ridge has occurred, scraping the ridge will not be necessary because the denture base will cover the ridge and support the teeth in the position the natural teeth originally occupied.

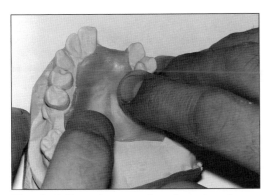

Fig 18-13 Baseplate wax is softened and contoured to fit the palatal portion of the cast.

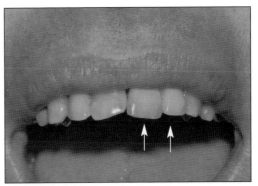

Fig 18-14 Once the denture teeth (arrows) are contoured and attached to the baseplate wax, the try-in denture is evaluated in the patient's mouth. Required changes then can be made.

The selection of one or more artificial teeth will be governed by the available restorative space and by comparison with the same teeth on the opposite side of the dental arch. If all anterior teeth are being replaced, the practitioner should apply guidelines used in complete denture construction. It is especially important to match the maxillary midline with the facial midline. A significant difference in these midlines will result in an artificial appearance.

The number of teeth used as replacements is also important. Every attempt should be made to place an appropriate number of anterior teeth (ie, one artificial tooth for each natural tooth that is missing). The number of posterior teeth is not important as long as occlusal harmony and function are restored.

One of the chief advantages in using plastic teeth is that reshaping is relatively simple. Contouring incisal edges can be accomplished to match or harmonize the prosthetic teeth with the natural teeth.

After the denture teeth have been properly positioned on the cast, a stone matrix should be made to retain the teeth during formation of the denture base. If a heat-activated material is to be used, a matrix is not necessary. The denture base can be waxed and the master cast invested and processed as with complete dentures.

### Esthetic try-in of anterior teeth

A try-in appointment should be used on a routine basis for interim partial dentures that will replace one or more anterior teeth. After the denture teeth have been positioned as desired, a double thickness of baseplate wax is adapted to the master cast (Fig 18-13). The wax is adapted to the lingual surfaces of the natural teeth and extended onto the palate, or to the lingual ridge of the mandibular arch, far enough to provide strength for the try-in appointment. The denture teeth are attached to the baseplate wax and the wax chilled. Obviously, care must be used in handling this temporary try-in partial denture, but if the patient is cautioned against attempting to function with the denture, an esthetic evaluation can be made (Fig 18-14). Any necessary changes in tooth position or shade can be accomplished with the patient present. When both the dentist and the patient are satisfied, a matrix can be constructed.

### Completing the interim partial denture

The majority of temporary partial dentures are constructed using chemically activated acrylic resin in conjunction with a sprinkle-on technique. For this reason, a stone matrix is necessary to maintain the position of the artificial teeth. The master cast must be soaked thoroughly in supernatant dental slurry and subsequently painted with a gypsum separating medium. The matrix should include the facial and incisal/occlusal surfaces of several teeth on each side of the artificial teeth. The matrix should extend onto the facial surface of the cast and should be positively indexed at this point. Several V-shaped notches may be prepared on the base of the cast to ensure that the matrix can be repositioned accurately (Fig 18-15).

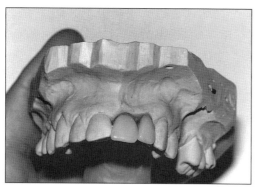

**Fig 18-15** Notches have been prepared on the base of the cast. These notches permit the removal and accurate replacement of a positional matrix.

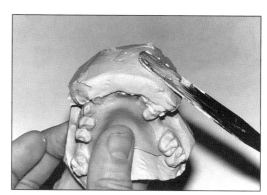

**Fig 18-16** A thick mix of accelerated stone is adapted to the labial surfaces of the cast and the artificial teeth.

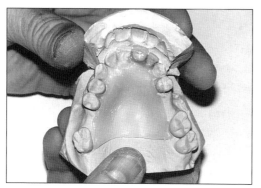

**Fig 18-17** The matrix is removed after the stone has set.

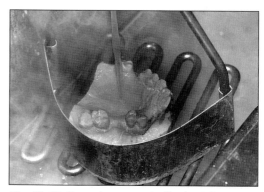

**Fig 18-18** Baseplate wax is flushed from the cast with boiling water.

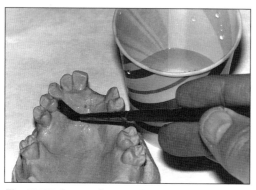

**Fig 18-19** Separating medium is painted onto the surface of the cast.

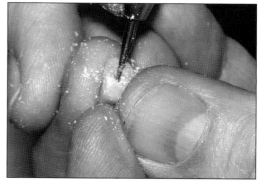

**Fig 18-20** Diatorics are prepared in the ridge lap portions of artificial teeth to provide mechanical retention.

A thick mix of accelerated dental stone is prepared and adapted to the cast and artificial teeth (Fig 18-16). The matrix should be 8 to 10 mm thick to provide adequate strength. When set, the matrix is carefully removed from the cast and trimmed (Fig 18-17). The wax that was used to support the denture teeth during matrix construction is removed from the cast using boiling water (Fig 18-18).

Two coats of an alginate separating medium are painted on the surface of the cast while it is still warm from the boil-out procedure (Fig 18-19). Diatorics, or retention channels, are prepared in the ridge lap por-

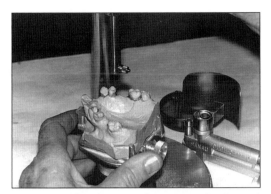

**Fig 18-21** After large undercuts on the lingual surfaces of the cast have been eliminated using baseplate wax, a dental surveyor is used to ensure that parallel blockout has been achieved.

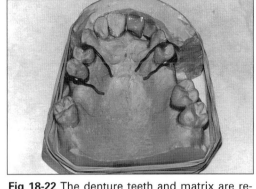

**Fig 18-22** The denture teeth and matrix are reassembled on the master cast. Rubber bands are used to hold the matrix in position.

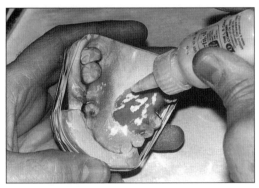

**Fig 18-23** Chemically activated acrylic resin is added using a sprinkle-on technique.

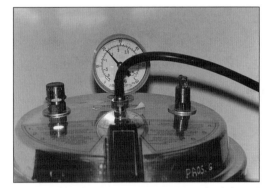

**Fig 18-24** Chemically activated resin is processed in a pressure pot (20 psi for 20 minutes).

tions of the teeth to provide mechanical retention (Fig 18-20). At this stage, the teeth are properly positioned in the matrix and secured with sticky wax. The sticky wax must not interfere with the adaptation of the matrix to the cast.

Before the denture base is formed, gross undercuts on the lingual surfaces of the cast should be eliminated using baseplate wax. A dental surveyor should be used to verify that parallel blockout has been achieved (Fig 18-21). It is important to note that slight undercuts on the teeth need not be eliminated because a certain amount of retention can be gained from them. Acrylic resin will engage the undercuts and provide some resistance to displacement.

When the necessary blockout has been accomplished, the stone matrix is secured to the cast using thick rubber bands (Fig 18-22). If a labial flange has been planned, the negative portion of the flange, seen in the surface of the matrix, should be partially filled with resin before the matrix is attached to the cast. When the matrix is attached,

the remainder of the denture base can be added either by using the sprinkle-on method or by guiding a thin mix of acrylic resin into the space with a brush (Fig 18-23).

The outline of the denture base for an interim removable partial denture in the maxillary arch will normally be that of a horseshoe major connector with the acrylic resin contacting the lingual surfaces of the remaining teeth. For the mandibular arch, the denture base will be in the form of lingual plating and should extend inferiorly as far as possible without encroaching on the movable tissues of the floor of the mouth. Posteriorly it also should extend at least to the distolingual surface of the first molar if anterior teeth are being replaced. This is required not only to distribute forces generated by the presence of the partial denture, but also to provide stability of the denture against anterior tipping forces.

After being formed, the denture base should be allowed to polymerize in a pressure pot at 20 psi for 20 minutes (Fig 18-24). If a pressure pot is not available,

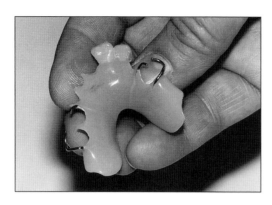

**Fig 18-25** The cameo surface of the interim removable partial denture is finished and polished.

polymerization should take place in an environment saturated with monomer. This can be accomplished by placing a cotton roll saturated with monomer adjacent to the dental cast and inverting a rubber mixing bowl over the cast and the cotton roll. The saturated environment prevents excessive loss of monomer from the denture base through evaporation and thus prevents porosity of the denture.

Following polymerization, the cast should be returned to the articulator to correct any occlusal errors that may have developed during denture base construction. This is accomplished using articulating paper and rotary instruments. The interim denture is then recovered from the cast, finished, and polished (Fig 18-25).

### Delivery of the interim partial denture

At the delivery appointment, the intaglio of the interim partial denture should be painted with pressure indicator paste before being seated (Fig 18-26). During the initial placement, little pressure should be applied. It is possible for the acrylic resin to spring over undercuts and become locked into place in the mouth. Removal of the prosthesis under these conditions can be trying for both the patient and the practitioner.

After identifying areas of the prosthesis that are interfering with placement, the denture base should be carefully reshaped using a laboratory bur in a low-speed handpiece (Fig 18-27). Adjustments at each insertion should be kept to a minimum. If a denture base flange is present, it also must be viewed as a possible area of interference and should be checked with

pressure indicator paste at each trial insertion. Blanching of the soft tissues indicates interference caused by the denture base flange. Intimate contact between the denture base and the soft tissue is desired, but excessive pressure must be avoided. The number of seatings that will be required before the denture goes into place will vary from prosthesis to prosthesis.

Since the majority of interim partial dentures will be used to replace anterior teeth, the goal of the artificial tooth position is to be free from contact with opposing teeth in centric relation or maximum intercuspation (Fig 18-28) and to have light contact in eccentric jaw positions.

When posterior teeth are being replaced, light occlusal contact is the goal in developing the prosthetic occlusion. If multiple posterior teeth are being replaced and normal occlusal contacts are necessary to provide the patient with a functional occlusion, some method of providing vertical support for the prosthesis may be necessary to prevent damage to the soft tissues and edentulous ridge. Rapid resorption of alveolar bone can take place if occlusal overloading is present. Occlusal rests can be incorporated into the interim partial denture if necessary. The simplest method of constructing occlusal rests is by bending a piece of wrought wire to engage the occlusal surfaces of at least one posterior tooth on each side of the arch (Fig 18-29). The wire must be positioned so that it does not interfere with the occlusion. The opposite end of the wire is bent to form several angles. The purpose of the angles is to provide a firm attachment to the denture base because this end of the wire will be embedded in acrylic resin. This type of occlusal rest

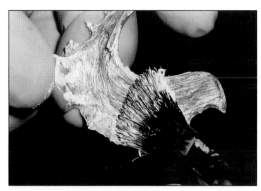

**Fig 18-26** Pressure indicator paste is applied to the intaglio of the prosthesis.

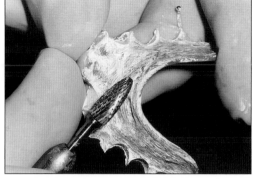

**Fig 18-27** Areas of excessive pressure are adjusted using rotary instruments.

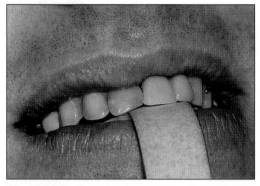

**Fig 18-28** In the anterior region, there should be no contact between the artificial teeth and the opposing natural teeth. Tissue paper should slide between opposing surfaces.

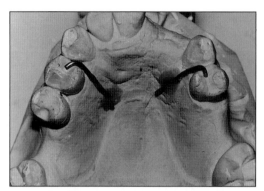

**Fig 18-29** Occlusal rests can be incorporated into temporary prostheses by adapting wrought wire to nonfunctioning fossae.

will provide sufficient resistance to protect the gingival tissues and alveolar bone from excessive trauma.

When all necessary occlusal corrections have been accomplished, the patient must be counseled regarding oral hygiene and care of the prosthesis. The prosthesis must not be worn continuously. Ideally, the denture should be removed at bedtime, allowing the tissues to recover over a prolonged period.

Before the patient is dismissed, a program for instituting definitive care should be established. To avoid possible legal difficulties, the patient must be informed that treatment rendered to this point must be considered temporary. If a long period must elapse before definitive treatment can be started, a periodic recall schedule must be established. Insertion of an interim partial denture should never be considered a termination to treatment.

## Transitional Partial Dentures

### Indications

A transitional denture is planned when some or all of the remaining teeth are beyond the point of restoration but immediate extractions are not indicated for physical or psychological reasons. In these instances, the teeth will be removed over a long period of time, and the patient must be provided with a functional prosthesis during treatment.

For an elderly patient or a patient suffering from a chronic debilitating disease where multiple extractions could exacerbate the basic illness, this treatment plan can be used effectively. By removing the hopeless teeth as adverse symptoms arise, the patient may be spared a major crisis in his or her physical condition.

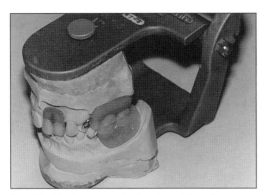

**Fig 18-30** Master casts for transitional removable partial dentures are mounted on an articulator and the artificial teeth arranged.

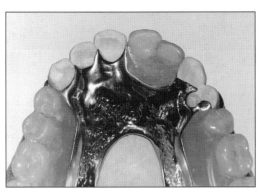

**Fig 18-31** The maxillary right central incisor is to be extracted and added to the transitional partial denture.

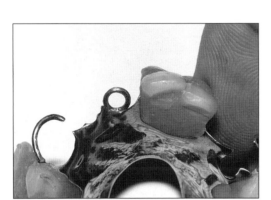

**Fig 18-32** A metal retentive loop is soldered onto the plating.

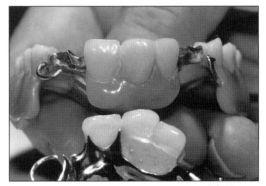

**Fig 18-33** Mirror view shows adaptation of artificial tooth to the lingual plate and addition of a labial flange.

Another group of patients who may be served with this treatment concept are those who are psychologically unable to accept the loss of teeth. In the minds of many people, the presence of teeth is related to youth and happiness, whereas the loss of teeth indicates the opposite. The dentist should not attempt to become an amateur psychologist, but should understand that the loss of a single tooth—especially the last one—can be a frightening emotional experience for some patients. Therefore, the dentist should attempt to gain some insight as to the value the patient places on the retention or the loss of teeth. If a patient is truly concerned over the loss of teeth, but the loss is inevitable, the treatment should be carried out over as long a period as possible. During treatment, the patient should be reassured as to the success of treatment and mentally prepared to accept the unavoidable result. This type of problem can be minimized if the dentist remembers to "meet the mind of the patient before meeting the mouth of the patient," as DeVan so aptly put it.[1]

## Clinical procedures

The clinical procedures for this and all temporary partial dentures remain basically the same. The practitioner must make accurate, properly extended alginate impressions. From these impressions, accurate casts must be made. Jaw relation records also may be required to mount the casts on an appropriate articulator (Fig 18-30).

If the transitional denture is not to be an immediate partial denture, the construction of the denture will be the same as that for the interim partial denture. The denture base will normally be constructed of acrylic resin. If the denture is to serve for a prolonged period, a cast metal framework may be used. When cast metal is planned, special design considerations

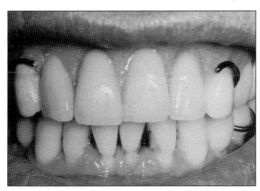

**Fig 18-34** A maxillary transitional partial denture that has been converted to a complete denture. Clasps have been left on the prosthesis to retain a natural appearance.

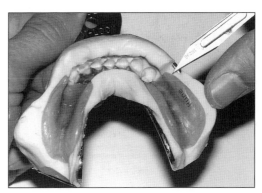

**Fig 18-35** Transitional denture is "picked up" in an alginate impression.

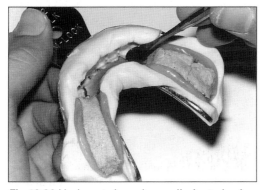

**Fig 18-36** Undercuts have been eliminated using wet paper towels. A thin film of wax is flowed onto the intaglio surface of the lingual plate.

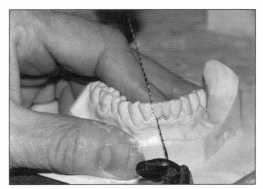

**Fig 18-37** Teeth that are to be extracted are removed from the cast.

must be used so that as natural teeth are lost, prosthetic teeth can be added to the metal framework. The design that most clearly satisfies this requirement generally includes lingual plating of the teeth most likely to be lost (Fig 18-31). As natural teeth are extracted, metal retention loops can be soldered to the lingual plating (Fig 18-32) and artificial teeth processed to the retention loops (Fig 18-33). With this form of treatment, the patient will never truly be without teeth.

The transitional partial denture concept of treatment can be used with preexisting partial dentures, provided the design will allow the placement of additional prosthetic teeth. When necessary, patients may be transitioned from a partially edentulous to a completely edentulous condition (Fig 18-34).

If the design of the existing partial denture is such that teeth may be added to it, following are the clinical procedures to add teeth to the denture. The removable partial denture is seated in the mouth. With a slightly oversized impression tray, an alginate impression is made over the denture (Fig 18-35). In a majority of cases, the partial denture will remain in the impression as it is removed from the mouth. If the denture does not remain in the impression as it is removed from the mouth, the denture must be repositioned in the impression.

Before the working cast is poured, any area of undercut in the denture base (or bases) must be blocked out. The blockout may be accomplished with baseplate wax, modeling clay, or wet paper towels (Fig 18-36). After the cast is poured, the removable partial denture must be recovered from the cast. In turn, the teeth that are to be extracted are removed from the cast (Fig 18-37). The initial cuts should be even with the surrounding gingival tissues. Simulated sockets

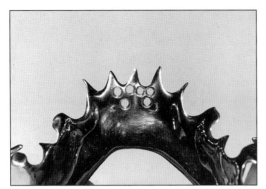

**Fig 18-38** Perforations in the lingual plating may be used to retain artificial teeth.

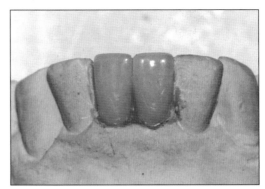

**Fig 18-39** Artificial teeth are contoured to fit the cast and the removable partial denture framework.

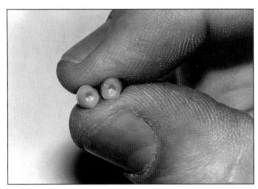

**Fig 18-40** Diatorics are prepared to provide mechanical retention.

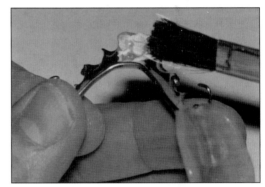

**Fig 18-41** Pressure indicator paste is used to identify pressure spots.

may then be created by preparing slight concavities, with each center 2 mm deeper than the periphery. If an anterior tooth is being replaced, the labial surface of the cast should be scraped lightly.

Some method of retention for the teeth to be added must be developed on the framework. The retention may be in the form of wire loops soldered to lingual plating or perforations through the plating (Fig 18-38).

With the partial denture seated on the cast, denture teeth are ground to fit the trimmed cast and the partial denture framework (Fig 18-39). If a denture flange is not present or planned, the necks of the teeth should be butted to the ridge. This is the reason the labial surface of the cast should be scraped before the denture tooth is contoured to fit the ridge. The light pressure of the tooth against the soft tissue in the mouth provides a more normal appearance.

At this stage, diatorics should be drilled into the teeth to provide additional mechanical retention (Fig

18-40). The denture teeth may then be attached to the framework using a chemically activated acrylic resin.

After the teeth have been added to the partial denture, the patient is prepared for the extractions. Following surgery, pressure indicator paste is painted onto the intaglio of the denture (Fig 18-41). The denture is then fully seated in the mouth. Upon removal of the prosthesis from the oral cavity, the internal surface is carefully examined and the necessary adjustments are made using appropriate laboratory burs.

The patient should be seen within 24 hours to monitor both surgical and prosthodontic procedures. Early recall and adjustment often will prevent significant difficulties.

Patients receiving transitional partial denture service should normally be placed on a routine recall system (at intervals not greater than 3 months) so that the questionable remaining teeth can be monitored closely. Deep periodontal pockets will frequently be

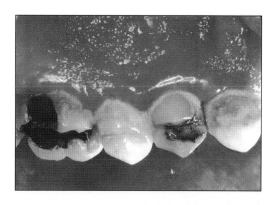

Fig 18-42 Marginal gingivitis may result from prolonged prosthesis wear in conjunction with inadequate oral hygiene.

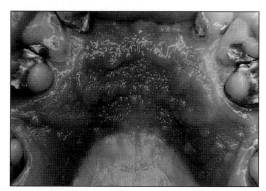

Fig 18-43 The palatal tissues are a frequent site of inflammatory hyperplasia.

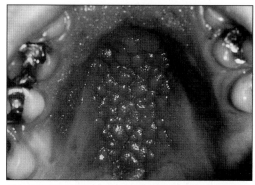

Fig 18-44 Papillary hyperplasia is often associated with ill-fitting major connectors and poor oral hygiene.

present, and acute exacerbation in the form of periodontal abscesses may be expected if adequate home and office care is not practiced.

## ▣ Treatment Partial Dentures

### Indications

A treatment partial denture may be used for a variety of purposes. In most instances, a treatment partial denture is used to carry tissue conditioner to abused oral tissues. Hence, the following discussion will be focused upon the treatment partial denture as a carrier for tissue conditioner.

### Vehicle for tissue conditioner

If a prosthesis causes excess force against the oral soft tissues, an adverse soft tissue reaction may take place. This is especially true if poor oral hygiene also is present.

The reaction can be in the form of simple erythema or hyperkeratinization, or it may be much more severe.

One of the most potentially dangerous soft tissue reactions is marginal gingivitis affecting the crevicular tissues (Fig 18-42). Prolonged marginal gingivitis can lead to chronic periodontal disease. This commonly occurs when temporary partial dentures are used for too long without adequate professional care.

Soft tissues, particularly gingival tissues, will respond in one of two ways if subjected to chronic irritation. Hyperplasia may occur, or the tissues may recede. In either event, the source of irritation must be identified and eliminated before the results of the irritation become irreversible.

A frequent site of inflammatory hyperplasia is beneath the major connector of a maxillary partial denture (Figs 18-43 and 18-44). The condition is referred to as *papillary hyperplasia*, or *papillomatosis*, and is most often seen on the palatal tissues beneath a complete denture. The acute infection and inflammation present in the hyperplastic tissues can be controlled by the local applica-

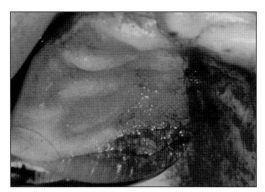

Fig 18-45 Elimination of hyperplastic tissues may be accomplished surgically.

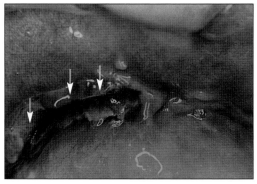

Fig 18-46 A denture epulis *(arrows)* caused by overextension of the associated denture base.

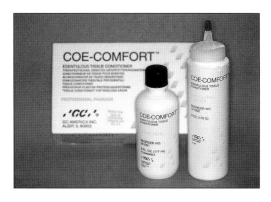

Fig 18-47 Tissue conditioners are used to treat unhealthy or abused soft tissues.

tion of a tissue conditioner, but in most instances the condition is not entirely reversible. As a result, surgical intervention is often required (Fig 18-45).

Two common factors can almost always be found associated with a hyperplastic tissue response: *(1)* the patient has been wearing the prosthesis continuously, without giving the tissues a chance to recover, and *(2)* oral hygiene habits, including cleansing of the prosthesis, are poor if not altogether absent.

Another abnormal tissue response that warrants treatment with a resilient conditioner is an epulis fissuratum or denture epulis. Epulis fissuratum is a hyperplastic response to the overextended border of a denture base (Fig 18-46). The overextension of the denture base is generally not so great as to produce pain, but is enough to cause proliferation of the irritated tissues. Simple shortening or adjustment of the denture base flange may result in a slow shrinkage of the hyperplastic tissues. Usually, however, treatment with a tissue conditioner will be needed to reverse the process. This treatment may be extended over several

weeks or months. If the tissue response is not satisfactory, surgery may be required.

## Tissue conditioner

Tissue conditioner (Fig 18-47) is a soft material that is applied to the intaglio of a complete or partial denture to allow a more equitable distribution of forces throughout the dental arch. The material is nonirritating and nontoxic. It is soft and elastic, so it does not undergo substantial permanent deformation. The softness and elasticity of most tissue conditioners last approximately 1 week, after which the material begins to harden and can itself become an irritant. To be effective in treating abused oral tissues, the conditioner must be changed every 3 to 5 days.

Tissue conditioner is usually supplied as a powder and a liquid. The powder is acrylic polymer, usually ethyl methacrylate, and the liquid is usually a mixture of ethyl alcohol and an aromatic ester. The two combine to form a gel that remains pliable for several days.

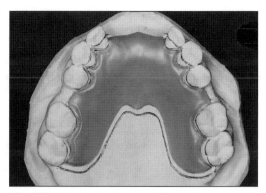

Fig 18-48 A single layer of baseplate wax is adapted to the cast over abused areas. The wax acts as a spacer for the tissue conditioner.

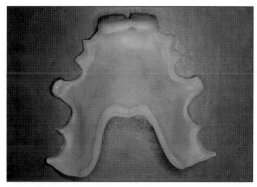

Fig 18-49 Upon completion of processing, the wax spacer is removed from the treatment denture.

The mechanism of action of the conditioner is a combination of improved force distribution and a short-term cushioning effect.

## Clinical procedures

If a new temporary partial denture is to be constructed solely to serve as a vehicle for the tissue conditioner, the clinical procedures will be exactly the same as for constructing an interim or transitional partial denture. The laboratory procedures will vary slightly.

If a serviceable prosthesis is available and if some relief space can be created or obtained on the tissue surface of the denture adjacent to the abused tissues, the prosthesis can be used as the vehicle to support tissue conditioner. If the tissue surface of the partial denture is metal, more difficulty will be encountered in using it as the vehicle since adequate relief cannot be obtained between the abused tissue and the metal, and sufficient thickness of tissue conditioner must be present in order to be effective.

## Laboratory procedures

After the casts have been mounted on an articulator, one thickness of baseplate wax is adapted to the area of the cast corresponding to the abused tissues (Fig 18-48). At this point, the treatment partial denture

can be constructed following the same technique used for an interim partial denture.

Upon completion of processing, the wax spacer is removed from the treatment partial denture (Fig 18-49). In turn, the cameo surface of the prosthesis is brought to a high polish to prevent plaque and other debris from collecting on its surface.

## Using the tissue conditioner

A treatment partial denture is fitted to the mouth using pressure indicator paste. The occlusion is checked and refined following normal procedures. The tissue conditioner is then applied as shown in Figs 18-50 to 18-52. Subsequently, the treatment partial denture with the tissue conditioner is seated in the mouth under light pressure (Fig 18-53). The pressure is maintained as the material flows. Border tissues should be manipulated to border mold the conditioner. For a mandibular removable partial denture, the tongue should be brought forward and forcibly placed into each cheek to define the lingual extension accurately. If posterior artificial teeth are present, the patient must close the teeth together while the conditioner is still capable of flowing in order to align the artificial teeth properly with the opposing occlusion. Once the denture has been seated and aligned, the patient should sit quietly for 4 to 5 minutes until the gel stage of the conditioner has been reached. At that time the denture should be removed

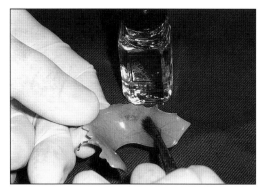

**Fig 18-50** The cameo surface of the prosthesis is painted with separator.

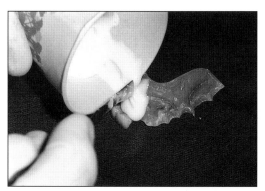

**Fig 18-51** After the tissue conditioner is mixed according to manufacturer's recommendations, it is flowed onto the intaglio of the denture.

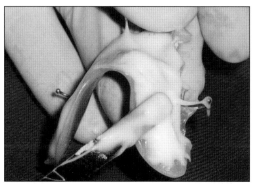

**Fig 18-52** Tissue conditioner is distributed evenly using a small spatula.

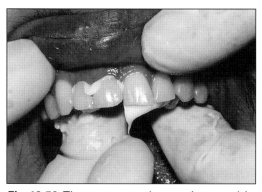

**Fig 18-53** The treatment denture is seated in the mouth.

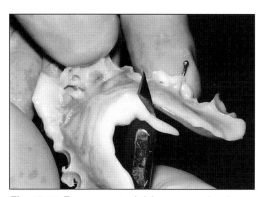

**Fig 18-54** Excess material is removed using a sharp blade.

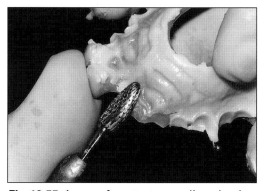

**Fig 18-55** Areas of contact are relieved using laboratory burs.

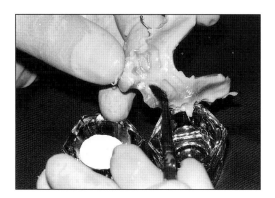

**Fig 18-56** Freshly mixed tissue conditioner is added to areas that have been relieved.

from the mouth and examined. Excess material should be trimmed from the partial denture using a sharp blade (Fig 18-54).

If the denture base is exposed through the treatment material, these areas should be relieved and new material added (Figs 18-55 and 18-56). The best way to relieve the denture base is by coating the surface of the treatment material with liquid soap and cutting away the exposed portion of the acrylic resin denture base with laboratory burs. The liquid soap prevents fragments from attaching to the surface of the tissue conditioner. The soap and grindings may then be washed from the denture and additional conditioner added. The denture must be reseated in the mouth while the conditioner is still capable of flowing.

The patient should be counseled regarding home care of the treatment partial denture. The tissue conditioner should not be allowed to dry. For those periods of time when the denture is not in the mouth, it must be submerged in water or cleansing solution.

## ▢ Reference

1. DeVan, MM. The transition from natural to artificial teeth. J Prosthet Dent 1961;11:677–688.

## ▢ Bibliography

Bennett CG. Transitional restorations for function and esthetics. J Prosthet Dent 1965;15:867–872.

Blatterfein L. Role of the removable partial denture in the restoration of lost vertical dimension. N Y Univ J Dent 1952;10:274–276.

Bolender CL, Swenson RD, Yamane G. Evaluation of treatment of inflammatory papillary hyperplasia of the palate. J Prosthet Dent 1965;15:1013–1022.

Bruce RW, Kobes P. Immediate removable partial dentures. J Prosthet Dent 1972;28:36–42.

DeVan MM. The additive partial denture: Its principles and design (partial dentures). Northwest Dent 1956;35:303–307.

Dreizin S. Nutritional changes in the oral cavity. J Prosthet Dent 1966;16:1144–1150.

Ettinger RL. The etiology of inflammatory papillary hyperplasia. J Prosthet Dent 1975;34:254–259.

Frank RP. Fabrication of temporary and treatment partial dentures. J Prosthet Dent 1973;30:215–221.

Harvey WL. A transitional prosthetic appliance. J Prosthet Dent 1964;14:60–70.

Lambson GO. Papillary hyperplasia of the palate. J Prosthet Dent 1966;16:636–645.

Reitz PV, Weiner MG. Fabrication of interim acrylic resin removable partial dentures with clasps. J Prosthet Dent 1978;40:686–688.

Schopper AF. Loss of vertical dimension: Causes and effects: Diagnosis and various recommended treatments. J Prosthet Dent 1959;9:428–431.

Thomas KH. Papillomatosis of the palate. Oral Surg Oral Med Oral Pathol 1952;5:214–218.

Waldron CA. Oral leukoplakia, carcinoma, and the prosthodontist. J Prosthet Dent 1965;15:367–376.

# Other Forms of Removable Partial Dentures

For the most part, this book describes the design, construction, and clinical appointments concerned with conventional, extracoronal, clasp-retained, removable partial dentures. Interim, transitional, and treatment partial dentures are also discussed.

However, other forms of removable partial dentures are available, some of which are considered here. The basic rules of design and construction apply no matter what the reason for use.

## ❑ Guide Plane Removable Partial Dentures

### Indications

One important use for removable partial dentures that has been alluded to previously in the text is stabilizing teeth that have lost supporting bone. The form of removable partial denture used for this purpose, termed a *guide plane removable partial denture*, differs from the normal concept of design and construction and yet still adheres to the basic design philosophy.

There have been many ways in which dental specialists and general practitioners have approached the problem of stabilizing weakened teeth. Lack of stability may have been brought about by natural destructive processes or as a result of therapy (Fig 19-1). The most definitive method of supporting these teeth is the use of fixed periodontal prostheses, which, barring contraindications, should be considered the treatment plan of choice (Fig 19-2). However, most people who have periodontally weakened teeth are in the fourth, fifth, or sixth decade of life, and many have major medical problems that contraindicate the extensive treatment necessary for multiple fixed prostheses. Such patients and those whose dental prognoses are limited at best are of particular interest here.

Physiologically, the periodontium permits a tooth to move in three different directions: vertically, mesiodistally, and buccolingually (Figs 19-3 to 19-5). A number of investigators have shown that excessive lateral, or buccolingual, force is the most destructive of the directional forces. This is the principal reason why splinting with fixed prostheses is often not the answer to stabilizing weakened teeth. Unless it encircles nearly the entire arch, a fixed splint will provide in-

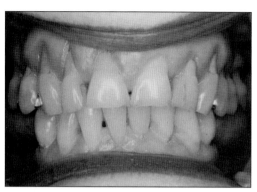

**Fig 19-1** Destructive processes often occur when excessive forces are concentrated on a few teeth. This patient exhibits gingival recession and bone loss related to occlusal trauma.

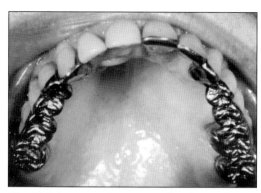

**Fig 19-2** In some instances, fixed prostheses may be used to splint periodontally compromised teeth.

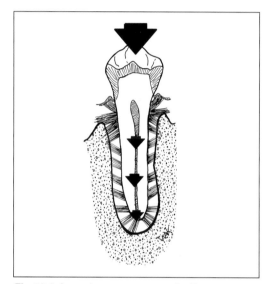

**Fig 19-3** A tooth may move vertically.

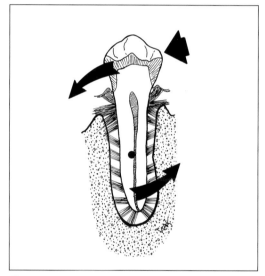

**Fig 19-4** A tooth may move mesiodistally.

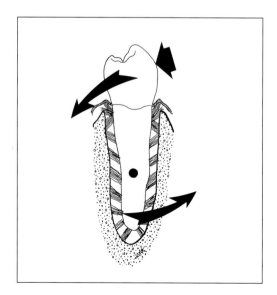

**Fig 19-5** A tooth may move buccolingually.

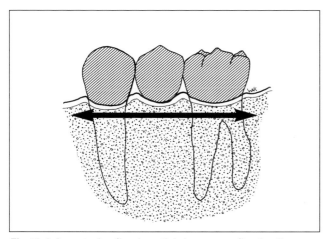

**Fig 19-6** A posterior fixed partial denture or fixed splint provides stabilization in an anteroposterior direction only *(arrow)*.

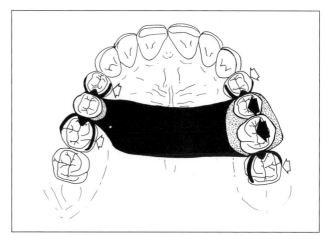

**Fig 19-7** A removable partial denture is capable of providing cross-arch stabilization. Occlusal forces *(solid arrows)* are resisted by abutments *(open arrows)* on both sides of the arch because of the rigidity of the framework.

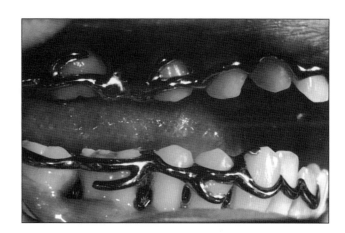

**Fig 19-8** A continuous loop removable splint rigidly supports weakened teeth.

creased resistance only to anteroposterior forces (Fig 19-6). Little or no additional support is gained in a buccolingual direction. A guide plane removable partial denture, being anchored on both sides of the arch and joined together with a rigid major connector, can provide cross-arch stabilization to forces operating in a buccolingual direction (Fig 19-7).

There have been many attempts to correlate the amount of tooth movement with periodontal health. In all reported cases in which the splint-type guide plane removable partial denture (Fig 19-8) has been worn, mobility of the teeth has remained the same or decreased. The basic concept in stabilizing weakened teeth is that the teeth must be held completely rigid. If

any movement is allowed, an increase in mobility is to be expected.

## Design

When the status of periodontally weakened teeth is evaluated, the following factors should be considered: *(1)* how the teeth can be protected from insult caused by continuous or intermittent movement, *(2)* how the gingival and interproximal tissues can be protected from abuse caused by the improper shunting and packing of food, and *(3)* how the forces of occlusion can be directed to prevent unnecessary trauma to supporting structures.

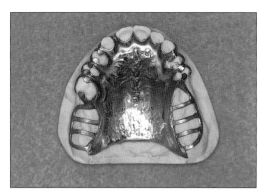

**Fig 19-9** The design for a stabilizing prosthesis follows the philosophy of broad stress distribution.

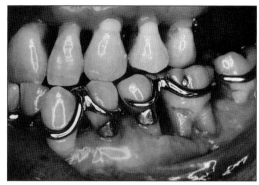

**Fig 19-10** There should never be more than two retentive clasp arms on one side of the arch. All other clasp arms should be positioned occlusal/incisal to the height of contour and should brace the remaining teeth.

The partial denture design philosophy of broad stress distribution is the best method of obtaining support for weakened teeth. The stress is distributed through the use of rigid major and minor connectors and multiple rests and clasps (Fig 19-9). It must be remembered that not all clasps will be retentive—many will be used only to prevent the tooth from being moved in a lateral direction. Mouth preparation before the construction of the denture is extremely important. Periodontally weakened teeth must be supported rigidly not only when the prosthesis is in place, but also while the partial denture is being inserted and withdrawn.

It must be remembered that before a retentive clasp tip engages the associated abutment, the reciprocal portion of that clasp, whether an arm, plate, or rest, should contact the opposite side of the tooth so that the retentive clasp tip will flex and not force the tooth to move (see chapter 3). The framework should be completely passive in the mouth. Prevention of lateral pressures being distributed to supporting teeth, important in the design and construction of all removable partial dentures, becomes of critical importance in the treatment of weakened teeth. As a result, the prosthesis will contact more teeth than normal, and multiple parallel guiding planes will be required. It may be difficult to prove that parallelism of these multiple surfaces has been achieved by visual inspection of the teeth. To make certain that the goal has been achieved or to locate surfaces that may need further correction, impressions of the arch should be made in irreversible hydrocolloid and casts should be poured using a fast-setting dental stone. Then these casts can be mounted on the surveyor and checked to be certain the guiding planes have been developed at the proper positions. Corrections can be made at the same appointment. Although intraoral paralleling devices are available, with experience the techniques described can be accomplished effectively and accurately.

In arches where bone loss is generalized and severe, each posterior tooth should receive support from both the buccal and lingual aspects. The support against movement in the buccal direction must come from buccal clasp arms. The use of multiple embrasure clasps, although not normally the most desirable form of clasping, is frequently necessary, particularly in arches where few teeth are missing. Removable splints may be made for arches with no missing teeth to provide support for the weakened teeth.

When multiple buccal clasp arms are designed, no more than two on each side of the arch should be retentive. The remainder should be rigid and designed to contact the tooth at or above the survey line (Fig 19-10). To gain as much mechanical advantage against tipping forces as possible, it is extremely important to recontour the buccal surfaces to move the survey line toward the gingival attachment. It is also possible to gain some esthetic advantage by keeping the clasps positioned as far apically as possible.

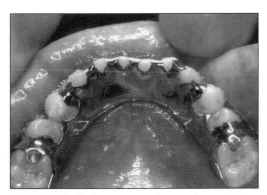

**Fig 19-11** Incisal rests may be used to stabilize weakened anterior teeth.

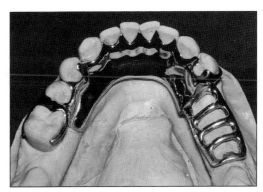

**Fig 19-12** A lingual plate provides cross-arch stabilization and lingual support for individual teeth.

If the patient under consideration for treatment is conscious of esthetics, the guide plane removable partial denture is not likely to prove satisfactory. A careful explanation should be offered to the patient that in order to maintain the natural teeth, some display of metal will be necessary. If the teeth have lost the majority of bony support, generally the only alternative to this form of treatment is a complete denture. Esthetic qualities can be maintained or improved through the use of the complete denture, but the long-term prognosis for maintenance of the residual ridges is not favorable unless the overdenture concept is followed.

## Role of the lingual plate

Weakened anterior teeth usually will not require support from the facial surfaces. The muscular action of the lips during speech and eating is sufficient to prevent anterior migration except when tongue-thrusting habits are present or when bone loss is severe. A decision is often made to maintain mandibular anterior teeth as long as possible even when severe bone loss is present. Under these conditions, it is possible to prepare mesial and distal incisal rests on the remaining anterior teeth and to engage these rest seats with projections from the lingual plating (Fig 19-11). This approach will hold the teeth rigidly. (Another technique for supporting weakened anterior teeth is provided by the Swing-Lock partial denture, which is described later in the chapter.) The lingual plate serves as the major connector for the

prosthesis and provides cross-arch stabilization, as well as lingual support for the individual teeth (Fig 19-12).

The role of the lingual plate is twofold: *(1)* to a major degree, it contributes horizontal stability to a removable partial denture, and *(2)* in the event that the removable partial denture is not used primarily to replace teeth but to act as a splint for the remaining natural teeth, it helps prevent the application of excessive lateral forces on the teeth.

The interproximal spaces for these weakened teeth will be larger than normal because of tissue recession around the necks of the teeth, so it is essential that the interproximal spaces lingual to the contact point be completely closed to prevent packing of food beneath the plate from an occlusal or incisal direction (Fig 19-13). Several periodontal groups have shown that the lingual plate can perform this secondary function. When the interproximal extensions of the lingual plate are constructed properly, the design of the plate in these areas will be needle shaped and sharp (Fig 19-14). From this pointed interproximal tip, the plate should fall away to a razor-thin edge and just cover the cingulum of an anterior tooth or lie just occlusal to the largest convexity of a posterior tooth. The plate should fit the cingulum as accurately as an inlay fits its preparation. Food that passes over this portion of the lingual plate should be shunted away from the margin of the major connector. If the joint between the plate and the tooth is too thick, food and other debris will collect, increasing the difficulty of maintaining proper

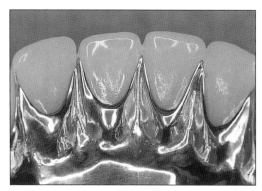

**Fig 19-13** A lingual plate must close the interproximal spaces. Note that the lingual plate presents a distinct "scalloped" appearance.

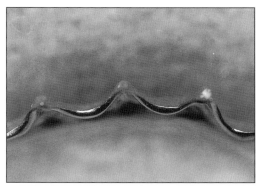

**Fig 19-14** A properly constructed lingual plate should be knife-edged when viewed from above.

oral hygiene and contributing to the discomfort of the patient.

### Fitting the framework

As for all removable partial dentures, it is imperative that the practitioner check the fit of the framework before completion. (This process is covered in detail in chapter 11.)

### Prognosis

The results of this form of treatment are encouraging. Clinical results have been consistently promising. Thus, carefully planned, constructed, and fitted guide plane removable partial dentures can be effective in stabilizing weakened teeth.

## ⌑ Swing-Lock Removable Partial Dentures

In the Swing-Lock removable partial denture, first described by Dr Joe J. Simmons in 1963,[1] all or several of the remaining teeth are used to retain and stabilize the prosthesis against vertical displacement. The prosthesis consists of a hinged buccal or labial bar attached to a conventional major connector (Figs 19-15 to 19-18). Retention and stabilization are provided by this bar.

The labial bar is generally designed with small vertical projection arms that contact the labial or buccal surfaces of the teeth gingival to the height of contour (Fig 19-19). These vertical arms look like I- or T-bars and provide both retention and stabilization for the prosthesis. The labial bars can also be designed with acrylic resin retention components (Fig 19-20), in which case retention and stability are provided by an acrylic resin denture base attached to the labial bar. This design is used if the vertical projection bars would produce a poor esthetic result or if extensive loss of gingival tissue has occurred and a resin gingival veneer is needed to improve appearance.

### Advantages

The primary advantage of the Swing-Lock concept is that it provides a relatively inexpensive method for using all or most of the remaining teeth for the retention and stabilization of a prosthesis. Alternatives to this type of treatment include (1) removal of the remaining teeth and (2) fixed splinting of the remaining teeth and construction of a conventional removable partial denture. The latter is relatively time consuming and expensive and presents problems if one of the splinted teeth fails. Loss of a splinted tooth could necessitate removal and reconstruction of a fixed splint, whereas a tooth can be removed and added to the major connector of a Swing-Lock prosthesis through a simple laboratory procedure.

Because the construction of a Swing-Lock removable partial denture is relatively simple and inexpensive, it can be used in situations in which more conventional types of treatment may appear hopeless.

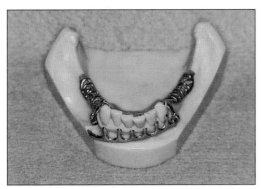

**Fig 19-15** A Swing-Lock removable denture exhibits a hinged labial bar.

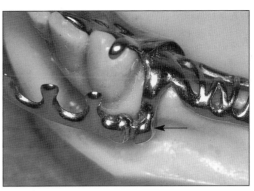

**Fig 19-16** The labial bar is attached to the framework by a hinge mechanism *(arrow)* that permits it to open and close like a gate.

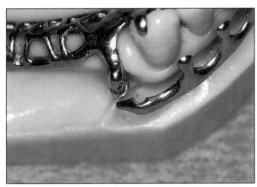

**Fig 19-17** Locking mechanism in the open position.

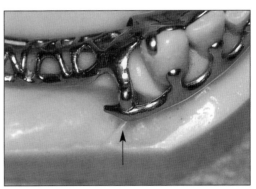

**Fig 19-18** Locking mechanism in the closed position *(arrow)*.

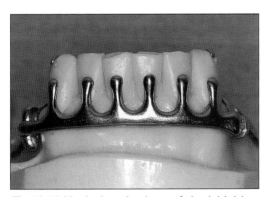

**Fig 19-19** Vertical projections of the labial bar contact the remaining teeth.

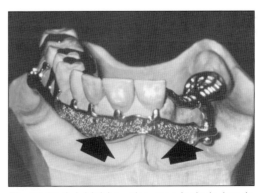

**Fig 19-20** A labial bar also may include beads *(arrows)* to permit attachment of an acrylic resin veneer.

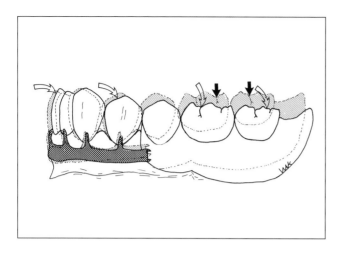

**Fig 19-21** Occlusal forces *(solid arrows)* applied to a distal extension Swing-Lock prosthesis may cause the denture base to move toward the soft tissues. This may produce distal rotation of the abutments *(open arrows).*

## Disadvantages

A Swing-Lock prosthesis can produce a relatively poor esthetic result for patients with short or extremely mobile lips. Obtaining perfect adaptation of a resin veneer is difficult because the path of insertion is dictated by the hinge movement of the labial bar.

The remaining teeth are grasped firmly by the prosthesis. A long distal extension base is likely to move toward the tissue under the forces of occlusion. This movement can tip the teeth grasped by the prosthesis (Fig 19-21).

## Indications

There are a number of indications for use of the Swing-Lock design in the treatment of partially edentulous patients:

1. Too few remaining natural teeth for a removable partial denture of conventional design
2. Remaining teeth too mobile to serve as abutment teeth for conventional design
3. Position of remaining teeth not favorable for a conventional design
4. Retention and stabilization needed for maxillofacial prostheses such as obturators for postsurgical patients
5. Retention of a prosthesis for patients who have lost large segments of teeth and alveolar ridge as a result of traumatic injury

## Selection of metal for Swing-Lock framework

Chrome alloys are the materials of choice for the metallic frameworks of Swing-Lock removable partial dentures. Gold is contraindicated because the hinge and lock mechanisms show noticeable wear in a relatively short time when gold is used. Moreover, to provide the necessary rigidity and strength, gold components must be more bulky than chrome components.

## Design

The path of insertion for a Swing-Lock prosthesis is from the lingual direction with the labial arm open. However, it is imperative that the cast be surveyed with the occlusal plane of the teeth parallel with the base of the surveyor (Figs 19-22 to 19-25). Most forces applied to the prosthesis will be directed perpendicular to the occlusal plane. Survey lines are drawn on all the remaining teeth. Lingual plating is positioned above the survey lines. With the gate closed, the lingual plating and the rests in definite rest seats resist movement toward the underlying tissues. The vertical projection extensions from the labial arm prevent occlusal movement. All teeth contacted by the framework act collectively to prevent movement. Such precautions against movement are essential because long distal extension bases can place tipping forces on all the teeth grasped by the prosthesis if the extension base moves toward the soft tissues.

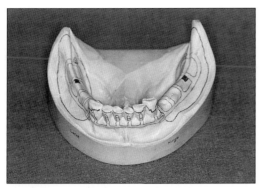

**Fig 19-22** The Swing-Lock prosthesis must be neatly and precisely drawn on the cast.

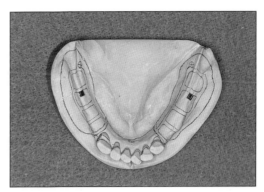

**Fig 19-23** Occlusal view of Swing-Lock design. In mandibular applications, a lingual plate major connector is used.

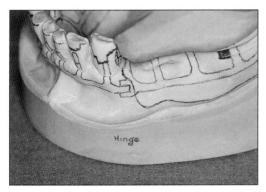

**Fig 19-24** The hinge must be properly located and clearly identified.

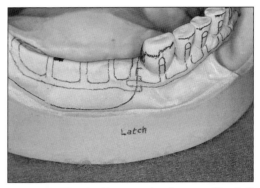

**Fig 19-25** The locking mechanism, or "latch," also must be appropriately located and clearly identified.

**Fig 19-26** A lingual plate major connector is commonly used in mandibular Swing-Lock applications. The lingual plate must be extremely well adapted to the remaining natural teeth.

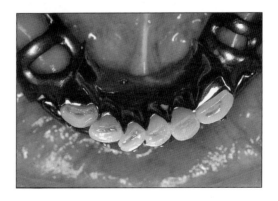

The lingual plate major connector is usually the connector of choice for the mandibular arch (Fig 19-26). A double lingual bar (Kennedy bar) can be used, but it has more disadvantages than advantages. The lingual plate major connector must be designed to provide rigidity and comfort. The active floor of the mouth is measured, and those measurements are transferred to the master cast to indicate the position of the inferior border of the major connector. The connector should be constructed with the same contour and size as a lingual bar, with lingual plating extending from the superior aspect of the bar to the correct position on the teeth. The lingual plating must be positioned above the survey line and scalloped with extensions to the contact point areas of the teeth.

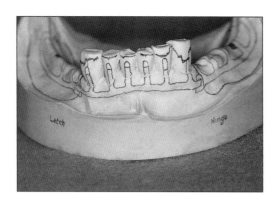

**Fig 19-27** The conventional Swing-Lock design consists of a labial arm with I- or T-bar vertical projections that contact the teeth apical to their survey lines. Esthetics may be improved by placing the vertical projections as apically as possible.

Major connectors for the maxillary arch should use as much of the palate as possible for support of the prosthesis. Full palatal coverage is generally indicated. An anteroposterior palatal strap design can also be used if anatomic considerations or patient desires indicate the need for an opening in the palatal coverage. The remaining teeth are plated on the lingual surfaces, with the plating extending above the survey line.

The labial arm can be designed in two ways. The conventional design consists of a labial arm with I- or T-bar vertical projections that contact the labial or buccal surfaces of the teeth below the survey line (Fig 19-27). An alternate approach is the use of acrylic resin retention loops on the labial arm and a processed resin veneer. This design is used if esthetics would be compromised by the show of metal or if a great loss of gingival tissue has occurred. The resin veneer design is usually used when the patient has mobile or short lips. The patient is asked to say words such as "sheriff" or "shepherd" to produce maximum movement of the lips and exposure of the teeth, and lines are drawn on the casts to indicate the position of maximum lip movement. If metal components would be visible and would be objectionable to the patient, the resin veneer is included in the design.

Although positioning of lingual plating above the survey line does prevent movement toward the tissues, well-designed rests in properly prepared rest seats ensure that the forces are directed along the long axes of the teeth. Rests are placed adjacent to edentulous areas. If teeth are present distal to the first premolar, an additional rest is placed on the mesio-occlusal surface of the first premolar or on the lingual or incisal surface of the canine.

Location of the hinge and locking mechanisms is determined by the patient's ability to open the lock. It is usually easier for a right-handed patient to open the locking mechanism if it is located on the right side of the prosthesis.

## Impressions

Alginate (irreversible hydrocolloid) is the impression material of choice for a Swing-Lock denture. Most patients who require this type of treatment have gingival recession and large gingival embrasures. Rubber base impression material is too tough and will lock into undercut embrasure areas. Alginate, however, will tear and release without excessive application of force. It also possesses an exceptional degree of accuracy if it is handled properly.

The extension of the impression into the buccal and labial vestibules is critical. Frequently, a custom tray must be constructed to record these areas accurately. This is particularly true if the anterior teeth are labially inclined. Modeling plastic is used to border mold the vestibular areas of the tray to provide the proper extension. A custom tray must be constructed with sufficient relief to provide 5 to 6 mm of space for alginate around the remaining teeth. The tray should be prepared with several holes to help retain the alginate in the tray. If a stock tray is used, the edentulous areas should be customized using modeling plastic. Alginate adhesive is applied to the tray and its borders.

Heavy-bodied alginate is used for making the impression. If this type of alginate is not available, less water should be used in mixing regular-bodied algi-

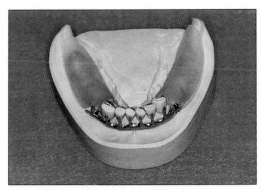

**Fig 19-28** Impression trays are added in preparation for corrected cast impression procedures.

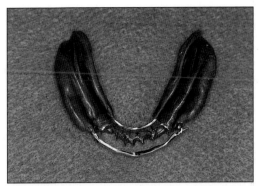

**Fig 19-29** After the impression trays have been border molded using modeling plastic, an impression is made using polysulfide rubber base impression material.

nate. Good technique should be followed in making the impression, including isolating the mouth with gauze and syringe or finger placement of impression material around the teeth and into the vestibular areas. The impression is allowed to remain in the mouth for 2 minutes more than usual. This allows the alginate time to develop maximum strength. The impression is removed with a single snap, with the force applied along the long axes of the remaining teeth.

The alginate will usually tear interproximally, particularly if open gingival embrasures are present. The torn surfaces are carefully approximated and luted in position with small amounts of sticky wax. The interproximal contours are important because the framework will extend into these areas because of the lingual path of insertion. The impression is cleaned, disinfected, and poured within 12 minutes using a Type III or IV dental stone.

## Fitting the framework

A critical procedure in the construction of a Swing-Lock prosthesis is the fitting of the framework to the teeth and to the opposing occlusion. Disclosing wax is added to all areas of the framework that contact the teeth with the exception of the labial arm, which is fitted later. The framework is then seated into position with the labial arm open. Closure of the labial arm should not be attempted until all other areas of the framework have been fitted. Pressure is applied in a vertical direction through pressure on the rests. The framework is removed and inspected for evidence of metal show-through. These areas are adjusted using a multifluted carbide bur in a high-

speed handpiece, and the procedure is repeated until the framework is completely seated.

Disclosing wax is then applied to all areas of the labial arm that will contact teeth. The framework is seated, and pressure is applied to the arm starting at the hinge area and progressing toward the lock. If there appears to be resistance to total closure, the framework is removed and inspected, and those areas impeding closure are relieved. This procedure is followed until the labial arm will close in the mouth with the same degree of force needed when the framework is on the cast. Care must always be exercised in closing the labial arm to avoid trapping and pinching the lip or cheek in the locking mechanism. Initially it may be necessary to use a blunt instrument to open the lock. After wearing the prosthesis for a short period, the patient will be able to open the locking mechanism with the thumbnail alone.

The occlusion must be checked and corrected to ensure that no part of the framework keeps the natural teeth apart.

## Corrected cast procedure

All mandibular distal extension removable partial denture situations require the making of corrected cast impressions (Figs 19-28 to 19-35). Optimum support from the residual ridge is critical to the success of a distal extension removable partial denture. Significant movement of the denture bases toward the soft tissues will quickly loosen the remaining teeth because the teeth are so firmly engaged by the framework.

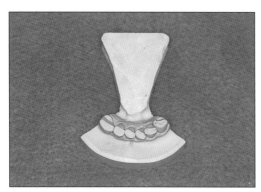

**Fig 19-30** The cast is modified to accept the corrected cast impression.

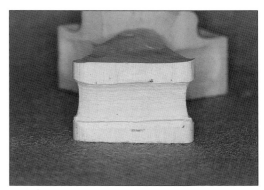

**Fig 19-31** A concavity is prepared on the vertical segments of the cast modification. This concavity takes the place of dovetails, but can only be used in bilateral applications.

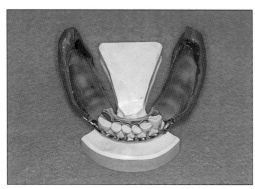

**Fig 19-32** The framework is seated on the modified cast. The practitioner must ensure that the framework is completely seated. Modeling plastic or sticky wax is used to affix the framework to the cast.

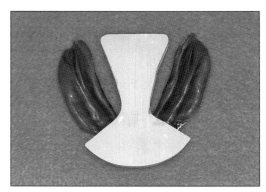

**Fig 19-33** The assembly is inverted in preparation for rimming and boxing procedures. The borders of each impression should be visible and should not bind against the modified cast.

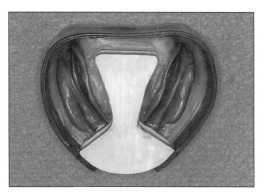

**Fig 19-34** The assembly is rimmed and boxed using the techniques described in chapter 12. Freshly mixed dental stone is poured into the prepared space.

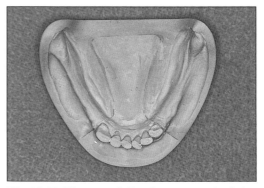

**Fig 19-35** The cast following removal of the framework/impression assembly and trimming.

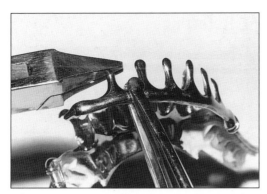

**Fig 19-36** Pliers may be used to adjust vertical projection arms. Adjustment should be kept to a minimum.

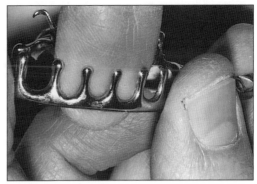

**Fig 19-37** The locking mechanism may be tightened by supporting the ends of the labial arm and applying pressure to its lingual or internal surface.

Overdisplacement of tissue and overextension of denture base borders can also contribute to early failure of the prosthesis. Almost continuous force will be applied to the remaining teeth if either of these conditions is present. Therefore, the selection of the corrected cast impression material and care in border molding procedures are critical factors in this phase of treatment.

## Development of occlusion

An occlusion that will minimize the lateral forces applied to the prosthesis should be developed. A "locked-in" occlusion with lateral interferences should be avoided. Simultaneous occlusal contact between both the natural and artificial teeth at the patient's occlusal vertical dimension is essential. Premature contact of artificial teeth on a distal extension base will hasten the loss of the remaining natural teeth.

## Placement of the completed prosthesis

Pressure indicator paste is used to locate pressure areas caused by the denture bases. The lingual path of insertion may cause insertion problems if the residual ridge is undercut on the buccal aspects. However, this is rarely a problem.

The occlusion is evaluated in centric and eccentric relations. Corrections are made if indicated.

If the Swing-Lock prosthesis is entirely tooth supported, the vertical struts of the labial arm can remain in intimate contact with the teeth for maximum retention. If long distal extension bases are involved or if the supporting tissues are easily displaced, maximum retention may be detrimental to the prognosis of the treatment. A plier can be used to adjust the vertical projection arms slightly (Fig 19-36). Reducing retention by bending the arms slightly out of contact with the tooth will allow some movement of the denture bases toward the tissue without placing tipping forces on the remaining natural teeth.

## Postinsertion care

Oral and prosthesis hygiene must be emphasized because the Swing-Lock denture's extensive tooth coverage complicates the maintenance of adequate hygiene. Frequent observation and maintenance are essential to the success of the treatment.

Distal extension denture bases must be relined if any appreciable resorption of the residual ridges occurs. The impression of the denture base areas should be made with the labial arm locked to ensure that the framework is in its correct position. The impression must be made with the teeth out of occlusion.

Occasionally, a locking mechanism may loosen. It can be tightened by adjusting the labial bar. The bar is stabilized at both ends, and a finger is used to apply slight pressure against the bar in the direction away from the side that contacts the teeth (Fig 19-37). This adjustment will usually necessitate slight adjustment of the vertical projection arms.

Teeth can be added to the Swing-Lock prosthesis as a relatively simple laboratory procedure. An alginate impression is made with the prosthesis in position and the labial arm unlocked. Usually the prosthesis will be retained in the impression. Undercuts in the denture base areas are blocked out, leaving only the borders exposed. A stone cast is poured. The labial arm will be enclosed by alginate, so special care should be taken in removing the impression from the cast. The safest procedure is to remove the tray from the impression material and cast and to peel the alginate away from the framework and cast. A retention loop can be soldered to the major connector and the replacement tooth attached with chemically activated acrylic resin.

## Prognosis

Clinical research has shown that teeth with unfavorable alveolar support can be retained for significant periods by the use of a well-constructed Swing-Lock prosthesis, provided the patient maintains an adequate level of oral hygiene.

## ☐ Reference

1. Simmons JJ. Swinglock stabilization and retention. Texas Dent J 1963;81:10–12.

## ☐ Bibliography

Antos EW Jr, Renner RP, Foerth D. The swing-lock partial denture: An alternative approach to conventional removable partial denture service. J Prosthet Dent 1978;40:257–262.

Beard CC, Clayton JA. Effects of occlusal splint therapy on TMJ dysfunction. J Prosthet Dent 1980;44:324–335.

Bergman B. Periodontal reactions related to removable partial dentures: A literature review. J Prosthet Dent 1987;58:454–458.

Fish EN. Periodontal diseases: Occlusal trauma and partial dentures. Br Dent J 1953;95:199–206.

Jordan LG. Treatment of advanced periodontal disease by prosthodontic procedures. J Prosthet Dent 1960;10:908–911.

McKinzie JS. Mutual problems of the periodontist and prosthodontist. J Prosthet Dent 1955;5:37–42.

Nevin RB. Periodontal aspects of partial denture prostheses. J Prosthet Dent 1955;5:215–219.

Rudd KD, O'Leary TJ. Stabilizing periodontally weakened teeth by using guide plane removable partial dentures. J Prosthet Dent 1966;16:721–727.

Schooper AF. Partial denture and its relation to periodontics. J Am Dent Assoc 1952;45:415–421.

Schulte JK, Smith DE. Clinical evaluation of swinglock removable partial dentures. J Prosthet Dent 1980;44:595–603.

Schuyler CH. The partial denture as a means of stabilizing abutment teeth. J Am Dent Assoc 1941;28:1121–1125.

Seeman S. A study of the relationship between periodontal disease and the wearing of partial dentures. Aust Dent J 1963;8:206–208.

Simmons JJ. Swinglock Clinical Manual. Dallas: Ideal Development, 1968.

Sprigg RH. Six year clinical evaluation of the Swing-Lock removable partial denture. The Haus Turkheim memorial lecture presented at the Anglo-Continental Dental Society, Spring 1970, London.

Stewart KL, Rudd KD. Stabilizing periodontally weakened teeth with removable partial dentures. J Prosthet Dent 1968;19:475–482.

Trapozzano VR, Winter GR. Periodontal aspects of partial denture design. J Prosthet Dent 1952;2:101–107.

# Attachments for Removable Partial Dentures

The removable partial denture components that engage abutments to resist dislodging forces are called *direct retainers*. Strict criteria guiding the design of direct retainers must be observed. When appropriately designed and constructed, direct retainers prevent a removable partial denture from being dislodged and limit the transfer of detrimental stresses to abutments and supporting tissues. In general, there are two types of direct retainers: intracoronal and extracoronal (Fig 20-1). In chapter 3, a thorough discussion of extracoronal clasp arm direct retainers was presented. Here, a review of intracoronal and extracoronal attachment direct retainers will be provided.

## ❏ Intracoronal Attachment Direct Retainers

Intracoronal attachment direct retainers were introduced in the late nineteenth century with substantial contributions from Dr Herman E. S. Chayes. Often referred to as simply "attachments," intracoronal direct retainers are composed of two closely fitting components. The first component, or *matrix*, is a metal receptacle or keyway. The matrix is positioned within the normal clinical contours of a cast restoration placed on the abutment. The second component, or *patrix*, is attached to the removable partial denture. When the removable partial denture is placed in the patient's mouth, the two components interlock in a sliding joint configuration. This sliding joint resides within the normal clinical contours of an abutment and functions to retain, support, and stabilize the removable partial denture (Figs 20-2 and 20-3).

Parallelism of multiple attachments must be carefully considered when designing a removable partial denture. The paths of engagement for the attachments, ie, the long axes of the attachments (Fig 20-4), must be parallel to each other and parallel to the path of prosthesis insertion. When parallelism is achieved, friction and binding between components occurs as forces act to dislodge the prosthesis. Binding that occurs between components secondary to a non-axial dislodging force is the major mechanical factor contributing to retention. The prosthesis can only be removed when force is intentionally applied to the removable partial denture parallel to the long axes of the attachments.

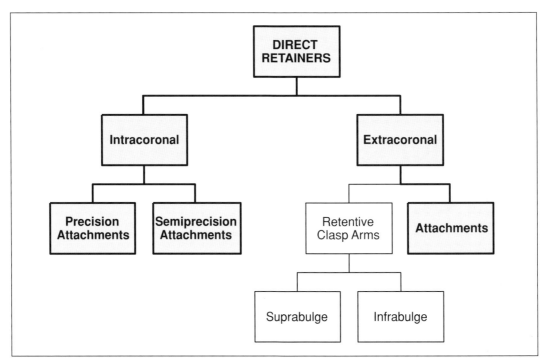

**Fig 20-1** Classification of direct retainers. Note the location of attachments in the overall scheme.

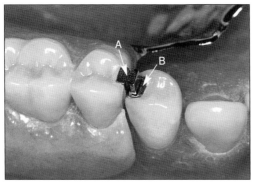

**Fig 20-2** An example of an intracoronal attachment direct retainer, including the patrix (A) and the matrix (B). The removable partial denture is not completely seated.

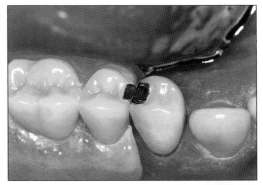

**Fig 20-3** With the removable partial denture completely seated, the interlocking configuration of the intracoronal attachment direct retainer is evident.

Intracoronal direct retainers are subdivided into two categories based on the method of fabrication and the tolerance of fit between components. If the components are fabricated in metal using low-tolerance, precision manufacturing techniques, the intracoronal direct retainers are considered *precision attachments* (Figs 20-5 and 20-6). Both the matrix and patrix of a precision attachment are machined from wear-compatible metals.

Attachments in the second category, *semiprecision attachments*, incorporate laboratory-fabricated components that typically involve a tapered wall geometry (Fig 20-7). Although components of semiprecision attachments may originate as prefabricated metal elements, the matrices and/or patrices of semiprecision attachments are usually cast from plastic or wax patterns (Fig 20-8). When accurately fabricated, semiprecision attachments demonstrate well-fitting components. How-

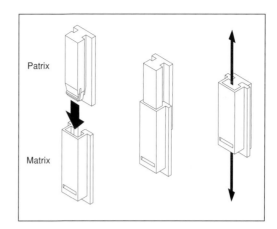

**Fig 20-4** A diagrammatic illustration of an intracoronal attachment. *Arrows* represent the path of engagement of the patrix into the matrix, as well as the long axis of the attachment.

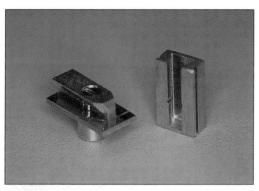

**Fig 20-5** An intracoronal attachment with the patrix *(left)* and matrix *(right)* separated. Note the precise machining used during fabrication of the attachment.

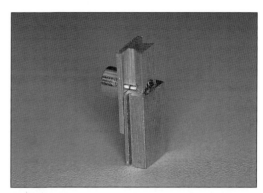

**Fig 20-6** The patrix and matrix of the attachment shown in Fig 20-5 are engaged and partially seated. Note the precise fit of this sliding joint.

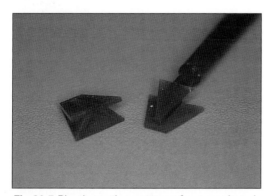

**Fig 20-7** Plastic casting patterns for a semiprecision intracoronal direct retainer. The matrix *(left)* and patrix *(right)* are separated. Note the straight projection extending from the patrix. This projection fits in a dental surveyor to assist in properly orienting the attachment during crown fabrication.

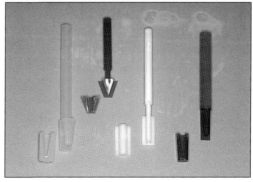

**Fig 20-8** A variety of plastic patterns are available for the fabrication of intracoronal semiprecision attachments.

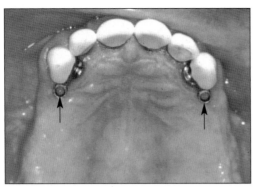

**Fig 20-9** The matrices of extracoronal attachment direct retainers *(arrows)* extend from the distal surfaces of crowns placed on the maxillary canines. (Courtesy of Dr W. Gardner, University of Texas Health Science Center, San Antonio).

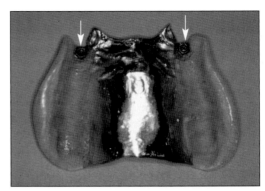

**Fig 20-10** A view of the intaglio of the removable partial denture for the patient depicted in Fig 20-9. The patrices are identified by *arrows*. (Courtesy of Dr W. Gardner, University of Texas Health Science Center, San Antonio).

ever, in the absence of computer-controlled machining processes, semiprecision attachments will always demonstrate greater fit discrepancies than will precision attachments.

## ⌑ Extracoronal Attachment Direct Retainers

Extracoronal direct retainers are mechanical devices that reside entirely outside the normal clinical contours of abutments. They serve to retain and stabilize removable partial dentures when dislodging forces are encountered. Extracoronal direct retainers may be divided into two categories: *extracoronal attachments* and *retentive clasp arms*. Of these, retentive clasp arms are by far the most common.

First introduced to dentistry in the early 1900s by Henry P. Boos and later modified by F. Ewing Roach, an extracoronal attachment provides a rigid, movable, or resilient connection between an abutment and a removable partial denture. Like its intracoronal counterpart, the extracoronal attachment is a sliding joint that derives its retentive characteristics from closely fitting components. Because mechanical connection resides outside the normal clinical contours of the abutment crown, this attachment is considered extracoronal (Figs 20-9 and 20-10). Many of these at-

tachments permit movement of the prosthesis during occlusal loading. This mechanical accommodation to functional movement is intended to minimize the transfer of potentially damaging forces to the abutments. This concept supports the "stress-breaking" philosophy of removable partial denture design.

## ⌑ Other Classification Systems

In addition to the aforementioned methods of classification, attachments may be categorized based on the stiffness of the resulting joint or geometric form.

### *Stiffness of resulting joint*

When metal-to-metal contact of the patrix and matrix restrict relative movement between the abutment and prosthesis during functional loading of the removable partial denture, the attachment is said to be *rigid*. On the other hand, many attachments are designed to permit movement of the denture base during functional loading. These attachments are considered *resilient* attachments. Functional movement of the prosthesis may be restricted to a defined vertical, horizontal, and/or rotational path (Figs 20-11 and 20-12), or omnidirectional displacement of the prosthesis may be permitted.

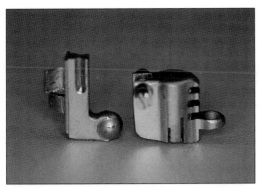

**Fig 20-11** The patrix *(left)* and matrix *(right)* of an extracoronal attachment. Note the spherical projection from the patrix. This configuration permits rotational movement of the removable partial denture in response to occlusal loading.

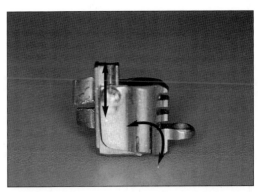

**Fig 20-12** The patrix and matrix of the extracoronal attachment depicted in Fig 20-11 are engaged. *Arrows* illustrate the sliding and rotational movements that are possible between the matrix and patrix.

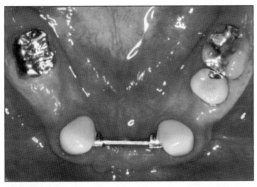

**Fig 20-13** This patient has been treated using a bar-and-clip attachment system. A Hader bar (Attachments International, San Mateo, CA) connects the mandibular canine crowns. The cross section shape of the bar permits a clip, which is fabricated in the removable partial denture, to fasten onto the bar and aid in prosthesis retention. (Courtesy of Dr W. Gardner, University of Texas Health Science Center, San Antonio.)

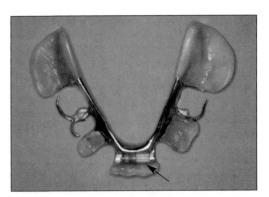

**Fig 20-14** A view of the intaglio of the removable partial denture for the patient depicted in Fig 20-13. The clip that will fasten to the bar is identified by the *arrow.* (Courtesy of Dr W. Gardner, University of Texas Health Science Center, San Antonio.)

## Geometric form

Another method of classification is based upon the overall geometric configuration and design of the attachment system. A wide variety of designs have been described in this classification method, including key and keyway, ball and socket, bar and clip (Figs 20-13 and 20-14), bar and sleeve, telescope, hinge, pushbutton, latch, interlock, and screw units.

## ◻ **Advantages and Indications**

Consideration must be given to retention, support, stability, comfort, and esthetics when designing a removable partial denture. In carefully selected patients, attachments may offer some advantages. Clasp arm direct retainers placed on canine and premolar abutments may be esthetically objectionable. The appro-

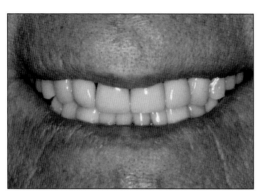

**Fig 20-15** Facial view of a patient wearing maxillary and mandibular attachment-retained removable partial dentures. Rather than placing clasp arm direct retainers on the canines, attachments were used. Elimination of clasps results in improved esthetics. (Courtesy of Dr W. Gardner, University of Texas Health Science Center, San Antonio.)

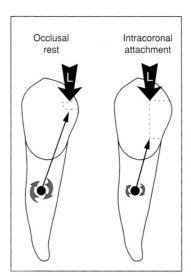

**Fig 20-16** When compared to occlusal rests, the apical extension of an intracoronal attachment reduces non-axial loading and diminishes rotational movement of the abutment. *L arrow* represents occlusal loading.

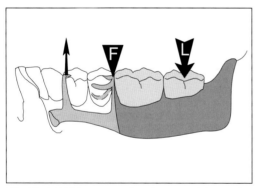

**Fig 20-17** With conventional removable partial denture design, clasp arm direct retainers must be sufficiently flexible to dissipate stresses originating from displacement of the extension bases during occlusal loading *(L arrow)*. *F* represents the fulcrum in this system.

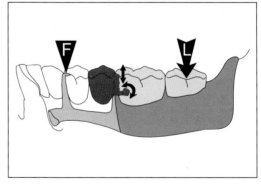

**Fig 20-18** With the broken stress philosophy, stress transfer to abutments is minimized during occlusal loading *(L arrow)* of extension bases. Extracoronal attachments permit relatively stress-free rotational and vertical movement *(small arrows)* between the removable partial denture and the abutments. *F* represents the fulcrum in this system.

priate use of attachments may eliminate the need for facial clasp arms while providing acceptable retention, support, and stability to the prosthesis. The result is both improved esthetic appearance (Fig 20-15) and elevated psychological acceptance of the prosthesis.

Intracoronal attachments may also have mechanical benefits. Because the attachment resides within the normal anatomic contours of the abutment, functional load transfer to the abutment may be directed more apically. Compared to conventional occlusal rests, the apical extension of an intracoronal attachment reduces non-axial loading and diminishes rotational movement of the abutment (Fig 20-16). Cross-arch load transfer and prosthesis stabilization may

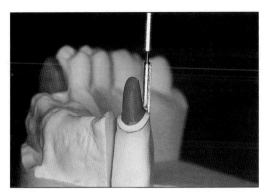

Fig 20-19 Aggressive tooth preparation of the distal surface of this canine was necessary to permit placement of the intracoronal precision attachment within the normal anatomic contours of the planned crown.

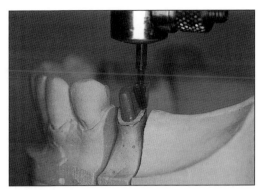

Fig 20-20 Aggressive and properly contoured tooth preparation permits placement of this intracoronal semiprecision attachment within the normal anatomic contours of the planned crown.

also be improved with attachments, particularly when rigid, precision attachments are used.

In general, the removable partial denture design philosophy discussed in this textbook follows the principles of *broad stress distribution*. That is, stress on the abutments is minimized by deriving optimal support from the edentulous ridges, developing harmonious occlusion, providing adequately flexible direct retainers, and constructing a rigid major connector. By following these concepts during prosthesis design, applied functional loads may be distributed throughout the dental arch so that no one area receives excessive stress.

A theoretically distinct concept, the *broken stress philosophy*, suggests that it is more appropriate to mechanically isolate the abutments from extension base movement during functional loading. To accomplish this isolation, mechanical devices or attachments must be positioned between abutments and extension bases within the removable partial denture framework (Figs 20-17 and 20-18). These attachments permit vertical, horizontal, and/or rotational movement of the denture bases relative to the abutments. A prosthesis incorporating a broken stress design is believed to limit the potentially damaging forces imparted to the abutments as the extension bases are mobilized during function. Much contention surrounds this philosophical approach to removable partial denture design, and its practical application is not typically considered the standard of care.

## ▢ Disadvantages and Contraindications

The most apparent disadvantages of attachment-retained removable partial dentures are complexity of design, fabrication, and clinical treatment. Abutments must be crowned in order to incorporate attachment components. Precise and structurally demanding tooth preparation must be accomplished so that attachment components can be housed within the normal anatomic contours of the abutments (Figs 20-19 and 20-20). It is not uncommon to encroach on the root canal space when attempting to adequately prepare abutments to receive attachments. Accurate handling of attachment components during all laboratory procedures is necessary to ensure that the path of attachment engagement corresponds to the planned path of insertion for the removable partial denture. This is particularly true when more than one attachment will be incorporated into the design.

Many commercially available attachment systems are contraindicated for short abutments. In order to facilitate an acceptable emergence profile, incorporate attachment components, and satisfy minimum vertical space requirements, a minimum abutment height of 4 to 6 mm is necessary, depending on the attachment system used. Shorter abutments may yield overcontoured coronal restorations or reduced frictional/

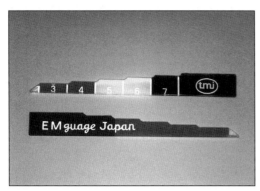

**Fig 20-21** The EM Gauge (TMJ Instrument, Santa Ana, CA) is used to measure available vertical space when considering the use of attachments during treatment planning.

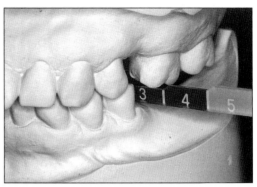

**Fig 20-22** Use of the EM Gauge to measure available space on the distal surface of this mandibular second premolar demonstrates inadequate vertical space (approximately 3 mm) to incorporate most forms of attachments.

binding retention of the attachments (Figs 20-21 and 20-22).

Increased complexity of both the laboratory and clinical procedures involved in the construction of attachment-retained removable partial dentures contribute dramatically to the overall cost of treatment. As with all mechanical devices, attachment components will wear over time and may require repair or replacement. Some attachment systems are fairly simple to repair, while others are more challenging. In all situations, attachment maintenance involves additional cost to the patient. Experience and knowledge on the part of the dentist and laboratory technician are essential to successful fabrication and maintenance of these relatively complex restorations.

More direct and definitive functional load transfer to the abutments can be expected with many of the attachments currently available. This is particularly true of intracoronal precision attachments. Therefore, poor periodontal health of the abutments (Fig 20-23), poor crown-to-root ratio, and compromised endodontic or restorative conditions may contraindicate the use of attachments. Optimizing and maintaining extension base support from the edentulous ridge is critical with attachment-retained removable partial dentures.

The use of attachments requires adequate understanding, cooperation, and manual dexterity on the part of the patient. Patients need to be aware of the potential problems and expected maintenance associated with attachments, not the least of which is the initial cost of the prosthesis and the estimated costs related to periodic maintenance and repair. Moreover, attachment-retained removable partial dentures usually are more difficult to insert and remove from the mouth. Patients who are visually or manually challenged may be better served with more conventional designs that are easier to manipulate.

Poor oral hygiene (Fig 20-24) due to poor motivation, inability to comprehend instructions, and inadequate manual dexterity normally contraindicate complicated restorative therapies. Several attachment systems render oral hygiene more challenging, thus increasing demands on oral hygiene performance. Less complicated removable partial denture therapies may be more appropriate for patients who demonstrate substandard hygiene practices.

In general, whenever a conventional clasp arm direct retainer can be used, it is the design of choice. The overwhelming popularity and consistent success associated with clasp arm direct retainers is based, in part, on practical experience and an understanding of the mechanical principles guiding their design and function.

## ⌨ Summary

Intracoronal and extracoronal attachments may be used in the treatment of partially edentulous patients

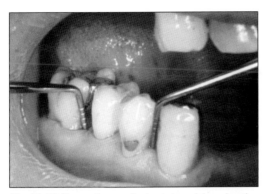

Fig 20-23 Excessive periodontal probing depths render this patient an unacceptable candidate for attachment-retained removable partial dentures.

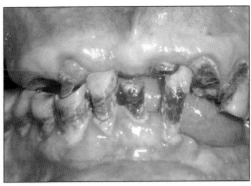

Fig 20-24 Poor oral hygiene habits dramatically increase the risk of failure when planning attachment-retained removable partial dentures.

requiring removable partial dentures. However, the highly specialized, and often complex, principles and procedures necessary to accomplish such therapies must be carefully considered. The esthetic advantages of attachments must be weighed against the difficulties associated with such restorations. Thorough and insightful treatment planning, a sound knowledge base, practical experience, and reliable technical support must be available in order to be successful with this removable partial denture design approach.

Attachments are not a panacea. They are costly, complicated, and require periodic repair and replacement. The practitioner and patient must be aware of the limitations and potential problems associated with attachment-retained removable partial dentures and be willing and able to accommodate these situations. However, by following sound principles of treatment planning, clinical therapy, and laboratory construction, attachment-based removable partial dentures can provide an excellent service for partially edentulous patients.

## 🖵 Bibliography

Baker JL, Goodkind RJ. A comparison of nonresilient and resilient attachments. The use of "stress directors." In: Theory and Practice of Precision Attachment Removable Partial Dentures. St. Louis: Mosby, 1981:190–197.

Baker JL, Goodkind RJ. Introduction to intracoronally retained removable partial denture prostheses. In: Theory and Practice of Precision Attachment Removable Partial Dentures. St. Louis: Mosby, 1981:1–9.

Baker JL, Goodkind RJ. Stress analysis in intracoronal removable partial denture prostheses. In: Theory and Practice of Precision Attachment Removable Partial Dentures. St. Louis: Mosby, 1981:18–26.

Becerra G, MacEntee M. A classification of precision attachments. J Prosthet Dent 1987;58:322–327.

Becker CM, Campbell HC, Williams DL. The Thompson dowel-rest system modified for chrome-cobalt removable partial denture frameworks. J Prosthet Dent 1978;39:384–391.

Blatterfein L . The use of the semiprecision rest in removable partial dentures. J Prosthet Dent 1969;22:307–332.

Boitel RH. Precision attachments: An overview. In: Tylman SD, Malone WFP (eds). Tylman's Theory and Practice of Fixed Prosthodontics, ed 7. St. Louis: Mosby, 1978:501–568.

Boos HP. The tube attachment. In: Nichols IG (ed). Prosthetic Dentistry—An Encyclopedia of Full and Partial Denture Prostheses. St. Louis: Mosby, 1930:599–618.

Burns DR, Ward JE. A review of attachments for removable partial denture design: Part 1. Classification and selection. Int J Prosthodont 1990;3:98–102.

Burns DR, Ward JE. A review of attachments for removable partial denture design: Part 2. Treatment planning and abutment selection. Int J Prosthodont 1990;3:169–174.

Caldarone CV. Attachments for partial dentures without clasps. J Prosthet Dent 1957;7:206–208.

Chayes HES. Bridgework conducive to health and the instrument for constructing it. Dent Items Interest 1939;37:267.

Chayes HES. Empiricism of bridgework. Dent Items Interest 1910; 32:745–755.

Chayes HES. Movable-Removable Bridgework. New York: Chayes System Laboratories, 1922.

Chayes HES. Principles, functions and construction of saddles in bridge work. Dent Items Interest 1915;37:831.

Chayes HES. The problem of the lower extension bridge and its rational solution. Dent Items Interest 1909;31:103–113.

Chayes HES. Removable bridge work by the use of the single-bar double-lock attachment. Dent Cosmos 1908;50:271–272.

Clayton JA. A stable base precision attachment removable partial denture (PARPD): Theories and principles. Dent Clin North Am 1980;24:3–29.

Cohn LA. The physiologic basis for tooth fixation in precision-attached partial dentures. J Prosthet Dent 1956;6:220–244.

Coye BR. Precision attachment removable partial dentures. J Calif Dent Assoc 1992;20:45–52.

Cunningham DM. Indications and contraindications for precision attachments. Dent Clin North Am 1970;14:595–601.

Dolder EJ. The bar joint mandibular denture. J Prosthet Dent 1961;11:689–707.

El Charkawi HG, El Wakad MT. Effect of splinting on load distribution of extracoronal attachments with distal extension prosthesis in vitro. J Prosthet Dent 1996;76:315–320.

Everhart R, Cavazos E. Evaluation of a fixed removable partial denture: Andrews bridge system. J Prosthet Dent 1983;50:180–184.

Gillings BRD. Magnetic retention for the overdenture. In: Brewer AA, Morrow RM (eds). Overdentures, ed 2. St. Louis: Mosby, 1980:376–397.

Goncalves A. A system of modified abutments for removable partial dentures. J Prosthet Dent 1955;5:649–662.

Goodkind RJ. Precision attachment removable partial dentures for the periodontally compromised patient. Dent Clin North Am 1984;28:327–336.

Grieder A, Cinotti WR. Case V: Terminal borderline case; internal clip bar technique, semiprecision attachment, and precision attachment removable partial dentures. In: Periodontal Prosthesis, vol 2. St. Louis: Mosby, 1968:602–660.

Grosser D. The dynamics of internal precision attachments. J Prosthet Dent 1953;3:393–401.

Handlers M, Lenchman NH, Weissman B. A retaining device for partial dentures. J Prosthet Dent 1957;7:483–488.

Harris FN. The precision dowel rest attachment. J Prosthet Dent 1955;5:43–48.

Hollenbach GM. The role of the precision attachment in partial denture prosthesis. J Am Dent Assoc 1950;41:173–182.

Isaacson G. Telescopic crown retainers for removable partial dentures. J Prosthet Dent 1969;22:436–448.

James AG. A self-locking posterior attachment for removable tooth-supported partial dentures. J Prosthet Dent 1955;5:200–205.

Koran A. Impression materials for recording the denture bearing mucosa. Dent Clin North Am 1980;24:97–111.

Kornfeld M. Precision removable partial dentures. In: Mouth Rehabilitation—Clinical and Laboratory Procedures, vol 2. St. Louis: Mosby, 1974:767–814.

Kotowicz WE. Clinical procedures in precision attachment removable partial denture construction. Dent Clin North Am 1980;24:142–164.

Kratovil JF, Thompson WD, Caputo AA. Photoelastic analysis of stress patterns on teeth and bone with attachment retainers for removable partial dentures. J Prosthet Dent 1981;46:21–28.

Landa LS. Diagnosis and management of partially edentulous cases with a minimal number of remaining teeth. Dent Clin North Am 1985;29:3–16.

Lee K. Double impression procedure for removable partial denture retained with semiprecision attachments: A clinical report. J Prosthet Dent 1996;75:583–587.

Lee RE. Mucostatics. Dent Clin North Am 1980;24:81–96.

Leff A. Precision attachment dentures. J Prosthet Dent 1952;2:84–91.

Leung T, Preiskel HW. Retention profiles of stud-type precision attachments. Int J Prosthodont 1991;4:175–179.

Lorencki SF. Planning precision attachment restorations. J Prosthet Dent 1969;21:506–508.

Lorey RE. Abutment considerations. Dent Clin North Am 1980;24:63–79.

Lucia VO. The removable partial denture with precision attachment retainers. Quintessence Int 1982;13:1193–1207.

Lucia VO. The removable partial denture with precision attachment retainers. In: Modern Gnathological Concepts—Updated. Chicago: Quintessence, 1983:237–269.

Mensor MC. Attachment fixation of the overdenture—The fail-safe implant! CDS Rev 1976;69(10):30–32.

Mensor MC. Attachments and semirigid connectors. In: Rhodes JE, Rudd KD, Morrow RM (eds). Dental Laboratory Procedures—Fixed Partial Dentures, vol 2. St. Louis: Mosby, 1986:331–366.

Mensor MC. Attachments for overdentures. In: Rudd KD, Morrow RM, JE Rhodes (eds). Dental Laboratory Procedures—Removable Partial Dentures, vol 3. St. Louis: Mosby, 1986:577–616.

Mensor MC. Attachments for the overdenture. In: Brewer AA, Morrow RM (eds). Overdentures, ed 2. St. Louis: Mosby, 1980:208–251.

Mensor MC Jr. Attachment fixation for overdentures. Part I. J Prosthet Dent 1977;37:366–373.

Mensor MC Jr. Attachment fixation of the overdenture. Part II. J Prosthet Dent 1978;39:16–20.

Mensor MC Jr. Attachment stabilization of the overdenture. Quintessence Int 1976;7(4):25–28.

Mensor MC Jr. Classification and selection of attachments. J Prosthet Dent 1973;29:494–497.

Mensor MC Jr. The rationale of resilient hinge-action stressbreakers. J Prosthet Dent 1968;20:204–215.

Morrison ML. Internal precision attachment retainers for partial dentures. J Am Dent Assoc 1962;64:209–215.

Moulding MB, Holland GA, Sulik WD. Photoelastic stress analysis of supporting alveolar bone as modified by non-rigid connectors. J Prosthet Dent 1988;59:263–274.

Mueninghoff L, Johnson M. Fixed-removable partial denture. J Prosthet Dent 1982;48:547–550.

Owall B. Precision attachment-retained removable partial dentures: I. Technical long-term study. Int J Prosthodont 1991;4:249–257.

Plotnick IJ. Internal attachment for fixed removable partial dentures. J Prosthet Dent 1958;8:85–93.

Preiskel H. The use of internal attachments. Br Dent J 1966;121: 564–567.

Preiskel HW. Precision attachments: Uses and abuses. J Prosthet Dent 1973;30:491–492.

Preiskel HW. Precision Attachments in Prosthodontics: Overdenture and Telescopic Prostheses, vol 1. Chicago: Quintessence, 1984.

Preiskel HW. Precision Attachments in Prosthodontics: Overdenture and Telescopic Prostheses, vol 2. Chicago: Quintessence, 1984.

Renner RP. Semiprecision attachment-retained removable partial dentures. Quintessence Dent Technol 1994;17:137–144.

Rhodes JE. The fixed-removable partial denture. J Prosthet Dent 1982;48:122–129.

Rhodes JE. Fixed-removable partial dentures. In: Rhodes JE, Rudd KD, Morrow RM (eds). Dental Laboratory Procedures—Fixed Partial Dentures, vol 2. St. Louis: Mosby, 1986:367–380.

Riedy SJ. The precision attachment removable partial denture. J Tenn Dent Assoc 1997;77:36–39.

Roach FE. Conserving the natural teeth in supplying partial dentures. Dent Cosmos 1908;50:17–23.

Rybeck SA. Simplicity in a distal extension partial denture. J Prosthet Dent 1954;4:87–92.

Schuyler CH. An analysis of the use and relative value of the precision attachment and the clasp in partial denture planning. J Prosthet Dent 1953;3:711–714.

Studer SP, Mader C, Stahel W, Scharer P. A retrospective study of combined fixed-removable reconstructions with their analysis of failures. J Oral Rehabil 1998;25:513–526.

Swepston JH. Frictional wall precision attachment partial prosthesis. In: Rudd KD, Morrow RM, Rhodes JE (eds). Dental Laboratory Procedures—Removable Partial Dentures, vol 3. St. Louis: Mosby, 1986:458–500.

Terrell WH. Specialized frictional attachments and their role in partial denture construction. J Prosthet Dent 1951;1: 337–350.

Tsuka T, Hamada T, Yamada S. Casting a gold alloy to embedded precision attachment metals. J Prosthet Dent 1979;42: 262–270.

Wichmann M, Kuntze W. Wear behavior of precision attachments. Int J Prosthodont 1999;12:409–414.

Williamson RT. Removable partial denture fabricated using extracoronal resilient attachments: A clinical report. J Prosthet Dent 1993;70:285–287.

Yalisove IL, Dietz JB. The crown and sleeve-coping prosthesis. In: Brewer AA, Morrow RM (eds). Overdentures, ed 2. St. Louis: Mosby, 1980:175–207.

Zahler JM. Intracoronal precision attachments. Dent Clin North Am 1980;24:131–141.

Zinner ID. Modification of the Thompson dowel rest for distal-extension removable partial dentures. J Prosthet Dent 1989; 61:374–378.

Zinner ID. Precision attachments. Dent Clin North Am 1987;31: 395–416.

Zinner ID, Miller RD, Parker HM, Panno FV. Prefabricated metal intracoronal attachments for removable partial dentures. Int J Prosthodont 1989;2:357–364.

# Index

Jeanette Novara.